Overweight
and
Weight
Management

The Health Professional's Guide to Understanding and Practice

Sharron Dalton, PhD, RD

Associate Professor
Department of Nutrition and Food Studies
New York University
New York, New York

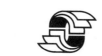

AN ASPEN PUBLICATION®
Aspen Publishers, Inc.
Gaithersburg, Maryland
1997

Library of Congress Cataloging-in-Publication Data

Dalton, Sharron.
Overweight and weight management: the health professional's guide
to understanding and treatment/Sharron Dalton.
p. cm.
Includes bibliographical references and index.
ISBN 0-8342-0636-6
1. Obesity. 2. Weight loss. I. Title.
[DNLM: 1. Obesity—prevention & control. WD 210 D152o 1997]
RC628.D13 1997
613.2'5—dc21
DNLM/DLC
for Library of Congress
97-6338
CIP

Aspen Publishers, Inc., grants permission for photocopying for limited personal or internal use. This consent does not extend to other kinds of copying, such as copying for general distribution, for advertising or promotional purposes, for creating new collective works, or for resale. For information, address Aspen Publishers, Inc., Permissions Department, 200 Orchard Ridge Drive, Suite 200, Gaithersburg, Maryland 20878.

Orders: (800) 638-8437
Customer Service: (800) 234-1660

About Aspen Publishers • For more than 35 years, Aspen has been a leading professional publisher in a variety of disciplines. Aspen's vast information resources are available in both print and electronic formats. We are committed to providing the highest quality information available in the most appropriate format for our customers. Visit Aspen's Internet site for more information resources, directories, articles, and a searchable version of Aspen's full catalog, including the most recent publications: **http://www.aspenpub.com**
  Aspen Publishers, Inc. • The hallmark of quality in publishing
Member of the worldwide Wolters Kluwer group.

Editorial Resources: Bill Fogle
Library of Congress Catalog Card Number: 97-6338
ISBN: 0-8342-0636-6

Printed in the United States of America

1 2 3 4 5

*To my students (the many) and
to my spouse (the one)
for their good ideas and
constant support.*

Table of Contents

Contributors

EDITOR

Sharron Dalton, PhD, RD
Associate Professor
Director, Graduate Program in
  Nutrition
Department of Nutrition and Food
  Studies
New York University
New York, NY

David B. Allison, PhD
Assistant Professor of Psychology in
  Psychiatry
Columbia University College of
  Physicians and Surgeons
and Associate Research Scientist
Obesity Research Center
St Luke's–Roosevelt Hospital Center
New York, NY

Nancy J. Aronoff, RD
Research Nutritionist
Obesity Research Center
St Luke's–Roosevelt Hospital Center
New York, NY

Claude Bouchard, PhD
Professor of Exercise Physiology
Director, Biology of Physical Activity
  Research Unit
Physical Activity Science Laboratory,
  PEPS
Laval University
Ste Foy, Quebec, Canada

Carol N. Boozer, DSc
Assistant Professor, Department of
  Medicine
College of Physicians and Surgeons
Columbia University
Obesity Research Center
St Luke's–Roosevelt Hospital Center
New York, NY

Debra K. Brown, MPH, RD
Pediatric Nutrition Specialist
Director, Kids Weight Down Weight
  Management Program
Department of Pediatrics
Maimonides Medical Center
Brooklyn, NY

Arthur L. Campfield, PhD
Distinguished Research Leader
Department of Metabolic Disease
  Research
Hoffmann-La Roche Inc
Nutley, NJ

Joseph C. Cappelleri, PhD, MPH
Assistant Professor of Medicine
Department of Medicine, New
  England Medical Center
and Tufts University School of
  Medicine
Boston, MA

Kenneth M. Carpenter, PhD
Psychologist and Post-Doctoral
  Research Fellow
Columbia University School of Public
  Health
Psychiatric Epidemiology Training
  Program
New York, NY

**Victoria Hammer Castellanos, PhD,
  RD**
Assistant Professor
Department of Dietetics and Nutrition
Florida International University
Miami, FL

Steven J. Danish, PhD
Professor of Psychology and
  Preventive Medicine
Director, Life Skills Center
Virginia Commonwealth University
Richmond, VA

Carol M. Devine, PhD, RD
Assistant Professor
Division of Nutritional Sciences
Cornell University
Ithaca, NY

Cara B. Ebbeling, MS
Research Assistant
Department of Nutritional Sciences
University of Connecticut
Storrs, CT

Myles S. Faith, PhD
Post-Doctoral Fellow
Obesity Research Center
St Luke's–Roosevelt Hospital Center
New York, NY

Jean-Pierre Flatt, PhD
Professor of Biochemistry
Department of Biochemistry and
  Molecular Biology
University of Massachusetts Medical
  School
Worcester, MA

Allan Geliebter, PhD
Associate Research Scientist
Department of Medicine and
  Psychiatry
St Luke's–Roosevelt Hospital Center
Columbia University College of
  Physicians and Surgeons
and Professor and Chair, Department
  of Psychology, Touro College
New York, NY

Janet K. Grommet, PhD, RD
Associate Professor
Long Island University/CW Post
  Campus
Department of Health Sciences,
  Programs in Nutrition
Brookville, NY

Harvey L. Katzeff, MD
Director, Diabetes and Lipid
 Treatment Program
Associate Professor of Medicine,
 Division of Endocrinology
New York University School of
 Medicine
North Shore Hospital
Manhasset, NY

Ruth Kava, PhD, RD
Director of Nutrition
American Council on Science and
 Health
New York, NY

**Shiriki K. Kumanyika, PhD, RD,
MPH**
Professor of Nutrition and
 Epidemiology
Head, Department of Human Nutrition
 and Dietetics
University of Illinois at Chicago
Chicago, IL

Idamarie Laquatra, PhD, RD
Nutrition Consultant
Pittsburgh, PA

Alice K. Lindeman, PhD, RD
Associate Professor in Applied Health
 Science
Department of Applied Health Science
Indiana University
Bloomington, IN

Carol A. Maggio, PhD
Research Associate
Obesity Research Center
St Luke's–Roosevelt Hospital
New York, NY

Wayne C. Miller, PhD
Assistant Professor, Exercise Science
Exercise Science Programs
The George Washington University
 School of Medicine
Washington, DC

Barbara J. Moore, PhD
President and CEO
Shape Up America!
Bethesda, MD

Christiaan B. Morssink
School of Public Health
University of Illinois at Chicago
Chicago, IL

Cathy Nonas, MS, RD, CDE
Director, Theodore B. Van Itallie
 Center for Nutrition and Weight
 Management
and Joslin Center for Diabetes
St Luke's–Roosevelt Hospital Center
New York, NY

Richard N. Pierson Jr., MD
Professor of Clinical Medicine
Columbia University College of
 Physicians and Surgeons
Director, Nutrition Research Center
St Luke's–Roosevelt Hospital Center
New York, NY

Nancy R. Rodriguez, PhD, RD
Assistant Professor
Department of Nutritional Sciences
University of Connecticut
Storrs, CT

Barbara J. Rolls, PhD
Professor and Guthrie Chair in
  Nutrition
Department of Nutrition
The Pennsylvania State University
University Park, PA

Lori J. Silverstein, PhD, RD
Assistant Professor of Clinical
  Medicine
Nutrition Education and Research
  Program
and Department of Family and
  Community Medicine
University of Nevada School of
  Medicine
Reno, NV

Jeffery Sobal, PhD
Associate Professor, Division of
  Nutritional Sciences
Cornell University
Ithaca, NY

Sachiko T. St. Jeor, PhD, RD
Professor, University of Nevada
  School of Medicine
Director, Nutrition Education and
  Research Program
Department of Internal Medicine and
  Family and Community Medicine
Reno, NV

Joseph R. Vasselli, PhD
Senior Research Associate
Obesity Research Center
St Luke's–Roosevelt Hospital Center
New York, NY

Jack Wang, MS
Associate Director, Body Composition
  Unit
St Luke's–Roosevelt Hospital Center
Columbia University, Department of
  Medicine
New York, NY

Preface

Compared to managing body weight, few contemporary human undertakings produce so little outcome for the effort put forth. This effort can be measured in several ways: individual emotional, physical, and social expenditures; collective time and expertise expenditures of health professionals; and amount of money spent by industry and consumers on weight-related products, services, and media.

In reviewing one of the many books on obesity, and responding to the vast amount of information published on this topic, a frustrated practitioner recently exclaimed, "What can we really do in the long run?" One answer was reported on the international news about the time this handbook was conceived.

Headlines August 8, 1994 in the leading newspaper of Nepal, the *Kathmandu Post,*[1(p1)] reported that "In weight, an ounce of prevention is better than a pound of cure." These research findings, presented at the seventh International Congress on Obesity in faraway Canada and beamed halfway around the world by Associated Press to this Himalayan kingdom, were news. As a Fulbright Scholar assigned to teach nutrition at the national university, I was struck by the Nepalese fascination with overweight among people in developed countries. The Nepalese were also fascinated by the notion that researchers would spend 10 years and one million dollars in government funds (that too was in the headline) on a study to learn that avoiding weight gain in middle-aged monkeys lowered their heart disease risk and prevented diabetes.[2] In contrast, of notable lesser interest in terms of prevention, to both Nepalese and participants in the international meeting, was diarrheal disease, the major killer of 80 out of every 1000 children in Nepal. Nonetheless, the trend in developing countries is clear. As individual income goes up, so does body weight. Overweight is a growing global problem.[3] Although this volume draws on data and experience largely from North America and Europe, professionals world-wide may also find this weight management guide useful.

One would hope that the *Kathmandu Post* headline becomes a motto for practitioners: "In weight, an ounce of prevention is better than a pound of cure." This book is intended to provide guidance for weight management, the goals of which are prevention of overweight and maintenance of a healthy weight. In practice, weight gain is a continual challenge. So is the cycle of gain, loss, and regain. Or, more likely, gain and more gain. The overall process of weight management is complex for both the practitioner and client. One new approach involves health promotion and maintenance at any weight, bringing up the question: Is it possible to be fit *and* fat? Another approach examines both perception and method, asking: Is it possible to manage weight without dieting?

This handbook advocates understanding, skills, and, perhaps, fresh approaches to a relentlessly enduring problem. This book is for the health professional and advanced students. The overall concept of weight management is developed by contributors who address multiple aspects of overweight: What is overweight? Who is overweight? Why are people overweight? How is overweight managed? How is the effectiveness of weight management programs measured? Their contributions provide both context and content for understanding and a great deal of guidance on weight management practice.

Thanks to all whose efforts have resulted in a fine outcome, especially Alice Conrad in the Department of Nutrition and Food Services at New York University.

REFERENCES

1. *Kathmandu Post.* August 27, 1994.
2. Hansen BC, Ortmeyer HK, Bodkin NL. Prevention of obesity in middle-aged monkeys: food intake during body weight clamp. *Obes Res.* 1995;3(suppl):199S–204S.
3. Van Itallie T. Global patterns and trends of obesity. *Pharmo Econ.* 1994;5(SI):1–7.

Introduction

By the year 2030, 100% of adults in the United States will be overweight if the current rate of gain continues.[1] This astonishing prospect is based on prevalence study data[2] from 1960 to 1991 that define overweight as a body mass index (BMI) of more than 27.8 for men and more than 27.3 for women. At least two responses have emerged to meet the challenge posed by this worrisome prediction: antiobesity agents (drugs) and antidieting philosophies. The antiobesity agent proponents support integrating diet, physical activity, and ongoing medication into a daily self-managed program with intermittent professional support. The antidieting proponents support less medicalization and encourage healthy weight at any body size through self-managed healthy lifestyles.

The topics discussed and the questions raised in this volume include these two approaches, their backgrounds, and how students and professionals may think about and use them. The underpinnings for these discussions of body weight and body fat are provided in chapters that review the studies and the role of genetics, energy regulation, interventions, treatments, treatment regulations, and guidelines for the practice of weight management among children and adults, including a chapter on women and reproduction.

A new philosophy among health professionals is called for that is based on studies of the change process itself and the results from studies of other behaviors such as smoking cessation. Effective change as an ongoing process requires new and renewed skills for all involved in weight management. Self-management with intermittent but lifelong support from professionals is discussed, an approach similar in some ways to management of other chronic diseases such as diabetes and hypertension. The issue of whether this may perpetuate medicalized patient dependency is also discussed. How do professionals determine the line between a controlling and a cooperative approach to weight management? Professionals and students are asked to consider "what's in it" for each party: the patient, the professional, the research community, and the health care and pharmaceutical industries.

New approaches that include anitobesity agents such as drugs and antidieting philosophies such as "healthier weights" do not necessarily advocate "throwing out the baby with the bathwater," but call for creative multidisciplinary management of overweight and "overfat."

Numerous volumes are brimming with research findings about obesity: theories, therapies, pathophysiology, psychology, and treatment. Yet, because the effort spent on managing weight is so great, we need reminders that, for some people, overweight is a chronic problem, requiring long-term management. For others, simply maintaining their current weight, rather than losing weight, is progress. Rather than wring our hands at the slow progress in basic research that may one day make a difference to those for whom losing and maintaining lost weight are elusive goals, there is a great need to understand what is currently known and not known, to promote healthy living at a variety of body weights, and to cope with the social and economic injuries dealt those with body sizes considered unacceptable. This handbook encourages professionals to develop a working philosophy about a major health condition that touches our attitudes, behaviors, and knowledge—our feelings, our actions, and our minds—as well as those of our clients and colleagues. We no longer set the goal as weight loss, but as weight management, which is a lifelong process with attention to the activities of choosing food, of bodily movement, and of accepting different body dimensions and shapes.

This handbook defines and documents what we know and do not know about overweight and weight management: What is it? Who has it? Why do we have it? What can we do about it, and how is our help limited? How as practitioners can we become part of the solution, and not part of the problem? In the long run we may:

- understand what is known and not known from current research
- question our weight management practices with individuals and groups
- apply and examine our skills, observe the results, and rethink our approach
- develop a philosophy about the nature of overweight and its management
- consider a new model of empowerment, facilitation, and/or self-management

Developing practical skills, a helpful attitude, and a working philosophy about overweight requires asking many questions. What is overweight? At what point, if any, is it a chronic disease? If so, should treatment involve lifelong management as with other chronic diseases? Should management be achieved through diet? Exercise? Drugs? Or through a non-diet approach aimed at improving physical and psychological well-being?

Because dietary control alone has a record of some success in weight loss and almost no success in maintaining weight loss, professionals are asking for ways to help their clients with coping skills, motivation techniques, and methods of behavior change.

We are in a remarkable era for health professionals concerned with healthy weight, dietary fat, and body fat. In late 1994 attention was focused on the Third National Health and Nutrition Examination Survey (NHANES III) findings: we are gaining body weight while eating less fat.[2] We were also eating 14% more calories per capita in 1990 compared with 1960.[3] It is worth noting that potato chip consumption was up 50% and alcoholic beverage consumption up 29% in that same time period.[4] By 1996 fat-free potato chips appeared on the market. A news report claimed that "Most Americans Are Overweight."[5] Other headlines read "New Scale Finds More Fat Adults."[6] The "new" scale is simply an application of the 1995 World Health Organization (WHO) definition of overweight: a BMI of greater than 25 rather than greater than 27. The same data was analyzed earlier with the result that over 30% of American adults were defined as overweight. Applying the WHO scale suggests that 59% of men and 49% of American women are overweight. Clearly, how we define overweight can vastly change our perception of its prevalence.

No matter what definition is used, the steady acceleration of excess weight is troubling. We are provided perspective from scientists who studied energy balance in 1930, 100 years earlier than when we shall all be, as predicted, "fat." "Excess energy is deposited as adipose tissue. This disproportion arises from a variety of conditions that may be thought of under two general headings. The first group includes the various human weaknesses such as over-indulgence and ignorance. The second group is composed of conditions that cause a decrease in the requirement for energy: such as lessened activity. If the long established food habits do not respond to this lessened demand, obesity is inevitable."[7]

The U.S. Department of Agriculture and U.S. Department of Health and Human Services provide a contemporary corollary recommendation for Americans: "Balance the food you eat with physical activity—maintain or improve your weight."

Old problem. Same advice. Will renewed understanding and new skills improve our professional practice of weight management? Henry David Thoreau observed that when improvement is desired, it is far better to give active assistance than abstract advice. The dietary guidelines provide the advice; providing assistance is the practitioner's challenge.

REFERENCES

1. Foreyt J, Goodrick K. The ultimate triumph of obesity. Commentary. *Lancet.* 1995;346:134–135.
2. Kuczarmarski RJ, Flegal KM, Cammpbell SM, Johnson CL. Increasing prevalence of overweight among US adults: the National Health and Nutrition Examination Surveys, 1960 to 1991. *JAMA.* 1994;272:205–211.

3. McDowell MA, Briefel RR, Alaimo K, et al. Energy and macronutrient intakes of persons ages 2 months and over in the United States: Third National Health and Nutrition Examination Survey. Phase 1, 1988–1991. *Advance Data from Vital and Health Statistics*; No 255. Hyattsville, MD: National Center for Health Statistics; 1994.

4. Stilling BR. Trends in foods. *Nutrition Today.* 1994;29:6–13.

5. Most Americans are overweight. *New York Times.* Oct. 16, 1996, p A11.

6. Cooke R. New scale finds more fat adults. *Newsday.* Oct. 16, 1996, p A25.

7. Newburgh LH, Johnston MW. Endogenous obesity—a misconception. *JAMA.* 1930;3:815–825.

Foreword

Over the past decade our understanding of the physiology of obesity and body weight regulation has vastly increased. Much of this new knowledge has been developed by authors of chapters in this book. At the same time, much new information has accumulated on environmental, behavioral, and psychological aspects of the disorder, and how best to treat it. Many experts have contributed to our understanding of the dietary, physical activity, and behavioral aspects of treatment. Since these developments have altered both our understanding of the etiology and pathogenesis of disorders of body weight and strategies for treating them, it is important for health professionals who care for patients with these problems to have the latest information in hand. *Overweight and Weight Management: The Health Professional's Guide to Understanding and Practice* is a valuable resource for all health professionals who deal with obesity and its sequellae, and will be welcome on the bookshelves of many offices, including my own.

Johanna Dwyer, D.Sc, RD
Professor of Medicine and Community Health
Tufts University Schools of Medicine and
Nutrition and Director, Frances Stern Nutrition Center
New England Medical Center Hospital

CHAPTER 1

Body Weight Terminology, Definitions, and Measurement

Sharron Dalton

A good definition gives a precise and clear meaning, denoting a point of reference. Defining a person in terms of body weight status can be done according to at least three different but related types of definitions. *Medical definitions* employ statistical analysis to measure mortality, using epidemiological data that relate longevity to weight. Medical definitions also include morbidity risk, which may be examined statistically by relating the disease risk factor (weight) and the health outcome. *Social and cultural definitions* are perceptual, based on the normative values of a specific ethnic or age or geographic group toward body size and shape. *Practical or operational definitions* are developed for therapeutic and management use and include functional considerations, such as a person's ability and desire to perform activities of daily living. A practical definition includes elements from each type of definition, some difficult to measure; yet applying an operational measurement of medical, social, and psychological aspects of body weight status is critical in order to distinguish effective weight management practices from ineffective ones.

The definition or classification of body weight standards is important to health professionals responsible for weight management of individuals and groups, to policymakers in establishing weight guidelines, and to the general public in making lifestyle choices about food, eating, exercise, and buying and using weight-related products and services. Scientifically valid guidelines for acceptable weights and degrees of fatness are especially important for practitioners when making decisions: Who needs professional guidance? What weight management approach is appropriate? Is the approach effective?

TERMINOLOGY: PROFESSIONAL AND POPULAR

Body weight terminology is not uniform among professionals or the public. Descriptors such as "big," or "large," are common in the popular media. "Fat" is often used pejoratively, although one may argue that with the exception of a few muscular athletes, the majority of overweight people may accurately be called fat because fat is what overweight people have "too much of." The scientific literature includes numerous definitions for a given category of weight such as moderate overweight, average weight, and mild obesity as shown in Table 1–1.[1-6]

An "acceptable" weight may describe a medically and socially defined size and shape. A "healthy" weight may refer to a low risk of weight-related disease as well as an attitude toward weight, and "optimal" is likely to represent a weight that is socially acceptable, free from disease, and promotes long life. In terms of weight management, an operational definition of optimal weight ought to be based on practical considerations: the weight that supports a high level of psychological and physical health at each stage of a person's long life.

Scientifically, *overweight* refers to an excess amount of total body weight that includes all tissues (e.g., fat, bone, and muscle) and water. *Obesity* refers to excess body fat. The definition of overweight does not distinguish between body fat and lean body tissue. An individual may be overweight without being obese, as in the case of bodybuilders who gain a large amount of muscle mass. One may also be obese without being overweight as with sedentary "couch potatoes" and some elderly persons. However, for practical purposes, most overweight people are also obese.[3]

From a social perspective, many people with excess adiposity or fatness think of themselves as overweight, not obese. For them, obesity is an uncomfortable concept, a disease that defies treatment, whereas overweight is familiar and wide-

Table 1–1 Classification of Relative Body Weight from Various Sources

USDA/DHHS[1]	NCHS[2]	IOM[3]
		Very severe obesity
	Severe overweight	Severe obesity
Severe overweight	Overweight	Moderate obesity
Moderate overweight	Average weight	Mild obesity
Healthy weight		

Van Itallie[4]	Krause[5]	Garrow[6]
	Super obese	
Morbid obesity	Morbidly obese	
Severe overweight	Medically significant obesity	Very obese
Moderate overweight	Obese	Obese
Mild overweight	Overweight	Overweight
Acceptable range	Ideal body weight	Acceptable
		Underweight

spread among acquaintances, a condition that responds to treatment. Others ask, "Over what weight? Overweight is just a polite term that implies that there is an ideal lower weight to which fat people should conform."[7] To others, "obese implies a medicalization of a body size, with the meta-message of pathology."[8(p28)]

Many organizations and government agencies in the United States and other countries are now expressing body weight according to the body mass index (BMI), which is based on body weight for a given height, or weight in kilograms/height in meters squared. The BMI makes interpretation of weight guidelines simpler and is helpful for cross-comparisons of weight recommendations and of average BMIs for groups sorted by age, gender, and geographic location (see Chapter 5).

However, comparisons are difficult when the BMI classification boundaries, the so-called "cut-points," vary. For example, prevalence of overweight is often expressed as a percentage of people who fall into a specific category such as 27 to 30 BMI, described as "moderate obesity" in the United States according to the 1995 Institute of Medicine report.[3(p51)] The corresponding category in the United Kingdom is marked by BMI cut-points of 25 to 30.[6] Comparing the percentage of overweight people in each country using these two categories is thus meaningless. Comparing the average BMI of two similar groups is more meaningful. The average BMI of females age 35 to 49 in the United Kingdom is 24.8;[9] the average BMI of U.S. females age 30 to 49 is 26.7.[10]

The BMI also appears to be a reasonable substitute for assessing percentage of body fat in epidemiological studies,[11(p127)] as it indicates the relative fatness of individuals. However, although the BMI correlates reasonably well with body fat percentage ($r = 0.70$),[12] using the BMI as the only measurement may lead to misclassification in some individuals. For example, Table 1–2 illustrates that when cross-classified, about 6.7% American men were found to be obese, while 10.2% were overweight, but not obese.

Among health professionals, overweight and obesity are terms that have distinct though related meanings and are often used interchangeably as illustrated in the following statements from the same report: "If the National Center for Health's BMI cutpoints are used, 33 percent of the U.S. population aged 20 and over is *overweight* and 14 percent is severely overweight. We believe that this large prevalence of *obesity* qualifies as an epidemic."[3(p46–47)]

A leader in British obesity research, John Garrow, suggests that one reason why obesity is not easily cured or prevented is its vagueness of definition. He claims it "makes nonsense of attempts to characterise obesity, or even to measure prevalence, because obesity, like baldness, is a continuum and dividing people into categories of say, obese and non-obese is impossible."[13(p2)] Perhaps choosing BMI cutoff points for weight definitions is similar to choosing democracy as a form of government. Winston Churchill observed that democracy is the worst form of government—except for all the rest. Given the other choices, carefully measured weight and height (BMI) remain the most easily performed and useful determi-

Table 1–2 Prevalence of Cross-Classification of Relative Body Weights (BMI) and Body Fat (Two Skinfold Measurements) of U.S. Adults

Categories	Cross-Classification Prevalence (%)	
	Men	Women
Underweight,[a] not obese[b]	18.1	17.8
Normal weight,[c] not obese	52.4	46.7
Normal weight, obese[d]	6.7	6.0
Overweight,[e] not obese	10.2	7.9
Overweight, obese	12.6	21.6

[a]Underweight: <15th percentile of the distribution of BMI (P = 2 for men; 1.5 for women).
[b]Not obese: <85th percentile of the distribution of triceps plus subscapular skinfold measurements.
[c]Normal weight: ≥15th to <85th percentile of the distribution of the BMI.
[d]Obese: ≥85th percentile of the distribution of triceps plus subscapular skinfold thickness.
[e]Overweight: ≥85th percentile of the distribution of the BMI.
Note: The reference population, on which the percentiles referred to were based, was made up of a representative sample of civilian noninstitutionalized U.S. men and nonpregnant women, age 20 to 29 years, who were examined during the first National Health and Nutrition Examination Survey (NHANES I), 1971–1974.
Source: Reprinted with permission from T.A. Van Itallie, Body Weight, Morbidity, and Longevity, In *Obesity,* P. Bjorntorp and B.N. Brodoff, eds., p. 362, © 1992, Lippincott-Raven Publishers.

nants of health and predictors of mortality for the general population.[11] The practical question remains: Where are the boundaries along the BMI continuum for an acceptable/unacceptable weight? A healthy/unhealthy weight? A brief historical review of body weight definitions and standards follows. History serves to remind us that the process of seeking answers in defining weight, as in many endeavors, resembles a spiral rather than a straight line. We often find that one answer leads to another more complex question.

HISTORY OF WEIGHT DEFINITIONS AND CLASSIFICATIONS

Historically, overweight people have been classified in several ways: causes (etiological factors); anatomical characteristics such as weight for height and the amount and location of fat cells; weight-related behavior; psychological and social characteristics; and health risk and longevity.

Endogenous/Exogenous Causes of Overweight and Obesity

In the 17th century, obesity was attributed to an imbalance of biochemical functions or a mechanical malfunction. In the 18th and 19th centuries, etiological or primary cause classification was attempted.[14] In the early 20th century, the term *endogenous obesity* was used to describe a condition of patients who failed to lose weight during a period of low-calorie diet observation. These patients were thought to be unfortunate victims of constitutional disease, an abnormality of one or more of the endocrine glands (hypophysis, thyroid, gonads). Such abnormalities unrelentingly caused a progressive deposition of adipose tissue, independent of activity or dietary habit (exogenous factors). This view was challenged in a classic paper by Newburgh and Johnston in 1930, "Endogenous Obesity—A Misconception," which concluded that "Obesity is always caused by an over abundant inflow of energy. The excess is deposited as adipose tissue."[15(p825)] Their work determined that the disproportion in energy inflow and outflow was caused by two general conditions: (1) human weaknesses such as overindulgence and ignorance, and (2) a decrease in the requirement for energy, such as lessened activity. They warned that "if the long established food habits do not respond to this lessened demand, obesity is inevitable."[15(p825)]

Anatomical Characteristics of Overweight and Obesity

Body composition was studied in 19th-century Germany and researchers suggested that obesity was due to an excessive number of fat cells. Physical measurements, called physiogamy or physical anthropology, were applied to populations. In Belgium, Quetelet developed an index of weight corrected for height based on measurements of "a moderate number of Belgians" and published his results in 1836.[16] The Quetelet Index is now referred to as the body mass index (W/H^2 Metric). In 1956, greater health hazards were suggested to be related to abdominal obesity, compared to lower-body obesity, which appeared more benign.[17] Classification according to regional fat distribution was thus established.

Social Classifications of Overweight and Obesity

Weight has had both positive and negative connotations in societies worldwide.[18] Historians have found overweight related to fertility, particularly citing prehistoric Venuses, statues of obese female figures, as symbols of womanhood and fertility.[19] In Elizabethan England (16th century), a moralistic approach was taken to obesity as illustrated by Shakespeare's character, Falstaff, who "sweats to death, And lards the lean earth as he walks along."[20] Both physical malfunction and overeating because of personality and temperament were related to obesity. By 1940, obese people were considered to have psychological problems. A 1952 *Newsweek* story read, "excess pounds are nothing more than a symptom of a personality out of kilter."[21(p110)] Based on her extensive work, Bruch identified two psychological types of obese people: those who ingest excess food as an emotional reaction to situations in the environment ("reactive obesity") and those who use food to reduce the feelings of emotional deprivation present since early childhood, caused perhaps by unstable parental relationship, need for autonomy, wariness of relationships, or conflicts over exhibitionism ("developmental obesity").[22] Attitudes of both professionals and the public have continued to define overweight, often negatively, in psychological, or behavioral, and cultural terms. See Chapters 3 and 13 on cultural and social aspects of body weight.

Medical Classifications of Overweight and Obesity

Medical definitions have traditionally reflected both positive and negative symptoms and characteristics related to overweight. Although Hippocrates observed that those who are naturally fat rather than lean more commonly suffer sudden death and infertility,[14] until the early 20th century most traditional cultures associated fatness with prosperity and good health, largely because low weight signified malnutrition and wasting diseases such as tuberculosis. The belief also prevailed in life insurance circles that weight above average represented a reserve that could be drawn upon in the event of disease, trauma, or emergency. Between 1900 and 1920 this relationship began to disappear in Western countries, particularly in the United States. A landmark analysis, published in 1908 as "The Influence of Overweight and Underweight on Vitality" by Brandreth Symonds, a leading figure of life insurance medicine, demonstrated statistically the relationship between weight and longevity and showed that overweight was a greater risk factor in reduced life span than underweight.[23] Symonds analyzed the 1843 to 1898 mortality experiences of average, overweight, and underweight men insured by his company, The Mutual Life Insurance Company of New York. Because of diseases such as tuberculosis and pneumonia, overweight of any magnitude until age 29 was associated with a lower-than-average mortality rate. However, with advancing age, the mortality rate for all overweight individuals increased to "bad" (moderate overweight) and "very bad" (excessive overweight).[16]

Ideal weights for women were published in 1942[24] and for men in 1943[25] by the Metropolitan Life Insurance Company. The concept of "ideal weight" was developed by Louis Dublin, a chief actuary, based on the proposition that mere averages did not provide appropriate body weight standards. "For adults, irrespective of age, the most favorable weights for health and longevity are probably close to the averages observed at ages 25 to 30."[24(p7)] Thus, these tables were not age specific, and did not allow for weight gain with age. Such gain was deemed undesirable, even dangerous to health and longevity. The 1942 Metropolitan *Statistical Bulletin* proclaimed that "Overweight is so common an impairment that it constitutes a national health problem of the first order."[24(p7)] In 1959, the Build and Blood Pressure Study[26] of several million people insured by 26 life insurance companies between 1935 and 1953 provided the basis for a revision of the Metropolitan tables. The 1959 Metropolitan tables of desirable weight presented weight ranges for three frame sizes of men and women of differing heights associated with the lowest mortality rate.[27]

The 1980 Recommended Dietary Allowances for weight were developed for men and women by recalculating mean weights from the 1959 Metropolitan tables to express weight ranges without frame size, heights without shoes, and weights without clothes.[28] A different set of desirable weight tables was published in 1979 by another government agency, the National Center for Health Statistics, based on data from the 1971–1974 National Health and Nutrition Examination Survey (NHANES I).[29] The weight gain found to accompany advancing age was considered undesirable and the mean weights of the early years of adulthood were used as the standard.

Based on the analysis of the 1979 Build Study,[30] the Metropolitan tables were revised in 1983. In this revision, weights were based on the lowest mortality for men and women ages 25 to 59, sorted by height and body frame. Although average weights of men and women had increased between 1959 and 1979, so had weights associated with the lowest mortality; the gap had narrowed between average weights and weights associated with the lowest mortality. Thus, the new tables showed increases in weights associated with the lowest mortality for some groups. Weight increases for tall men and women were not as large as those for short persons or for those of medium height. The weights associated with the lowest mortality were no longer called "desirable" or "ideal." Simply called "height-weight tables," the 1983 tables only "indicate the weights at which people should have the greatest longevity."[31(p9)] The 1983 tables were presented by Metropolitan Life with disclaimers that indicated current related social and cultural issues: "These weights are not used in computation of insurance premiums, nor do they minimize illness, nor optimize job performance, nor are they the weights for the best appearance." They were presented as a "health education tool—a guideline."[31(p9)] Nonetheless, these tables not only spawned an entire body of research literature on frame size and shape measurement,[32–35] but also served to define weight throughout a decade of unprecedented weight gain among Americans.[10] See Chapter 5 on prevalence of overweight.

Because the 1983 Metropolitan tables presented increased weight over a broad age range (25 to 59 years), an argument was set in motion that continued through the release of the third (1990)[36] and fourth (1995)[1] editions of the *Dietary Guidelines for Americans*. Is weight gain with increasing age harmful, or not? The hypothesis underlying the argument that it is not harmful: Minimal mortality occurs at progressively increasing body weight from 20 through 69 years. Accepting this proposition is a major departure from the notion that weight at age 25 to 30 is desirable for life. Support for this argument was spearheaded by Rubin Andres at the Institute on Aging[37] when the data from the 1979 Build Study[30] became available and was reanalyzed. Based on this analysis as well as data relating weight and height to both morbidity and mortality for nearly all Norwegians (1.7 million),[38] the National Research Council proposed BMI ranges in relation to age.[39(p564)] In turn, the 1990 Dietary Guidelines included two sets of suggested weights for height for adults according to age: 19 to 34 years and 35 years and over.[36] The outcry from the research community led by Walter Willett, a lead researcher of the nationwide U.S. Nurses Health Study, claimed these weight guidelines were not justified, and were "fundamentally invalid, there is no biological rationale for recommending that persons increase their weight as they grow older; indeed, there is much evidence to the contrary."[40(p1102)] The evidence cited included two reports from the Nurses Health Study[41–42] showing weight gain associated with increased risk of diabetes and blood pressure and reduction in high-density lipoprotein concentrations.

The social and cultural aspects of the argument were illustrated by the media and the courts. *Consumer Reports Magazine* reported "by a small margin, our nutrition experts prefer the weight table presented in the 1990 Dietary Guidelines for Americans, which allows higher weights for people age 35 and above."[43(p8)] *Health* magazine reported in "The Great Weight Debate" the story of a 50 year old "compact and muscular" 5 ft 4 in, 150 lb flight attendant who had been given an ultimatum by the airline to "shed 17 pounds or lose your job." In September 1991 the airline settled weight discrimination lawsuits filed against it by the flight attendants' union. Among the documents used in pleading their case was the government's 1990 Dietary Guidelines for Americans, allowing the flight attendant to weigh as much as 157 pounds.[44]

The 1995 Dietary Guidelines Advisory Committee[45] dropped the higher age category. They cited studies that they claimed demonstrated that mortality increases significantly above a BMI of 25[46–48] and that morbidity, particularly diabetes, begins to increase well below a BMI of 25.[49,50] The committee concluded that because mortality is the most significant and reliable consequence of a disease, the use of a BMI of 25 to define the upper boundary of healthy weight appeared the most reasonable definition. The 1995 Dietary Guidelines for "healthy weight" therefore encompass a narrower range than the 1990 suggested weights for adults and do not allow any increase in weight with age. Opposing reports and controversy about the recommended weight range continued in 1996. A 1996 analysis of 19 studies reported that mortality increased with low BMI ≤23 and high BMI ≥28 when subjects entered the study without evidence of disease, suggesting a higher upper limit, especially for men.[51] One commentary opposed the decision to remove the weight increase after age 35 and quoted several researchers who agreed. "BMIs associated with minimum mortality have generally been high in studies of older persons." "The old saw that one's best weight is that achieved at age 20 or 25 needs to be discarded."[52(p53)]

Prior to the publication of the 1995 guidelines, other scientific groups had discussed and presented comments that were considered by the Dietary Guidelines

Committee and that continue to inform discussions about specific weight guidelines. The American Institute of Nutrition (AIN) recommended that weight guidelines be directed at healthy nonpregnant adults age 21 and over, primarily for the *prevention* of obesity and obesity-related complications and that a separate document be created for the management of overweight persons whose weight falls outside the weight guidelines.[53] The American Health Foundation brought together a panel of experts who were charged with developing a public health recommendation, aimed at disease prevention, for a "healthy weight." The panel represented authorities on chronic disease, lifestyle components, and communications for motivating changes in health behavior. Panel recommendations were made for both a healthy weight target and a specific weight loss to reduce disease risk.[54] Recommendations from these two groups are discussed later in this chapter.

Nearly as much new research on overweight and obesity was produced in the mid-1980s to mid-1990s as in the previous 50 years.[55] The history of defining body weight status and developing guidelines for healthy body weight has swollen in tandem with other weight-related research. Health practitioners must keep up with current research and results.

TYPES OF BODY WEIGHT DEFINITIONS

Because all definitions require professional judgment when applied in individual cases, understanding the development of each definition and the procedures for their use offers the health professional an opportunity to not only choose and apply useful and current definitions in practice but to develop an overall philosophy toward weight management. The types of definitions for use in assessing and managing overweight and obesity are presented according to their purpose and measurement method in Table 1–3. Each type is then discussed according to its data source, reference standard, and procedure for use.

A medical/statistical definition is generally based on physical (anthropometric) and biochemical measures that indicate health risk; medical and food history information is useful in making a clinical judgment but may actually reduce the precision of definition. A purely statistical definition simply selects the overweight persons who fall in the upper 5% or 15% of whatever criterion is being used. A social and psychological/behavioral definition is sometimes determined using psychological and perceptual measurement tools; interview and observation may be helpful to the practitioner but may allow bias in interpreting perceptions of weight. The practical (operational) definition is the least precise, incorporating elements of medical, social, and psychological definitions, but is the most important in determining current weight status and evaluating change, both positive and negative, in weight status. Change in a person's weight status may involve physical change, psychological change, or social change.

Table 1–3 Types of Definitions, Measurement Components, and Tools

| Measurement | Definition Type | | |
	Medical/ Statistical	Social/ Psychological	Practical/Operational
Component	Morbidity Mortality	Motivation Coping Body image Diet readiness	Biological/statistical Social/psychological plus Functional (sick days, fitness)
Source/Tools	Disease risk BMI Body fat Waist/hip ratio	Questionnaire Scales	plus Individual goals

Medical and statistical definitions of weight are usually based on three physical measurements: weight for height, body fat, and regional body fat distribution.

Weight for Height Definitions

Body mass index (BMI), or weight in kilograms divided by height in meters squared, is correctly called the Quetelet index; other "weight-corrected-for-height" indexes using different exponential power to relate body mass (weight) and stature (height) are the Ponderal ($wt/ht^{1/3}$), Khosla-Lowe (wt/ht^3), and Benn's (wt/ht^p). Ideally an index should indicate body weight regardless of how tall or short a person is and should correlate with estimates of body fatness. BMI reference standards with criterion values or "cut-points" are established using evidence from both mortality and morbidity data. Figure 1–1 presents the recommended BMI for adults published by various government and research organizations. The reference sources and procedures for using the recommendations are discussed in this section. BMI may be determined from weight and height by reference to Table 1–4 or Figure 1–2.

Ideal body weight (IBW) is commonly used in dietetic practice and appears in many clinical manuals. Also called the Hamwi "rule of thumb"[56] this method for determining IBW was first published in 1964 and is based on a formula developed to calculate weight for height similar to the 1959 Metropolitan Desirable Weight Table. Table 1–5 indicates that compared to the 1983 Metropolitan Height and

Table 1-4 Body Weights in Pounds According to Height and Body Mass Index*

Height (in.)	Body Mass Index (kg/m²)													
	19	20	21	22	23	24	25	26	27	28	29	30	35	40
	Body Weight (lb)													
58	91	96	100	105	110	115	119	124	129	134	138	143	167	191
59	94	99	104	109	114	119	124	128	133	138	143	148	173	198
60	97	102	107	112	118	123	128	133	138	143	148	153	179	204
61	100	106	111	116	122	127	132	137	143	148	153	158	185	211
62	104	109	115	120	126	131	136	142	147	153	158	164	191	218
63	107	113	118	124	130	135	141	146	152	158	163	169	197	225
64	110	116	122	128	134	140	145	151	157	163	169	174	204	232
65	114	120	126	132	138	144	150	156	162	168	174	180	210	240
66	118	124	130	136	142	148	155	161	167	173	179	186	216	247
67	121	127	134	140	146	153	159	166	172	178	185	191	223	255
68	125	131	138	144	151	158	164	171	177	184	190	197	230	262
69	128	135	142	149	155	162	169	176	182	189	196	203	236	270
70	132	139	146	153	160	167	174	181	188	195	202	207	243	278
71	136	143	150	157	165	172	179	186	193	200	208	215	250	286
72	140	147	154	162	169	177	184	191	199	206	213	221	258	294
73	144	151	159	166	174	182	189	197	204	212	219	227	265	302
74	148	155	163	171	179	186	194	202	210	218	225	233	272	311
75	152	160	168	176	184	192	200	208	216	224	232	240	279	319
76	156	164	172	180	189	197	205	213	221	230	238	246	287	328

*Each entry gives the body weight in pounds (lb) for a person of a given height and body mass index. Pounds have been rounded off. To use the table, find the appropriate height in the left-hand column. Move across the row to a given weight. The number at the top of the column is the body mass index for the height and weight.

Source: Reprinted by permission of *The Western Journal of Medicine*, G.A. Bray and D.S. Gray, Obesity, Part I, Pathogenesis, 1988, Vol. 149, pp. 429–441.

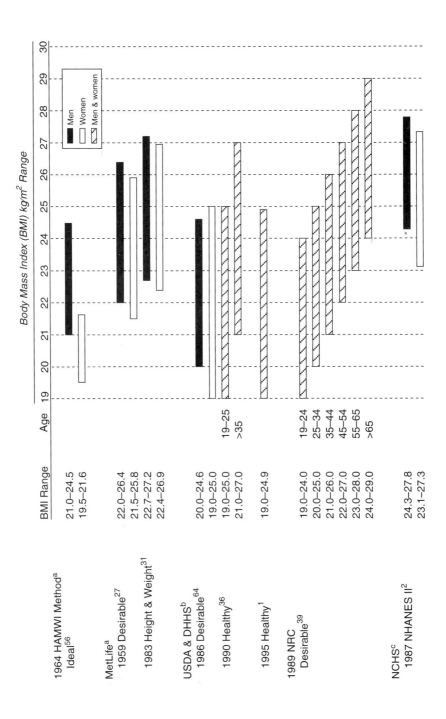

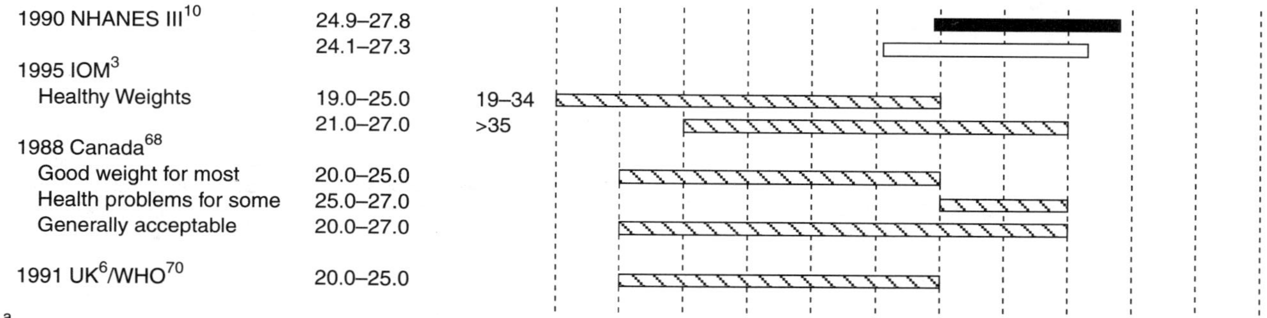

1990 NHANES III[10]   24.9–27.8

1995 IOM[3]   24.1–27.3

Healthy Weights   19.0–25.0   19–34
                       21.0–27.0   >35

1988 Canada[68]
Good weight for most   20.0–25.0
Health problems for some 25.0–27.0
Generally acceptable   20.0–27.0

1991 UK[6]/WHO[70]   20.0–25.0

[a]Range calculated as ideal weight for medium frame women 5–6 ft and medium frame men 5–6 ft 3 in. (Also see Table 1–4).
[b]Range calculated as midpoint and 120% of midpoint of medium frame for adults.
[c]50th–80th percentile for NHANES III; NHANES III, phase I, range calculated as 50th percentile and BMI values consistent with NHANES II upper cutoff.

Figure 1–1 Body mass index range frequently used to define recommended weight for adults.

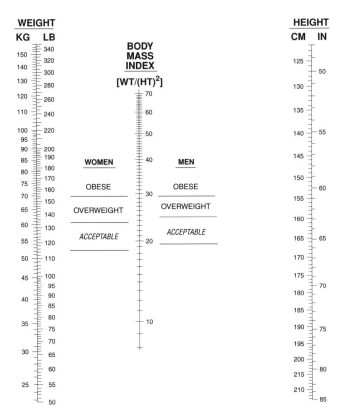

Figure 1–2 Nomogram for determining body mass index. Place a straightedge between the column for weight and the column for height. The BMI value is indicated at the point the straightedge crosses the body mass index line. *Source:* Copyright George A. Bray, 1978.

Weight Tables midpoint of medium frame, this method underestimates IBW for short and tall men and women, and medium height men.[57]

Although frame size was included in the original formula, determining frame size in practice may pose problems when classifying individuals because the original life insurance data did not include objective frame size measurement. The procedure for calculating IBW (medium frame): For women, allow 100 lbs for the first 5 ft of height; add 5 lbs/in for each inch over 5 ft. For men, allow 106 lbs for the first 5 ft of height; add 6 lbs/in for each inch over 5 ft. Subtract 10% of calculated weight for small frame; add 10% of calculated weight for large frame.[58(p29)]

The Metropolitan Life Insurance Company (MetLife) tables have been the most widely used references for healthy adult men and women since the 1940s. Based

Table 1–5 Comparison of Metropolitan Midpoint Weight (MMW) and Ideal Body
Weight (IBW) or Hamwi ("rule of thumb") Method

Height (in)	Metropolitan 1983 MMW (lb)[a]	Hamwi Method[b] lb	% MMW
Women			
57	112	NA	NA
58	114	NA	NA
59	116.5	NA	NA
60	119	100	84.0
61	122	105	86.1
62	125	110	88.0
63	128	115	89.8
64	131	120	91.6
65	134	125	93.3
66	137	130	94.9
67	140	135	96.4
68	143	140	97.9
69	146	145	99.3
70	149	150	100.7
71	152	155	102.0
Men			
60	NA	106	NA
61	131	112	85.5
62	133	118	88.7
63	135	124	92.9
64	137.5	130	94.5
65	140	136	97.1
66	143	142	99.3
67	146	148	101.4
68	149	154	103.4
69	152	160	105.3
70	155	166	107.1
71	158.5	172	108.5
72	162	178	109.9
73	166	184	110.8
74	169.5	190	112.1
75	174	196	112.6

[a]MMW = Metropolitan Life midpoint weight: midpoint frame range for adults 25 to 29 years adjusted for clothing (less 1 in for heels; less 3 lb clothing for women and less 5 lb clothing for men).
[b]Hamwi method = women: 100 lb for first 5 ft plus 5 lb for each additional inch; men: 106 lb for first 5 ft plus 6 lb for each additional inch. (For medium frame.)
Source: J.H. Roth, What Is Optimum Body Weight? Copyright The American Dietetic Association. Reprinted by permission from *Journal of the American Dietetic Association,* Vol. 95, p. 856, © 1995.

on weights associated with the lowest mortality from actuarial studies[26,30] of weight and stature among insured individuals that provide data on nearly 5 million people, they suffer from a self-selection bias of including only those who choose to take out life insurance; the insured tend to have a longer life expectancy, to be healthier, and, on average, to weigh less than the general population. Other criticisms of the height-weight tables have diminished their application to the population as a whole: underrepresentation of the lower socioeconomic classes, minorities, and the elderly; arbitrary definition of body frame size; reference to populations instead of individuals; and failure to eliminate early mortality from the overall analysis.[59,11,60] Desirable or recommended weight is commonly set between 90% and 110%, overweight generally at 110% to 120%, and obesity at >120% of the midpoint weight of medium frame for height of an individual by sex. Relative weight is a term sometimes used with the Metropolitan Height and Weight Tables. Relative weight is defined as actual weight divided by some reference weight and multiplied by 100 to express percentage. The Framingham Heart Study, for example, used the midpoint of the desirable weight range for a person of medium frame as the reference weight. Relative weight in this case was called Metropolitan relative weight.

Procedure for using the 1959 Metropolitan Desirable Weights of Men and Women: Measure height with shoes and weight with indoor clothing. Select frame size and determine weight range according to height. Male indoor clothing is assumed to weigh 7 lbs, including shoes; female clothing 4 lbs, including shoes. A 1-in heel height is assumed for men and a 2-in for women. Procedure for 1983 Metropolitan Height and Weight of Men and Women: Measure height of men and women with 1 in heels. Measure weight in indoor clothing weighing 5 lb for men, 3 lb for women. To make an approximation of frame size, extend the arm and bend the forearm upward at a 90-degree angle. Place the thumb and index finger of your other hand on the two prominent bones on either side of elbow. Measure the space between your fingers against a ruler. Compare the measurement with the table of elbow measurements. The table is presented in the *Statistical Bulletin*[31(p5)] and on pocket-size cards; a plastic sliding gauge is also available from Metropolitan Insurance Company. Although the 1983 tables provided this technique for determining frame size, apparently the classification of frame size relied upon subject self-appraisal in the original data.[61(p47)] Many methods of estimating frame size have been proposed,[35] but the increased use of weight for height indexes such as the BMI and a lack of data on the relationship of frame size to body weight make this measure less useful in practice. (Note: The "cut-points" in Figure 1–1 for the 1959 and 1983 MetLife recommendations were adjusted to the BMI categories presented in the 1988 Surgeon General's report,[62(p283)] which were adjusted for medium frame, without shoes or clothing [1959] and with shoes and light clothes [1983]).

The United States Department of Agriculture and Department of Health and Human Services (USDA/DHHS) Dietary Guidelines for Americans contain a weight guidelines in each of the four editions: maintain ideal weight, first edition, 1980[63]; maintain desirable weight, second edition, 1986[64]; maintain healthy weight, third edition, 1990[36]; balance the food you eat with physical activity—maintain or improve your weight, fourth edition, 1995.[1] The first three editions included weight for height tables. The source given for the weight ranges in the first two editions was the 1959 Metropolitan Desirable Weight Table. The third edition table of Suggested Weights for Adults (Table 1–6) presented two age categories, 19 to 34 years and 35 years and over, and was derived from the National Research Council (NRC) 1989 Diet and Health report, which proposed desirable body mass index increases in relation to age[39] (see NRC discussion below and in Figure 1–1).

Table 1–6 1990 Dietary Guidelines: Suggested Weights for Adults

| Height[1] | Weight in Pounds[2] | |
	19–34 Years	35 Years and Over
5'0"	97–128[3]	108–138
5'1"	101–132	111–143
5'2"	104–137	115–148
5'3"	107–141	119–152
5'4"	111–146	122–157
5'5"	114–150	126–162
5'6"	118–155	130–167
5'7"	121–160	134–172
5'8"	125–164	138–178
5'9"	129–169	142–183
5'10"	132–174	146–188
5'11"	136–179	151–194
6'0"	140–184	155–199
6'1"	144–189	159–205
6'2"	148–195	164–210
6'3"	152–200	168–216
6'4"	156–205	173–222
6'5"	160–211	177–228
6'6"	164–216	182–234

[1]Without shoes.
[2]Without clothes.
[3]The higher weights in the ranges generally apply to men, who tend to have more muscle and bone; the lower weights more often apply to women, who have less muscle and bone.
Source: Reprinted from the United States Department of Agriculture—Department of Health and Human Services.

Procedure for the 1990 Dietary Guidelines of Suggested Weights for Adults: As noted in Table 1–6, heights are without shoes and weights without clothes. Although sex is not distinguished, instructions state that higher weights in the ranges generally apply to men; the lower weights apply to women. The text explains that "The table shows higher weights for people 35 years and above than for younger adults. This is because recent research suggests that people can be a little heavier as they grow older without added risk to health."[36(pp8–9)]

The source given for the 1995 Dietary Guidelines for Americans is the report of the Dietary Guidelines Advisory Committee 1995,[45] which cites three studies relating weight and longevity,[46,47,38] four studies relating weight to diabetes and coronary heart disease,[36,46,47] and several studies relating fat distribution to disease risk.[48,49,65,66] Compared to the 1990 guidelines, the weight ranges set in 1995 are more narrow and do not allow any increase with age. The report states that "the cutoff point of 25 BMI to define the upper boundary of healthy weight is higher than that indicated by morbidity data such as diabetes, but was chosen, in part, because the designation of obesity at a point below a BMI of 25 will label well over half of the population obese."[45(p24)] Procedure for the fourth edition of the Dietary Guidelines: A graphic titled "Are you Overweight?" is presented to determine healthy weight (Figure 1–3).

Instructions state "See where your weight falls on the chart for people of your height. The health risks due to excess weight appear to be the same for older as for young adults. Weight ranges are shown in the chart because people of the same height may have equal amounts of body fat but different amounts of muscle and bone. However, the ranges do not mean that it is healthy to gain weight, even within the same weight range."[1(p17)] A graphic rather than a BMI chart was selected as consistent with an increased "dose effect" of a rising BMI. This suggests a graded risk for increasing BMI above 25 rather than that a given weight for height is either healthy or unhealthy.

The National Research Council (NRC) 1989 report, *Diet and Health: Implications for Reducing Chronic Disease Risk*,[39] proposed ranges for BMI in relation to age based on the reanalysis of data from the 1979 Build Study[30] and a study conducted in Norway of 1.7 million people that related weight and height to morbidity and mortality, and included a five-year follow-up.[38] The ranges overlap so that, for example, the highest cut-point for 10- to 24-year-olds is the lowest for people over 65.

The National Center for Health Statistics (NCHS) conducts National Health and Nutrition Examination Surveys (NHANES) designed to provide nationally representative reference data and prevalence estimates for a variety of health measures including height, weight, and skinfolds (see next section in this chapter). From 1960 to 1991 the NCHS conducted five surveys, including the Hispanic Health and Nutrition Examination Survey (HHANES), which targeted three Hispanic subgroups. The NCHS BMI ranges presented in Figure 1–1 are based on the

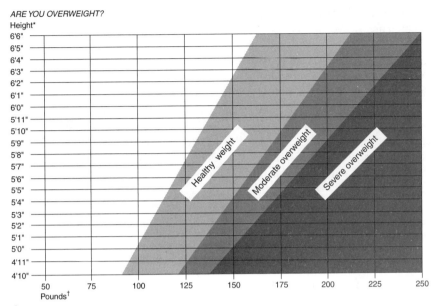

Figure 1–3 Dietary guidelines for Americans. *Source:* Reprinted from *Dietary Guidelines for Americans,* p. 18, 1995, USDA/DHHS.

normal distribution of weight in relation to height, with overweight defined at the 85th percentile using the reference weights of men and women aged 20 through 29 years from NHANES II (1976 to 1980).[2] Overweight was thus defined as BMI cutoffs of ≥27.8 for men and ≥27.3 for women, which were 85th percentile values for men and women aged 20 through 29 from NHANES II data. In order to compare data from NHANES III, the same cutoffs were used to define overweight.[10] Two problems with such a definition are that average weight may not be the weight of optimal health, and that as a population gains weight, so too will the weight rise at the 85th percentile. The BMI cut-point at which overweight begins thus varies with population weight change. The use of percentiles as the cutoff points to define obesity entails at least three assumptions: (1) that overweight, as measured by BMI, is an appropriate measure of adiposity; (2) that 15% of U.S. adults 20 to 29 years are overweight; and (3) that standards derived from young adults are appropriate for older adults. The NCHS BMI cutoff values represent approximately 124% of desirable weight for men and 120% of desirable weight for women defined as the midpoint of the range of weights for a medium frame from the 1983 Metropolitan Height and Weight Tables, after adjustments for clothing and shoes.

The NCHS defines overweight as a BMI at or higher than the 85th percentile for men and women age 20 to 29 years studied between 1976 and 1980. The NCHS defines severe overweight as a BMI at or higher than the 95th percentile of the same 20- to 29-year-old reference group.

The Institute of Medicine (IOM) Committee to Develop Criteria for Evaluating the Outcomes of Approaches to Prevent and Treat Obesity defines healthy weight as a BMI ≤25 through age 34 and a BMI ≤27 beyond age 34.[3] The same definition is recommended by the National Institutes of Health (NIH) National Task Force on Prevention and Treatment of Obesity.[67] The recommendation implies that weight gain with age is acceptable.

Canadian guidelines for healthy weight were determined by an expert committee based on national health surveys[68] and allow flexibility in the upper limit. A BMI of 20 to 25 is called a "good weight for most people" and a more lenient range of 20 to 27 is allowed as a "generally acceptable range." These ranges are not age-specific, in contrast to the 1990 U.S. Dietary Guidelines and the IOM weight recommendations for Americans, which allow the upper limit of 27 BMI only for people 35 years and older.

The United Kingdom Nutrition and Physical Activity Task Forces[6] adopted their classifications of overweight and obesity from Garrow[13]: underweight, acceptable, overweight, obese, and very obese, based on five-unit BMI increments. Reasons for choosing the range of 20 to 25 as the zone associated with minimum mortality are based on evidence from mortality data in U.S. and U.K. life insurance reports and "because of lack of evidence that a BMI of 25 is better or worse than 22.5."[13(p4)]

The World Health Organization (WHO) expert committee on the use and interpretation of anthropometry to determine physical status examined weight and health data from worldwide reports[69] and weight recommendations and in 1995 recommended the same guidelines as the United Kingdom.[70]

Healthy weight was also defined by an expert panel convened by the American Health Foundation in 1994.[54] The panel proposed a BMI of 25 as a generous upper limit to protect against development of chronic diseases. Various healthy body weight targets based on morbidity and mortality risks of chronic diseases are presented in Table 1–7.

Maximum healthy weight targets were offered as the best standard for people not yet overweight. Because the healthy weight target is already exceeded by one in three American adults, a different weight target for overweight people was also proposed, called a "healthier-weight goal."[71] See Table 1–8.

For people who exceed a BMI of 25, a weight loss of 10% was proposed as sufficient to reduce disease risks associated with overweight and also to address the problem of weight regain. The panel's recommendations are meant to highlight the health advantages of sustaining a stable healthy weight throughout life;

Table 1–7 Healthy Body Weight (BMI) Targets Based on Mordibity and Mortality Risks of Chronic Diseases

	Target Weight (BMI)	
Disease	*Men*	*Women*
Cardiovascular	22.6	21.1
Blood pressure regulation	if ≥25, ↓3–5 kg	
Non–insulin-dependent diabetes	≤25	≤25
Osteoarthritis	if ≥25, ↓≈5 kg	
Osteoporosis	≈25 (26–28 limited protection)	
Endometrial and breast cancers		≤27
Colon cancer	stable weight	

Source: Data from J.G. Meisler et al., *American Journal of Clinical Nutrition*, Vol. 63 (supplement), pp. 409S–477S, © 1996, the American Society for Clinical Nutrition.

setting modest, rather than unrealistic, weight loss goals supports the likehood of stabilizing weight after weight loss. Thus, two essential criteria were considered in developing the healthier-weight goal: the goal must be reasonable to achieve and possible to maintain. The proposed healthier-weight goal is approximately two BMI units of weight loss for height as shown in Table 1–8.[71]

What is a healthy body weight? Is it based on mortality, morbidity, ability to function, or on the reality of current average weight? The great range of recommended BMIs in Figure 1–1 suggests the underlying differences and debates about the sources of the data, their interpretation, and their impact on the public and the individual.

Body Fat Definitions

Because obesity, in contrast to overweight, describes excess body fat, measuring the size and number of fat cells would provide one way to define obesity. However, outside of the research laboratory, the procedures for obtaining fat cells are impractical and other measurements of body fat are used. Excess fat accumulation is associated with increased fat cell size, called hypertrophic obesity. In hypercellular obesity fat cell numbers are also increased. The number may increase to three to five times the normal number in people who exceed a BMI of 24 to 25 by approximately 75%.[72] See Chapter 2 for discussion of increased lean body mass in obesity.

Definitions of body fatness or obesity, like definitions of overweight, imply that a specific degree of fatness, or adiposity, is excessive. Adiposity simply reflects an individual's degree of fatness on a continuum of body composition. Just as BMI standards for healthy weight are related to mortality and morbidity risks, so are body

Table 1–8 Healthy Weight Targets (Maximum for Height)* for Adults and Healthier-Weight Goals (Loss in lbs)** for Adults above Healthy Weight Targets

Healthy Weight Target		Healthier Weight Goal	
Height (in)	Weight Maximum (lb)	Height (in)	Weight Loss (lb)
58	119	58	10
59	124	59	10
60	128	60	10
61	132	61	11
62	136	62	11
63	141	63	11
64	145	64	12
65	150	65	12
66	155	66	12
67	159	67	13
68	164	68	13
69	169	69	14
70	174	70	14
71	179	71	14
72	184	72	15
73	189	73	15
74	194	74	16
75	200	75	16
76	205	76	16

*Derived from a body mass index of 25.
**Derived from about two-unit equivalents of the body mass index.
Source: Reprinted with permission from J.G. Meisler and S. St. Jeor, Summary and Recommendations from the American Health Foundation's Expert Panel on Healthy Weight, *American Journal of Clinical Nutrition,* Vol. 63, p. 467S, © 1996, American Society for Clinical Nutrition.

fat standards for "healthy fatness" related to chances of longer life and absence of disease. Criteria for such standards of excess fatness include blood pressure, metabolic homeostasis, and cosmetic concerns. In terms of body fat, obesity is thus defined clinically by the presence of adverse metabolic or cardiovascular consequences corresponding to varying degrees of body fat. As pointed out in Chapter 2, desirable levels of fatness set by experts in sports medicine tend to use lower percentages of body fat than are used in weight management. Classification and standards for body fatness recommended by four researchers are presented in Table 1–9.

For men, 10% to 20% and for women, 17% to 25% are suggested as optimal or normal body fat ranges for Americans.[73–76] As discussed in the first section of this

Table 1–9 Suggested Percent Body Fat Standards for Adults

Classification	Percent Body Fat	
	Males	Females
Neiman[73]		
Lean	<8	<15
Optimal health	8–15	15–22
Slightly overweight	16–20	23–26
Fat	21–24	27–32
Obese (overfat)	≥25	≥32
Wilmore[74]		
Borderline obesity	20–25	30–35
Obesity	≥25	≥35
Lohman[75]		
Not recommended	≤5	≤14
Optimal	10–20	17–25
Obesity	≥25	≥32
Weisner[76]		
Normal	12–20	20–30
Borderline	21–25	31–33
Obese	≥25	≥33

chapter, *overweight* and *overfat* are commonly used interchangeably and, in fact, most overweight people are also overfat. However, the examples of misclassfication presented in Table 1–2 are important to bear in mind when measuring body weight and fatness because the meanings attached to classifications of overweight and obesity are emotionally charged among both professionals and clients in the practice of weight management.

Measurement procedure for body fat: The two common methods for fat estimation in weight management settings are measurements of fat skinfolds (tricep and subscapular) and circumference (waist, thigh, hips), which are then calculated using formulas derived from data obtained by laboratory and field measurements. The classic table used for estimating body fat from skinfolds at four different sites (Table 1–10) was developed on a Scottish population by Durnin and Womersley in 1974[77] and is commonly used although the Scottish standards have not been applied to other populations.[39(p565)]

Triceps and subscapular skinfolds were measured in the NCHS surveys, but since no other measures of body fat were collected, the measurements have not been used to establish standards for fatness. As with BMI distributions, the cutoff points for fatness at, say, the 85th percentile would vary along with the fatness

Table 1–10 Equivalent Fat Content, as Percentage of Body Weight, for a Range of Values for the Sum of Four Skinfolds

Skin-folds (mm)	Men (age in years)				Women (age in years)			
	17–29	30–39	40–49	50+	16–29	30–39	40–49	50+
15	4.8				10.5			
20	8.1	12.2	12.2	12.6	14.1	17.0	19.8	21.4
25	10.5	14.2	15.0	15.6	16.8	19.4	22.2	24.0
30	12.9	16.2	17.7	18.6	19.5	21.8	24.5	26.6
35	14.7	17.7	19.6	20.8	21.5	23.7	26.4	28.5
40	16.4	19.2	21.4	22.9	23.4	25.5	28.2	30.3
45	17.7	20.4	23.0	24.7	25.0	26.9	29.6	31.9
50	19.0	21.5	24.6	26.5	26.5	28.2	31.0	33.4
55	20.1	22.5	25.9	27.9	27.8	29.4	32.1	34.6
60	21.2	23.5	27.1	29.2	29.1	30.6	33.2	35.7
65	22.2	24.3	28.2	30.4	30.2	31.6	34.1	36.7
70	23.1	25.1	29.3	31.6	31.2	32.5	35.0	37.7
75	24.0	25.9	30.3	32.7	32.2	33.4	35.9	38.7
80	24.8	26.6	31.2	33.8	33.1	34.3	36.7	39.6
85	25.5	27.2	32.1	34.8	34.0	35.1	37.5	40.4
90	26.2	27.8	33.0	35.8	34.8	35.8	38.3	41.2
95	26.9	28.4	33.7	36.6	35.6	36.5	39.0	41.9
100	27.6	29.0	34.4	37.4	36.4	37.2	39.7	42.6
105	28.2	29.6	35.1	38.2	37.1	37.9	40.4	43.3
110	28.8	30.1	35.8	39.0	37.8	38.6	41.0	43.9
115	29.4	30.6	36.4	39.7	38.4	39.1	41.5	44.5
120	30.0	31.1	37.0	40.4	39.0	39.6	42.0	45.1
125	31.0	31.5	37.6	41.1	39.6	40.1	42.5	45.7
130	31.5	31.9	38.2	41.8	40.2	40.6	43.0	46.2
135	32.0	32.3	38.7	42.4	40.8	41.1	43.5	46.7
140	32.5	32.7	39.2	43.0	41.3	41.6	44.0	47.2
145	32.9	33.1	39.7	43.6	41.8	42.1	44.5	47.7
150	33.3	33.5	40.2	44.1	42.3	42.6	45.0	48.2
155	33.7	33.9	40.7	44.6	42.8	43.1	45.4	48.7
160	34.1	34.3	41.2	45.1	43.3	43.6	45.8	49.2
165	34.5	34.6	41.6	45.6	43.7	44.0	46.2	49.6
170	34.9	34.8	42.0	46.1	44.1	44.4	46.6	50.0
175	35.3					44.8	47.0	50.4
180	35.6					45.2	47.4	50.8
185	35.9					45.6	47.8	51.2
190						45.9	48.2	51.6
195						46.2	48.5	52.0
200						46.5	48.8	52.4
205							49.1	52.7
210							49.4	53.0

Note: Biceps, triceps, subscapular, and suprailiac of men and women of different ages.

Source: Reprinted with permission from Durnin and Womersley, Biceps, Triceps, Subscapular, and Suprailiac of Men and Women of Different Ages, *British Journal of Nutrition,* Vol. 32, pp. 77–97, © 1974, Cambridge University Press.

level of the American population. Because average weight is increasing[10] and physical fitness level decreasing[78] body fatness must surely also be increasing. Therefore setting a standard based on a percentile for 85% of the population would be misleading. A comprehensive review of body composition measurements, specifically body fat, is presented in Chapter 2.

Regional Fat Distribution

Fat distribution refers to patterns of body fat located in different regions of the body, both central and truncal locations. Persons with central (abdominal) fat are commonly referred to as "apple shaped" or android (male). Those with truncal (gluteofemoral) or peripheral fat are called "pear shaped" or gynoid (female) (Figure 1–4). Regional fat can be estimated by skinfold measurements, by waist-to-hip circumference ratios, or methods such as computed tomography.

Recommendations for "healthy" fat distribution patterns are generally based on the relationship between the waist-to-hip ratio (WHR) and a variety of health outcomes.[48,49,65,66] At least one study found that using the waist measurement alone predicts diabetes risk.[49] Studies that relate health risks and regional fat distribution are increasing because of the growing use of computed tomography (CT) and magnetic resonance imaging (MRI) technology. (See Chapter 2.) Worth noting

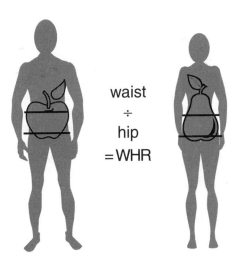

Figure 1–4 Method for determining waist to hip circumference ratio (WHR) of "apple" (left) and "pear" (right) types of fat distribution.

also is that the BMI does not delineate central and truncal locations of excess body fat, and the different health risks associated with them.

In order to use new information in assessing health risks related to overweight, practitioners will benefit from learning clinical methods that accurately measure body circumferences yet use inexpensive equipment. Many studies report using tape measures; however, the measurement site for the waist, in particular, is not consistent among studies.[79,80]

Most regional fat research is based on the hypothesis that central obesity is hazardous to health while truncal obesity is more benign. Central fat is of two kinds: subcutaneous and visceral. Truncal fat is mostly subcutaneous. The visceral fat in the central region seems to have a much more rapid turnover than the sluggish subcutaneous fat in the truncal region, which suggests the mechanism for the increased risk of central obesity. Increased free fatty acids (FFAs) from the increased amount and turnover of visceral fat is thought to generate most of the established risk factors for cardiovascular disease, stroke, and non–insulin-dependent diabetes.[81]

Standards for levels of fat distribution that may indicate risk were developed from the Canadian Fitness Surveys.[82] The IOM states that a WHR of more than 1.0 in males and 0.8 in females suggests a weight distribution that poses increased risks to health compared to excess weight alone.[3(p45)] However, critics claim that these values are based primarily on mortality data from Europeans and may not be appropriate for all age and ethnic groups in the United States.[79] A higher WHR among older people[83] and African American women[84] are two other reported differences. The criteria for risk in various studies is reported to range from >0.95 for men and >0.80 for women and >0.85, >1.00, or >0.90 for both male and females.[79]

The USDA/DHHS 1995 Dietary Guidelines do not give a specific cutoff point at which the WHR may indicate increased health risk; less emphasis is on how fat distribution should be determined and more emphasis on factors that increase central fat distribution such as smoking, stress, and alcohol use.[1]

In addition to central and truncal fat, CT scan images distinguish visceral (intraabdominal) and subcutaneous fat in the abdominal region. Figure 1–5 shows their relationship to WHR. Higher ratios may indicate a higher risk for a clustering of factors known as "syndrome X" or the "metabolic syndrome." Some of the factors are hyperlipidemia, hypertension, and insulin resistance or glucose intolerance.[85,86]

Procedures for Regional Fat Measurements

Waist-to-hip ratio (WHR) or abdominal-to-gluteal circumference ratio (AGR) is calculated by dividing waist girth by hip girth (Figure 1–4). Most researchers follow the procedure of measuring waist and hip circumferences of the subject while standing, using a cloth tape measure at the waist and the hip. The measurement site of the waist is variously described as the "minimal,"[87] "smallest,"[65,88]

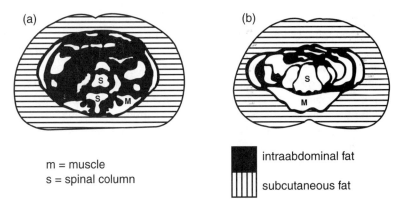

m = muscle
s = spinal column

intraabdominal fat

subcutaneous fat

Figure 1–5 Representative CT scans of (a) women with high WHR and (b) women with low WHR.

"narrowest,"[89,90] or "circumference at the umbilicus."[48,49] A measurement at the umbilicus results in a higher ratio than a measurement at the minimal abdominal girth. However, the level of the umbilicus is often the greatest anterior extension of the abdomen and may be a better indicator of abdominal obesity than the natural waist, which is often the smallest circumference of the torso.[80]

Waist measurement at the umbilicus has been used to collect data in surveys by the National Center for Health Statistics (NCHS) as reported in NHANES II. However, for NHANES III a revised NCHS protocol for measurement of abdominal circumference was developed using a well-defined bony landmark rather than the umbilicus landmark in an attempt to facilitate standardized instructions and reliable measurements. The revised protocol avoids the problem of a displaced umbilicus, common in obese persons. "Specifically, the abdominal circumference in the current NHANES III is taken in a horizontal plane, parallel to the floor at a point palpated and marked just above the right ilium on the midaxillary line."[80(p12)] A video demonstrating this method is now available from: Superintendent of Documents, Box 371954, Pittsburgh, PA 15250-7954. Stock number 017-022-0133505. Critics have pointed out problems of changing techniques in comparing measurements in longitudinal studies.[90] Of course, noting the difference in measurement technique is vital in comparing related disease risks and incidence of elevated WHR among studies.

The hip measurement site appears to be more universally agreed to be the largest circumference or the maximum posterior extension between the iliac crest and buttocks. However, some definitions of the hip site vary from the nearest inch at the maximum point between iliac crest and buttocks to the nearest centimeter at the iliac crest.[79]

Another measure, the abdominal diameter in the sagittal plane, is reported as a marginally better indicator of health risk than WHR.[3(p45)] The basis for this indicator is work in Sweden that found that the sagittal diameter specifically measures visceral rather than subcutaneous abdominal fat when compared to computed tomography measurements. The sagittal diameter is measured when the person lies facing up. A carpenter's level is placed horizontally on the abdomen at the iliac crest. After a normal breath expiration, the sagittal diameter is measured as the distance from table to the horizontal level. The visceral fat should remain in position; the subcutaneous fat tends to fall to the side. Equations for interpreting this measurement in relation to risk are being developed for clinical use.[91]

Medical Definitions

Medical (clinical) definitions of overweight are based on metabolic indicators of disease risk (morbidities) that have been found to be related to various levels of BMI, body fat, and regional fat distribution. The risk factors are commonly called comorbidities when combined with elevated body weight. Figure 1–6 illustrates health risks at various BMI levels considering comorbidities and WHR.

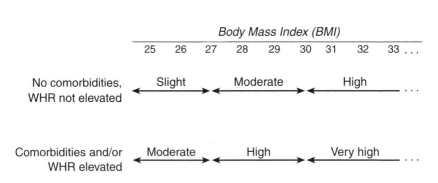

The risks are increased when adipose tissue is concentrated in the abdominal or visceral region (clinically assessed by calculating the waist-to-hip ratio [>1.0 for males and >0.8 for females]) and the presence of comorbidities such as high blood pressure (>140/90), lipid concentrations (cholesterol >200 mg/dl; triglycerides >225 mg/dl), non–insulin-dependent diabetes mellitus, osteoarthritis, sleep apnea, and premature death in the family from coronary heart disease. This figure presents general guidelines; each person requires individual evaluation.

Figure 1–6 Health risk of overweight according to body mass index. *Source:* Adapted with permission from *Weighing the Options: Criteria for Evaluating Weight Management Program,* p. 38, © 1995, National Academy Press.

The term "morbid obesity" usually indicates a level of obesity above a BMI of 30 accompanied by one or more risk factors.[4,5] Table 1–1 illustrates the lack of consistency in the medical descriptors of overweight people used by health professionals.

An ideal medical definition of obesity would be the point above which either excess weight or fat contributes to an increase in risk factors. The problem is that this point is currently unknown, and if it were, differences among individuals, such as genetics and physical activity, would not allow its universal application.[92] The BMI range recommended by one group of experts as a healthy weight in relation to risk factors for seven diseases is presented in Table 1–7. The target weights are suggested as reasonable goals to lower risk based on reviews of clinical and epidemiological studies.[54]

Is it harmful to be overweight? Within the range of "normal" weights, is it better to be thinner? Is it unhealthy if weight changes over time, as happens with repeated fluctuation (weight cycling)? Does it matter if weight increases gradually with age? Most of the research seeks answers by studying disease risk and longevity related to each question in epidemiologic, clinical, and animal studies.

Is it possible to be fit *and* fat? A question of growing importance because of the increased number of Americans who are overweight, or predicted to become so, is whether health risks can be reduced through physical activity in spite of overweight status. One study followed over 25,000 men initially tested for physical fitness. The results suggest that moderate and high levels of physical fitness are associated with lower risk of mortality in overweight and normal-weight men when compared with their low-fit peers.[93] Although physical activity or exercise training may not make all people lean, an active way of life may have important health benefits, even for those who remain overweight.

Overweight is also defined as a medical risk according to other indicators such as the number of hospitalizations,[94] excessive physician visits, work-loss days, and restricted activity days.[95] This type of functional definition is obviously statistically valuable in estimating health care costs. But it is also important when assigning a risk level in the clinical setting because a definition of overweight based on the ability to function in activities of daily living or on the degree of economic and social costs may be more important to an individual than a definition based on longevity.

Another medical definition is "metabolic fitness," proposed as medically oriented goals or outcomes for treatment to replace the focus on weight goals. (See Chapter 18.) Four suggested goal levels in metabolic fitness are:

1. medically significant reduction of risk factors
2. restoration of abnormal risk factors to normal ranges
3. reversal of "high normal" or "borderline" parameters
4. prevention of risk factors in overweight individuals

Metabolic fitness may be independent of weight loss but related to increased healthy behaviors such as increased physical activity, changes in diet such as reduction in fat, saturated fat, or total calories, and increased fruit and vegetable consumption.

Procedures for defining overweight in medical terms include a weight-related medical history, a diet history, physical examination, and biochemical information including a lipid profile and glucose tolerance and insulin sensitivity indicators. Medical risks evaluated by a physician include high blood pressure, insulin resistance or diabetes, low high-density lipoprotein cholesterol (HDL-C)/low-density lipoprotein cholesterol (LDL-C) ratio, left ventricular hypertrophy (LVH), sleep apnea, and hirsutism. A medical evaluation may also include signs of hypothalmic obesity resulting from trauma, malignancy, or inflammatory diseases, and endocrine disorders such as Cushing's disease, polycystic ovary syndrome, hypogonadism, and growth hormone deficiency. Some rare diseases, suggesting genetic factors, may be associated with obesity including Bardet-Biedl, Cohen, and Prader-Willi Syndromes.[96]

A thorough assessment of food and liquid consumption based on food recalls, food records, and food frequency reports is essential in the medical definition of overweight. Estimations of food intake by a registered dietitian or a person trained in determining food portion sizes and nutrient composition of foods may estimate food intake adequately[97] and food diaries do have a valuable role in goal setting and tracking progress in weight management.[98] However, self-reports do not generally represent accurate amounts of food consumption.[99,100] Epidemiological studies that relate food intake and weight generally use a food intake assessment method that has been calibrated with another method in the specific study population. Studies requiring more accurate energy balance information use metabolic laboratory methods of precise food measurement with constant surveillance of the subjects or the doubly labeled water method among free-living subjects, which is a combination of two isotopes taken by mouth and traced in urine. The ratio between them indicates energy consumed. These methods are described in Chapter 2.

Overconsumption of energy, especially from high-fat foods, is a major contributor to overweight in the United States.[101,102] The growing portion size of food servings appears to match growing girth. Discrepancies between expected weight change from survey data and reported energy consumed may result from a changing perception of "normal" portion sizes.[103]

In sum, a medical definition of overweight is based on physical and biochemical measurements that indicate morbidity and mortality risk, disease and diet history information, functional ability, and goals. The medical definition is mostly determined through estimates of risk. Relative risk is calculated from morbidity rates, expressed as incidence rates. Some medical practitioners suggest explaining risk to patients in order to encourage cooperative weight management.[4] For example, if diabetes among overweight individuals 20 to 45 years old is 40 per 1,000 but only 10 per 1,000 among nonoverweight but otherwise comparable individuals in the same population, then the relative incidence of diabetes among the overweight group is 4.0 or 400%. Overweight persons who belong to a group with similar age, sex, and race characteristics may be able to conceptualize risk related to their weight if they are told that within the population group of which they are members, a nonoverweight person's risk of dying or developing a weight-related illness is very much lower than theirs. An individual determination of overweight risk must, of course, consider the number of comorbidities or "risk enhancers" present (Figure 1–6).

Social, Cultural, and Psychological Definitions of Overweight

A comprehensive definition of overweight requires assessment of social, cultural, and psychological aspects of an individual or group. Perceived body image is a defining characteristic of weight management for many people whose goals are weight reduction, weight maintenance, or chronic dieting management. Because obese, overweight, and normal-weight people are evaluated and often evaluate themselves in terms of socially acceptable body size and shape, body size satisfaction can be crucial in defining a person's weight status, setting goals, and evaluating progress in weight management. See Figure 1–7.

Procedures for measuring body size satisfaction: Tools to assess body size and shape satisfaction need only elicit "I look like this" and "I'd like to look like that." Series of line drawing silhouettes have been developed for men and women[104,105] and for children.[106] Intensity of dissatisfaction is indicated by comparing the distance between current and desired silhouettes. Body shape[107] and global body satisfaction questionaires[108,109] are also useful. See Chapter 3 for a discussion of cultural definitions and Chapter 12 for social definitions. Also useful is a collection of case studies of the social aspect of obesity that describes the Nauru people of the Pacific who consider a large body size as a very positive attribute and the importance of understanding social factors on the part of those concerned about medical aspects of overweight.[110] Another study of African American teenagers defines body weight as less important than "attitude."[111]

Measurements of psychological and emotional aspects of overweight are also important components of a person's definition of body weight status. Several measurements are described in Chapter 4 on binge eating and night-eating and in Chapter 18 on emotional measures related to food behavior and body weight. Measures of motivational readiness are helpful in practice,[112] as are assessments of dieting readiness.[113] See Chapter 14 for a discussion of behavior change and measurement. Measures of social definition including discrimination regarding overweight, are discussed in Chapter 13. The practitioner will benefit from assessing several dimensions of weight status in the process of developing an operational definition with each client.

Please answer the following questions by comparing yourself to these figures.

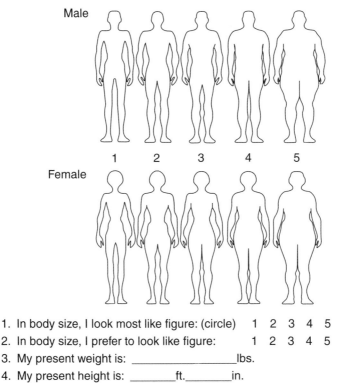

1. In body size, I look most like figure: (circle)   1   2   3   4   5
2. In body size, I prefer to look like figure: 1   2   3   4   5
3. My present weight is: _____lbs.
4. My present height is: _____ft._____in.

Figure 1–7 Example of a silhouette scale to determine perception of body size and shape.

Operational Definitions for the Practitioner

Medical and statistical definitions based on mortality and morbidity data provide only the first step in weight management. The operational definition used by the practitioner depends on the operational definition used by the client. Weight management requires problem solving: identifying, measuring, and addressing a person's main weight-related concerns in order to achieve or maintain a healthy weight. Practitioners may then define or classify overweight clients according to the likely outcome of management, the type of management, or the ability to function economically, psychologically, and socially. Attempts to develop broad-based characterization systems of overweight and obesity that can be applied clinically have had limited progress to date because of the extreme diversity among overfat people.[114]

Yet, the need for cross-disciplinary operating definitions has been demonstrated in successful weight maintenance and prevention of relapse by including coping skills and social support in overall weight management.[115] In Chapter 13, Gromett suggests the need to change the focus of weight management and a method for doing so.

MEASURING OUTCOMES OF WEIGHT MANAGEMENT

In calling for a redefinition of success in obesity intervention, some experts contend that measuring success by the amount of weight lost during a relatively short, predetermined period is "scientifically invalid, inappropriate from a behavioral perspective, and ethically unacceptable." They claim that "long-term amelioration of medical problems and health risk and improved quality of life, with or without weight loss, are the most important measures of success."[116] They, and others,[117,118] state that more appropriate measures than weight or fat loss are increased physical activity, qualitative changes in food consumption, and change in smoking behavior.[119] In turn, these lifestyle changes would be expected to blunt age-related increases in total and central body fatness.[87] Total weight management includes a concern for a healthy quality of life, regardless of weight. Measuring success of obese people in shedding their shame and accepting responsibility for making the difficult countercultural changes to improve their health regardless of weight are also important outcomes. In weight management, baseline and continued measurement of multiple aspects of weight status are essential.[120]

REFERENCES

1. US Department of Agriculture and US Department of Health and Human Services. *Dietary Guidelines for Americans.* 4th ed. Washington, DC: US GPO; 1995. Home and Garden Bull 232.

2. *Anthropometric Reference Data and Prevalence of Overweight, United States 1976–1980.* Hyattsville, MD: NCHS. 1987. DHHS Publ (PHS) 87-1688.

3. Institute of Medicine. *Weighing the Options: Criteria for Evaluating Weight-Management Programs.* Washington, DC: National Academy Press; 1995.

4. Van Itallie TA. Body weight, morbidity, and longevity. In: Bjorntorp P, Brodoff BN, eds. *Obesity.* Philadelphia: JB Lippincott Co; 1992:361–370.

5. Mahan LK, Escott-Stump S. *Krause's Food, Nutrition & Diet Therapy.* 9th ed. Philadelphia: WB Saunders Co; 1996.

6. Department of Health. *The Health of the Nation: Reversing the Increasing Problem of Obesity in England. A Report from the Nutrition and Physical Activity Task Forces.* London: HMSO; 1995.

7. Lyons P, Burgard D. *Great Shape.* Palo Alto, CA: Bull Publishing; 1989.

8. Brown LS. *Overcoming Fear of Fat.* Binghamton, NY: Harrington/Haworth Press; 1989.

9. Gregory J, Foster K, Tyler H, Wiseman M. *The Dietary and Nutritional Survey of British Adults.* London: Office of Population and Census Surveys. HMSO; 1990.

10. Kuczmarski RJ, Flegal KM, Campbell SM, Johnson CL. Increasing prevalence of overweight among US adults. *JAMA.* 1994;272:205–211.

11. Kushner RF. Body weight and mortality. *Nutr Rev.* 1993;51:127–136.

12. Smalley KJ, Knerr AN, Kendrick ZV, Colliver JA, Owen OE. Reassessment of body mass indices. *Am J Clin Nutr.* 1990;52:405–408.

13. Garrow JS. *Treat Obesity Seriously: A Clinical Manual.* Edinburgh, Scotland: Churchill Livingstone; 1981.

14. Bray GA. Obesity: Historical development of scientific and cultural ideas. *Int J Obes.* 1990;14:909–926.

15. Newburgh LH, Johnston MW. Endogenous obesity—a misconception. *JAMA.* 1930;3:815–825.

16. Weigley ES. Average? Ideal? Desirable? A brief overview of height-weight tables in the United States. *J Am Diet Assoc.* 1984;84:417–423.

17. Vague J. The degree of masculine differentiation of obesities: a factor determining predisposition to diabetes, atherosclerosis, gout, and uric calculus. *Am J Clin Nutr.* 1956;4:20–34.

18. Brown PJ. The biocultural evolution of obesity: an anthropological view. In: Bjorntorp P, Brodoff BN, eds. *Obesity.* Philadelphia: JB Lippincott Co; 1992:320–329.

19. Rice P. Prehistoric Venuses: symbols of motherhood or womanhood. *J Anthropol Res.* 1981;37:402–409.

20. Shakespeare W. *Henry IV,* Part One, Act II, Scene 2.

21. Fat personality. *Newsweek.* Nov 17, 1952:110.

22. Bruch H. *Eating Disorders: Obesity, Anorexia Nervosa and the Person Within.* New York: Basic Books; 1973.

23. Symonds B. The influence of overweight and underweight on vitality. *Med Soc NJ.* 1908;5:159–165.

24. Metropolitan Life Insurance Company. Ideal weights for women. *Stat Bull Metrop Insur Co.* 1942;23:6–8.

25. Metropolitan Life Insurance Company. Ideal weights for men. *Stat Bull Metrop Insur Co.* 1943;24:6–8.

26. Society of Actuaries. *Build and Blood Pressure Study.* Vol 1. Chicago: Society of Actuaries; 1959.

27. Metropolitan Life Insurance Company. New weight standards for men and women. *Stat Bull Metrop Insur Co.* 1959;40:1–5.

28. National Research Council. *Recommended Dietary Allowances.* Washington, DC: National Academy Press; 1980.

29. *Advance Data, Overweight Adults in the United States.* Hyattsville, MD: National Center for Health Statistics; 1979. DHEW Publ (PHS) 79-1250.

30. Society of Actuaries. *Build Study 1979.* Chicago: Society of Actuaries, Association of Life Insurance, Medical Directors of America; 1980.

31. Metropolitan Life Insurance Company. 1983 Height and weight tables. *Stat Bull Metrop Insur Co.* 1984;64:2–9.

32. Frisancho R, Flegel PN. Elbow breadth as a measure of frame size for US males and females. *Am J Clin Nutr.* 1983;37:311–314.

33. Katch VL, Freedson PS. Body size and shape: derivation of the "HAT" frame size model. *Am J Clin Nutr.* 1982;36:669–675.

34. Katch VL, Freedson PS, Katch FI, Smith L. Body frame size: validity of self-appraisal. *Am J Clin Nutr.* 1982;36:676–679.

35. Novascone MA, Smith EP. Frame size estimation: a comparative analysis of methods based on height, wrist circumference, and elbow breadth. *J Am Diet Assoc.* 1989;89:964–966.

36. US Department of Agriculture and US Department of Health and Human Services. *Dietary Guidelines for Americans.* 3rd ed. Washington, DC: US GPO-273-930; 1990. Home and Garden Bull 232.

37. Andres R, Elahi D, Tobin JD, Muller DC, Brant L. Impact of age on weight goals. *Ann Intern Med.* 1985;103:1030–1033.

38. Waaler HT. Height, weight and mortality: The Norwegian experience. *Acta Med Scand Suppl.* 1984;679:1–56.

39. National Research Council Committee on Diet and Health. *Diet and Health: Implications for Reducing Chronic Disease Risk.* Washington, DC: National Academy Press; 1989.

40. Willett WC, Stampfer M, Manson J, VanItallie T. New weight guidelines for Americans: justified or injudicious? *Am J Clin Nutr.* 1991;53:1102–1103.

41. Colditz GA, Willett WC, Stampfer MJ, et al. Weight as a risk factor for clinical diabetes in women. *Am J Epidemiol.* 1990;132:501–513.

42. Manson JE, Colditz GA, Stampfer MJ, Willett WC. A prospective study of obesity and risk of coronary heart disease in women. *N Engl J Med.* 1990;322:882–889.

43. Consumers Union. Are you eating right? *Consumer Reports Magazine.* 1992;Oct:RO119.

44. Long P. The great weight debate. *Health.* 1992;Feb/Mar:42–47.

45. US Department of Agriculture, Dietary Guidelines Advisory Committee. *Report of the Dietary Guidelines Advisory Committee on the Dietary Guidelines for Americans, 1995.* To the Secretary of Health and Human Services and the Secretary of Agriculture. Beltsville, MD: Agricultural Research Service; 1995.

46. Willett WC, Manson JE, Stampfer MF. Weight, weight change, and coronary heart disease in women. *JAMA.* 1995;273:461–465.

47. Lee RD, Nieman DC. *Nutritional Assessment.* Madison, WI: Brown and Benchmark; 1993.

48. Rimm EB, Stampfer MJ, Giovannucci E, Ascherio A, Spiegelman D, Colditz GA, Willett WC. Body size and fat distribution as predictors of coronary heart disease among middle-aged and older US men. *Am J Epidemiol.* 1995;141:1117–1127.

49. Chan JM, Rimm EB, Colditz GA, Stampfer MJ, Willett WC. Obesity, fat distribution, and weight gain as risk factors for clinical diabetes in men. *Diabetes Care.* 1994;17:961–969.

50. Colditz GA, Willett WC, Rotnitzky A, Manson JE. Weight gain as risk factor for clinical diabetes mellitus in women. *Ann Intern Med.* 1995;122:548–549.

51. Troiano R, Frongillo E, Sobal J, Levitsky D. Relationship between body weight and mortality. *Int J Obesity.* 1996;20:63–75.

52. Berg FM. New guidelines given for "healthy weight." *Healthy Weight J.* 1996;May/June:53–54,57.

53. American Institute of Nutrition. Report of the American Institute of Nutrition (AIN) Steering Committee on healthy weight. *J Nutr.* 1994;124:2240–2243.

54. American Health Foundation Roundtable on Healthy Weight. Report of an expert panel discussion. *Am J Clin Nutr.* 1996;63:409S–477S.

55. Stunkard AJ. Introduction and overview. In: Stunkard AJ, Wadden TA, eds. *Obesity: Theory and Therapy.* New York: Raven Press; 1993.

56. Hamwi GJ. Therapy changing dietary concepts. In: Danowski TS, ed. *Diabetes Mellitus: Diagnosis and Treatment.* Vol 1. New York: American Diabetes Association; 1964:73–78.

57. Roth JH. What is optimum body weight? *J Am Diet Assoc.* 1995;95:856–857.

58. Powers MA, ed. *Nutrition Guide for Professionals.* Chicago: American Diabetes Assoc and American Dietetic Assoc; 1988.

59. Knapp TR. A methodological critique of the "ideal weight" concept. *JAMA.* 1983;250:508–512.

60. Manson JE, Stampfer MJ, Hennekens CH, Willett WC. Body weight and longevity: a reassessment. *JAMA.* 1987;257:353–358.

61. Frisancho AR. *Anthropometric Standards for the Assessment of Growth and Nutritional Status.* Ann Arbor, MI: University of Michigan Press; 1990.

62. US Department of Health and Human Services, Public Health Service. *The Surgeon General's Report on Nutrition and Health.* Washington, DC: US GPO; 1988. Pub. no. 88-50210.

63. US Department of Agriculture and US Department of Health and Human Services. *Dietary Guidelines for Americans.* Washington, DC: US GPO; 1980. Home and Garden Bull 232.

64. US Department of Agriculture and US Department of Health and Human Services. *Dietary Guidelines for Americans.* 2nd ed. Washington, DC: US GPO; 1986. Home and Garden Bull 232-2.

65. Wing RR, Matthews KA, Kuller LH, Meilahn EN, Plantinga P. Waist to hip ratio in middle-aged women: associations with behavioral and psychosocial factors and with changes in cardiovascular risk factors. *Arterio Thrombosis.* 1991;11:1250–1257.

66. Troisi RJ, Heinold JW, Vokonos PS, Weiss ST. Cigarette smoking, dietary intake, and physical activity: effects on body fat distribution—the normative aging study. *Am J Clin Nutr.* 1991;53:1104–1111.

67. National Institute of Diabetes and Digestive and Kidney Diseases (NIDDK). *Understanding Adult Obesity.* Rockville, MD: National Institutes of Health; 1993. NIH Pub. No. 94-34-3680.

68. Minister of National Health and Welfare (Canada). *Canadian Guidelines for Healthy Weights: Report of an Expert Group.* Ottawa, Canada: Minister of Supply and Services; 1988.

69. World Health Organization. *Report of a WHO Study Group: Diet, Nutrition, and the Prevention of Chronic Diseases.* Geneva, Switzerland: WHO; 1990. WHO Tech Rep Series 797.

70. World Health Organization. *Physical Status: The Use and Interpretation of Anthropometry: Report of a WHO Expert Committee.* Geneva, Switzerland: WHO; 1995. WHO Technical Report Series 854.

71. Meisler JG, St Jeor S. Summary and recommendations from the American Health Foundation's Expert Panel on Healthy Weight. *Am J Clin Nutr.* 1996;63(suppl):474S–477S.

72. Hirsch J, Batchelor B. Adipose tissue cellularity in human obesity. *Clin Endocrinol Metab.* 1976;5:299–311.

73. Neiman DC. *Fitness and Sports Medicine: An Introduction.* Palo Alto, CA: Bull Publishing Co; 1990.

74. Wilmore JH. Body composition. In Brownell KD, Fairburn CG, eds. *Eating Disorders and Obesity.* New York: Guilford Press; 1995:42–45.

75. Lohman TG. Measurement of body energy stores. In: Brownell KD, Fairburn CG, eds. *Eating Disorders and Obesity.* New York: Guilford Press; 1995:95–99.

76. Weisner RL. Clinical assessment of obese patients. In: Brownell KD, Fairburn CG, eds. *Eating Disorders and Obesity.* New York: Guilford Press; 1995:463–468.

77. Durnin JV, Womersley J. Body fat assessed from total body density and its estimation from skinfold thickness: measurements on 481 men and women aged from 16–72 years. *Br J Nutr.* 1974;32:77–97.

78. US Department of Health and Human Services, Public Health Service. *Healthy People 2000: Midcourse Review and 1995 Revisions.* Hyattsville, MD: DHHS; 1996. (PHS) 96-1232-2.

79. Croft JB, Keenan NL, Sheridan DP, Wheeler FC, Speers MA. Waist-to-hip ratio in a biracial population: measurement, implications, and cautions for using guidelines to define high risk for cardiovascular disease. *J Am Diet Assoc.* 1995;95:60–64.

80. Chumlea WC, Kuczmarski RJ. Using a bony landmark to measure waist circumference. *J Am Diet Assoc.* 1995;95:12.

81. Bjorntorp P. Regional obesity. In: Bjorntorp P, Brodoff BN, eds. *Obesity.* Philadelphia: JB Lippincott Co; 1992:579–586.

82. Minister of State, Fitness and Amateur Sport. Canadian Standardized Test of Fitness (for 15 to 69 years of age). 3rd ed. *Operations Manual.* Ottawa, Ontario: Government of Canada; 1986. FAS 7378.

83. Folsom AR, Burke GL, Byer CL, et al. Implications of obesity for cardiovascular disease in blacks: the CARDIA and ARIC studies. *Am J Clin Nutr.* 1991;53:1604S–1611S.

84. Lackland DT, Orchard TJ, Keil JE, Saunders DE, et al. Are race differences and the prevalence of hypertension explained by body mass and fat distribution? A survey in a biracial population. *Int J Epidemiol.* 1992;21:238–245.

85. Bjorntorp P. Abdominal obesity and the development of noninsulin-dependent diabetes mellitus. *Diabetes Metab Rev.* 1988;4:615–622.

86. Matsuzawa Y, Shimomura I, Nakamura T, Keno Y, Kotani K, Tokunage K. Pathophysiology and pathogenesis of visceral fat obesity. *Obes Res.* 1995;3:187S–194S.

87. Poehlman ET, Roth MJ, Bunyard LB, et al. Physiological predictors of increasing total and central adiposity in aging men and women. *Arch Intern Med.* 1995;155:2443–2448.

88. Lapidus L, Bengtsson C, Hallstrom T, Bjorntorp P. Obesity, adipose tissue distribution and health in women: results from a population study in Gothenburg, Sweden. *Appetite.* 1989;13:25–35.

89. Young TK, Gelskey DE. Is noncentral obesity metabolically benign? *JAMA.* 1995;274:1939–1941.

90. Carson CA, Meilahn EN, Caggiula AW. Comparison of waist measurements: a methodologic issue in longitudinal studies. *J Am Diet Assoc.* 1994;94:771–772.

91. Sjostrom L. Impacts of body weight, body composition, and adipose tissue distribution on morbidity and mortality. In: Stunkard AJ, Wadden TA, eds. *Obesity: Theory and Therapy.* New York: Raven Press; 1993.

92. US Department of Health and Human Services, Public Health Service. *Healthy People 2000: National Health Promotion and Disease Prevention Objectives.* Hyattsville, MD: DHHS; 1990. (PHS) 88-50210.

93. Barlow CE, Kohl HW, Gibbons LW, Blair SN. Physical fitness, mortality and obesity. *Int J Obesity.* 1995;19:S41–S44.

94. Sichieri R, Everhart JE, Hubbard VS. Relative weight classifications in the assessment of underweight and overweight in the United States. *Int J Obes.* 1992;16:303–312.

95. Wolf AM, Colditz GA. Social and economic effects of body weight in the United States. *Am J Clin Nutr.* 1996;63(suppl):466S–469S.

96. Bray GA. Etiology and prevalence of obesity. In: Bouchard C, ed. *The Genetics of Obesity.* Boca Raton, FL: CRC; 1994:17–33.

97. Dwyer JT. Dietary assessment. In: Shils ME, Olson JA, Shike M, eds. *Modern Nutrition in Health and Disease.* 8th ed. Philadelphia: Lea & Febiger; 1993:842–860.

98. Streit KJ, Stevens NH, Stevens VJ. Food records: a predictor and modifier of weight change in a long-term weight loss program. *J Am Diet Assoc.* 1991;91:213–216.

99. Lichtman SW, Pisarska K, Berman ER, et al. Discrepancy between self-reported and actual calorie intake and exercise in obese subjects. *N Engl J Med.* 1992;327:1893–1898.

100. Heymsfield SB, Darby PC, Muhlheim LS, Gallagher D, Wolper C, Allison DB. The calorie: myth, measurement, and reality. *Am J Clin Nutr.* 1995;62(suppl):1034S–1041S.

101. Pi-Sunyar FX. The fattening of America. *JAMA.* 1994;272:238–239.

102. McDowell MA, Briefel RR, Alaimo K, et al. *Energy and Macronutrient Intakes of Persons Ages 2 Months and Over in the United States: Third National Health and Nutrition Examination Survey, Phase 1, 1988–91.* Hyattsville, MD: National Center for Health Statistics: AdvanceData; 1994. DHHS Publ 255 (PHS) 95-1250.

103. Young LR, Nestle M. Portion sizes in dietary assessment: issues and policy implications. *Nutr Rev.* 1995;53:149–158.

104. Stunkard A, Sorenson T, Schlusinger F. Use of the Davish Adoption Register for the study of obesity and thinness. In: Kety S, Rowland LP, Sidman RL, Matthysse, eds. *The Genetics of Neurological and Psychiatric Disorders.* New York: Raven; 1983:115–120.

105. Williamson DA, Davis CJ, Bennett SM, Goreczny AJ, Gleaves DH. Development of a simple procedure for assessing body image disturbances. *Behavioral Assessment.* 1989;11:433–446.

106. Collins ME. Body figure perceptions and preferences among preadolescent children. *Int J Eating Dis.* 1991;10:199–208.

107. Cooper PJ, Taylor MJ, Cooper Z, Fairburn CG. The development and validation of the Body Shape Questionnaire. *Int J Eating Dis.* 1987;6:485–494.

108. Slade PD, Dewey ME, Newton T, Brodie D, Kiemle G. Development and preliminary validation of the Body Satisfaction Scale (BSS). *Psychology and Health.* 1990;4:213–220.

109. Thompson JK, Fabian LJ, Moulton DO, Dunn MF, Altabe MN. Development and validation of the physical appearance related testing scale. *J Per Assess.* 1991;56:512–521.

110. Pollock NJ. Social fattening patterns in the Pacific—the positive side of obesity. A Nauru case study. In: de Garine I, Pollock NJ, eds. *Social Aspects of Obesity.* Amsterdam: Bordon and Breach Science Publishers; 1995:87–109.

111. Parker S, Nichter M, Nichter M, Vuckovic N, Sims C, Ritenbaugh C. Body image and weight concerns among African American and White adolescent females: differences that make a difference. *Human Org.* 1995;54:103–114.

112. Rossi JS, Rossi SR, Velicer WF, Prochaska JO. Motivational readiness to control weight. In: Allison, ed. *Handbook of Assessment Methods for Eating Behaviors and Weight-Related Problems.* Thousand Oaks, CA: Sage Publications; 1995:387–430.

113. Brownell KD. The Dieting Readiness Test. *The Weight Control Digest.* 1990;1:6–8. Reproduced in IOM, *Weighing the Options: Criteria for Evaluating Weight-Management Programs.* Washington, DC: National Academy Press; 1995, 198–205.

114. Parham ES. Nutrition education research in weight management among adults. *J Nutr Ed.* 1993;25:258–268.

115. Kayman S, Bruvold W, Stern JS. Maintenance and relapse after weight loss in women: behavioral aspects. *Am J Clin Nutr.* 1990;52:800–807.

116. Robison JI, Hoerr SL, Petersmarck KA, Anderson JV. Redefining success in obesity intervention: the new paradigm. *J Am Diet Assoc.* 1995;95:422–423.

117. Atkinson RL. Proposed standards for judging the success of the treatment of obesity. *Ann Intern Med.* 1993;119:677–680.

118. Abernathy RP, Black DR. Is adipose tissue oversold as a health risk? *J Am Diet Assoc.* 1994;94:641–644.

119. Seidell JC, Verschuren VMM, VanLeer EM, Kromhout D. Overweight, underweight, and mortality. *Arch Intern Med.* 1996;156:958–963.

120. Sullivan M, Karlsson J, Sjöstrom L, et al. Swedish obese subjects (SOS)—an intervention study of obesity. Baseline evaluation of health and psychosocial functioning in the first 1743 subjects examined. *Int J Obes.* 1993;17:503–512.

CHAPTER 2

Body Composition and Resting Metabolic Rate: New and Traditional Measurement Methods

Richard N. Pierson Jr.
Jack Wang
Carol N. Boozer

INTRODUCTION

Measurements of body composition and metabolism are fundamental to scientific approaches in the diagnosis of a few diseases, and to the management of many of the interventions that have during this century changed medicine from a descriptive art to an interventional science. One of the early Christian disciples and saints, Doubting Thomas, is depicted in a statue measuring the depth of the crucifixial wounds of Christ, in order to judge the truth of the subsequent miracle of the resurrection, and to provide credibility to disciples who would tell the story to an audience of citizens taught by their experience to be skeptical. In the modern era, the skeptical citizens are replaced by the Food and Drug Administration (FDA), or by our colleagues seeking better titration of doses of drugs with a small margin of therapeutic/toxic ratio. The principle is comparable: measurements must be appropriate as well as accurate. Height, weight, and external widths and circumferences can be measured with an accuracy that can almost arbitrarily be extended beyond the range of usefulness. Thus several tissue masses, not only the adipose tissue, are abnormal in obesity, and obesity and its treatment cannot be easily understood unless measurements are carried beyond those of fat alone. For example, in acquired immune deficiency syndrome (AIDS), the epiphenomena of shrinking body cell mass, loss of body fat, and fluctuating extracellular water each affect body weight, but when each can be precisely measured, effective interventions can be discriminated from harmful ones. In managing obesity, understanding the contribution of each tissue to weight, and the homeostatic mechanisms controlling adipose tissue, may benefit both the clinician and the patient.

A BRIEF HISTORY OF BODY COMPOSITION METHODOLOGIES

The fundamental studies of body composition earlier in this century were chemical. Small numbers of chemistry-based analyses of cadavers carried out by Forbes in the 1950s were important extensions of the techniques of chemical analysis first applied to cadavers in Germany a century previously.[1] Chemical analysis is a direct and potentially precise method for the analysis of body composition at the molecular level. However, there are three inherent problems that interfere with the utility of these anatomic/chemical measurements. First, each of these investigations was based on tedious and remarkable efforts to control the calculations required in aliquoting large masses of tissue. Difficult dissections at times required arbitrary separations, and large volume multiplication factors of concentrations measured by chemical analyses had to be applied to measurements with a margin of error in the range of ±2%. Second, the health status of subjects becoming available as cadavers as appropriate surrogates for normal populations is inherently uncertain. Third, body composition varies by sex, age, and occupation, making "average" body composition as irrelevant to the clinician faced with a particular patient, as the post-Platonic philosophers found Socrates' "theory of the Forms" to be applicable to the problems of the agora.

In the middle of this century, three basic techniques for measuring body composition were added to the armamentarium of the modern analogues of doubting Thomas. These methods, hydrodensitometry, body water, and body potassium, are often described as the "traditional methods." Each depends on the simplification, or the "model," that the body consists of two components: fat and lean body mass. By this model, if one of these two components is measured by some technique, the other component can be inferred by subtraction, since body weight is readily and accurately measured. Body water in the Pace method,[2] body density in the Behnke method,[3] and body potassium in the Forbes method[4] all produce an estimate of lean body mass, depending on the assumption that water, density, or potassium are constant in the fat-free mass. At about the same time, stimulated by the problems of management of a large number of burn victims, the surgeon Francis Moore[5] began a series of "pools and volumes" measurements in which multiple body components, or compartments, were measured simultaneously by isotope dilution. In the same wartime decade, Brozek et al[6] studied starvation and refeeding by multiple techniques simultaneously. By 1963, when an epochal symposium on body composition was convened by the New York Academy of Sciences,[7] the groundwork for multi-compartmental analysis had been well developed.

Physical anthropometry, the measurement of height, weight, widths, circumferences, and skinfold thicknesses, was developed over the same period, providing nutritionists, epidemiologists, and physicians studying and caring for larger populations with field-level tools to study growth, development, and malnutrition in circumstances when field surveys, or remote populations, required inexpensive and noninvasive methods. These methods have often been calibrated and validated when more laboratory-intensive methods were available.[8]

The techniques developed and refined in the 1960s and 1970s were applied widely enough to turn up problems, and to stimulate the development of the current generation of methods. All of these methods depend on assumptions of the constancy of a measured element or characteristic, usually an element of the "lean body," an entity that we prefer to redefine as the "fat-free mass," because this definition recognizes that the adipocyte is a member of the body cell mass. However, virtually every study in which the assumed constancies have been carefully measured has shown that gender, age, fatness, and ethnicity are potent variables affecting these "constants," which are therefore in fact not constant at anything like the margin of error of ±2% to 5% we now expect of our measurements. These variables thus render incorrect, or at least only approximate, the body composition measurements derived from them.

As a result of these observations, reflection on their implications for the study of body composition, researchers must turn to a new generation of methods that are free of the constancy assumptions that, although the mainstay of measurement science in obesity for the past 30 years, can provide only approximate, "first decimal place" accuracy. This chapter provides a review of the traditional methods, since most of the literature in body composition requires that they be understood. It is clear that the "constancy assumption" methods of body composition can provide highly useful approximations, but not precise understanding of compartment changes, particularly when a disease process (and obesity is a disease process) distorts some of the intercompartmental ratios that are less variable in normals. Approximation in science has an honorable history: Copernican astronomy could predict the courses of the stars and planets with sufficient precision for open-air navigation to discover new continents, but was supplanted by the precision of Newtonian mechanics.

COMPARTMENTAL MODELS OF HUMAN ANATOMY

It is convenient to describe the components of body composition by using numbers from a "standard" man and woman. Figure 2–1 shows the "four-compartment" model, an arrangement of molecular components according to structural *compartments,* which provides a convenient, powerful, and integrated understanding of the physiologic relationships among them. The four compartments are the body cell mass (BCM), the extracellular water (ECW), skeletal components, and the adipose tissue (AT). Most of the intercompartmental homeostatic mechanisms operate at the level of the *components* of the four compartments, and most of the measurement systems involve measuring or accounting for these contents. Figure 2–1 shows these four compartments in a structure diagram, scaled by weight in a healthy young man, which we shall apply throughout this chapter.

The body cell mass consists of all the living cells. The BCM makes up from 20% to 50% of body weight in health, more in males and less in females due to the larger skeletal muscle mass in males. All cellular metabolism, anabolic and catabolic, occurs only in this compartment, providing the "purpose" for which the other compartments exist. Since body composition measurements, at the whole-body level, are restricted to considering the average body cell, the measured cell mass will be a composite of average body cells, an abstraction that is occasionally useful. Since the cells of individual organs differ greatly in their contents according to their individual functions, the body cell mass components that can be measured by whole-body techniques will be dominated by the contents of the large organs, of which the skeletal muscle mass is by far the largest, comprising from 50% to 80% of the total cell mass.

Intracellular water (ICW) accounts for approximately 80% of the body cell mass. Cells receive their special attributes according to their proteins, which are organized into specialized molecular and structural configurations according to the organs where they are found. These proteins carry out every aspect of the control of cellular composition, and determine every aspect of cell function. The other chemical components of the cell are lipids, primarily in the cell membrane; the electrolytes, partially in solution in the intracellular water, where they play an electrochemical role; and carbohydrates, which are largely sources of highly available energy.

Specialized Organs of the Body Cell Mass

Nerve and muscle include those cells that function by depolarizing and repolarizing their membranes, resulting in contraction and relaxation in the case of muscle, and transmitting impulses in the case of the nervous system. These cells depend on specialized membranes that respond to triggering messages by quickly passing ions of sodium (Na) into, and potassium (K) out of the cell. Since the membrane potential of the cells is created by the potassium and sodium gradients (K_{IN} to K_{OUT}, and Na_{OUT} to Na_{IN}), the result of a successful depolarization and repolarization is associated with loss of the membrane potential, which varies among cell types from about -90 MeV in muscle cells to about -50 MeV in intestinal cells, a potential that is described by the Nernst equation.

The body cell mass is the sum of many disparate organs of different specialized components including, in most analytic systems, the viscera. The BCM is measured

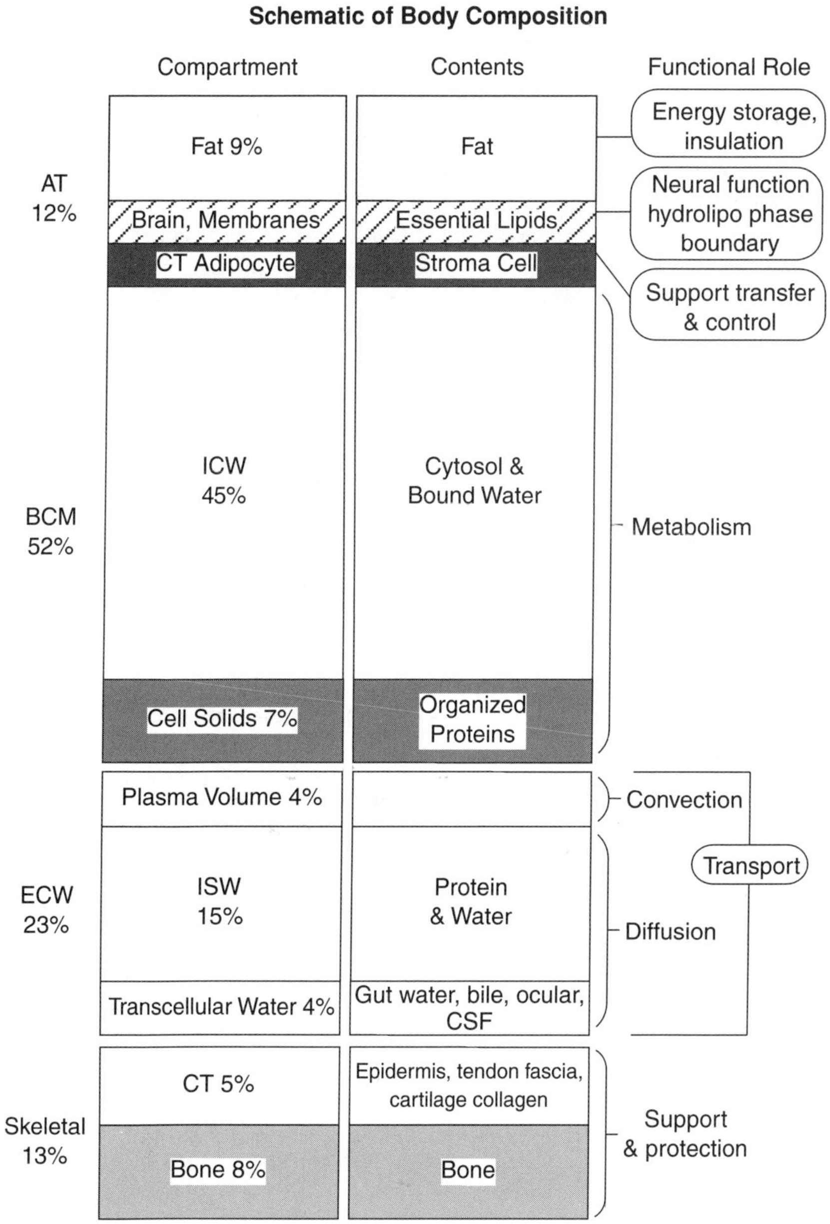

Schematic of Body Composition

Figure 2–1 Principal contents and functional roles of the four compartments scaled by weight in a healthy young man.

as a physiologic compartment, which is the volume of distribution of the principal intracellular cation potassium, after subtraction of the $2 \pm 0.5\%$ of body K, which is in the extracellular water. The measurement of body potassium is described later in this chapter. While this is an important technique among methods of determining body composition, only highly specialized laboratories have this capability. This method should be considered an important capability for any body composition laboratory because it marks better than any other method the body cell mass, and provides a measurement of the integrity or quality of this central compartment.

Extracellular fluid (ECF) accounts for 22% to 28% of body weight, and is the principal component of the vascular, the lymphatic, and the interstitial spaces. The largest component of the ECF, the extracellular water, makes up 95% of the volume of the ECF. It serves as the transport vehicle for plasma proteins (5% by weight), ions, gases, carbohydrates, lipids, and metabolites by mass transfer in the vascular spaces, and by diffusion in the interstitial spaces and at the cell membranes. Active metabolism transfers solutes and ions across the cell membranes according to individual organ system requirements, and whole-body setpoints control the osmotic and ionic balances, largely at the glomeruli and loop systems in the kidney.

Plasma volume is a subset of the ECF, at about 4% of body weight, serving as the transport fluid within the vascular spaces, and also as a vehicle for the red cell mass, about 3% of weight, and the other mobile cells of the granulocyte, lymphocyte, and platelet series.

Water spaces are measured by tracer dilution according to the principles of indicator dilution theory. Total body water (TBW) is readily measured by the prompt (1 to 3 hours) dilution of any of several tracers, based on the fact that there is no barrier to the free diffusion of water at most cell membranes. The margin of error of the measurement for TBW is about 1%. The size of the measured ECW is dependent on the molecular species of the tracer chosen; the smaller the molecule, the larger the measured space. Choice of tracer is influenced by safety (radiation is associated with several of the most effective tracers), convenience, ease of measurement, and cost. Different tracers produce different measured ECW spaces. The plasma volume and the red cell mass are readily measured by tracer dilution; when a solid, iodinated human serum albumin, is used as the tracer, it is the smaller ECF that is measured rather than the 5% larger ECW, which is measured by a molecular tracer such as sulfate.

Skeletal compartment components are the bone organ, about 8% of body weight, and the non-vital portions of connective tissues (CT), tendons, ligaments, CT adipocytes, and the external, non-vital layers of the epidermis.

THE TRADITIONAL METHODS: TWO-COMPARTMENT MODELS

All models provide simplifications that are used for teaching or research purposes. The older two-compartment models are so basic to many current teachings that they must be placed into the framework of any text. We do so in Figure 2–2, which indicates the relationships between the two- and the four-compartment models. All two-compartment systems divide the body into fat and fat-free, and all depend on an attribute of the fat-free body. The body water, body density, and body potassium methods each measure the fat-free component, and infer the fat mass by subtraction. It should first be made clear that there is a difference between fat-free mass (FFM) and lean body mass (LBM). These two terms are often used interchangeably in spite of their different meanings. The lean body mass refers to fat-free tissue in a living organism and includes a small amount of essential fat (perhaps as much as 3%) within

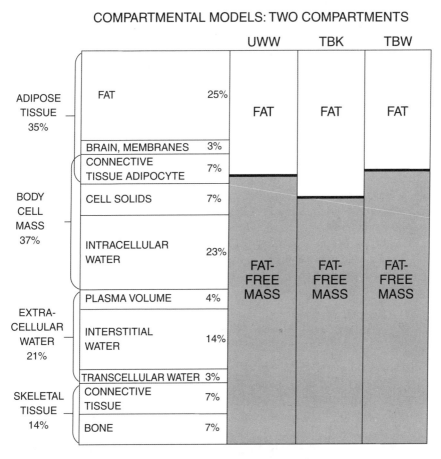

Figure 2–2 The left panel shows four body composition compartments in a healthy young woman. The three right-side panels provide simplified approximations according to the indicated fat measurements, but no information concerning the fat-free mass.

internal organs, bone marrow, and all neural tissues, mainly the central nervous system (CNS). In contrast, fat-free mass implies tissue devoid of all extractable fat, a compartment that can only be measured through direct chemical analysis. The LBM sums the non-adipose tissue components of a living organism (determined by indirect methods, and containing a small amount of essential fat). In fact, the LBM is made up of many organs that differ widely in hydration, density, and potassium content. However, this is considered by many to be a useful term, and with the newer methods of measuring organ volumes by the sum of image slices, it may be considered a "measurable" compartment.

BODY COMPOSITION MEASUREMENT METHODS

Densitometry (Hydrostatic Weighing)

The use of densitometry to determine body composition is based on the fact that at normal body temperature (37°C or 98.6°F), the density of body fat is 0.901×10 kg/m^3 and the average density of the FFM is 1.097×10 kg/m. When body density is measured, the percent of body weight as fat can be calculated from prediction equations given by Siri,[9] Brozek et al,[6] and others.

Body density is most commonly estimated from hydrostatic weighing by applying Archimedes' principle. The subject is asked to submerge, expire maximally, and remain as motionless as possible for a few seconds while underwater weight is recorded. Because any air remaining in the lungs, and gases trapped in the gastrointestinal tract, sinuses, etc., at the time of underwater weighing contribute to buoyancy, these volumes must be corrected for. In general, gas other than in the lungs is small in quantity and can be ignored. However, residual lung volume is large and therefore must be measured and subtracted from the total body volume. It is usually estimated by means of the closed-circuit nitrogen dilution technique with 100% oxygen as the tracer gas.[10] Body density and percentage of body fat can then be calculated as follows:

Body density = Mass/Volume
        = (Wt in air)/[(Wt in air – Wt in water)/(Residual volume – Density of water)]
% Body fat   = [(4.95/Body density) – 4.501] × 100

This method is well established and is commonly accepted as the "gold standard" in the study of body composition. However, the procedure is not without problems. The errors of body density are approximately 0.003 g/cc for children and 0.008 g/cc for adults. As calculated by Roche,[11] this measurement error corresponds to 0.6 kg for children, 0.4 to 1.8 kg for men, and 2.3 kg for women with average body fat. Furthermore, the percentage of fat may vary considerably depending on the prediction equation used. In a study of the body composition of young women, Young and Munro[12] employed five formulas to calculate fat content and found the value varied from 25% to 29% depending on the formula used. This finding is consistent with the observation of Lim and Luft[13] who studied a group of male adults. They found that the Siri formula yielded results for fat content some 6% to 7% higher than did the Keys-Brozek formula. If the average fat content for young men is 20%, then the discrepancy between the two methods of calculation is approximately 30%.

Although densitometry seems simple in theory, in practice there are a number of obstacles to overcome. First, one must convince subjects to submerge and remain underwater calmly until their underwater weight is recorded. This is particularly difficult if the subject is obese and therefore more buoyant, and it is also difficult with young children and the aged, whose cooperation is difficult to ensure, especially for those who have never learned to swim. The procedure also requires an experienced operator with subjective but accurate judgment to perform the underwater weighing and residual lung volume determinations.

Air-Displacement Methods for Body Volume

Methods of measuring body density by helium dilution in a plethysmographic "body box" were evaluated by Siri and others in the 1960s.[7] A modern version of the closed-box instrument using air displacement has recently been made available,[14] using modern bioengineering techniques to simplify this method, with the attractive advantage that corrections for lung volume are unnecessary in a system in which the air in the lungs is in equilibration with the air in the plethysmographic box, and is (appropriately) not considered a part of the body in measuring its volume. This leaves only the much smaller intestinal gas component as an unmeasured low-density element for which an arbitrary correction factor is required. This instrument may become widely used for this purpose.

Total Body Water

Estimating body fat using measurement of total body water (TBW) requires the assumption that fat is stored in anhydrous form, and that all the water in the body exists in fat-free tissue in a constant proportion. Direct chemical analysis of cadavers has revealed that fat-free weight contains 67.4% to 77.5% water, with a mean of 72.5%. This mean value is similar to the 73.2% water content obtained from chemical analysis of 50 eviscerated guinea pigs.[2] Thus, if TBW is known, body fat content can be estimated as follows:

$$\text{FFM (kg)} = \text{TBW (l)}/0.732$$
$$\text{Body fat (kg)} = \text{Body weight (kg)} - \text{FFM (kg)}$$

TBW is commonly determined by an isotopic dilution using either deuterium (D_2O), tritium (^3H_2O), or ^{18}O as a tracer. After the ingestion (or injection) of a known quantity of the tracer, from 1 to 3 hours is needed for the tracer to equilibrate in the body. Any loss of the tracer through excretion should be collected and subtracted from intake.

Although TBW can be measured quite accurately, with a measurement error of ±0.5% to 2%, the accuracy of estimating FFM from a TBW determination is affected by any disturbance in normal hydration such as dehydration, fluid retention, or the disproportional increase in extracellular water that is associated with obesity. Furthermore, the estimate of TBW by dilution techniques may overestimate TBW by up to 5.2% because of the exchange of tracer hydrogen with the nonaqueous (labile) hydrogen in the body, a readily correctable error.[15] Generally the TBW method yields values for FFM greater than those obtained from underwater weighing in obese people. It seems fair to conclude that the TBW procedure alone is not a suitable method for measuring body composition in obese patients or for determining changes in body composition during weight reduction.

Combination of Total Body Water and Densitometry

In order to obtain a more reliable estimate of body composition a prediction equation was developed by Siri[16] that combines body water and density measurements:

$$\% \text{ Fat} = (2.057/\text{Body density}) - (0.786 \times \text{TBW}/\text{Body weight}) - 1.286$$

The rationale for the combined use of TBW and body density is that the combination of methods corrects for variations in hydration and thereby reduces the error that derives from uncertainty about the hydration of FFM. But, as Siri[16] pointed out, this combination really does not eliminate the uncertainty about fundamental assumptions. Segal et al[17] measured the fat content of 75 people and found that the percentage of body fat calculated from the combination of density and TBW did not differ from that determined by density alone. This is not surprising because their subjects were normal healthy volunteers with normal hydration. It would be more interesting to test this formula in a population who varied in hydration of FFM.

Total Body Potassium

On the assumptions that 98% of potassium (K) in the body resides in fat-free tissue, and that fat-free tissue has a constant potassium content, it is possible to estimate the quantity of fat-free tissue if the total body potassium (TBK) is measured.[4] Then, body fat can be readily calculated by the difference between body weight and fat-free tissue.

Fat-free tissue (kg) = TBK/(Potassium concentration/kg of fat-free tissue)

Based on direct chemical analyses of four cadavers, Forbes[4] proposed a constant of 68.1 mmol of potassium for each kilogram of human fat-free tissue. However, based on in vivo measurement by TBK counting and densitometry, Womersley[18] suggested 64.4 and 59.7 mmol of potassium per kilogram of fat-free tissue for men and women, respectively. Later, when potassium counting was corrected for body geometry, higher values of millimoles of potassium, 71.8 for men and 60.8 for women, were reported by Pierson et al.[19]

The TBK can be measured in two ways: (1) by the ^{42}K dilution technique, which requires administration of a radioisotope (^{42}K), or (2) by a more convenient and rapid procedure using a whole-body scintillation counter. The use of the whole-body counter to measure TBK depends on the fact that the principal gamma ray activity in humans comes from a naturally occurring radioactive isotope of ^{40}K. It is also known that ^{40}K constitutes 0.0118% of total potassium, regardless of its origin, which is composed of three isotopes: ^{39}K (93.2%), ^{40}K (0.012%), and ^{42}K (6.8%). Thus, it is possible to calculate TBK from ^{40}K measurement by a body counter. The counter varies from a single crystal detector (the least accurate) to 2 π (180°) and 4 π (360°) (the most accurate) whole-body liquid scintillation counters. All whole-body counters must use formulas that recognize gamma ray "self-absorption" within the body, the failure of gamma rays originating within the body to escape the mass of the subject's tissues.

The whole-body liquid scintillation counter is an expensive and intricate instrument, available in only a dozen sites in the world. The procedure of measuring subjects is rapid, convenient, and objective, and requires minimal cooperation from the patient, who must simply lie down in the counter for 10 to 30 minutes. However, its application in obese patients needs special attention; Colt et al[20] reported that ^{40}K radiation is attenuated by all tissues, causing a reduction in the counting efficiency for TBK measurement, which is greater in obese patients. Appropriate corrections should be made for the geometry of the subjects by use of a calibration equation derived from measurement of ^{42}K. The error of the TBK measurement varies, according to the instrument used, from ±1.2% to 10%.

The TBK method has another limitation because of its assumption of the constancy of potassium content in fat-free tissue. Potassium content is not uniform in different types of fat-free tissue, and is affected by the subject's health, nutritional status, and age. Since potassium is highest in skeletal muscle, which accounts for 60% to 80% of the potassium in the body, the measurement is affected by the state of development of the skeletal muscle mass, which is highly influenced by gender, slightly influenced by race, and declines with age. Tables of normal values are available in the literature; see Pierson et al.[19]

Anthropometric Measurements

Total body fat content can be estimated from measurements of circumferences and skinfold thicknesses at various strategic sites of the body using measuring tape and skinfold calipers. Anthropometry is based on the assumption that a major depot of body fat, which is accumulated under the skin as subcutaneous fat, will either be the dominant fat depot, or that it will have a close correlation to the other major depot, visceral fat. The assumption is more accurate at young ages; by the middle of the fourth decade subcutaneous fat as percentage of total fat begins to decline, until at about age 60 the visceral fat is dominant, and the atrophy of the subcutaneous fat depots is impressive.

The procedure for measuring skinfold thickness is to grasp a fold of skin and subcutaneous fat firmly with the thumb and forefinger, pulling it away from the underlying muscular tissue following the natural contour of the fatfold, after which the calipers are applied. The thickness of the double layer of skin and subcutaneous tissues is then read directly from the caliper dial and recorded in millimeters.

The most common places for measuring skinfold thickness are at the triceps, subscapular, suprailiac, abdomen, and upper thigh sites. All measurements are customarily made on the right side of the body, with the subject standing. A minimum of two measurements are made at each site, and the average value is the score for that site.

Numerous prediction equations have been developed to estimate the total body fat content from anthropometric data using either skinfolds alone or in conjunction with circumference measurements. Some investigators[21] have claimed that measuring one or two skinfold thicknesses at particular site(s) is as good as measuring multiple sites in estimating total body fat content. Conversely, other investigators[22] consider that as many as 12 measurements (4 skinfolds, 6 circumferences, and 2 lengths) in addition to height and weight are necessary to obtain accurate estimations of body fat content. Since many of the anthropometric prediction formulae were developed with data collected from the normal-weight population,[23] their applicability to obese people may be questionable.

Durnin and Womersley[21] reported a linear relation between body density and the logarithm of the sum of the skinfold thicknesses of triceps, biceps, subscapular, and suprailiac. This relation was discovered in their studies of 272 women and 209 men varying widely in age (16 to 72 years), body weight (51 to 122 kg), and body fat content (5% to 61%). From these findings, Durnin and Womersley constructed a table in which percentage of body fat corresponded to differing values for the total of the four skinfold thicknesses (biceps, triceps, subscapular, and suprailiac). The table is subdivided for sex and age. The highest percentage of fat content in the table was 46% for men and 53% for women. The estimated error was within ±3.5% of body weight as fat for women and ±5% for men. At the present time, this table may be one of the best tools for estimation of body fat of the obese population in clinical settings if accurate measurements of skinfold thickness at the four sites can be obtained. See Chapter 1, Table 1–10.

The equipment for this procedure is economical and can be easily used in clinical settings. Only minimal cooperation is required from the subject. However, the wide variation (low reproducibility) of the measurement at the same site by different operators, and also with the same operator performing repeated measurements, is common and most criticized. Its low reproducibility makes the data collected less trustworthy. As with densitometry, skinfold thickness measurements also require careful technique by an experienced operator. Moreover, measurements of skinfold thickness in grossly obese patients can be impossible, as quite often the thickness of the skinfold is greater than the capability of the jaws of the calipers.

To overcome this problem, ultrasonography was adapted to measure skinfold thickness. A lightweight portable ultrasound meter is commercially available to measure the distance between the skin and fat-muscle layer. Therefore the measurement is of a single fatfold, unlike that with calipers, which measure a double fold.

The probe (transducer) of the ultrasound meter is placed on the skin surface of the site. It emits pulses of high-frequency sound waves that penetrate the skin surface. The sound waves pass through adipose tissue until the muscle layer is reached; the sound waves are then reflected from the fat-muscle interface to produce an echo that returns to the ultrasound unit. The time for sound wave transmission through the tissues and back to the receiver is converted to a distance score and displayed on a light-emitting diode (LED) scale. Although the ultrasound meter has no limit in measuring the thickness of fatfold and is based on proven scientific principles, it too requires an operator's experienced judgment for accurate and reliable readings. But because of its portability, and its basis in sound scientific theory, with additional technical refinement to overcome the problems posed by "layers" of fat separated by connective tissue, it may become the preferred choice over calipers for skinfold thickness measurement.

Body Mass Index (BMI)

Ideally, obesity should be assessed by direct measures of the degree of fatness. However, all the in vivo methods for body composition discussed above are indirect, cumbersome, and, with the exception of anthropometric measurements, impractical to implement in a clinical setting. Accordingly, a BMI derived from weight (W) and height (H) is frequently used as an indirect correlate of obesity in human subjects. Frisancho and Flegel,[24] using data from the U.S. National Health and Nutritional Examination Survey (NHANES I), 1971–1974,[25] compared the age-adjusted correlation coefficient of weight and various indexes of obesity (W/H^2, W/H^3, W/H^p) where the exponent may vary, with skinfold thickness at triceps and subscapula, and the sum of skinfolds for adults. It was found that W/H^2 or W/H^p explained 60% of the variability in body fat.

BMI has been used as an index and classification of obesity. Recently, the correlation between BMI (weight [kg]/height [m]^2) and total body fat (kg) was examined in 104 women and 24 men aged 14 to 60 years. Total body fat was determined by densitometry, TBW, and TBK. In both sexes, density, water, and potassium gave progressively higher estimates of body fat (kg), and there were significant differences among the values obtained by the different methods. The average of the estimates by these three methods was taken to be the "true" value for each person. Regression of fat/H^2 on W/H^2 was 0.9555 for women and 0.943 for men. Prediction equations were developed based on these findings. Fat (kg) can be calculated from height and weight as follows:

$$\text{Women: Fat (kg)} = (0.713 \ W/H^2 - 9.74) \ H^2$$
$$\text{Men: Fat (kg)} = (0.715 \ W/H^2 - 12.1) \ H^2$$

The authors found that the measurement error was approximately 4.2 and 5.8 kg of fat for women and men, respectively. Thus the BMI as an index of fatness is quite approximate, useful "on average," but quite misleading in individuals who have either hypertrophied or atrophied their skeletal muscle mass, this being the other major contributor to weight.[26] See Chapter 1 for definitions of weight for height and body fat; also Table 1–2.

This magnitude of error is similar to that obtained with densitometry, TBW, and TBK. The prediction of body fat may be inaccurate in special groups, such as older people and very muscular athletes, but these are not groups for whom obesity is an important clinical problem. If these predictive equations prove to be valid, they will enable economic and simple evaluation of a patient's fatness.

NEWER METHODS OF BODY COMPOSITION MEASUREMENT

In the 30 years since the aggregation and compilation of these reports, a series of new methods have appeared: bioimpedance analysis, dual photon absorptiometry, in vivo neutron activation analysis, and computerized tomography and magnetic resonance imaging. This chapter describes these techniques in some detail, and provides guidance for their application in studies of different types. The new measurements are of four types.

Computerized tomography (CT) and magnetic resonance imaging (MRI) provide data by summing a number of individual images, or "slices," of the body, which may be as many as 42 slices,[27] or as few as 4 or 9 slices. Analysis by solid geometry reconstructions well-supported by sophisticated mathematics and complex computer algorithms for recognizing tissues and tissue boundaries provides a "body composition by volumes summary" that is richer in regional information than any other method. Accurate measurements for both subcutaneous and visceral fat masses is readily accomplished by these three-dimensional techniques. The well-validated CT and MRI methods are just beginning to be applied in the necessary range of subjects, accounting for age, gender, and race as dominant variables among normals. The task of studying ill subjects, both to profile the disease states and changes in body composition with interventions, will provide the principal basis for a new criterion method in body composition in the next century. Because of radiation dose with CT, and procedure costs of between $250 and $1000 (1996) with both methods, these techniques are only relevant to the research or the clinical environments.

Neutron activation analysis[28] for the whole-body contents of the elements C, N, Na, P, Cl, and Ca, in conjunction with measurements of body potassium by counting the naturally occurring tracer radioactive ^{40}K, requires three separate activation procedures, and a substantial radiation dose, comparable to an upper gastrointestinal series, a CT scan of the abdomen, or an intravenous pyelogram. In vivo neutron activiation analysis requires expensive instruments, special construction, and highly skilled laboratory staff. It is available at only a few specialized research centers, where it is used as a criterion method to validate simpler and more practical surrogate methods, such as those described elsewhere in this chapter.

Dual energy X-ray absorptiometry (DXA) is at the other end of the scale of measurement complexity. It has become a prominent contender as a primary measurement method for body composition.[29] Invented to measure bone density, the principle of differential absorptiometry uses two precisely known X-ray energies, which can be produced with a margin of error less than 0.5%, to probe tissues of unknown composition. The X-rays, being of different energies, are absorbed differently by chemical elements of different electron density, such that the ratio of transmitted X-rays will provide information concerning the elements in the unknown tissue. This technique was found to be very successful and precise for measuring bone density differences between healthy and osteoporotic bone. The ratios of absorption in soft tissue were observed to map the relative components of low-density fat and higher-density fat-free cellular tissues (largely muscle) with almost as high a precision as for bone.[29] This technique is region-specific, but not organ-specific, except for the appendicular skeletal muscle organ, for which it will probably be well accepted.[30] Introduced in 1981 to evaluate bone calcification and osteoporosis, DXA promises wide application in the study of obesity, measuring both regional and total body fat content, enabling study of the regional distribution of fat. Its vaunted margin of error of about 1% for bone measurements applies within ranges of thickness from 10 to 20 cm. Precision for fat measurements falls off rapidly at thicknesses greater than 25 cm. (Precisions are better maintained for bone, which has much greater density differences than fat/lean soft tissue gradients.) While further software developments may reduce the "thickness problem," very precise measurements are often clinically irrelevant in the very obese. Underwater weighing has been replaced by DXA in many laboratories.

Bioimpedance analysis (BIA) is a widely performed method. This noninvasive method requires only the application of four electrodes (similar to electrocardiogram [ECG] electrodes) on wrist and foot, and the recording of a tiny current, which is unnoticed and harmless. Completed in five minutes, it can be applied in almost any population, age, physical condition, and field condition. BIA is a "black-box" method, the direct output being simply a number for resistance and a number for reactance. These are entered into empirical formulas, derived by many investigators and quite different from one study to another to provide estimates for body water and body fat. Other compartments, the body cell mass and the fat-free mass, are secondarily derived from the estimate for body water, based on the traditional assumptions described above. The numerous articles about measurements made with BIA do not identify any underlying logical connection between an electrical signal and a result labeled "body fat" or "fat-free mass."[31]

For such uses as sports and fitness centers, and bariatrician's offices, where a number suffices, these measurements are very popular. Some sophisticated research groups have declared faith in the BIA,[31] showing regression equations that match changes in BIA readings with other more direct methods such as body water or fatness derived from DXA. In obesity, initial studies have given results consistent with other techniques,[28] but later studies document the limitations of BIA for assessment of body fat in severe obesity[29] and in serial measurements in critical illness.[32]

Single-frequency BIA has limitations of data collection that are completely bypassed by BIA spectroscopy, the taking of data at several or many frequencies, which could separately assess the extra- and intracellular water volumes. So far these have failed to give consistent results.[32] Since better equations may be written based on subsequent research, this intriguing technique will remain under study.

INFREQUENTLY USED METHOD OF BODY COMPOSITION MEASUREMENT

Total body electrical conductivity (TOBEC) is an electrical method applied to the assessment of body composition. Like BIA, it relies on the fact that fat-free tissue is far more electrically conductive than fat tissue in the body owing to the rich electrolyte content in fat-free tissue.

The TOBEC instrument (DJ Medical Instrument Corp) is an open-ended cylinder type of body counter surrounded by a large solenoidal coil driven by a 2.5-MHz oscillating radio frequency current. The difference between impedance when the subject is inside the coil and when the coil is empty corresponds to the electrical conductivity of the subject, which is proportional to the FFM. The measurement can be completed in about five minutes.

A high correlation has been reported between TOBEC scores (signals of conductivity) and FFM estimated from body density. Segal et al[33] measured the body composition of 75 men and women varying widely in body weight (49 to 133 kg) and fat (5% to 55%), using densitometry, TBK, TBW, TOBEC, and BIA methods. A strong correlation ($r = 0.962$) was found between the percent of fat obtained by densitometry and by TOBEC. The validity of the TOBEC method for determining body composition in healthy human subjects has been confirmed on repeated occasions. The lower initial cost of the BIA instrument and the greater simplicity of the method make it likely that of the two methods based on body electrolyte content, BIA will be more widely used.

APPLICATIONS OF MEASUREMENTS

Body Weight and Frame Size

Many published tables provide ideal or desirable weight for a person based on height and gender. Attributable in large part to publications from the Metropolitan Life Insurance Company, there is a widespread belief that body weight norms in adults should be related to frame size. Frame size is an ill-defined concept. Katch et al[34] found a significant difference between self-reported frame size and that appraised by investigators. An index of frame size should have no relation to adiposity since tall people are not necessarily fatter than short people, large frame size is not correlated with fatness. We consider that "frame size" has passed from utility as a useful concept in the study of body composition, and we include it for historical interest.

Anthropometrics

Frisancho and Flegel[24] examined the data of the U.S. National Health and Nutritional Examination Survey I of 1971–1974. They found that elbow breadth, as compared with bitrochanteric breadth, and body weight, as compared with sum of skinfolds (triceps and subscapular), had the lowest correlation with adiposity and a low correlation with age regardless of sex or race. It seems that elbow breadth is the best indicator of frame size. A table of small, medium, and large categories of elbow breadth was established for adults depending on whether the elbow breadth was below the 15th (small), between the 15th and the 85th (medium), or above the 85th (large) sex-, age-, and race-specific percentiles for elbow breadth.[24] In general, the elbow breadth of blacks is greater than that of whites in each frame category, and, as expected, men have significantly greater elbow breadth than either black or white women.

Elbow breadth can be measured with the spreading caliper. The examinee's right arm is extended forward perpendicular to the body. With the arm bent so that the angle at the elbow is 90°, with the fingers pointing up and the dorsal part of the wrist toward the examiner, the greatest breadth across the elbow is measured.

APPLICATIONS OF BODY COMPOSITION RESEARCH IN WEIGHT MANAGEMENT

The clinician could face a difficult task in recommending an "appropriate" or "desirable" body fat content for the patient. Values for desirable average percentage of body fat reported in the literature vary depending on the type of research performed by the investigator. Scientists who are interested in sports medicine tend to set a lower average percentage of body fat than the ones who treat obesity. In the general population, body fat may range from 5% of body weight in wrestlers ready for competition to 50% or more in very obese people. Male athletes in peak condition have 5% to 15% body weight as fat; the female equivalent may have 15% to 20%. Hannon and Lohman[35] suggest the upper end of this range, 15% for men and 22% for women, to represent the ideal body fatness for the average American. However, comparing body composition of obese and non-obese people, most investigators included subjects who had body fat up to 20% for men and 25% for women in the control, non-obese groups. It may be reasonable to consider body fat of up to 20% for men and 25% for women as acceptable, average values for normal-weight people. See Chapter 1, Table 1–9.

Weight Gain, Weight Loss, and the Lean Body Mass

Although obesity is generally defined as an excessive accumulation of fat, as obesity develops, fat-free tissue also increases. In 1964 Forbes[36] reported that fat-free tissue in obese children is greater than in non-obese peers. Subsequently, Drenick et al[37] also found an increase in fat-free tissue, as evidenced by the higher TBK content (calibrated with ^{42}K self-absorption) in 49 obese adults (body weight ranging from 78 to 238 kg) over age- and height-matched non-obese control subjects.

James et al[38] assessed the body composition of 71 obese people (11 men and 61 women) and 26 normal-weight control subjects by skinfold thickness and TBK (calibrated with ^{42}K). They concluded that the excess weight accumulated by the obese over the normal-weight subjects was not pure fat, but was composed of 32% to 38% FFM and 62% to 68% fat. These numbers differ slightly from those reported by others. Webster et al[39] measured the body composition of 104 obese and normal-weight women by densitometry, and reported that the excess weight accumulated by the obese over the non-obese women consisted of 22% to 30% lean and 70% to 78% fat. They therefore proposed that, in the treatment of obesity, fat-free tissue loss should not contribute more than 22% of total weight lost.[39]

Forbes and Welle[40] examined data on FFM in their own and other published reports to address the question of whether obese children and adults have increased FFM. Because the amount of fat-free tissue is closely related to stature, the data were expressed as a lean:height ratio and compared. Their own data indicated that 75% of the obese had a lean:height ratio that exceeded one standard deviation (SD) of the mean for normal-weight subjects, and more than half of them exceeded two SD. Extensive review of the literature confirmed that, on average, obese subjects have a larger fat-free tissue mass than their non-obese peers, and that the lean component of the body accounts for a mean of 29% of the excess weight. This mean value is between the estimates of James and Webster.

Body Fat Distribution and Weight Change

Changes in body fat distribution have been found to accompany weight loss. Subjects with greater upper-body obesity tend to achieve greater reductions in the waist-to-hip ratio (WHR) and upper body than those with lower-body obesity who tend to lose large amounts of fat from both upper and lower fat depots. Five circumference measurements were correlated with fat loss in this study.[41] Other work evaluating effects of weight loss on regional fat distribution in premenopausal women comparing WHR and CT measurements reported "changes in body weight over the entire period (16 weeks on a low-energy diet) correlated with initial body weight and with total and subcutaneous abdominal fat, but not with visceral abdominal fat."[42] Asians have been found to have lower BMI, but greater body fat than whites of both sexes. Asians had more subcutaneous fat, particularly upper-body fat, than did whites and had different fat distributions than whites, indicated by greater WHRs in a study of 445 white and 242 Asian adults.[43]

Ethnic variations have been studied extensively in the late 1980s and 1990s. A distinction between *biological* and *sociocultural* ethnic influences is usually difficult, since low income and obesity have a well-recognized high correlation, and historically black and Hispanic subjects studied in the United States have been of lower socioeconomic status than whites or Asians. Increased fatness stimulates increased bone density and mass in all ethnic groups, an interaction between body compartments for which both hormonal and antigravity functional correlations related to activity levels have been shown. It is not yet possible to dissect away the socioeconomic influence, but several trends are well established: blacks have bone masses and bone densities about 10% higher than whites, Hispanics, or Asians at all ages, after all available normalizations for age, height, and fatness have been considered. They also have slightly higher skeletal muscle mass. Inability to measure physical activity level with precision represents a major methodological flaw in these determinations, since it is clear that being sedentary is associated with loss of muscle and increase of fat, the converse also being readily demonstrable, as the correlation between form and function is maintained.

RESTING METABOLIC RATE

Definition of Resting Metabolic Rate

The minimal metabolic rate is that during sleep. Basal metabolic rate (BMR) is the minimal metabolic rate of an awake individual. It is equivalent to the energy needed to maintain vital functions (heart, liver, kidney, and other organs and cellular metabolic processes) plus the energy cost of arousal from sleep. It is usually measured under the following conditions:

- 12 to 18 hours after the last intake of food
- patient lying awake and quiet in a thermally neutral environment
- patient relaxed and emotionally calm

Because it is difficult to obtain these true basal conditions, resting metabolism is often measured instead of basal metabolism, and is determined two to four hours after a light breakfast. This resting metabolism is somewhat different from that defined in the Recommended Daily Allowances (RDA).[44] In the RDA, resting metabolic rate (RMR) represents the average energy metabolism of a person resting in a comfortable environment, not engaged in any physical activities. This rate may be measured at any time of the day and includes the thermic effect of food.

Most laboratories continue to measure RMR under the conditions specified for BMR, but term it the RMR with the understanding that true basal conditions under which the metabolic rates are assessed are standardized to some extent. The advantage of such standardization is obvious: it makes the comparison of results obtained from sequential measurements in a patient, or from one laboratory to another, possible and more interpretable.

Measurement of Resting Metabolic Rate

Although the RMR can be determined by a direct calorimeter, which directly measures heat production (changes in temperature), it is commonly measured by indirect calorimetry. The preference for indirect over direct calorimetry is attributable to the cost and unavailability of direct calorimeters (only a few exist in the United States). In addition, direct calorimetry requires extensive time for equilibration and measurement.

Indirect calorimetry measures oxygen consumption and/or carbon dioxide production. From the rate of oxygen consumed and carbon dioxide produced, one can calculate the corresponding energy expenditure. The Benedict-Roth respirometer apparatus, which is a closed-circuit system, has been used since the turn of this century. In this method, a known volume of pure oxygen is supplied to the subject, and carbon dioxide is constantly removed as it passes through soda lime without being measured. The decrease in the gas volume in this closed system is related to the rate of oxygen consumption, from which the metabolic rate is then calculated.

The commonly used indirect calorimeters are open-circuit systems. Several machines for indirect calorimetry have been developed and are commercially available. The subject inspires room air, and expired air is collected and analyzed for oxygen and carbon dioxide content. Normally, room air contains 20.93% oxygen and 0.003% carbon dioxide. The difference in content between room air and expired air is assumed to be consumed or produced by the subject. Newer systems are computer driven, allowing the measurement of RMR in a short time. The most difficult task in obtaining reliable RMRs is proper preparation of the patient in a relaxed, postabsorptive condition.

All indirect calorimetry methods necessitate the collection and analysis of expired air. The use of a mouthpiece to collect the expired air requires less equilibration time, but has been criticized for causing discomfort. Such discomfort has been reported to cause higher metabolic rates than with a hood system or a respiration chamber.[45] However, others found no significant differences between results obtained using a mouthpiece, a mask, or a hood system to measure metabolic rate of young men.[46]

Many factors may affect the RMR. For example, RMR decreases with age, and men have a higher RMR than women matched for age, height, and weight. Other factors such as body weight, body composition, diet, temperature, hormones, drugs, stress, and exercise may also affect the RMR. Discussion here focuses on RMR with respect to body composition.

Expression of Resting Metabolic Rate

It is difficult to know the best way to express RMR. The problem lies in part in comparing the RMR of subjects of differing body size, and in part in defining what is "normal." Most workers in the field propose the FFM, which is an approximation of the respiring tissue mass. Other factors, such as body weight to the two-thirds power (another estimate of metabolically active tissue), body surface area, and total body weight have been used as the denominator to relate oxygen consumption to body size.

Generally, metabolic rate is reported either as an absolute value (kcal/24 hr) or in relation to body surface area ($kcal/m^2$) so that it can be compared with reference values, discussed below. A RMR within 15% of the predicted reference value is usually considered "normal," although there is a wide variation in RMRs in obese as well as non-obese people.

Standardization by FFM has been advocated by several groups.[47,48] Expressing RMR in terms of FFM reduces the observed differences between men and women and the apparent diminution of RMR with age in normal-weight people.[49,50] Recently, it has been shown that organ mass is an even better basis for expression of metabolic rate.[51]

Surface Area

Rubner[52] found that when he expressed the metabolic rates of dogs of different sizes in terms of their body surface area, the rates became remarkably similar. The "surface law" had an enormous influence on the energy metabolism field, leading to the development of equations to predict surface area from height and weight.[53] These formulas were developed from measurements of surface area of one cadaver and nine subjects who had a wide range of age, adiposity, and health status. Other predictive formulas based on larger numbers of subjects were subsequently developed,[54] but all of these equations had limitations that led to inaccuracies too great for application to individuals (see Elia for review[55]). In addition to the difficulties in predicting surface area, its use to express metabolic rate failed to provide the universal basis that was sought when it could not account for differences due to age, sex, and body composition. Consideration therefore has turned to expression of metabolic rate in terms of heat production rather than heat loss.

Fat-Free Body Mass

Since fat-free body mass (FFM) accounts for the most metabolically active tissue, expression of metabolic rate in relation to FFM eliminates some of the limitations of surface area expression. Generally, its use reduces differences between males and females, old and young, and lean and obese. While considered more universal as a basis for metabolic rate, FFM is also not easy to determine accurately. Predictive equations for estimating FFM have been developed using skinfold thicknesses, total body potassium, water dilution, and densitometry. Differences in laboratories and techniques lead to wide variability in estimates. Variability can be reduced by use of multiple methods for assessing FFM in the same individual, but only large research centers have such a variety of methods available. Astrup et al[56] have proposed prediction formulas for energy expenditure based on lean body mass determined by bioimpedance measurement. Using these formulas, Astrup's group was able to predict energy expenditure with a high degree of precision in normal-weight subjects. If similar levels of precision can be obtained with other groups, this technique might provide an inexpensive but precise method for determining FFM and predicting metabolic rate.

Organ Mass

Even when expressed per unit of FFM, the metabolic rate of adults is found to be significantly lower than that for young children. This difference is attributed to the decreasing ratio of organs to muscle with age. Organs such as brain, heart, liver, and kidney have metabolic rates 15 to 40 times that of muscle and 50 to 100 times that of adipose tissue.[57] In infants, the brain, with a high rate of metabolic activity, requires almost half of the total body energy expenditure while muscle requires very little. In adults, however, the relative requirement for the brain is only 20% while that for muscle is 30% to 40%. Therefore, metabolic rate expressed per unit of surface area or body weight decreases with age, but when expressed in relation to organ weight is relatively constant over the life span. The concept of expressing metabolic rate in terms of organ size also has implications for explaining energy requirements during various nutritional and disease states. A study in lambs found that energy restriction decreased whole-body oxygen consumption by about one third and decreased the proportional requirement for liver by one half compared to non-restricted control animals.[57] Diets that reduce the proportion of organ to muscle, as do low-protein diets[58,59] or total starvation,[60] might therefore be expected to reduce energy consumption to a greater extent than energy-restricted diets that preserve the ratio. Little is known about the contribution of alterations in organ sizes to energy requirements during disease, an important area requiring further research.

Reference Standards for Resting Metabolic Rate

A number of reference standards for metabolic rate have been developed. These vary widely in terms of the basis for expression and in the source of data used to derive the standards. The Harris-Benedict standards[61] based on height and weight were derived from data for 239 individuals from 15 to 73 years of age and included men and women, athletes and non-athletes, and obese and lean. These standards continue to be widely used despite evidence that they overestimate energy requirements by about 5%. The Mayo Clinic standards on 80,000 individuals are expressed in terms of surface area.[61] Other standards using surface area are those by Robertson and Reid[62] and by Fleish.[63] The Schofield standards[64] are among the few that use data from a variety of races and countries. The results obtained when metabolic rate for a given individual is computed using these and other standards have been compared and found to vary considerably. This variability can be ascribed to differences in methodology as well as to differences in the populations used to establish the standards in terms of gender, race, obesity, and age. In addition to these variables, errors associated with estimating surface area increase the error of metabolic rate estimation when those standards using surface area are applied.

More recently, equations have been derived to predict metabolic rate from FFM. A typical equation is: Metabolic rate $= k_1 + k_2$ FFM. An equation recently proposed by Nelson[65] replaces the k_2 FFM term with three terms, one for organ mass, one for skeletal muscle mass, and one for adipose tissue mass. Although inclusion of a term for FM is controversial,[66] due to its very low metabolic activity it may not be a significant contributor to metabolic rate until it becomes very large. The inclusion of the constant, k_1, a number greater than zero, in the equation indicates that the relationship between RMR and FFM has a positive intercept. The implication of this is that RMR expressed per unit of FFM will tend to be lower for larger individuals. Ravussin and Bogardus[67] have proposed that appropriate comparisons of metabolic rate data can be made by comparing the slopes of the lines derived using multiple regression analyses for different subject groups. Another approach would be to add the value for k_1 to the metabolic rate divided by FFM. The value for k_1, determined to be 18 kg by Ravussin's group, should be determined for each laboratory.[38]

While expression of metabolic rate in relation to FFM or organ and skeletal muscle mass is more accurate than measurement using body surface area, these too depend upon the accuracy of the techniques used to determine the denominator. These techniques all have inherent error. The importance of the error in estimating energy requirement depends on the application. For research purposes a high error rate would be unacceptable but could be reduced by utilizing multiple sophisticated techniques to assess body composition and by repeated tests of the individual. Such techniques, however, are not widely available. For many clinical applications, overestimation of energy requirement from use of the traditional reference values may not be problematic because the objective is generally to provide more than minimal energy requirements and the patient is closely monitored to allow for constant adjustments. Until accurate, inexpensive methods for assessing FFM or organ mass are available, it may be necessary to rely on such estimates of "normal" as within ±15% to 20% (mean ±2 SD) of the value from one of the reference sets discussed above, with recognition of the errors involved in such comparisons.[38,67]

Obesity and Resting Metabolic Rate

Numerous attempts have been made to establish whether obese patients have a metabolic abnormality that contributes to their obesity, or accounts for their difficulty in weight reduction. The findings reported in the literature are varied and support all possible claims, that obese patients have low, normal, or high RMR, depending on how the comparison is made. A perception of reduced RMR in obese subjects may be due in part to the underestimation of RMR in obese compared with normal-weight individuals when expressed in terms of FFM, as discussed above. Ravussin et al[68] found that increased total energy expenditure (TEE), but not RMR, was predictive of subsequent weight gain in Pima Indians. In the Baltimore Longitudinal Study of Aging,[69] neither RMR nor deviations from predicted RMR were related to weight change. Studies of postobese adults have also found no evidence for a relationship between low RMR and subsequent weight gain. Similar to the results for Pima adults, Saltzman and Roberts[70] found that low TEE but not RMR was related to subsequent weight gain in infants. Thus the data currently available suggest that obesity may be related to reduced total energy expenditure, due perhaps in part to reduced physical activity, but probably not due to a decreased resting energy requirement.

Effect of Weight Change on Resting Metabolic Rate

A continuing controversy in the field of energy metabolism concerns the question of whether changes in energy expenditure subsequent to overfeeding or underfeeding are disproportionate and thereby represent mechanisms to return the body to its usual weight. In a recent review of this subject, Saltzman and Roberts[70] analyzed the data from 20 recent studies assessing RMR following overfeeding or underfeeding. Both by regression analysis and by comparison with cross-sectional data, the reported changes in RMRs were disproportionately altered in the direction to oppose the weight change. However, when Saltzman and Roberts estimated the energy costs of increased protein turnover that would be associated with increased protein deposition following overfeeding, they found that they could account for nearly all of the measured increase in RMR. A similar analysis, however, showed that the expected decrease in RMR due to decreased protein turnover in underfeeding was significantly less than that observed in the studies.[70] They conclude that the increase in RMR with overfeeding is not greater than can be accounted for due to changes in body composition. However, the disproportionately greater decrease in RMR with underfeeding than can be attributed to body composition changes, may represent an adaptive energy conserving mechanism. While this analysis is in agreement with others on the subject,[70] it does conflict with a recent report by Leibel et al[71] of compensatory alterations in energy expenditure subsequent to overfeeding as well as underfeeding.

Another question addressed by Saltzman and Roberts[70] is whether the additional decrease in RMR with underfeeding beyond that attributed to changes in body composition persists beyond the period of energy restriction. Of seven studies that addressed this question by measuring RMR after a period of weight stabilization following weight loss, five reported persistently decreased RMR relative to FFM.[70] However, three studies that compared RMRs of weight-stable postobese with weight-matched controls all reported no differences.[70] One might conclude from these comparisons that the weight stability periods of the former studies were insufficiently long to allow for normalization of RMR. However, Saltzman and Roberts point out that it is also possible that the postobese included in the latter studies may not be representative because very few postobese are successful in maintaining stable weight subsequent to weight loss.

While many questions remain regarding the relationship between metabolic rate and energy balance, it does appear that the body is better adapted to defend itself against energy deficiency than against energy excess.

Resting Metabolic Rate and Exercise

It was reported in 1980 that exercise prevents the decrease of RMR that occurs during dieting in normal-weight volunteers consuming 800 kcal/day.[72] Since this report, exercise programs have been avidly promoted in the treatment of obesity. It was thought that the addition of exercise to the program of weight control may favorably modify the composition of weight loss and/or prevent the excessive reduction in RMR. Studies of the effectiveness of exercise in maintaining FFM and thereby attenuating the decrease in RMR during weight loss have had mixed results. In a review of these studies, Calles-Escandon and Horton[73] found more evidence for preservation or increase[74–76] than decrease[77] in RMR with exercise during moderate energy restriction. Exercise is less effective in preserving RMR during severe dietary restriction.[78–80] Comparison of such studies is difficult because in some cases the energy cost of the exercise is additional to the dietary restriction, and in other studies it is not. The additional energy deficit resulting from exercise may be insignificant during moderate caloric restriction but significant during severe restriction. The response may also depend on initial body composition, since loss of FFM is greater in lean than obese individuals for a given amount of body weight loss.[40]

CONCLUSION

Most methods for in vivo determination of body composition are indirect and based on the assumption of certain constants, such as hydration of tissue, density of fat, etc. These factors, however, are not constant: they vary from tissue to tissue and change according to individual health status. In addition, each method has its own associated measurement errors. Thus, none of the methods currently used including densitometry, the commonly accepted gold standard, is error-free.

When reviewing data on body composition, especially in comparing differences between groups or between sequential measurements, one should keep in mind the magnitude of measurement error of the method used and be cautious in drawing conclusions about whether the differences are clinically significant.

The choice of methods and facilities for body composition measurement in a clinical setting is rather limited. It is unlikely that a typical clinic could afford to install an underwater weighing facility or other large or technically demanding equipment. There is a need to validate and/or develop procedures that can be easily used in a clinical setting, and that can provide noninvasive, simple, convenient, and accurate measurements.

It is clear that "healthy" obesity is associated with increased FFM, which accounts for a mean of 23% to 29% of the excess weight that obese people accumulate over the normal-weight population. It is therefore recommended that in the treatment of obesity FFM should not constitute more than this proportion of total weight loss. This may be accomplished by a slower rate of weight loss.

The majority of obese people have RMRs that are appropriate for their obese weight but elevated when compared with predicted rates for height-matched non-obese people. This discrepancy diminishes when the metabolic rate is expressed per unit of FFM or organ mass. The choice of units for expressing metabolic rates depends largely on the intention of the clinician; total calories may be more useful than calories based on body weight (kcal/kg) or FFM (kcal/kg of FFM) in estimating energy expenditure and prescribing diets. On the other hand, when one compares metabolic rates in people of different body weights, the slopes of lines obtained from multiple regression analysis should be used, or alternatively, a constant obtained by regression analysis should be added to the value to avoid bias due to size. The RMR (kcal/day) accounts for 70% to 80% of daily energy expenditure of obese, sedentary people. It decreases with weight loss during the treatment of obesity and thereby makes it more difficult to lose weight. Exercise in conjunction with diet may attenuate this decrease, particularly when caloric restriction is not severe.

REFERENCES

1. Forbes RM, Mitchell HH, Cooper AR. Further studies on the gross composition and mineral elements of the adult human body. *J Biol Chem.* 1956;223:969–975.

2. Pace N, Rathbun EN. Studies on body composition: body water and chemically combined nitrogen content in relation to fat content. *J Biol Chem.* 1945;158:685–691.

3. Behnke AR, Feen BG, Welham WC. Specific gravity of healthy man. *JAMA.* 1942;118:495–498.

4. Forbes GB, Gallup J, Hursch JB. Estimation of total body fat from ^{40}K content. *Science.* 1961;133:101–102.

5. Moore FD, Olesen KH, McMurrey JD, Parker JHV. *The Body Cell Mass and Its Supporting Environment: Body Composition in Health and Disease.* Philadelphia-London: WB Saunders Co; 1963.

6. Brozek J, Grand F, Anderson JT, Keys A. Densitometric analysis of body composition from girth measurement: revision of some quantitative assumptions. *Ann NY Acad Sci.* 1963;110:113–140.

7. Body composition. *Ann NY Acad Sci.* 1963;110:1–5.

8. Roche AF. Anthropometric methods: New and old, what they tell us. *Int J Obes.* 1984;8:509–523.

9. Siri WE. Body composition from fluid spaces and density: analysis of methods. In: Brozek J, Henschel A, eds. *Techniques for Measuring Body Composition.* Washington, DC: National Academy of Sciences; 1969:223–244.

10. Wilmore JH. A simplified method for determination of residual lung volumes. *J Appl Physiol.* 1969;27:96–100.

11. Roche AF. *Body Composition Assessments in Youth and Adults.* Columbus, OH: Ross Laboratories; 1985.

12. Young VR, Munro HN. N-methylhistidine (3-methylhistidine) and muscle protein turnover. An overview. *Fed Proc.* 1978;37:2291–3000.

13. Lim TPK, Luft UC. Body density, fat and fat-free weight. *Am J Med.* 1961;30:825–832.

14. McCrory MA, Gomez TD, Bernauer EM, Mole PA. *Med SC Sports Ex.* 1995:1686–1692.

15. Culebras JM, Moore FD. Total body water and exchangeable hydrogen. A theoretical calculation of non-aqueous exchangeable hydrogen in man. *Am J Physiol.* 1977;232:R54–R59.

16. Siri WE. The gross composition of the body. *Adv in Biol and Med Phys.* 1956;49:239–280.

17. Segal KR, Van Loan M, Fitzgerald PI, Hodgdon AJ, Van Itallie TB. Lean body mass estimation by bioelectrical impedance analysis: a four-site cross-validation study. *Am J Clin Nutr.* 1988;47:7–14.

18. Womersley J, Durnin JVGA, Boddy K, Mahaffy M. Influence of muscular development, obesity, and age on the fat-free mass in adults. *J Appl Physiol.* 1976;41:223–229.

19. Pierson RN Jr, Lin DHY, Phillips RA. Total body potassium in health: the effects of age, sex, height, and fat. *Am J Physiol.* 1974;226:206–212.

20. Colt EW, Wang J, Stallone F, Van Itallie TB, Pierson RN Jr. A possible low intracellular potassium in obesity. *Am J Clin Nutr.* 1981;34:367–372.

21. Durnin JGVA, Womersley J. Body fat assessed from total body density and its estimation from skinfold thickness: measurements on 481 men and women aged from 16 to 72 years. *Br J Nutr.* 1974;32:77–97.

22. Steinkamp RC, Cohen NL, Gaffey WR, Siri WB, Sargent W, Walsh HE. Measures of body fat and related factors in normals. II. A simple clinical method to estimate body fat and lean body mass. *J Chron Dis.* 1965;18:1291–1307.

23. Steinkamp RC, Cohen NL, Siri WB, et al. Measurement of body fat and related factors in normal adults. I. Introduction and methodology. *J Chron Dis.* 1965;18:1279–1291.

24. Frisancho AR, Flegel PN. Relative merits of old and new indices of body mass with reference to skinfold thickness. *Am J Clin Nutr.* 1982;36:676–679.

25. Johnson CL, Fullwood R, Abraham S. Basic data on anthropometric measurements and angular measurements of hip and knee for selected age groups 1–74 years of age: United States, 1971–1975. *Vital and Health Survey No. 219.* Hyattsville, MD: National Center for Health Statistics; 1981. US Dept of Health and Human Services publication (PHS) 81-1669.

26. Smalley KJ, Knerr AN, Kendrick ZV, Colliver JA, Owen OE. Reassessment of body mass indices. *Am J Clin Nutr.* 1990;52:405–408.

27. Sjostrom L, Kvist H, Cederblad A, Tylen U. Determination of total adipose tissue and body fat in women by computed tomography, ^{40}K, and tritium. *Am J Physiol.* 1986;250:E736–E745.

28. Cohn SH. In vivo neutron activation analysis: State of the art and future prospects. *Med Phys.* 1981;8:145–154.

29. Heymsfield SB, Gallagher D, Wang ZM, et al. Theoretical foundation of dual energy X-ray absorptiometry soft tissue estimates: validation in situ and in vivo. Submitted.

30. Heymsfield SB, Smith R, Aulet M. Appendicular skeletal muscle mass: measurement by dual-photon absorptiometry. *Am J Clin Nutr.* 1990;52:214–218.

31. Deurenberg P. Limitations of the bioelectrical impedance method for the assessment of body fat in severe obesity. *Am J Clin Nutr.* 1996;64(suppl):4495–4525.

32. Heymsfield SB, Wang ZM, Visser M, Gallagher D, Pierson R. Techniques used in the measurement of body composition: an overview with emphasis on bioelectrical impedance analysis. *Am J Clin Nutr.* 1996;64(suppl):478S–484S.

33. Segal KR, Gutin B, Presta E, Wang J, Van Itallie TB. Estimation of human body composition by electrical impedance methods: a comparative study. *J Appl Physiol.* 1985;58:1565–1571.

34. Katch VL, Freedson PS, Katch FL, et al. Body frame size: validity of self-appraisal. *Am J Clin Nutr.* 1982;36:676–679.

35. Hannon BM, Lohman TG. The energy cost of overweight in the United States. *Am J Public Health.* 1978;68:765–767.

36. Forbes GB. Lean body mass and fat in obese children. *Pediatrics.* 1964;34:308–314.

37. Drenick EJ, Blahd WH, Singer FR, et al. Body potassium content in obese subjects and potassium depletion during prolonged fasting. *Am J Clin Nutr.* 1966;18:278–285.

38. James WPT, Bailes J, Daives JL, et al. Elevated metabolic rates in obesity. *Lancet.* 1981;1:1122–1125.

39. Webster JD, Hesp R, Garrow JS. The composition of excess weight in obese women estimated by body density, total body water and total body potassium. *Hum Nutr Clin Nutr.* 1984;38C:299–306.

40. Forbes GB, Welle SL. Lean body mass in obesity. *Int J Obes.* 1983;7:99–107.

41. Wadden TA, Stunkard AJ, Johnston FE, Wang J, Pierson RN. *Am J Clin Nutr.* 1988;47:229–234.

42. Zamboni M, Armellini F, Turcat E, et al. Effect of weight loss on regional body fat distribution in premenopausal women. *Am J Clin Nutr.* 1993;58:29–34.

43. Wang J, Thornton JC, Russell M, Burastero S, Heymsfield S, Pierson RN. Asians have lower body mass index but higher percent body fat than do whites: comparisons of anthropometric measurements. *Am J Clin Nutr.* 1994;60:23–28.

44. National Research Council. *Recommended Dietary Allowances.* Washington, DC: National Academy of Sciences; 1989.

45. Tremoliere J, Carre L, Naon R. Interrelations between body weight level of vigilance and energy expenditure in subjects on various diets. In: Apelbaum M, ed. *Energy Balance in Man.* Paris: 1973.

46. Segal KR. Comparison of indirect calorimetric measurement of resting energy expenditure with a ventilated hood, face mask, and mouthpiece. *Am J Clin Nutr.* 1987;45:1420–1423.

47. Keys A, Taylor HL, Grande F. Basal metabolism and age of adult man. *Metabolism.* 1973;22:579–587.

48. Miller ATJ, Blyth CS. Lean body mass as metabolic reference standard. *J Appl Physiol.* 1953;5:311–316.

49. Tzankoff SP, Norris AH. Effect of muscle mass decrease on age-related BMR changes. *J Appl Physiol.* 1977;43:1001–1006.

50. Cunningham JJ. A reanalysis of the factors influencing basal metabolic rate in normal adults. *Am J Clin Nutr.* 1980;33:2372–2374.

51. Elia M. Organ and tissue contribution to metabolic rate. In: Kinney JM, Tucker HN, eds. *Energy Metabolism: Tissue Determinants and Cellular Corollaries.* New York: Raven Press; 1992:61–80.

52. Rubner M. Uber den Einfluss der Korpergrosse auf Stoff-und Kraft-wechsel. *Z Biol.* 1883;19:535–562.

53. Dubois D, Dubois EF. A formula to estimate the approximate surface area if height and weight be known. *Arch Intern Med.* 1916;17:863–871.

54. Isaksson B. A simple formula for the mental arithmetic of the human body surface area. *Scand J Clin Lab Inv.* 1958;10:283–289.

55. Elia M. Energy expenditure in the whole body. In: Kinney JM, Tucker HN, eds. *Energy Metabolism: Tissue Determinants and Cellular Corollaries.* New York: Raven Press; 1992:19–60.

56. Astrup A, Thorbek G, Lind J, Isaksson B. Prediction of 24-h energy expenditure and its components from physical characteristics and body composition in normal-weight humans. *Am J Clin Nutr.* 1990;52:777–783.

57. Burrin DG, Ferrel CL, Eisemann JH, Britton RA, Nienaber JA. Effect of nutrition on splanchnic blood flow and oxygen consumption in sheep. *Br J Nutr.* 1989;62:23–34.

58. Coward WA, Whitehead RG, Lunn PG. Reasons why hypoalbuminaemia may not appear in protein-energy malnutrition. *Br J Nutr.* 1977;38:115–126.

59. Lunn PG, Whitehead RG, Baker BA, Austin S. The effect of corticosterone acetate on the course of development of experimental protein energy malnutrition in rats. *Br J Nutr.* 1976;36:537–550.

60. Addis T, Poo LJ, Lew W. The quantities of protein lost by the various organs and tissues of the body during a fast. *J Biol Chem.* 1936;115:111–116.

61. Boothby WM, Berkson J, Dunn HL. Studies of the energy of metabolism of normal individuals: a standard for basal metabolism, with a nomogram for clinical application. *Am J Physiol.* 1936;116:468–484.

62. Robertson JD, Reid DD. Standards for the basal metabolism of normal people in Britain. *Lancet.* 1952;1:940–943.

63. Fleish PA. La metabolisme basal standard et sa determination au moyen du "metabocalculator." *Helv Acta.* 1951;18:23–44.

64. Schofield. Predicting basal metabolic rate, new standards and review of previous work. *Hum Nutr Clin Nutr.* 1985;39C:5–91.

65. Nelson KM, Weinsier RL, Long CL, Schutz Y. Prediction of resting energy expenditure from fat-free mass and fat mass. *Am J Clin Nutr.* 1992;56:848–856.

66. Ferraro R, Ravussin E. Fat mass in predicting resting metabolic rate. *Am J Clin Nutr.* 1992;56:460–461.

67. Ravussin E, Bogardus C. Relationship of genetics, age, and physical fitness to daily energy expenditure and fuel utilization. *Am J Clin Nutr.* 1989;49:968–975.

68. Ravussin E, Lillioja S, Knowler W. Reduced rate of energy expenditure as a risk factor for body-weight gain. *N Engl J Med.* 1988;318:467–472.

69. Seidell JC, Muller DC, Sorkin JD, Andres R. Fasting respiratory exchange ratio and resting metabolic rate as predictors of weight gain: the Baltimore Longitudinal Study on Aging. *Int J Obes.* 1992;16:667–674.

70. Saltzman E, Roberts SB. The role of energy expenditure in energy regulation: findings from a decade of research. *Nutr Rev.* 1995;53:209–220.

71. Leibel RL, Rosenbaum M, Hirsch J. Changes in energy expenditure resulting from altered body weight. *N Engl J Med.* 1995;332:621–628.

72. Stern JS, Schultz C, Mole P, et al. Effect of caloric restriction and exercise on basal metabolism and thyroid hormone. *Alim Nutr Metab.* 1980;1:361. Abstract.

73. Calles-Escandon J, Horton ES. The thermogenic role of exercise in the treatment of morbid obesity: a critical evaluation. *Am J Clin Nutr.* 1992;55:533S–537S.

74. Tremblay A, Fontaine E, Poehlman ET, et al. The effect of exercise-training on resting metabolic rate in lean and moderately obese individuals. *Int J Obes.* 1986;10:511–517.

75. Nieman DC, Haigh JL, De Guia ED, Register UD. Reducing diet and exercise training effects on resting metabolic rates in mildly obese women. *J Sports Med Phys Fit.* 1988;28:79–88.

76. Belko AZ, Van Loan M, Barbieri TF, Mayclin P. Diet, exercise, weight loss, and energy expenditure in moderately obese women. *Int J Obes.* 1987;11:93–104.

77. Heymsfield SB, Casper K, Hearn J, et al. Rate of weight loss during underfeeding: relation to level of physical activity. 1995. Abstract.

78. Hill JO, Sparling PB, Shields TW, Heller PA. Effects of exercise and food restriction on body composition and metabolic rate in obese women. *Am J Clin Nutr.* 1987;46:622–630.

79. Forbes GB. Exercise and lean weight: the influence of body weight. *Nutr Rev.* 1992;157–161.

80. Webster JD, Hesp R, Garrow JS. The composition of excess weight in obese women estimated by body density, total body water and total body potassium. In: *Human Nutrition: Clinical Nutrition.* 1996:299–306.

CHAPTER 3

Cultural Appropriateness of Weight Management Programs

Shiriki K. Kumanyika
Christiaan B. Morssink

INTRODUCTION

Cultural issues are at the core of many aspects of obesity treatment. The prevalence of obesity varies by ethnicity and social class, both within and across populations.[1-4] Cultural norms about body size, which can be powerfully positive or negative, vary over time, within and across societies, and apply differently to individuals (e.g., men and women, young and old, rich and poor) within a given society.[5-7] Thus, underlying cultural factors within the larger society influence whether and how individuals attempt to control their weight and how they judge the success of these efforts.

This chapter addresses concepts and issues relevant to health professionals' understanding of cultural influences on obesity and weight management programs—using the term "weight management programs" broadly to cover various types of health behavior change programs, nutrition education/counseling programs, or clinical nutrition programs that focus on weight reduction or weight control.[8] The material in this chapter is particularly relevant to *cross-cultural* treatment situations, i.e., situations in which the providers and clients have different cultural backgrounds and in which the clients are members of a racial or ethnic minority population. Many health professionals (but certainly not only health professionals) who have been educated in the school of thought that everyone is (or is trying to be) pretty much the same are attempting to reorient themselves and their work to the perspective that diversity is an important factor to be considered and to explore, pragmatically, how cultural factors can be taken into account. The guidance offered is intended to be useful both to established practitioners seeking insights related to the specifically cultural elements of obesity treatment programming and also to new practitioners who wish to develop their skills in a manner that will be effective with culturally diverse populations.

The first part of the chapter provides background for considering cultural influences that may have an impact on obesity and weight management. The second part discusses incorporating cultural considerations into program design and implementation. This chapter is not a "cookbook" for undertaking cultural adaptations of weight management programs. Cookbook approaches cannot work, because the availability and nature of various "ingredients" of a weight management program are not static, generalizable variables that can be characterized and specified as fixed elements of a program design. Cultural adaptation is an iterative process that allows continual assessment of and response to manifestations of cultural factors among providers and clients, and in program dynamics.

WHAT ARE CULTURAL INFLUENCES?

Societal Guidelines

It is well established that culture influences all human behavior and that it shapes social institutions and social interactions among populations, groups, and individuals.[9] Culture can be defined as "a set of guidelines (both explicit and implicit) that individuals inherit as members of a particular society, and tells them how to view the world, how to experience it emotionally, and how to behave in it in relation to other people, to supernatural forces or gods, and to the natural environment."[10(p3)] Cultures are identifiable and transmitted from one generation to the next through distinctive symbols, language, and rituals. People who grow up in a particular society "slowly acquire the cultural 'lens' of that society"[10(p3)] and to that extent view the world in a similar manner.[11] The gradual nature of the acquisition (or loss) of a given cultural perspective in conjunction with the commonality of perspective within the reference group renders cultural factors invisible to those influenced by them. In other words, people do not usually notice that they are looking at the world through a specific lens or set of lenses. Their outlook may seem universal. The social practices through which cultural perspectives are applied or implemented seem normal, right, and non-negotiable. "Culture" is often visible only as a characteristic of those who are "different" on some variable that becomes apparent because there is a contrast in beliefs, expectations, or values (as when beliefs or customs expressed by a client are not congruent with those held by service providers).

Demographic Groups

All societies seem to use social categories to subdivide their population, e.g., by gender (boys or girls; men or women); by age (children or adults; young, middle-aged, or older people); by division of labor, skills, training, or education; by kin (blood-relatives or in-laws, family or non-family); by class, caste, or estate (nobility, elite, masses, homeless, Fortune 500); or health status (able or disabled; healthy or sick). This social stratification justifies pre-existing beliefs and expectations about people in these categories, creating a system of knowledge or paradigm that functions as the lens through which to interpret social reality and therefore interactions with others. Subdivisions may also evolve within cultures to the extent that distinctive attributes are established. These distinctive attributes may include language or language usage, attitudes, behaviors, dietary patterns, or other aspects of the way the world is viewed or survival is effected.

Using this broad description of cultures and subcultures, it is evident that virtually all societies are, to a degree, multicultural in the sense that numerous cultures coexist and develop within them.[10] In the United States, cultural diversity and development are acknowledged in many ways. For example, differences by age, race, region of the country, household composition, income level, and social values are openly acknowledged and utilized in the advertising field.[12] Cultural designations are sometimes used to differentiate subpopulations by country of origin (e.g., German-, Italian-, Polish-, or Irish-American), religion (e.g., Catholic, Protestant, Jewish, Muslim), or region of U.S. residence (e.g., Southerner or Northerner).

In the obesity literature, the term "cultural" is also often used narrowly to refer to cultural attitudes about physical attractiveness and ideal body size for women in a society.[13,14] Changing views of gender equity have heightened concerns about this double standard of physical attractiveness and its contribution to the disproportionate amount of weight- or eating-related psychosocial morbidity in women[15] (see Chapter 12).

Racial and Ethnic Minorities

Civil rights, women's rights, and affirmative action laws foster attention to and visibility of cultural factors that are defined by race/ethnicity or gender, or both. This attention has included recognition of numerous health disparities among racial/ethnic minority populations such as black Americans; Mexican; Puerto Rican; Cuban, or other Hispanic Americans; American Indians or Alaskan Natives; Asian Americans; or Pacific Islander Americans compared to the white population.[16,17] These health disparities include a striking excess of obesity in many minority populations.[2]

Increased concern for minority issues in the United States is also linked to the increased size of the aggregate minority population, now approaching 25% of the population,[18] particularly with respect to in-migration of persons from Spanish-speaking or Asian countries. Thus, the interest in minority issues is part cause and part effect of a changing view of diversity in American society. The current, plu-ralistic view of diversity is one in which the value to individuals and to society of preserving cultural differences is recognized. Health professionals are now ex-pected to deliver services in a manner compatible with the client's cultural and social framework. The former, unidirectional and overarching view was one of a "melting pot" in which diverse cultures would mix and blend in the direction of an Anglo-Saxon–oriented reference culture.[19] In this case the role of a health profes-sional would have been to foster assimilation: stimulate adoption of mainstream attitudes and behaviors, which implies compliance with instructions given by health professionals who represent the values of the majority population.

"Cultural" may be used by health professionals to refer only to cultural vari-ables affecting the delivery of services to minority individuals or communities. Those involved in educational or behavioral change interventions may focus par-ticularly on attitudes or behaviors that are thought to contribute to health dispari-ties between minorities and whites. The similarity across many minority groups in the disproportionate prevalence of obesity, diabetes, and other health problems tends to support the joint consideration of health problems of diverse groups as "minority health issues." It is important to recognize, however, that perspectives on population groups as minority populations are influenced more by political than by cultural considerations. Whereas ethnic designations derive their legiti-macy by reference to another country or distinct culture, minority status derives from a lesser position vis-à-vis a majority population (in this case a non-Hispanic, Caucasian majority). Minority group cultural perspectives focus on the "non-whiteness" of certain behaviors with respect to what is considered conventional (mainstream) American behavior. Conceptualizations of minority cultures may, therefore, be relatively non-specific with respect to the reference cultures of those minority group members.

The comparative emphasis on the "non-white" characteristics of minority popu-lations is aggravated by the tendency, for statistical reasons, to count people from different regions and cultures in a single category. For example, counting Spanish-speaking individuals from the Caribbean region (Puerto Rico and Cuba), Spain, South America, and the American Southwest (Mexican American) as "Hispanic" de-emphasizes numerous cultural differences between these groups. Counting people from anywhere on the Asian continent or the Pacific Islands as "Asian–Pacific Islander Americans" may imply to the uninformed health professional that cultural differences among people from places as diverse as Samoa, India, China, Japan, or Cambodia are relatively trivial.[20] The difficulty of separating the effect of the "minority" factor from socioeconomic factors is an additional problem lim-iting the utility of the "minority group" perspective on cultural adaptation. In short, to state this labeling problem brings up the question: Is a weight manage-ment program that is culturally appropriate for women from a lower socioeconomic African American community equally appropriate for African American women from a higher socioeconomic level?

CULTURAL INFLUENCES ON WEIGHT STATUS

Levels of Influence

Levels and types of cultural influences on weight status are shown in Figure 3–1. Cultural factors as such are societal-level forces—forces arising from the social systems and from strategies adopted by people in order to survive in and (depending on one's culture) to adapt to or to control the environment. Cultural influences incorporate experiences accrued over many generations and provide the common perspectives that shape the norms, values, beliefs, and behaviors of individuals within the group (socialization). Figure 3–1 distinguishes societal-level cultural factors from derivative attitudes and behaviors expressed by the individuals within a society (in this case the attitudes and behaviors that ultimately determine caloric intake and expenditure). However, as shown by the bi-directional arrows, attitudes and behaviors of individuals within the society feed back into the culture. Culture evolves over time, sometimes rapidly, sometimes almost imperceptibly in comparison to social, technical, or market changes. Cultural perspectives may lag behind attitudinal, structural, and situational changes within the population—and may sometimes yield only after wars or other major social upheavals.

Whereas behavior change programs can address individual knowledge and attitudes, and medical interventions such as drug treatment or surgery can alter physiological state, to address culture requires public health interventions, for example, public policies and mass education that either alter or circumvent societal patterns that perpetuate a health problem. The movement to change the cultural context for cigarette smoking through anti-smoking laws and taxation is an obvious example of an intervention at the societal level.[21] A counterpart intervention for obesity might affect the food environment (e.g., supply, accessibility of fat and calories) or to access and demand factors related to physical activity (e.g., modes of transportation, type and amount of occupational activity, or hours of access to television). In contrast, weight management programs (even those implemented in community rather than clinical settings) address individual-level factors and attempt to alter the behavior of individuals rather than characteristics of their environment.

This distinction is critical for understanding what is a feasible process of cultural adaptation and what is not feasible. Thus, this approach to cultural adaptation of weight management programs relates to variables that are influenced by culture, rather than to cultural variables as such. This relatively functional view is the only perspective on cultural adaptation that is workable for current programmatic approaches. As in the anti-smoking campaign, a critical mass of aggregate indi-

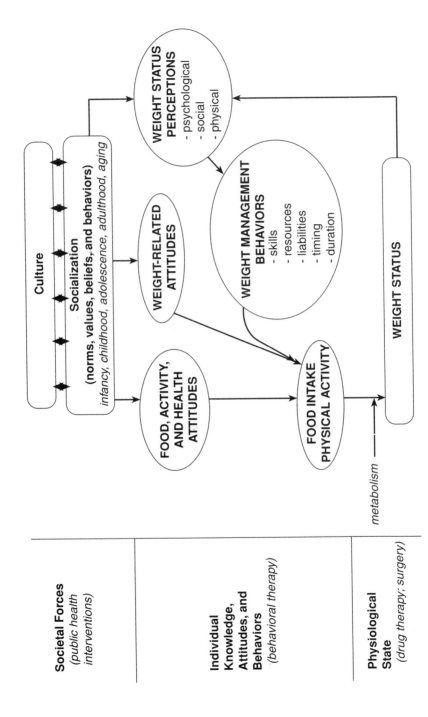

Figure 3–1 Levels and types of cultural influences on weight status.

vidual behavior and attitude change is needed before these changes lead to changes in the underlying cultural framework.

Types of Influence

Obesity cannot occur unless an individual has access to an ample amount of food or can be physically inactive (barring the small number of people who develop certain genetically determined forms of obesity). In terms of human history, obesity is a relatively modern problem[22] associated with increasing food abundance in a society, an increased caloric density of the foods available, transitions from agricultural to industrialized to post-industrial societies, increased reliance on labor-saving devices for transportation in the workplace and at home, and a predominance of sedentary forms of work and recreational activity such as watching television. Historically, the activities needed for survival and daily living and food acquisition (hunting, gathering, farming, and walking) in conditions of scarce food resources and periodic famine, and the prevalence of infectious diseases, prevented positive energy balance at the environmental level and shaped individual behaviors toward the avoidance of a negative energy balance or undernutrition. The current situation in developed and many developing countries where obesity is becoming more prevalent is the opposite: societal forces related to food availability and physical activity patterns promote a positive energy balance. Obesity then results from the inability or disinclination of the individual to either maintain energy balance or periodically create a negative energy balance, in opposition to these environmental forces. As evidenced by the substantial and increasing prevalence of obesity in the United States and elsewhere, the obesity-promoting environmental forces are often dominant. Given the slowness of biological evolution, these obesity-promoting forces find a ready substrate in a human species still metabolically geared to overcoming hunger and food scarcity.[22]

As shown in Figure 3–1 and elaborated further in Table 3–1, cultural factors influence obesity and weight gain through several attitudinal and behavioral pathways that converge in food intake and energy output. Cultural factors (in the United States the most obvious of these are ethnic and regional traditions) determine an individual's pattern of eating and activity (e.g., food preferences, social uses of food, style of food preparation, activity preferences, and attitudes toward fasting and feasting) and beliefs about food and health[23-25] both during development and throughout the life course. Cultural influences also include the translation of functional patterns (i.e., daily routines related to income level, neighborhood characteristics, environmental demands, occupation) into attitudes about eating (for example, eating a large breakfast before a day of physical work) or activity (resting at the end of a day of physical work) that may persist long after these functional patterns change. Cultural factors based on the historical availabil-

Table 3–1 Examples of Culturally Influenced Attitudes and Perceptions Related to Weight Status

Knowledge and Attitudes Related to Food, Activity, and Health	Weight-Related Attitudes	Weight Status Perceptions
• Beliefs about medicinal or health-promoting properties of food or about health-related food restrictions • Symbolic meanings and social uses of food (status foods, special ethnic foods, holiday foods, dieting foods) • Preferences for foods or flavors • Aversions to foods or flavors • Attitudes about feasting or overindulgence • Attitudes about fasting and food deprivation • Beliefs about interrelations of exercise, rest, psychological stress, and physical stress • Beliefs about appropriate activities by gender, age, or social roles, especially work roles • Preferred types of leisure time activity	• Ideal body size and shape • Importance of body size and shape • Relationship of body image to self-concept • Priority given to weight management • Attitudes and beliefs about ways to lose or gain weight or influence body shape • Attitudes about dieting • Fear of being fat • Positive or negative values for thinness or fatness • Attitudes about exercise to lose weight	• Self-perception of body size or shape • Self-perception of physical attractiveness • Self-perception of weight in comparison to others in reference group • Perceived social pressure to lose or gain weight • Perceived social or physical advantages of being at a given weight level • Perceived health or functional value associated with being at a given weight • Perceived determinants of weight status

ity of food in the environment or the association of thinness with malnutrition and female infertility influence societal standards of beauty, physical attractiveness, fitness,[5,6] and explanations for illness and disease[10] and thereby determine cultural views about body size and shape, the relationship of body image to self-concept and the priority given to weight management.[13,26] These same factors influence weight status perceptions—the type of psychological and social feedback perceived by those who are overweight or thin—and the extent to which various health or social problems are attributed to their weight status.[7] Cultural core (socialization) variables such as world view, religion, and hierarchies of social and material values influence variables such as intrafamilial and community relationships, sense of personal dependency or independence, attitudes toward cigarette and alcohol use, personal belief and value systems, and use of time.[27,28] These variables constitute the context for response to interventions that attempt to alter eating and activity behaviors and body weight.[29]

Cross-cultural variation, or differences in the nature of these cultural influences among coexisting ethnic groups (or among gender, age, income, or other socially differentiated groups), may result in either blending or polarization of attitudes and behaviors. What occurs and to what extent may depend on the history of interaction with the mainstream culture, whether the individuals in question are seeking to retain or relinquish their own culture, and what options they have, for example, whether their attempts at operating in either or both cultures are generally successful or unsuccessful.[30–32]

Evidence of Ethnic Differences in Weight-Related Attitudes and Behaviors

The potential for a contrast in attitudes toward heavier body size between developing countries with limited food supplies and prevalent undernutrition (more positive attitudes) compared to industrialized countries with ample food availability (more negative attitudes)[33] may be more readily apparent than for differences among cultural groups within the United States. However, the social forces shaping weight-related perspectives of ethnic and socioeconomic status (SES) subgroups differ, and they evolve slowly. Thus, a diversity of attitudes can be expected among U.S. populations. Evidence documenting culturally mediated differences in dieting motivations, body image, and dieting practices is considerable, particularly for contrasts between African Americans and whites. Indicative findings covering various age and sex groups are summarized in the following pages. The substantial detail reflects a need to demonstrate both the nature of the differences and the difficulty of making generalizations about the implications of these differences for programming purposes.

Body Image and Weight Control Motivations

Within a general picture of the relatively high level of weight preoccupation among females in the United States, differences in various dimensions of weight-related socialization and body image have been documented between black and white girls and women from pre-adolescence through aging, and some differences have also been noted in males. In a survey of adults ages 18 to 96 years, Rand and Kuldau[34] found that among both men and women who were more than 20 lbs overweight, black respondents were more likely than white respondents of the same sex to consider themselves as having "no weight problem": 55% vs 34% of black vs white men and 29% vs 6% of black vs white women. Rosen and Gross[35] reported that, among public high school students in the northeastern United States, black girls at all social class levels were more likely to be trying to gain and less likely to be trying to lose weight compared to white girls. These racial differences were unrelated to objectively measured weight status. Findings were less clear-cut in boys because of the difference in weight goals among boys in this age range (weight gaining and body building predominate over weight reduction).[35]

Based on questionnaires administered to convenience (non-random) samples of midwestern inner-city, primarily low-income high school students, Desmond et al[36] reported that only 40% of overweight black females perceived themselves as heavy, whereas all (100%) of the overweight white female students perceived themselves as heavy. Among girls aged 13 to 19 years studied by Kemper et al,[37] black females (who had a somewhat higher mean body mass index than the white girls) (1) selected a larger ideal body size; (2) were over twice as likely to perceive themselves as thinner than other girls their age; (3) were three times as likely to describe themselves as thin; (4) were seven times as likely to report that they were not overweight, compared to white girls; (5) perceived a larger normative body size in their social environment; and (6) were more likely to perceive that their friends and family evaluated them as thin and wanted them to gain weight.

Rucker and Cash[38] reported significant differences on numerous dimensions of body image among black and white women of college age, indicating that black women had, overall, less negative attitudes toward their bodies, less effort to conceal their body size, less concern about dieting, less drive to be thin, and less fear of fatness. Wing et al[39] found that, among women at both northern and southern U.S. colleges, black women were heavier but less likely to exhibit chronic dietary restraint than white women. These black-white differences were not observed among the men in this study.

Age differences in attitudes toward obesity involving a decreasing level of concern with being overweight have been suggested[40] and data consistent with this interpretation were reported by Rand and Kuldau[41]: the degree of overweight among those who considered themselves to have no weight problem tended to increase with age. Stevens et al[42,43] reported more positive attitudes toward obesity among blacks than among whites, and among both older women (ages 66 to 105) and older men (ages 55 to 98) in the Charleston Heart Study Cohort. Among the African American women, for example, the proportion who rated their figures attractive or somewhat attractive was unrelated to being overweight, whereas among the white women only half as many overweight vs not overweight gave this response.[43] Black women in this cohort were more satisfied with their weights and had a higher ideal weight than the white women. Among the men, significantly more of the white than the black men reported ever having dieted and the black men had a significantly higher ideal body size compared to the white men.[42]

A qualitative study of body size values among low- and high-income women suggests different and more multidimensional attitudes about body size and weight among black than among white women.[44] Black women were less likely to link body size to health and more likely than white women to discuss large body size in terms of positive physical attributes such as strength, stamina, and solidness. Black women also made a distinction between the type of obesity or overweight characterized by being flabby and that associated with being shapely, dressing stylishly, and having an attractive physical presence.

Most racial/ethnic comparisons of obesity-related attitudes include blacks and whites, although a few can be identified that focus on or include other ethnic minority populations. Some of these studies are consistent with the impression that these other ethnic groups also have a lesser preoccupation with dieting or less strict attitudes toward larger body size. Stern et al[45] reported that Mexican American men and women living in either ethnically mixed or predominantly Anglo neighborhoods in San Antonio, Texas, although heavier than the Anglo American comparison group, were much more likely to have the attitude that Americans in general are too concerned about losing weight. Wilkinson's findings in a comparison of Western Samoan adult women with overweight Caucasian women in Australia were similar to the impression obtained from some of the data for black women.[46] Samoan women who were objectively classified as overweight were as likely as the Australian women to perceive themselves as fat, but the importance of being fat and negativity toward it were much less than in the overweight Australian women. The large Samoan women were more likely than the Australian women to consider themselves attractive, fit, stronger, and better equipped for life. As observed for African American women in the Charleston Heart Study[43] and suggested by the qualitative data of Allan et al[44] for the low-income African American women, feelings of attractiveness were correlated with body size in the Australian women but not the Samoan women. In a large study of Native American adolescents,[47] almost one third of the girls with a high body mass index perceived themselves as being of normal weight; American Indian girls were less likely to have ever dieted when compared to teenage girls in rural Minnesota.

Thus, body image perspectives of various ethnic groups may be different from or more multidimensional than those in the mainstream culture, while reflecting some aspects of the mainstream view. Or, the same spectrum of attitudes might exist but on a different scale: a much greater degree of overweight may be needed to elicit certain negative views in some cultures. It would be erroneous to oversimplify these attitudinal differences as either positive or negative, and to equate attitudes that do not fit the expected negative view with completely favorable attitudes or with a complacency or lack of concern about obesity.

It is also erroneous to assume that, in other cultures, those who are overweight do not recognize this. Self-perception as overweight, when defined by the usual standards, tends to be relatively accurate for overweight persons in most populations surveyed. For example, body dissatisfaction and concerns related to being overweight were more prevalent among Native American adolescents than among a comparison group of whites in rural Minnesota, among both girls and boys.[47] Native American and Hispanic youths in the Southwest were more likely to be "always terrified of gaining weight" than comparison white youths.[48] Minority vs majority group differences in the validity of self-perception as overweight appear to be more evident among those who are not overweight than among those who are. Several of the above-cited studies suggest that among whites, compared to minorities, normal-weight or thin individuals were more likely to be dissatisfied with their bodies and to consider themselves to be too fat. Thus, overweight persons in all groups are likely to perceive themselves as overweight, while normal-weight whites report more body dissatisfaction than normal-weight persons in other cultural groups.

The actual prevalence of dieting, which is evidence of a certain level of weight control motivation, is very high among women in most populations surveyed and is often similar for Hispanics and whites, while being somewhat lower for blacks in some data sources. Among female respondents in the 1990 National Health Interview Survey, approximately 60% of overweight black women in the 18- to 64-year age range were currently trying to lose weight.[49] The percentage for Hispanics was somewhat higher than 60, very similar to that in non-Hispanic white women.[49] Similar proportions of persons trying to lose or maintain weight across race/ethnicity were reported from the 1989 Behavioral Risk Factor Survey.[50] However, the starting weights for weight loss attempts were 15 to 20 lbs heavier in black, compared to white or Hispanic women; the average amount of weight loss desired was more similar across race/ethnicity. A significant difference in the prevalence of long-term weight loss attempts (lower prevalence in black than white women) may reflect a difference in the intensity of motivation for weight loss between the black and white women.

As noted previously, cultural variables in racial/ethnic minority populations also incorporate socioeconomic factors. However, an inverse socioeconomic gradient in weight is commonly observed among women regardless of ethnicity.[1,30,41] Attitudes toward being overweight are thought to be more negative as social class increases, and the prevalence of dieting among overweight women is higher at higher levels of income or education.[49] Patterns observed by race and SES may be dependent in part on the samples involved in the study. In some cases, black-white differences in obesity-related attitudes appear to be confined to or more pronounced among women in the lower socioeconomic status stratum. For example, Allan et al[44] noted that low-income black women were different from both low- and higher-income white women as well as the higher-income black women with respect to expressing more positive values for being heavy.

Dieting Approaches and Exercise Practices

Variation in patterns of disordered eating or undesirable dieting practices by race/ethnicity suggest that the interaction of body image variables with specific dieting and exercise behaviors may also be culturally influenced. For example, among 13- to 19-year-olds studied by Emmons,[51] white girls practiced self-induced vomiting significantly more than black girls, while black girls used laxatives and diuretics significantly more than white girls. In a study of high school students in Memphis, Camp et al[52] reported that substantial percentages of white students, particularly girls, but no black students used smoking as a weight control strategy (60% vs 0%). Gritz and Crane[53] reported that, in a survey of high school seniors, blacks were less likely to use smoking, diet pills, or amphetamines for weight control. Wing et al[39] noted that college-age women from northern states scored higher measures on eating disorders than women from the South with no difference between African Americans and whites in this respect, or among men.

Story et al[47] reported a higher prevalence of binge eating and self-induced vomiting among Native American girls compared to a sample of rural Minnesota white girls but a lower prevalence of laxative and diuretic use. A study comparing Native American, Hispanic, and white youths (mean age 15) in the Southwest[48] also reported a higher prevalence of binge eating and induced vomiting in Native American compared to white girls.

Dieting by fasting tends to be relatively more prevalent than behaviors such as self-induced vomiting or use of laxatives, diuretics, or appetite suppressants. Differences in fasting by ethnicity are not consistent across studies. Emmons[51] reported a similar frequency of fasting in black and white girls, but other reports indicate that blacks and Hispanics are more likely to fast than whites.[48,54] The higher prevalence of fasting overall may relate to its cultural acceptability or familiarity based on rituals in many religions. In a cultural milieu in which other extreme behaviors for weight control purposes may be frowned upon, fasting may not draw criticism and may even be viewed favorably. Similarly, episodes of overeating or binging may be less noteworthy in cultures where feasting is socially acceptable.

Less prevalent or less intense exercise behaviors in black and low SES populations have been reported frequently.[55] These patterns may also be influenced by cultural attitudes. For example, persons in lower-paying jobs or who, from a cultural perspective, have traditionally held these types of jobs, may have higher levels of physical activity at work and view leisure time as an opportunity for compensating or psychological decompression through rest and sedentary pursuits rather than vigorous activity.[56] The opportunity for occupational and some sorts of recreational physical activity may decrease with age and with upward social mobility, so that maintaining or adopting physical activity becomes a leisure time pursuit of those so motivated and for whom the time and associated costs are affordable and feasible. Circumstances or schedules may preclude or limit adoption of activity for weight control purposes in some communities or social strata. In addition, from an attitudinal perspective, labor-saving devices, sedentary jobs, and leisure activities are associated with higher social status and may therefore be preferred by upwardly mobile individuals.

What are the ultimate implications of these cultural differences in weight-related attitudes and behaviors for obesity prevention and treatment? Health professionals familiar with the negative psychosocial consequences of the obsession with thinness have expressed the concern that an increased emphasis on weight control in minority communities will simply cause minorities to join the majority[48] in the vicious cycle of dieting preoccupation, disordered eating, and weight cycling. Some may even advocate, simplistically, to preserve the cultural milieu that apparently fosters some protection from the prevailing obesity stigmatization.[57,58] However, one cannot overlook the desire for more effective weight control among many in minority populations,[59] especially from a health perspective, given the marked prevalence of obesity and related diseases in minority populations.[2] When these potentially conflicting aspects of culturally related variables are understood, the difficulties of preventing and treating obesity in minority populations become particularly challenging and complex.

CULTURAL ISSUES IN OBESITY PREVENTION AND TREATMENT PROGRAMS

Overview

Cultural variables exist at the level of the community rather than the individual. Individuals in one particular societal group may be more likely than those in a different group to exhibit certain attitudes or behaviors that can be tied to cultural norms, values, or beliefs about health and diet. However, the outcome of these particular cultural forces is not uniform among members of a particular group. Attitudes and behaviors vary considerably among members of a group because the impact of cultural factors to which they are exposed is subject to a range of individual-level psychosocial filters. The influence of culture is usually recognized by inference when some incongruence arises with respect to an issue that is culturally determined. It is not possible to know in advance how much any given individual's behavior will fit the group's cultural perspective. One can, however, align the program with these cultural background variables so that it fits as well as possible with the social environment in which the individual lives, under the assumption that a poor fit will diminish the likelihood of a favorable long-term outcome.

Kumanyika et al[29] have characterized this concept of the need for a cultural match using the model shown in Figure 3–2. In this model, the five main elements of an obesity treatment program are the program, client, interaction between the program and the client, external events that may influence either the program or clients, and group dynamics that may influence the program-client interaction. The program and client are both viewed as being in equilibrium with their reference cultural context—equilibrium in the sense that everything they do will make sense to them in that context and will not put them in major conflict with their reference group. (We are fully aware that cultures change, can have an impact on conflict, and can be very heterogeneous. However, this is not directly relevant to our explanatory model, which is set in a hypothetical, culturally stable time cross section.) For example, in situations in which the client and institution/staff offering the program are from the same general reference culture (i.e., middle-class, white American), the reference culture as an intervening variable may be factored out—taken for granted—because everyone generally speaks the same language and has a similar spectrum of expectations and values. A key principle in this model is that when the client and the program have different reference cultures, the effect of the program will normally not be sufficient to alienate the client from his or her reference groups and culture. Aspects of learning that the person cannot fit within his or her own cultural and social context will then be short-lived in their effects.

Having said this, the tasks of identifying those characteristics of a program that make it culturally appropriate, and modifying programs so that they become culturally appropriate are far from straightforward. However, the need for guidance in this arena has become urgent. In the United States (and many other countries) we are now deeply involved in diversity issues that demand attention to cultural and cross-cultural variables, while the ability to address these variables has been grossly underdeveloped in the evolution of mainstream health behavior change theory.[60] A review of theoretical development in health behavior change indicates that the core is built upon individual psychology with peripheral attention to the familial and social context in which the individual operates.[61–63] This may reflect the dominance of an individualistically oriented cultural perspective among those engaged in theoretical development, in which cultural factors are considered subordinate to the individual's will. However, even the most self-centered individuals are influenced by their surrounding cultural values and norms.

It is not clear that individually oriented behavioral change models can be fully effective for any population other than white, middle-class Americans until cultural considerations have also been addressed more deliberately. The limitations of current approaches even for the mainstream population may be reflected in the significant increase in the prevalence of obesity in the total U.S. population during a period when applications of the conventional strategies had high visibility.[64,65] However, assuming that it is not feasible to begin anew to develop behavior

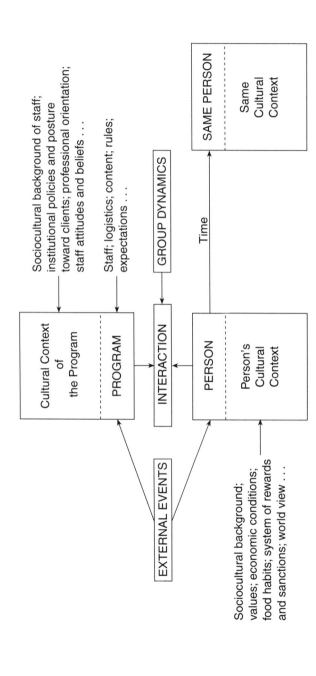

Figure 3–2 Areas of cultural impact on the interaction between program and client. *Source:* Adapted with permission from S. Kumanyika, C. Morssink, and T. Agurs, Models for Dietary and Weight Change in African-American Women: Identifying Cultural Components, *Ethnicity and Disease*, Vol. 2, p. 170, © 1992.

change theories and programmatic approaches in a more multidisciplinary perspective that includes recognition of cultural factors as essential, a practical strategy is to attempt to incorporate relevant cultural dimensions into current models.

Where Cultural Variables Enter the Process

An overall sense of where cultural factors might be considered as influences on program outcomes can be obtained from Figure 3–3. This figure depicts various phases of a weight change program, highlighting points at which cultural factors might affect outcomes. The cultural influences across the top of the drawing in Figure 3–3 are background variables that can be assessed for their impact, but not necessarily influenced by the counselor. For example, desired body size or perceived social pressure to lose weight or remain at a given body size may determine motivation to join a weight management program or readiness to lose weight. Maintaining motivation and acting upon it by regular attendance at classes or appointments may reflect culturally influenced reactions to what happens during participation: Does the person feel comfortable coming to the place where services are offered? Are the staff competent in cross-cultural communication? If groups are involved, are things said or implied by other participants that make people feel that they are among friends and peers with whom they can enjoy interacting, or are there awkward or unfamiliar aspects that limit motivation for coming back?

Given attendance (or possession of written or audiovisual educational materials), whether participants absorb and master what the program has to offer (learning and skill acquisition) may depend on whether the information and experiential learning components are in terms and concepts they can understand and are presented in a manner that makes clear the relevance to the participant's daily living situation. The terminology or skill-building activities that seem relevant and that foster learning will be partly determined by the context in which the person lives. Obvious examples are whether the foods, preparation methods, and proportionate amounts used in a proposed menu are familiar and acceptable to those being counseled.

Finally, behavioral adherence and success in translating knowledge and skills gained into actual weight loss will be influenced by the actual cultural and personal relevance of what is learned to the individual's life and by the extent to which the targeted behaviors are modeled by, acceptable to, and reinforced by others in the person's environment. Cultural influences relevant at this phase may be the most powerful. They may range from explicit cultural beliefs that contradict information provided within the program (about health-promoting properties of food or about the health benefits vs risks associated with exercise, for example) to more subtly conveyed attitudes that may either support or resist the individual's behavior change efforts. For example, when attempting to introduce a recipe at home, a person may pick up signals that certain social uses of food are not accept-

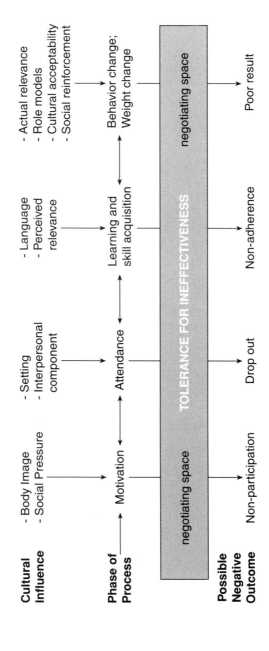

Figure 3–3 Schematic illustration of how cultural factors might influence participation and outcomes at various phases of the program.

able or accessible to change (serving salads for dinner, perhaps), or that certain foods or preparation styles associated with ethnic identity or principle should be defended against changes proposed by outsiders like the health professional. Efforts to season foods or to use foods in new ways at home or work may also be derailed by negative reactions of family members or peers to unfamiliar, nontraditional combinations of familiar foods or flavors. Or, family members may find frequent occasions to suspend weight loss considerations with respect to social meals or celebrations on the grounds that certain cultural foods are "off limits" for restrictions or modifications that may change their value or character.

Women or men in ethnic groups where obesity, or being heavy, is very common and perhaps, in some ways, positively valued may have difficulty maintaining adherence to dietary or physical activity regimens if they sense a potential for losing a peer group (if everyone else in the family is overweight) or losing social mooring (e.g., as a nurturer [women] or as a protector [men]) by not being heavy. People in working-class communities may have problems adhering to an exercise routine if there are strong cultural values indicating that activity should be undertaken more for social or functional than health purposes or that rest is more appropriate than exercise for restoring energy or health.

As shown in Figure 3–3, the nature of the cultural influences at each stage of the process of program participation can be somewhat different. Ineffectiveness also looks different depending on the stage at which it occurs. A poor weight loss result may be observed because the person: (1) never signed up, (2) dropped out, (3) came but didn't learn, or (4) learned but didn't do. This schema is not meant to imply that only cultural influences lead to ineffectiveness. Rather, it shows the types of cultural variables that may influence client-provider interactions at different phases of the process, along with other variables (not shown) to which practitioners may already be attuned.

Attempting to achieve cultural appropriateness of a program can, therefore, be viewed as an inexact process that leaves room for trial and error as long as one remains focused on the goals. This principle is illustrated by the relatively wide shaded area in Figure 3–3, labeled "tolerance for ineffectiveness." The concept, adapted from the organizational behavior concept of a "zone of indifference" in employee-supervisor relationships,[66] emphasizes that the professional and client give each other considerable latitude or negotiating space for things not to work before negative feedback registers or a negative outcome occurs.

Another concept from the organizational behavior literature is also relevant here to emphasize that the client's and perhaps the counselor's trial and error processes are not necessarily geared to finding the best solution in an absolute sense. Simon[67] proposes that a truly rational decision-making process that leads to selection of the best alternative takes place only within strict limitations, and that people may consider only a small amount of information or number of alternatives to come to a decision that is considered good enough to solve the immediate problem (termed "satisficing"). For clients whose social environment or cultural context is very different from that presumed by the program (e.g., for those who will have the most difficulty implementing the solution at home, or who have to juggle a multitude of social roles and responsibilities), the solution that is "good enough" may be good enough to save face in the group setting (by seeming to be in step with the others) or good enough to give a short-term sense of personal accomplishment, i.e., through sacrificing for a few days.

Trying to See the Invisible

Trying to identify cultural factors in behavioral change paradigms and programs is a little like trying to see the invisible, because the paradigms and program designs are embedded in our own cultures. The relatively limited racial/ethnic, social class, and even gender diversity among professionals engaged in weight management theory or program development limits the likelihood that contrasting cultural perspectives will emerge within institutional or professional ranks. In addition, health professionals, at least in the United States, may have a general awkwardness about cultural issues if they were raised or educated during the "melting pot" era or in less diverse regions of the country. They may have been taught (by way of denial) that racial or ethnic characteristics were to be overlooked, circumvented, or not talked about, among whites, or—if members of a minority group—denied or de-emphasized and reserved for special cultural or private occasions.[68]

The spontaneous recognition of cultural variables within the field of weight management has been limited to reactions to client attitudes or behaviors that are different from what is commonly assumed: the evidence that being thin is less important to members of many ethnic minority groups, compared to whites, even among those who may want to lose weight and that intrafamilial or intergenerational relations seem to be different in some cultures compared to what white Americans expect. An interesting example of the latter type of insight can be found in an article by Wadden et al[69] reporting results of an obesity treatment program in which black adolescent girls and their parents were either treated together or in separate, parallel groups or where the girls were treated alone without parental involvement. The level of maternal involvement was positively related to the treatment effect among the black girls, in contrast to a finding from a similar study of white girls reported by Brownell et al.[70] In reporting this finding, Wadden et al commented: "Brownell et al reported that participation of mothers and daughters in the same group *inhibited* [emphasis ours] both parties. We did not observe this tendency in our study of black adolescents. Group meetings of the mother-child together condition tended to be, if anything, more animated, fun, and supportive than were meetings of the child alone or mother-child separately. Children and mothers appeared comfortable in the same group."[69(p245)]

Descriptions of cultural differences between African Americans and whites often emphasize the greater extended family and community embeddedness of African Americans in comparison to the greater isolation of the individual and nuclear family in the white or mainstream community[27,71] (see Figure 3–4). This difference in the orientation toward family might explain the difference observed by Wadden and would be a potential basis for using a different set of assumptions when deciding whether and how to involve family members in weight control programs for African American girls.

Cultural differences may also be uncovered upon probing why certain negative program outcomes such as non-participation, non-attendance, non-adherence, or poor weight loss results are observed to occur disproportionately for certain ethnic or socioeconomic status groups. For example, Brill et al[72] reported that black employees were significantly less likely to enroll in a worksite wellness program and that those who did enroll were significantly more likely to drop out. Are there cultural factors that might explain why this occurred? Brill et al[72] observed no racial difference in mean weight lost by blacks and whites who completed the program. However, in risk-reduction trials in which there were relatively few drop outs per se (follow-up rates maintained for purposes of blood pressure measurement were very high), a racial difference in program effectiveness was suggested by the observation of significantly lower average weight losses among black participants.[73,74] Other authors have also reported lower average weight losses among black compared to white patients, apparently related to behavioral adherence.[75,76]

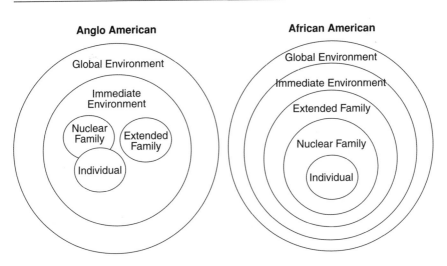

Figure 3–4 Differences in world view from Anglo American and African American perspectives.

Kumanyika et al[29] have suggested that these racial differences in weight loss may be explained in part by a cultural "mismatch" between elements of typical behavioral counseling programs. Various factors may prevent participants for whom the program is not a good match from dropping out, but other adherence may be limited by cultural incompatibility. As explained below, the factors limiting the relevance or appropriateness of a behavioral weight loss program for a particular group may be paradigmatic or may involve any of numerous aspects of the way the program is designed and implemented over time.

Behavioral Change Paradigms

Reference has already been made to two assumptions underlying behavioral change paradigms that may be unworkable for some or all cultural subgroups: (1) that the individual is the appropriate unit of treatment, perhaps supported by significant others, and (2) that the surface attitudes and behaviors of the individual can be addressed without direct attention to reference group factors (i.e., age, ethnicity, income level) that are underlying influences on these attitudes and behaviors. The previous analysis of behavioral change paradigms by Kumanyika et al[29] concluded that the cultural basis for these two assumptions is essentially Anglo American. Programs are being conducted within a cultural context in which the overriding hierarchy of values is that of an ideal typical white male. For example, conventional behavioral treatment strategies emphasize interpersonal control, personal autonomy, assertiveness, self-management, and goal setting—all of which are compatible with the prototypical white, middle-class U.S. businessman who is self-oriented, self-directed, task-centered, has an achievement-oriented perspective, and considers competition the most constructive way to organize human relations.[77] These characteristics and ideals are qualitatively and quantitatively different from aspects of African American culture and many other cultures (including some European cultures) that place relatively less emphasis on the individual and on mastery over the environment and more emphasis on extended family relations, adaptability to the environment, and cooperation rather than competition.[27,28,71,78] In some respects these characteristics are also different from those associated with Anglo American females,[79] although, within a culture, females may accept the characteristics of males as those for which to strive.[80]

If this analysis is correct, that is, if the underlying paradigms are culturally unsuitable for people from some cultures and would require that people think or act in ways that are alien to themselves and to their environments, then it is possible that adaptations of aspects of program implementation to meet the needs of a specific cultural group will fall short of the mark. For example, qualitative research on African American foodways[81] has supported the inference that coping mechanisms involve responsiveness to the demands of the environment and of the life circumstances (rather than dominating them) in which one finds oneself and that this responsiveness includes eating what is environmentally available. This type of "making the best of it" or "rolling with the punches" approach may have developed based on the practicalities of dealing with enslavement and segregation. However, there may also be more fundamental cultural principles favoring the achievement of equilibrium with one's environment, emanating from the African tradition.[28,82] From this perspective, the assumption that an individual participating in a behavioral change program can be trained to adopt a way of eating (e.g., low-calorie or low-fat) that is out of synchronization with the predominant food environment (e.g., high-calorie or high-fat) or that affects the food environment from a consumer demand perspective may be less valid for individuals influenced more by an Afrocentric perspective. Such individuals might expect to evolve eating patterns in concert with changes in the food environment.

Much more and a different line of research will be needed to guide cultural adaptation approaches that will be effective in diverse groups. Adaptations of implementation—hiring staff from the same cultural background—may not be sufficient to overcome such a fundamental problem.

Program Characteristics

What are the elements of a program for which cultural factors may be particularly important background variables? From the model in Figure 3–2, several routes of programmatic cultural influences can be identified: certain institutional- and staff-related background factors that set the context for the program, the specific format and content of the program, programmatically influenced aspects of the interaction with clients, and dynamics among groups of clients. Some questions that can serve as guides for assessing the possible cultural influences associated with these factors are given in Appendix 3–A.

Many institutional and staff factors are relatively fixed, for example, the image of the institution in the community and the professional orientation or ethnic and social class characteristics of the staff, and so cannot be adapted (at least not without a major effort of long duration) to a set of clients or their circumstances. However, it is especially important to recognize the potential impact these variables have on what is offered, expected, and considered acceptable by the program and how it is offered and evaluated.

In contrast to relatively fixed institutional or staff characteristics, various aspects of the program content and format often provide for flexibility. These constitute the usual foci for adaptation to the cultural perspectives of the client group(s). It is certainly appropriate and in many ways essential to modify these program variables. However, it is equally important to shape aspects of the provider-client interaction and group dynamics for effectiveness in a given cultural or multi-cultural context. As discussed in the next section, to do so requires not only endorsement from those in authority, but also the professional's willingness as well as sufficient cross-cultural (e.g., cross-ethnic, -class, -gender, or -age) knowledge, understanding, and communication skills. These cross-cultural skills are in addition to the already recognized requisite competencies in nutrition education, behavioral counseling, and group facilitation.

Program Planning and Implementation

The "Hard-to-Reach" Professional

Although clients from cultural backgrounds that are different from those of the mainstream population are often termed "hard-to-reach," this designation may be equally applicable to health workers who fail to approach cultural adaptation from a holistic perspective. Staff may have an existing program they wish to adapt for a particular group by making relatively minimal modifications in format or content. The presumed validity of this approach may rest in a desire to preserve the elements perceived to be core to their program, in an assumed need to standardize the program for dissemination and replication, or in a pragmatic view that beginning from scratch for every new client population is simply impossible.

The interest in having a fixed program may also be perpetuated because it is administratively useful as well as comfortable from the perspective of professionals trained in a medical model. One problem with this approach to cultural adaptation is that it establishes an adversarial situation in which the program, as designed for and possibly effective with some other client group, becomes the standard by which the clients are judged. Inevitably, those for whom it appears to work, who fit the program, are positively evaluated and those who do not fit are considered problematic. A standardized program approach also may be counterproductive, over the long term, even for those clients who appear to be a good fit for the program, because the dynamic may predispose clients to adopt temporary behavioral strategies in order to accommodate explicit or implicit staff wishes or to feel a sense of mastery.

In addition, attempts to culturally adapt programs based on relatively superficial modifications to content or format (for example, translating text, changing recipes, using ethnic illustrations) are particularly vulnerable to the pitfalls of stereotyping. In this context stereotyping can be defined as the inappropriate interpretation of group characteristics as applying to individuals; it may also involve an overly simplistic characterization of cultural attitudes and beliefs. An example of such stereotyping might be the interpretation that "soul food" is the core cuisine of the African American community, ignoring the historical context or overestimating the social-psychological dimensions. Another example might be the recognition of the importance of the family in the Mexican American community but then applying the Western nuclear family model in adapting the program.

Process Rather than Task Orientation

Rather than a task orientation—something one does to a part of a program—cultural adaptation is more appropriately viewed as an integrated part of the full instructional design, program planning, and implementation process (see Appendix 3–A). Programmers cannot second guess the needs and wants of the client or client group. They need to have a core of knowledge about the clients' attitudes, preferences, and lifestyles in order to develop possible intervention strategies, then obtain feedback on the effectiveness of various approaches and have the flexibility to revise as necessary. In this sense, cultural adaptation is a methodological and more complex extension of client-centered or consumer-friendly approaches.

Weight control or exercise programs that have been culturally adapted for African American communities[83-90] or Mexican American communities[91] reflect numerous strategies. Many go far beyond the obvious approaches of incorporating ethnic recipes, using a community location, or hiring staff from the same ethnic group. A program in Baltimore[83] integrated the program into the existing framework of black churches. This required specific accommodations to the social setting of the church, implying selectivity by membership, age, and gender. However, for those who participated, this approach grounded their weight control efforts directly in the ongoing support system that was inherent in their church membership and enabled them to integrate these efforts within their existing lifestyle. The Community Health Assessment and Promotion Project (CHAPP) in Atlanta[84] used a community center in a neighborhood housing project as the setting for instituting a weight control program. While this did not provide a social support context as such, it did provide a social context in which it was convenient for people with common socioeconomic circumstances and experiences to participate. However, note that compared to churches, which are cultural institutions as such,[92] it may be less safe to assume that the social characteristics of housing developments (which may not function as community institutions) will be different and possibly less favorable from a behavioral intervention program perspective.[85] Each community setting requires evaluation in relation to cultural and social dynamics as perceived by those who will be involved in a program.

Other features of the program adjustments that evolved in the most community-oriented programs were: (1) staff participation in the program along with clients; (2) home visits to build support for the program among family members not directly involved and to encourage their participation in the program; (3) interim telephone calls to individualize attention to participants in group-based interventions; (4) participant choice of program topics and activities; (5) ongoing modifications of various aspects of the program initiated by participants; (6) choice of name or program theme by participants; and (7) training participants to become peer leaders. In CHAPP, participant involvement led to a more holistic focus that included cultural events, field trips, and advice on make-up, wardrobe, and fashion analysis.

Attempting to culturally adapt a program presumes a willingness to examine various program elements, identify points where there is flexibility, consider alternative strategies, and try out these strategies to see if they work. Trying out various approaches can be costly and seemingly inefficient and may even result in apparent program failure, at least in the short-term. For this reason it is useful to "stack the deck" in favor of the potential for success of whatever is attempted. Guidelines for the appropriate preliminary steps are available[77,93–95] as are resources for learning about ethnic foodways and their origins[24] and the art of cross-cultural communication.[96] Technically oriented professionals should accept that some important aspects of cultural knowledge and perceptions of others (by ethnicity, age, gender, social class) cannot be learned from any reference books, especially as they apply to individuals. However, when setting and tone are right, additional necessary knowledge and insights will develop through direct, repeated interactions among those involved.

Evaluation Issues

Weight management professionals are far from knowing whether solid cultural adaptations of weight management programs will increase their acceptability to and effectiveness with diverse cultural groups. What cultural adaptation is or is not is still relatively undefined. The validity of attending to cultural influences can be logically established, drawing upon basic knowledge from anthropology and sociology. However, success in cultural adaptation is inherently difficult to evaluate.

Inclusion of some culturally oriented accommodations in a program format or setting can be evaluated directly, through changing the physical setting, serving different cultural foods, hiring staff from the same ethnic group, using educational materials written in the client's preferred language, or including family members as primary participants vs focusing primarily on only one family member. However, the salience of these changes from the client's perspective is much less measurable. Salient cultural influences may be difficult to articulate because they are tied to subtle symbolic meanings learned through affective rather than rational mechanisms. Also, the unit of measurement may be a problem. The usual intervention protocol and evaluation models focus on assessment of the individual as such, not the individual as a member of a social network or family, and not the family or network itself. However, effects that take place in the family or social network may be appropriate primary or at least secondary outcomes of interest in programs for some cultural groups.

If a certain level of cultural appropriateness is a minimum standard for any program, then it is unethical to conduct studies in which culturally inappropriate protocols are used as the basis for comparison. In addition, it is impractical to directly compare effectiveness of programs adapted for different groups because the characteristics of the programs and the participants in them will be different. However, taking note of differences in the way client groups respond to various program features can be informative. The Wadden et al[69] program for adolescent African American girls, cited previously, was specifically designed to meet their needs and interests but had a similar format for maternal involvement to a study in rural white girls[70] and could, therefore, be compared on this aspect.

Historical comparisons, although complicated by program variables other than those of interest and by secular trends, may be one alternative for evaluating the impact of changes made to achieve cultural relevance. For example, long-term weight losses achieved to date by state-of-the-art programs implemented in an ethnic minority group could be taken as the reference point against which to compare outcomes of future programs in which careful attention has been paid to a comprehensive set of cultural issues. A focus on long-term results is of particular importance: short-term results may reflect various short cuts or temporary behaviors, while long-term results reflect the extent to which treatment-related attitudes and behaviors were incorporated into the individual's overall cultural context (see Figure 3–3).

Another possible approach for estimating the validity of cultural adaptations is to review participant feedback from programs that are or are not culturally adapted or that are intracultural or cross-cultural. The objective would be to identify those aspects that are most or least well-received or that are requested by members of the client population of interest under these various conditions. The inferences of Kumanyika et al[29] about the possible cultural mismatch of behavioral treatment approaches with the cultural perspectives of African American women were based in part on participant evaluation data and semi-structured retrospective individual interviews with African American and white women who had participated in a conventional, i.e., not culturally adapted, weight control program. The program as received by clients may be as diverse as the cultural perspectives in the client group, making it difficult to generalize about what worked. Thus, ultimately, the key principle of cultural relevance may rest in the flexibility and responsiveness of the program to client perspectives as they evolve with exposure to the intervention. It may be feasible to measure programs in terms of flexibility and responsiveness to client feedback and to tie these to measures of individual or group behavior change.

Ethical Issues: What Not To Change

Some students of the topic of cultural adaptation of health programs or health services highlight the tendency of health workers from a dominant culture to impose their views and values on those of the client population, particularly in an international context but also across cultures within the same society. For example, Leininger[97] has described *cultural imposition:* "the tendency for health

personnel to impose their beliefs, practices, and values upon another culture because they believe that their ideas are superior to those of another person or
group."[97(p36)] The tendency for people to view their own cultural perspectives as
central and to see their way of doing things as the only way to do them is termed
ethnocentrism. Cultural imposition and ethnocentrism are particularly associated
with cross-cultural interactions in the context of political domination (i.e., majority vs minority population; industrialized countries vs developing countries).
However, they also apply to social status (middle and upper vs lower social class;
professional vs non-professional or professional vs client).

This chapter promotes cultural relativism, the idea that different approaches
that may have merit in a given culture or subculture are potentially acceptable;
each culture or subculture is judged on its own terms; and validity of views is
based on the members' own perceptions and feelings and rationales.[96] This view
requires a pluralistic outlook in which many cultures can coexist. This does not
imply that people should take a relative approach to their own culture. Accepting
and working with the cultural perspective held by a client does not mean that this
culture then becomes the perspective of the professional in question. In fact, working with people from another culture may heighten one's awareness and appreciation of one's own culture.

As a guide for health workers in taking a more relativistic approach,
Airhihenbuwa[98] has proposed the PEN-3 model in which two dimensions involve
classifying the nature of the attitudes and behaviors to be addressed as Perceptions,
Enablers, or Nurturers—each of which may be Positive, Exotic, or Negative. In this
framework the nurturance achieved through symbolism and social values of food
would be positively valued, fostered, and preserved in a culturally appropriate intervention. An intervention program might attempt to work around other exotic (unusual to the observer) food practices or folk beliefs that, although not necessarily
positive, have no identifiable negative health consequences.

Uncritical application of the concept of cultural relativism or cultural appropriateness may lead health workers into ethical dilemmas. It will then be difficult to
distinguish cultural imposition, to use Leininger's term, from fully justified attempts to change cultural practices that are objectively harmful to health (smoking
to prevent obesity).[99] A full discussion of these issues is far beyond the scope of
this chapter. The intent here is to make readers aware that these types of ethical
issues may arise and will need to be addressed.

CONCLUSION

Issues of cultural appropriateness arise in conjunction with nutrition and health
programs because of the belief that attending to cultural factors will allow for
services that are better aligned with the client's needs and circumstances and are

thus more effective and sensitive. Considering the marked gender differences in cultural perspectives on weight as well as age and socioeconomic status differences, cultural appropriateness issues should be viewed along all relevant dimensions, not just those relevant to "minority" populations.

Cultural factors influence obesity and weight gain through several attitudinal and behavioral pathways that converge in food intake and energy output. Differences in weight-related attitudes and practices can be readily documented among ethnic groups in the United States. Compared to middle-class whites, some population groups in which obesity is very prevalent have more tolerant views about obesity. How one preserves the psychologically healthier aspects of body image that may be present while stressing the potential health problems associated with overweight is unclear.

Cultural adaptation is not something one does at the level of the individual client. It is essentially an attempt to align a program with cultural background variables so that, for clients of the program, the "fit" with their ways of thinking and doing things is as close as possible. Identifying the characteristics of a program that make it culturally appropriate and modifying programs so that they become culturally appropriate are not easy, and what needs to be done differs at various phases of a program. As indicated by the guiding questions provided in Appendix 3–A, this is an inexact, iterative process that allows for continual assessment of and response to manifestations of cultural factors on providers, clients, and program dynamics. Several routes of programmatic cultural influences can be identified, including certain relatively fixed institutional- and staff-related background factors that set the context for the program as well as more modifiable factors such as the program setting, content, and format, and the tenor and quality of interactions of staff with clients and among clients in groups.

The program as received by clients may be as diverse as the individual perspectives in the client group, making it difficult to generalize about what works. Evaluation strategies should focus on the degree to which the program process allows for responsiveness to clients and for evolution over time as it relates to outcomes.

ACKNOWLEDGMENT

The authors are grateful to Joanne Caulfield for her assistance with manuscript preparation.

REFERENCES

1. Sobal J, Stunkard AJ. Socioeconomic status and obesity: a review of the literature. *Psychol Bull.* 1989;105:260–275.
2. Kumanyika S. Obesity in minority populations. An epidemiologic assessment. *Obes Res.* 1994;2:166–182.

3. Epstein FH, Higgins M. Epidemiology of obesity. In: Bjorntorp P, Bordoff BN, eds. *Obesity.* Philadelphia: JB Lippincott Co; 1992:330–342.

4. Gurney M, Gorstein J. The global prevalence of obesity: an initial overview of available data. *World Health Stat Q.* 1988;41:251–254.

5. Ritenbaugh C. Obesity as a culture-bound syndrome. *Cult Med Psychiatry.* 1982;6:347–364.

6. Brown PJ, Konner M. An anthropological perspective on obesity. *Ann NY Acad Sci.* 1987;499:29–46.

7. Cassel JA. Social anthropology and nutrition: a different look at obesity in America. *J Am Diet Assoc.* 1995;95:424–427.

8. Thomas PR. *Weighing the Options.* Washington, DC: National Academy Press; 1995.

9. Keesing FM. *Cultural Anthropology: The Science of Custom.* New York: Holt, Reinhart, and Winston; 1965.

10. Helman CF. *Culture, Health and Illness: An Introduction for Health Professionals.* Boston, MA: Wright; 1990.

11. Kuhn TS. *The Structure of Scientific Revolutions.* Chicago: University of Chicago Press; 1970.

12. Novelli WD. Applying social marketing to health promotion and disease prevention. In: Glanz K, Lewis FM, Rimer BK, eds. *Health Behavior and Health Education: Theory, Research and Practice.* San Francisco: Jossey-Bass Publishers; 1990:342–369.

13. Rodin J. Cultural and psychosocial determinants of weight concerns. *Ann Intern Med.* 1993;119:643–635.

14. Kumanyika S. Cultural factors in desirable body shapes and their impact on weight loss and maintenance. In: Allison DB, Pi-Sunyer FX, eds. *Obesity Treatment.* New York: Plenum Press; 1995:79–82.

15. Nichter M, Nichter M. Hype and weight. *Med Anthropol.* 1991;13:249–284.

16. *Report of the Secretary's Task Force on Minority Health.* Washington, DC: US Department of Health and Human Services, August 1985. Executive Summary Volume I.

17. Kumanyika SK. Diet and nutrition as influences on the morbidity/mortality gap. *Ann Epidemiol.* 1993;3:154–158.

18. O'Hare WP. America's minorities: the demographics of diversity. *Population Bulletin.* 1992;47:1–46.

19. Luhman R, Gilman S. *Race and Ethnic Relations: The Social and Political Experience of Minority Groups.* Belmont, CA: Wadsworth; 1980.

20. Yu ESH, Liu WT. US National Health Data on Asian Americans and Pacific Islanders. A research agenda for the 1990s. *Am J Public Health.* 1992;82:1645–1652.

21. Shopland DR, Burns DM, Samet JM, Gritz ER, eds. *Strategies To Control Tobacco Use in the United States: A Blueprint for Public Health Action in the 1990's.* Washington, DC: US Department of Health and Human Services; 1991. NIH Publication No. 92-3316.

22. Brown PJ. The biocultural evolution of obesity. An anthropological view. In: Bjorntorp P, Bordoff BN, eds. *Obesity.* Philadelphia: JB Lippincott Co; 1992:320–329.

23. Axelson ML. The impact of culture on food-related behavior. *Ann Rev Nutr.* 1986;6:345–363.

24. Kittler PG, Sucher K. *Food and Culture in America.* New York: Van Nostrand Reinhold; 1989.

25. Murcott A. Sociological and social anthropological approaches to food and eating. *World Rev Nutr Diet.* 1988;55:1–40.

26. Sobal J. Obesity and socioeconomic status: a framework for examining relationships between physical and social variables. *Med Anthropol.* 1991;13:231–247.

27. Leininger MM. Selected culture care findings of diverse culture using culture care theory and ethnomethods. In: Leininger MM, ed. *Culture Care Diversity and Universality: A Theory of Nursing.* New York: National League for Nursing Press; 1991:345–371.

28. Baldwin JA, Hopkins R. African-American and European-American cultural differences as assessed by the worldview paradigm: an empirical analysis. *The Western Journal of Black Studies.* 1990;14:38–52.

29. Kumanyika SK, Morssink C, Agurs T. Models for dietary and weight change in African-American women: identifying cultural components. *Ethn Dis.* 1992;2:166–175.

30. Hazuda HP, Mitchell BD, Haffner SM, Stern MP. Obesity in Mexican American subgroups. Findings from the San Antonio Heart Study. *Am J Clin Nutr.* 1991;53:1529S–1534S.

31. Jaynes GD, Williams RM Jr, eds. *A Common Destiny: Blacks and American Society.* Washington, DC: National Academy Press; 1989.

32. Wallendorf M, Reilly MD. Ethnic migration, assimilation and consumption. *J Consumer Research* 1983;10:292–302.

33. Brown PJ. Cultural perspectives on the etiology and treatment of obesity. In: Stunkard AJ, Wadden TA, eds. *Obesity: Theory and Therapy.* 2nd ed. New York: Raven Press Ltd; 1993:179–193.

34. Rand CSW, Kuldau JM. The epidemiology of obesity and self-defined weight problems in the general population: Gender, race, age, and social class. *Int J Eating Dis.* 1990;9:329–343.

35. Rosen JT, Gross J. Prevalence of weight reducing and weight gaining in adolescent girls and boys. *Health Psychol.* 1987;6:131–147.

36. Desmond SM, Price JH, Hallinan C, Smith D. Black and white adolescents' perceptions of their weight. *J Sch Health.* 1989;59:353–358.

37. Kemper KA, Sargent RG, Drane JW, Valois RF, Hussey JR. Black and white females' perceptions of ideal body size and social norms. *Obes Res.* 1994;2:117–126.

38. Rucker CE III, Cash TF. Body image, body-size perceptions, and eating behaviors among African-American and white college women. *Int J Eating Dis.* 1992;12:291–299.

39. Wing RR, Adams-Campbell LL, Marcus MD, Janney CA. Effect of ethnicity and geographical location on body weight, dietary restraint, and abnormal eating attitudes. *Obes Res.* 1993;1:193–198.

40. Harris MB, Furukawa C. Attitudes toward obesity in an elderly sample. *J Obesity & Weight Regulation.* 1986;5:5–16.

41. Rand CSW, Kuldau JM. The epidemiology of obesity and self-defined weight problem in the general population: gender, race, age, and social class. *Int J Eating Dis.* 1990;9:329–343.

42. Stevens J, Kumanyika S, Keil JE, Seibert L. Body size perceptions and eating attitudes in elderly men. *Obes Res.* 1994;2:127–134.

43. Stevens J, Kumanyika SK, Keil JE. Attitudes toward body size and dieting: differences between elderly black and white women. *Am J Public Health.* 1994;84:1322–1325.

44. Allan JD, Mayo K, Michel Y. Body size values of white and black women. *Res Nurs Health.* 1993;16:323–333.

45. Stern MP, Pugh JA, Gaskill SP, Hazuda HP. Knowledge, attitudes, and behavior related to obesity and dieting in Mexican Americans and Anglos: The San Antonio Heart Study. *Am J Epidemiol.* 1982;115:917–928.

46. Wilkinson JY, Ben-Tovim DI, Walker MK. An insight into the personal and cultural significance of weight and shape in large Samoan women. *Int J Obes Relat Metab Disord.* 1994;18:602–606.

47. Story M, Hauck FR, Broussard BA, White LL, Resnick MD, Blum RW. Weight perceptions and weight control practices in American Indian and Alaska Native adolescents. *Arch Pediatr Adolesc Med.* 1994;148:567–571.

48. Smith JE, Krejci J. Minorities join the majority: eating disturbances among Hispanic and Native American youth. *J Eating Dis.* 1991;10:179–186.

49. Piani A, Schoenborn C. Health promotion and disease prevention: United States, 1990. Hyattsville, MD: National Center for Health Statistics. *Vital Health Stat.* 1993;10(185).

50. Williamson DF, Serdula MK, Anda RF, Levy A, Byers T. Weight loss attempts in adults: goals, duration, and rate of weight loss. *Am J Public Health.* 1992;82:1251–1257.

51. Emmons L. Predisposing factors differentiating adolescent dieters and nondieters. *J Am Diet Assoc.* 1994;94:725–728.

52. Camp DE, Klesges RC, Relyea G. The relationship between body weight concerns and adolescent smoking. *Health Psychol.* 1993;12:24–32.

53. Gritz ER, Crane LA. Use of diet pills and amphetamines to lose weight among smoking and non-smoking high school seniors. *Health Psychol.* 1991;10:330–335.

54. Serdula MK, Williamson DF, Anda RF, Levy A, Heaton A, Byers T. Weight control practices in adults: results of a multistate telephone survey. *Am J Public Health.* 1994;84:1821–1824.

55. King AC, Blair SN, Bild DE, et al. Determinants of physical activity and interventions in adults. *Med Sci Sports Exerc.* 1992;24:S221–S236.

56. Airhihenbuwa C, Kumanyika S, Agurs TD, Lowe A, Saunders D. Perceptions and beliefs about physical activity, exercise, and rest among African-Americans. *Am J Health Promo.* 1995;9:426–429.

57. Kumanyika SK, Wilson JF, Davenport MG. Weight-related attitudes and behaviors of black women. *J Am Diet Assoc.* 1993;93:416–422.

58. Ikeda JP. Effective weight loss strategies for black women. Letter. *J Am Diet Assoc.* 1993;93:1252.

59. Kumanyika SK, Wilson JF, Davenport MG. Effective weight loss strategies for black women. Reply to J Ikeda. *J Am Diet Assoc.* 1993;93:1252.

60. Levine S, Sorenson JR. Social and cultural factors in health promotion. In: Matarazzo JD, Weiss SM, Herd JA, Miller NE, Weiss SM, eds. *Behavioral Health: A Handbook of Health Enhancement and Disease Prevention.* New York: John Wiley & Sons; 1984:222–229.

61. Rimer BK. Perspectives on intrapersonal theories in health education and health behavior. In: Glanz K, Lewis FM, Rimer BK, eds. *Health Behavior and Health Education: Theory, Research and Practice.* San Francisco: Jossey-Bass Publishers; 1990:140–157.

62. Perry CL, Baranowski T, Parcel GS. How individuals, environments, and health behavior interact: social learning theory. In: Glanz K, Lewis FM, Rimer BK, eds. *Health Behavior and Health Education: Theory, Research and Practice.* San Francisco: Jossey-Bass Publishers; 1990:161–186.

63. Ewart CK. Social action theory for a public health psychology. *Am Psychol.* 1991;46:931–946.

64. Kuczmarski RJ, Flegal KM, Campbell SM, Johnson DL. Increasing prevalence of overweight among U.S. adults. The national health and nutrition examination surveys, 1960 to 1991. *JAMA.* 1994;272:205–211.

65. Pi-Sunyer FX. Medical hazards of obesity. *Ann Intern Med.* 1993;119:655–660.

66. Gist JR. Decision making in public administration. In: Rabin J, Holdreth WB, Miller GJ. *Handbook of Public Administration.* New York: Marcel Dekker Inc; 1989:225–251.

67. Simon HA. *Administrative Behavior.* New York: Free Press; 1976.

68. Farley JE. *Majority-Minority Relations.* 2nd ed. Englewood Cliffs, NJ: Prentice Hall; 1988.

69. Wadden TA, Stunkard AJ, Rich L, Rubin CJ, Sweidel G, McKinney S. Obesity in black adolescent girls: a controlled clinical trial of treatment by diet, behavior modification, and parental support. *Pediatrics.* 1990;85:345–352.

70. Brownell KD, Kelman JH, Stunkard AJ. Treatment of obese children with and without their mothers: changes in weight and blood pressure. *Pediatrics.* 1983;71:515–523.

71. Boykin AW. The triple quandary and the schooling of Afro-American children. In: Neisser U, ed. *The School Achievement of Minority Children: New Perspectives.* Hillsdale, NJ: Lawrence Erlbaum Associates; 1986:82–103.

72. Brill PA, Kohl HW, Rogers T, Collingwood TR, Sterling CL, Blair SN. The relationships between sociodemographic characteristics and recruitment, retention, health improvements in a worksite health promotion program. *Am J Health Promo.* 1991;5:215–221.

73. Kumanyika SK, Obarzanek E, Stevens VJ, Hebert PR, Whelton PK. Weight loss experience of black and white participants in NHLBI-sponsored clinical trials. *Am J Clin Nutr.* 1991;53:1631S–1638S.

74. Wylie-Rosett J, Wassertheil-Smoller S, Blaufox DM, et al. Trial of antihypertensive intervention and management: greater efficacy with weight reduction than with a sodium-potassium intervention. *J Am Diet Assoc.* 1993;93:408–415.

75. Sugerman HJ, Londrey GL, Kellum JM, et al. Weight loss with vertical banded gastroplasty and roux-y gastric bypass for morbid obesity with selective versus random assignment. *Am J Surg.* 1989;157:93–102.

76. Darga LL, Holden JH, Olson SM, Lucas CP. Comparison of cardiovascular risk factors in obese blacks and whites. *Obes Res.* 1994;2:239–245.

77. Harris PR, Moran RT. *Managing Cultural Differences: High Performance Strategies for Today's Global Manager.* 2nd ed. Houston, TX: Gulf Publishing; 1987.

78. Mithun JS. The role of the family in acculturation and assimilation in America. A psychocultural dimension. In: McCready WC, ed. *Culture, Ethnicity, and Identity. Current Issues in Research.* New York: Academic Press; 1983:209–232.

79. Finch J. "It's great to have someone to talk to": ethics and politics of interviewing women. In: Hammersley M, ed. *Social Research: Philosophy, Politics and Practice.* London: Sage Publications; 1993:166–180.

80. Barrett NS. Women. In: Hornbeck DW, Salamon LM, eds. *Human Capital and America's Future.* Baltimore, MD: The Johns Hopkins University Press; 1991:69–94.

81. Airhihenbuwa CO, Kumanyika S, Agurs TD, Lowe A, Saunders D, Morssink CB. Cultural aspects of African-American eating patterns. *Ethnicity and Health.* 1996;1:245–260.

82. Airhihenbuwa CO. *Health and Culture: Beyond the Western Paradigm.* Thousand Oaks, CA: Sage Publications; 1995.

83. Kumanyika SK, Charleston JB. Lose weight and win: a church-based weight loss program for blood pressure control among black women. *Patient Educ Couns.* February 1992;19:19–32.

84. Lasco RA, Curry RH, Dickson VJ, Powers J, Menes S, Merritt RK. Participation rates, weight loss, and blood pressure changes among obese women in a nutrition-exercise program. *Public Health Rep.* 1989;104:640–646.

85. Lewis CE, Raczynski JM, Heath GW, Levinson R, Hilyer JC, Cutter GR. Promoting physical activity in low-income African-American communities: the PARR Project. *Ethn Dis.* 1993;3:106–118.

86. McNabb WL, Quinn MT, Rosing L. Weight loss program for innner-city black women with non-insulin-dependent diabetes mellitus: PATHWAYS. *J Am Diet Assoc.* 1993;93:75–77.

87. Domel SB, Alford BB, Cattlett HN. Weight control for black women. *J Am Diet Assoc.* 1992;92:346–347.

88. Pleas J. Long-term effects of a lifestyle-change obesity treatment program with minorities. *J Natl Med Assoc.* 1988;80:747–752.

89. Sullivan J, Carter JP. A nutrition-physical fitness intervention program for low-income black parents. *J Natl Med Assoc.* 1985;77:39–43.

90. Kanders BS, Ullmann-Joy P, Foreyt JP, et al. The black American lifestyle intervention (BALI): the design of a weight loss program for working-class African-American women. *J Am Diet Assoc.* 1994;94:310–312.

91. Cousins JH, Rubovits DS, Dunn JK, Reeves RS, Ramirez AG, Foreyt JP. Family versus individually oriented intervention for weight loss in Mexican American women. *Public Health Rep.* 1992;107:549–555.

92. Eng E, Hatch J, Callan A. Institutionalizing social support through the church and into the community. *Health Ed Q.* 1985;12:81–92.

93. Kumanyika SK, Morssink C. Working effectively in cross-cultural and multicultural settings. In: Frankle R, Owen A, eds. *Nutrition in the Community.* 3rd ed. St. Louis: Mosby; 1993:78–95.

94. Elaides DC, Suitor CW. *Celebrating Diversity: Approaching Families through Their Food.* Arlington, VA: National Center for Education in Maternal and Child Health; 1994.

95. Gonzalez VM, Gonzalez JT, Freeman V, Howard-Pitney B. *Health Promotion in Diverse Cultural Communities.* Palo Alto, CA: Stanford Center for Research in Disease Prevention; 1991.

96. Kavanaugh KH, Kennedy PH. *Promoting Cultural Diversity. Strategies for Health Professionals.* Newbury Park, CA: Sage Publications Inc; 1992.

97. Leininger M. Becoming aware of types of health practitioners and cultural imposition. *J Transcult Nurs.* 1991;2:36.

98. Airhihenbuwa CO. Health promotion and disease prevention strategies for African Americans. A conceptual model. In: Braithwaite RL, Taylor SE, eds. *Health Issues in the Black Community.* San Francisco: Jossey-Bass; 1992:267–280.

99. Bayer R. AIDS prevention and cultural sensitivity: are they compatible? *Am J Public Health* 1994;84:895–898.

Assessing Cultural Influences on Program Design, Implementation, and Participation

CULTURAL CONTEXT OF PROGRAM

- To what extent are the cultural characteristics of the client population represented among those of the the institutional decision makers and gatekeepers?
- Are persons from the same cultural background as the client visible within the institution or program? If so, in what roles (decision-making roles? professional staff? custodial staff?)? Might this influence the way clients from these ethnic groups are treated in the institution or perceived by staff?
- What are the historical cultural characteristics of the physical environment of the sponsoring institution (predominantly white neighborhood? inner city? middle-class or suburban area? low-income community?). What is the nature of relationships between the institution and its surrounding community? Are the clients of the weight control program from the surrounding community or culturally similar to persons in this community? What attitudes does the client community have toward the institution?
- What logistical or funding constraints are in effect that may limit flexibility in responding to client needs? For example, if people want or need to bring their family members or friends to classes in order to achieve success, is there space for them? Are there sufficient funds to provide materials or refreshments for family members? Will they have to pay? If clients need individual attention in addition to or instead of group counseling, is there sufficient staff time to provide this? Will administration view this as inefficient?
- Are there staff who believe that being overweight is bad and that clients should have attitudes similar to their own? How might this be manifested?

PROGRAM SETTING, CONTENT, AND FORMAT

- Is the setting in which the program is offered familiar to the client or client group? If so, what connotations does the setting have? Is it associated with:
  1. work identities, relationships or "pecking orders"? (worksite)
  2. having fun or participating in recreational activities? (community center)
  3. religious principles? (church center)
  4. voluntary social networks? (church center)
  5. neighborhood, tenant, or homeowner issues? (housing community)
  6. being "experimented on"? (research institution or teaching hospital)
  7. having medical problems, needing medical help? (any medical setting)
  8. health (fitness center or health club)
- Are the connotations of the setting neutral, supportive, or constraining of an atmosphere that is conducive to the education or behavior change goals of the program, in relation to:
  1. eating; eating with others
  2. making personal disclosures
  3. revealing ignorance or vulnerability
  4. helping others
  5. competing with others
  6. learning technical information
  7. trusting others
  8. feeling safe
  9. perceiving staff or other participants as authority figures
  10. feeling understood by others
  11. admitting failure
  12. learning from others
  13. needing to connect with others
  Are these connotations similar for all clients?
- What are the assumptions about clients' preferred learning styles? Is there a requirement that all clients adopt the same style, for example, a cognitively oriented, intellectual approach?
- How broad or narrow is the program scope in relation to other health or social needs in this client population? Does the program artificially isolate weight control issues from related issues such as basic nutrition, food purchasing, psychosocial stress, time management, health problems, and social life?
- What decisions about the program are made by the clients? For example, can clients decide how long the program continues? What topics to cover or in what order? Are they asked to help identify the experts who provide information? Do they decide when and with whom the exercise sessions take place (for example, Saturday morning in the park [and which park], along with

friends or family members, or at dinner time on a weekday with other class members)?
- What levels of reading and comprehension are needed for effective participation in the program? In what language? Are there any program aspects with a substantially higher or lower literacy demand? Language requirement?
- What practice in skill building or new experiences are offered within the program session or counseling visits? How relevant are these to experiences these clients would have on a typical day? Are themes used that some members of the group may be unable or unlikely to identify with at all?
- Which aspects of the program have been deliberately geared to the clients' cultural framework(s)? How have these been selected and implemented? How much cross-validation effort has been put into this?

INTERACTION BETWEEN STAFF AND CLIENT(S)

- How frequent are individual, face-to-face contacts with clients? Is there flexibility to increase or decrease frequency according to client preferences? Are clients given a choice about whether to have group or individual counseling? Are staff aware of cultural differences in "personal space"? privacy issues? assertiveness issues?
- How motivated and enthusiastic are the staff about implementing the program? Do they appear to like the clients as people? Do the clients appear to like the staff?
- What are the "rules" about how clients relate to the staff? What happens when clients want to be more or less dependent or emotional than is intended?
- Once the program has begun, how much and in what ways is the staff willing and able to adjust the program to meet the expressed needs and desires of the clients?
- What mechanisms are built in to identify the clients' views and needs and their implications for program changes?
- How is feedback on acceptability and relevance obtained and incorporated into the program?

GROUP DYNAMICS

- How diverse is the group in terms of ethnicity, social class, gender, age, and level of obesity? If very diverse, does the group incorporate this diversity directly or simply attempt to proceed in spite of it?
- Are there any obvious aspects of group dynamics that may influence problems for the intended group process (supervisors and supervisees in the same

group? people who persistently make, wittingly or unwittingly, biased or eth-nocentric remarks?)?

- Are there previously developed social interactions among members of the group? Among the group as a whole? For example, is this a program offered to an existing social group or to people who know each other well (work-place, church, neighborhood organization, social club, or another instruc-tional setting)? If so, have these prior relationships been incorporated into the behavioral change paradigm?
- What aspects of group dynamics might elicit defense mechanisms from indi-viduals who have experienced discrimination on the basis of race, gender, poverty, or stigmatization related to weight and thereby constrain their ability to participate in the group in the intended manner?
- What are the expectations about how the group will evolve and interact over time and the implications of these expectations for group members? For ex-ample, is the group a "class" in which people interact primarily with the group leader or instructor or is the intent that members become mutually sup-portive and develop friendships? Is the group closed and geared to evolve trust among members over time or does membership or attendance at sessions vary from occasion to occasion?
- Are there group exercises in which each member must actually use certain language, reading, or calculation skills while others are watching and listen-ing (inadvertently revealing low literacy skills)?
- When members of a diverse group have to participate in group activities, are teams assigned, based on the incidental seating arrangement, or voluntarily selected?

CHAPTER 4

Obesity-Related Eating Patterns: Binge Eating Disorder and the Night-Eating Syndrome

Nancy J. Aronoff

INTRODUCTION

More than 35 years ago, Stunkard[1] identified three distinct patterns of overeating among obese patients seeking weight control treatment. Based on patient interview and observation, he was able to define these eating patterns in terms of the following three variables: (1) the presence or absence of self-condemnation associated with the eating pattern, (2) the degree of personal meaning attached to the eating pattern, and (3) the degree of stress to which the patient is subjected at the time the unusual eating pattern occurs (Table 4–1). While Stunkard acknowledged the existence of unusual eating patterns in normal-weight and underweight individuals as well, he described the frequency and regularity with which they occurred in his obese patients as follows: "when a pattern does enter into the eating behavior of an obese person, it does so with some consistency and may well make a significant contribution to the production and maintenance of his obesity."[1(p287)] Binge eating, or consumption of large amounts of food in relatively short periods of time, and the night-eating syndrome (NES), characterized by morning anorexia, nocturnal hyperphagia, and insomnia, were among the patterns he most commonly observed. These eating patterns are currently being reconsidered in terms of their potential roles in attaining and maintaining varying degrees of overweight.

Like obesity itself, the establishment of a particular eating pattern is probably multifactorial in nature. It is also likely that certain individuals will demonstrate either combinations or varying degrees of deviant eating patterns depending on the physiological, psychological, and environmental conditions prevailing at the time they present for treatment. With the staggering prevalence of obesity in this country, identification of specific eating patterns with which to characterize dis-

Table 4–1 Characteristics of Three Eating Patterns of Obese Human Subjects Studied in 1959

	Periodicity	Brain Damage	Relation to Stress	Apparent Personal Meaning	Associated Self-Condemnation
Night eating	X	O	X	O	O
Binge eating	O	O	X	X	X
Eating without satiation	O	probably	O	O	O

Source: Reprinted with permission from A.J. Stunkard, Eating Patterns and Obesity, *Psychiatry,* Vol. 33, p. 287, © 1959, Guilford Press.

tinct subsets of overweight individuals could prove highly valuable in terms of potential treatment options. This chapter focuses on binge eating and the night-eating syndrome in terms of established criteria, prevalence, identification and assessment, clinical characteristics, and current and future treatment methods.

BINGE EATING AND OBESITY: HISTORY, DEFINITION, CRITERIA, AND PREVALENCE

As Stunkard points out,[2] "binge eating," a relatively recent term, evolved from the ancient ingestive behavior of bulimia, or uncontrolled eating in response to an insatiable appetite.[3] Until very recently, reports of this behavior have focused on normal-weight females who engage in frequent episodes of overeating followed by compensatory behaviors such as purging to prevent or minimize weight gain (bulimia nervosa). Attempts to clearly describe binge eating in the literature have been plagued by an inability to operationally define the term "binge." Identification of overeating as the single most important behavioral characteristic of bulimia nervosa[4] led to the first attempts to address this ambiguity. "Binge eating," an integral part of the DSM-III criteria for bulimia nervosa, was originally defined as "rapid consumption of a large amount of food in a discrete period of time, usually less than two hours" (Exhibit 4–1).[5] Other essential features of this disorder included "fear of not being able to stop eating voluntarily" (i.e., loss of control), and post-binge dysphoria.[5,6]

In the early 1980s, when binge eating became more widely recognized as a distinct obese eating pattern, it was this set of criteria that was initially used for diagnosis. Based on a loose interpretation of these criteria, Loro and Orleans[7] were among the first to report on the prevalence of obese binge eating. Using self-report questionnaires and clinical records, they identified "consumption of large or enor-

Exhibit 4–1 Diagnostic Criteria for Bulimia Nervosa (DSM-III)

A. Recurrent episodes of binge eating (rapid consumption of a large amount of food in a discrete period of time, usually less than two hours).
B. At least three of the following:
   (1) consumption of high-caloric, easily ingested food during a binge
   (2) inconspicuous eating during a binge
   (3) termination of such eating episodes by abdominal pain, sleep, social interruption, or self-induced vomiting
   (4) Repeated attempts to lose weight by severely restrictive diets, self-induced vomiting, or use of cathartics or diuretics
   (5) Frequent weight fluctuations greater than ten pounds due to alternating binges and fasts
C. Awareness that the eating pattern is abnormal and fear of not being able to stop eating voluntarily.
D. Depressed mood and self-deprecating thoughts following eating binges.
E. The bulimic episodes are not due to Anorexia Nervosa or any known physical disorder.

Source: Reprinted with permission from the American Psychiatric Association: *Diagnostic and Statistical Manual of Mental Disorders, Third Edition,* Washington, DC, American Psychiatric Association, 1980.

---

mous quantities of food in short periods of time," occuring at least twice weekly, in 28.6% of 280 overweight or obese patients seeking treatment for weight control. Unfortunately, wide acceptance of these criteria was limited by two factors: (1) they did not differentiate between obese binge eaters and those with other types of eating disorders, and (2) they lent little insight into the severity of the binge behavior.

Recognizing these limitations, Gormally et al[6] developed the Binge Eating Scale (BES) to confirm the presence of binge eating and assess the severity of this disorder in obese individuals. The specific purpose of the BES was to identify behaviors associated with binge episodes, as well as thoughts that might trigger or follow binges. At the same time, they designed a Cognitive Factors Scale (CFS) to examine whether binge severity among overweight individuals (as determined from BES results) was linked to a tendency to set extremely high dieting standards while maintaining very low compliancy expectations. Significant correlations with regard to binge severity and ability to adhere to self-imposed diet restrictions were obtained. Development of these scales was a valuable first step in helping to distinguish obese binge eating from that which was previously described.

Over the next few years, use of the BES in conjunction with the DSM-III criteria for bulimia nervosa greatly enhanced the rate at which prevalence data emerged. Reports of binge eating prevalence among obese individuals seeking weight control treatment ranged from 20% to 46%.[6,8–11] While Gormally et al[6] reported serious binge eating in 23% of 112 patients applying to a weight control program, Marcus et al[9] identified this behavior in a strikingly high 46% of 432 women seeking behavioral treatment for obesity. In 1987, the DSM-III criteria for bulimia nervosa were revised to (1) exclude the two-hour time period in which overeating was supposed to occur to be defined as a binge, and (2) redefine "loss of control" as "a feeling of lack of control over eating behavior during the eating binges" (Exhibit 4–2).[12] Unfortunately, these revisions still failed to provide for the seemingly large population of binge eaters who chose not to engage in post-binge compensatory behaviors, but instead, eventually sought out weight control treatment. Bulimia nervosa remained as the only widely accepted binge eating disorder. Various adaptations of both the DSM-III[5] and DSM-III-R[12] criteria may have contributed to the wide range of prevalence data reported at this time. Groups reporting the lowest prevalence of binge eating in obese subjects[8] often required more stringent adaptation of the DSM-III-R criteria than those with higher rates.

The early 1990s marked a turning point in the recognition of obesity-related binge eating as a prevalent and distinct disorder. In response to both experimental and clinical evidence, aggressive attempts to establish specific criteria to define this behavior were undertaken.[13,14] Among the leaders in this effort were a group of experts in the fields of eating disorders and obesity who, in collaboration with members of the Eating Disorders Work Group of the DSM-IV Task Force, devel-

---

Exhibit 4–2 Diagnostic Criteria for Bulimia Nervosa (DSM-III-R)

A. Recurrent episodes of binge eating (rapid consumption of a large amount of food in a discrete period of time).
B. A feeling of lack of control over eating behavior during the eating binges.
C. The person regularly engages in either self-induced vomiting, use of laxatives or diuretics, strict dieting or fasting, or vigorous exercise in order to prevent weight gain.
D. A minimum average of two binge eating episodes a week for at least three months.
E. Persistent overconcern with body shape and weight.

Source: Reprinted with permission from the American Psychiatric Association: *Diagnostic and Statistical Manual of Mental Disorders, Third Edition, Revised,* Washington, DC, American Psychiatric Association, 1987.

oped a set of preliminary diagnostic criteria to define binge eating disorder (BED). The salient features ascribed to BED were recurrent binge eating associated with feelings of loss of control, but without the compensatory behaviors demonstrated in bulimia nervosa. Based on these characteristics, it was felt that BED would encompass both the subset of overweight individuals who engage in such behavior, and the understudied population of individuals who occasionally overeat but are able to maintain normal weights.[10] The proposed BED attempted to identify and/or quantify the following diagnostic criteria: (1) episodic overeating; (2) loss of control; (3) associated symptoms (eating rapidly, eating without physical hunger, etc.); (4) feelings of distress post-binge; (5) duration and frequency of binge eating; and (6) lack of compensatory behaviors observed in bulimia nervosa (Exhibit 4–3).

Exhibit 4–3 Research Criteria for Binge Eating Disorder

A. Recurrent episodes of binge eating. An episode of binge eating is characterized by both of the following:
   (1) eating, in a discrete period of time (e.g., within any two-hour period), an amount of food that is definitely larger than most people would eat in a similar period of time under similar circumstances
   (2) a sense of lack of control over eating during the episode (e.g., a feeling that one cannot stop eating or control what or how much one is eating)
B. The binge eating episodes are associated with three (or more) of the following:
   (1) eating much more rapidly than normal
   (2) eating until feeling uncomfortably full
   (3) eating large amounts of food when not feeling physically hungry
   (4) eating alone because of being embarrassed by how much one is eating
   (5) feeling disgusted with oneself, depressed, or very guilty after overeating
C. Marked distress regarding binge eating is present.
D. The binge eating occurs, on average, at least two days a week for six months. **Note:** The method of determining frequency differs from that used for Bulimia Nervosa; future research should address whether the preferred method of setting a frequency threshold is counting the number of days on which binges occur or counting the number of episodes of binge eating.
E. The binge eating is not associated with the regular use of inappropriate compensatory behaviors (e.g., purging, fasting, excessive exercise) and does not occur exclusively during the course of Anorexia Nervosa or Bulimia Nervosa.

Source: Reprinted with permission from the American Psychiatric Association: *Diagnostic and Statistical Manual of Mental Disorders, Fourth Edition,* Washington, DC, American Psychiatric Association, 1994.

The proposed criteria for BED have been tested and validated in two very large multisite field trials[10,11] and have recently been included in an appendix of the DSM-IV[15] as a proposed diagnostic category requiring further investigation. Unlike previous studies in this area, these trials involved very large samples of obese individuals taken from a wide variety of weight control programs across the country. Smaller samples included for data comparison were subjects from nonpatient community groups, college students, and people with bulimia nervosa. Obese subjects were identified as engaging in varying degrees of binge eating based on responses to a self-report questionnaire. Combined prevalence data from both multisite studies revealed the presence of recurrent binge eating in 29% to 30% of the overweight individuals seeking weight control treatment, compared with a prevalence of less than 5% in the nonpatient community sample. Both studies noted that BED was somewhat more common in overweight females than in males seeking treatment, but occurred similarly among males and females in the nonpatient community sample. BED was also equally common among both white and nonwhite subjects in the weight control sample.

IDENTIFICATION OF OBESE BINGE EATERS

An experienced clinician can often identify the presence of binge eating by asking certain probing questions in a non-accusatory fashion. A 24-hour food recall obtained on an initial visit may indicate an individual's willingness to confront a destructive eating pattern. Weight gain should be deemed highly suspicious when dietary recalls suggest an intake significantly below maintenance energy expenditure (MEE), assuming physiological causes for obesity (e.g., untreated thyroid disease) have been ruled out. Inaccurate reporting suggests that a patient is having difficulty (1) accurately assessing daily intake; (2) accepting the presence of an eating disorder (i.e., binge eating); or (3) some combination of (1) and (2). Such patients should be encouraged to bring daily food records to subsequent visits to ascertain whether a more reliable account of daily intake can be provided in writing compared to a face-to-face report.

Food records have repeatedly been criticized as an unreliable method of assessing total daily food intake in overweight individuals.[16–18] Nonetheless, careful analysis of records to determine the source of their inaccuracy can provide valuable information in terms of potential treatment. For example, weekly records reporting a fairly regular consumption pattern, a wide variety of both high- and low-calorie foods, and a few obvious overeating episodes, may indicate inaccurate estimation of portion sizes. This type of underreporting is quite common in moderately overweight, sedentary, nutritionally naive individuals. These patients are often non-bingers who incur weight loss setbacks with the addition of a few hundred extra calories each day. Treatment that focuses on portion control, basic

nutritional food choices, and increased physical activity can prove highly beneficial to this type of patient. On the other hand, food records that consistently report
a limited intake of low-energy foods, little or no dietary indiscretion, and a daily
caloric intake grossly below that required for weight maintenance, suggest that
entire eating episodes, often binges, are being omitted from the records. This type
of underreporting is often observed in obese individuals entering new weight
treatment programs. Such patients often feel vulnerable revealing the extent of
their eating problem to an unfamiliar practitioner. While inaccurate records can be
excellent indicators of an individual's prior nutrition education and notion of an
ideal diet, they reveal little in terms of actual food consumption. In this type of
obese patient, measurement of the basal energy expenditure (BEE), or the number
of calories expended at rest/24 hrs, generally confirms the presence of a
normometabolic state, often more than 1000 calories above what the individual is
reporting in food records. The caloric discrepancy information between the measured BEE and daily reported food intake can be used to counter any preconceived
ideas patients have in terms of a metabolic basis for their obesity. Once the metabolic facts are established, an experienced practitioner should be able to elicit
more details as to times of day or night when an individual tends to omit particular
eating episodes from food records. These patients are often relieved to acknowledge the presence of previously unreported eating bouts, and such an admission is
often the first step toward appropriate treatment.

   It might be an oversimplification to suggest that obese individuals who, when
self-reporting, fail to recall significant eating episodes are most likely to be binge
eaters. A more realistic view might propose that most overweight individuals both
underestimate the portions of the foods they do report, and occasionally omit certain eating episodes, resulting in extremely inaccurate records. Yet, over 40 years
ago, Stunkard et al[19] considered the likelihood that many morbidly obese individuals accurately report a daily mealtime intake of approximately 1200 calories, but
that this reporting fails to account for the thousands of calories they consume at
other times of the day or night. He suggested that such individuals were actually in
a caloric deficit for many hours a day, and that a few calorically dense overeating
bouts (binges) might account for their excessive obesity. Such behavior is consistent with that reported by many obese bingers who present to clinics with "perfectly accurate" food records. Aronoff et al[20] reported on one such patient who
experienced chronic weight gain, had a measured BEE of 2800 calories/24 hrs,
and consistently reported a daily food intake of between 1000 and 1200 calories.
In time, the patient admitted to completely omitting two or three highly caloric
night-eating binges from his food records. When his food record accuracy improved, he lost significant weight. Lichtman et al[18] described an interesting group
of overweight "diet-resistant" individuals who underestimated energy intake by
almost 50% (below predicted expenditure). Unfortunately, the authors did not re-

port whether the most prevalent problem was portion underestimation or complete food omission. The data was not analyzed in terms of binge and non-binge eaters. Of note are data from Yanovski and Sebring,[21] which indicate that obese bingers self-report food intake with much greater accuracy than obese non-bingers (95% vs 60% of predicted energy expenditure). Others have suggested that obese bingers who identify their problem as an eating disorder rather than a weight problem are more willing to offer accurate accounts of the content and frequency of their binges. Obese non-bingers who significantly underreport food intake represent a very challenging population: When do they consume the excess calories not accounted for by self-report? While underreporting of food intake generally results in a weight plateau or steady gain, the clinical characteristics and potential courses of treatment associated with specific reporting behaviors may be quite different.

Clinical Characteristics of Obese Binge Eaters

Multiple attempts to identify specific demographic, behavioral, psychological, and physiological traits that might distinguish between obese bingers, obese non-bingers, and other individuals who engage in binge eating behavior (i.e., purging bulimics) have been made over the past 15 years.[6-11,21-26] Such studies suggest that the presence of certain behaviors or characteristics, along a continuum, can be highly indicative of the frequency and severity with which binge eating occurs. A brief review of popular psychometric instruments used to identify and assess binge eating and its associated traits will be followed by a review of the literature that best demonstrates the existence of such relationships.

Eating Disorder Assessment Scales

Over the past 20 years, a number of psychometric instruments have been constructed and redesigned to identify and assess the presence of characteristics and behaviors associated with various types of human eating behavior. Though many were designed for use in patients with anorexia or bulimia nervosa, most have been adapted for identification and characterization of obese binge eaters.

While Hawkins and Clement[27] designed the original Binge Scale to identify this behavior in various populations, Gormally's Binge Eating Scale (BES)[6] was the first to specifically identify and assess the severity of binge eating in an obese population. The BES is a 16-item scale constructed to identify both behaviors and feelings associated with a binge episode. BES scores are frequently used to determine the relationship between binge severity and the degree to which various other characteristics and behaviors are expressed in obese binge eaters (i.e., weight, eating behaviors, depression). This scale has been well-validated and is most often used in conjunction with other instruments.

In 1981, Stunkard[28] designed the Eating Inventory (EI), a 58-item self-report questionnaire designed to assess an individual's tendency to restrict food intake. This questionnaire incorporated most of the items found in Herman and Mack's Restraint Scale,[29] and attempted to identify levels of cognitive restraint, disinhibition/emotional lability, and perceived hunger in eating-disordered and control individuals. In 1985, Stunkard and Messick[30] constructed the Three-Factor Eating Questionnaire (TFEQ) from two existing questionnaires that had separately sought to measure "restrained eating" and "latent obesity."[29,31] The TFEQ is a 51-item questionnaire that was also designed to assess the presence and degree of cognitive restraint, disinhibition, and hunger among groups of individuals who exhibited extreme eating behaviors. More recently, Cooper and Fairburn[32] designed the Eating Disorder Examination (EDE), a semi-structured clinical interview designed to assess a full range of psychopathologies and behaviors specific to eating disorders. The EDE focuses on restraint, overeating, shape concerns, weight concerns, eating concerns, and binge eating behavior during the four weeks prior to its administration.

The Beck Depression Inventory (BDI),[33] the Minnesota Multiphasic Personality Inventory (MMPI), and Derogatis's Brief Symptom Index[34] have recently been utilized to identify levels of depression and other relevant personality patterns and psychopathology in obese persons.[21,35,36] The BDI specifically identifies and assesses depressive symptomatology, while the MMPI assesses both personality characteristics and degree of emotional disturbance that might exist. Both have been used effectively in conjunction with Gormally's BES. The Derogatis Brief Symptom Index is a 53-item general measure of current psychopathology. See Chapter 17 for further discussion of emotional eating assessment and management.

Most recently, an original and a revised version of the Questionnaire on Eating and Weight Patterns (QEWP and QEWP-R)[10,21] were developed for use in the BED Diagnostic Criteria Multisite Field Trials. Both are self-administered questionnaires that combine general questions on demographic variables and clinical characteristics, with inquiries specifically related to the individual components, duration, and frequency requirements of BED.

Binge Eating and Age of Onset

A number of reports suggest that obese binge eaters have an earlier age of onset of obesity than those who do not binge. In 1981, Loro and Orleans[7] reported a highly significant positive association between binge eating and age of obesity onset. Male and female subjects with either childhood or adolescent onset of obesity reported more problems with severity and frequency of binge eating than those with adult-onset obesity. Marcus et al[35] recently reported either childhood or adolescent onset of obesity in the majority of females presenting for treatment of binge eating behavior. Using the QEWP, the BED multisite trials[10,11] identified 16 and 20 years as the average ages of onset of obesity in males and females with and without BED, respectively. While a clear relationship between age of onset of dieting and binge eating severity has not been established, recent reports have identified frequent weight loss bouts (with losses of 5 to 10 kg followed by subsequent regain) as indicative of binge eating severity.[10,35]

Binge Eating and Weight

Degree of obesity has been considered as a potential determinant of both binge eating prevalence and severity in obese bingers compared to non-bingers. In a sample of 432 women seeking obesity treatment, binge eating severity was significantly correlated with weight and percentage overweight.[9] Moderate and serious bingers (as determined by BES scores) weighed significantly more than obese subjects with little or no binge problem. Using self-report data, Telch et al[37] also found binge eating to be significantly more prevalent as body mass index (BMI) levels increased. In a multisite BED field trial, Spitzer et al[10] found that obese subjects seeking weight control treatment were an average of 16.4 lbs heavier than those without BED, at their maximum adult weight. Conversely, Wilson et al[26] found no significant differences in mean weight or percentage body fat in obese male and female bingers and non-bingers entering a weight control program. Based on BES results, Marcus et al[35] have also identified a strong family history of obesity (i.e., one or more obese parents) as suggestive of binge eating severity in a group of obese females.

Binge Eating and Psychopathology

Binge eating in both obese and normal-weight individuals has been associated with the presence of depression, personality or affective disorders, and other dysfunctional behavior.[1,7,24-26,36,38-40] In 1959, Stunkard[1] identified the presence of "expressions of self-condemnation" in association with the binge eating described by certain of his obese patients. In the early 1980s, Loro and Orleans[7] and others suggested an association between binge eating and negative mood states that might trigger and/or follow binge eating episodes. More recently, Lingswiler et al[38] reported that binge eaters, regardless of weight, experienced greater daily emotional reactivity, especially in association with binge eating episodes, than non-bingers. Kolotkin et al[36] have identified a significant relationship between binge severity (based on BES scores) and certain MMPI scores in obese women seeking weight control treatment. Their results suggest that binge severity increases with psychological disturbance. The most recent literature suggests the presence of more psychiatric symptomology and affective disorder in obese binge eaters than in their non-binging counterparts,[25,39,40] but less than in individuals with purging bulimia nervosa. Further research is needed to clarify any relationships between binge eating and a history of addictive behaviors (alcohol, gambling, drugs), sexual abuse, or obsessive-compulsive disorders in obese individuals with BED.[11,25,26,41]

Food Intake Behaviors of Obese Binge Eaters

Notable differences have been observed when comparing the presence and severity of certain dietary cognitions and food intake behaviors in obese bingers, obese non-bingers, and normal-weight people with purging bulimia.

Which Came First? Strict Dieting or Binge Eating?

Early reports supported the view that strict dieting, followed by feelings of deprivation and hunger, was responsible for the establishment of binge eating behavior.[6,7] Gormally[6] felt that self-imposed, excessively rigid dietary standards coupled with low expectations for diet compliancy, strongly contributed to the establishment of binge eating in the obese. While this sequence (dieting followed by binging) may reflect the etiology of binging in normal-weight bulimic individuals, it has not been supported for obese binge eaters. In a recent study, less than 9% of obese bingers entering a weight control program reported having been on a "strict diet" at the point when binge eating began, and 64% indicated that binge eating had preceded their obesity.[26] In the BED multisite field trials, 49% of obese individuals with BED indicated that their binging preceded any attempts to lose weight by dieting, while 37% percent reported the converse.[11]

Dietary Restraint

Dietary restraint, or the tendency of some individuals to restrict food intake to control body weight,[29,30,42] has long been proposed as an important factor in the etiology of binge eating. Yet, its specific role in either promoting or perpetuating binging remains unclear. Based on BES and EI scores, Marcus et al[9] reported a positive association between binge severity and measures of total dietary restraint, disinhibition, and perceived hunger in 432 obese women seeking weight control treatment. Cognitive restraint (a third EI subscale) was not, however, associated with binge eating severity. Most subsequent studies using the TFEQ have obtained similar results, with cognitive restraint scores that were either the same or lower and hunger and disinhibition scores that were higher, in obese bingers vs non-bingers.[21,23] Guss et al[43] reported higher TFEQ scores for both restraint and disinhibition in obese bingers vs non-bingers following a multi-item meal in a laboratory setting. The fact that women with bulimia nervosa generally score higher on all three TFEQ subscales than either obese bingers or non-bingers is perhaps indicative of a more severe disturbance of eating behavior than that observed in the obese.[44] Marcus et al[35] recently reported that obese bingers scored significantly lower on the EDE restraint subscale than normal-weight bulimic patients. Scores on the overeating, eating concern, shape concern, and weight concern subscales did not differ significantly.

It has been suggested that the lower cognitive restraint scores observed for obese bingers might reflect years of repeated dieting failures and a lack of belief that they will ever be able to comply with dietary standards deemed necessary for long-term weight loss. Yanovski and Sebring[21] suggest that disinhibition, or a loss of control following various types of stimuli, rather than restraint, is the major contributor to the disordered eating observed in obese bingers. They noted that three months post–very-low-calorie diet (VLCD), obese bingers reported significantly reduced levels of food intake and higher levels of cognitive restraint than before weight loss, although binge frequency was similar. These results again oppose the notion that short-term stringent dieting promotes or exacerbates obese binge eating. Guss et al[43] similarly implicated disinhibition by obese bingers, in response to very specific external food cues (i.e., multiple item meals) as an important feature that distinguishes them from their non-binging counterparts.

Food Intake

A significant obstacle in binge eating research has been a lack of consensus as to when an eating episode should be defined as a "binge." Beglin and Fairburn[45] recently suggested that the lay community places greater emphasis on feelings associated with binge behavior (i.e., loss of control), while the scientific community apparently seeks a quantitative definition, such as the actual amount of calories consumed, for the term "binge." The EDE has attempted to address this discrepancy by defining and identifying both objective and subjective binges.[32] Objective binges are defined as those associated with both consumption of a large amount of calories and feelings of loss of control, and subjective binges as those during which the subject reportedly feels out of control, yet does not exhibit excessive calorie intake. Unfortunately, these definitions may fail to address those individuals described as "episodic overeaters"[46] who consume objectively large amounts of food, yet fail to describe the loss of control generally associated with a binge. Such individuals may either be in denial of their eating disorder, or may not have experienced significant physical or psychological symptomology to recognize their eating behavior as out of control. Since binge eating behavior occurs on a continuum, these "non-bingers" may become bingers when they perceive their eating behavior as a threat to their quality of life. This revelation may or may not be associated with an increase in food intake. Both feelings associated with binge eating and general binge size were considered in the recently established BED criteria.[10,11,15]

Until recently, estimates of binge size in both normal-weight bulimic and obese individuals were limited by a preponderance of self-report data. Self-reports of food intake during binges by normal-weight bulimics have ranged from 45 to 55,000 calories, with average binge size ranging from 1400 to 4800 calories.[22]

Anecdotal reports of binge size by obese individuals have ranged from 1,000 to 20,000 calories.[1,7] Self-reported binge intake in a group of non-purging bulimics ranged from 25 to 6,048 calories, with an average binge size of 602 calories.[47] While Yanovski and Sebring[21] recently reported that obese women with BED consume more calories during both binge and non-binge eating situations than obese women without BED consume during binges, the accuracy of the self-report data in the non-BED group must be questioned. A comparison of self-reported food intake data with predicted energy expenditure (PEE), in obese women with and without BED before weight loss, revealed that those with BED reported food intake much more accurately (94% PEE) than those without BED (64% PEE).[21] This suggests that despite the wide range of binge intake data reported in the past, and the questionable reliability of self-reported intake data, certain obese patients may actually report food intake with surprisingly high accuracy.

Recent attempts to evaluate food intake in the laboratory have revealed considerable differences between obese subjects with and without BED, normal-weight bulimic subjects, and normal-weight controls.[43,48,49] These studies reported that obese subjects with BED consume significantly more calories than obese subjects without BED, when asked to binge on a multiple-item (buffet style) meal in a laboratory setting. Despite the use of identical foods and portions, Yanovski's obese bingers[48] consumed considerably more calories during their multiple-item binge meals than obese subjects in more recent laboratory studies.[43,49] This may be due to the higher mean BMI level of her subjects with BED (39.5 kg/m²) compared with those in the latter studies (32.5 and 33.4 kg/m²).[9,37] Interestingly, the latter studies[43,49] also reported that BED and non-BED obese subjects consumed similar amounts of a single-item (ice cream) binge meal. Guss et al[43] reported that ice cream intake in the BED and non-BED groups (762 kcal) was significantly less than that of normal-weight bulimics (1307 kcal) and significantly more than normal-weight controls (308 kcal). The differences in intake observed between obese bingers and non-bingers in the multiple- vs single-item meals again suggest the likely role of external factors such as types or amounts of food in triggering disordered eating behavior.

Binge eaters, regardless of weight, often report an increased eating rate during binge episodes.[47] Ninety-seven percent of a group of obese female binge eaters reported eating rapidly during binges.[39] Nonetheless, increased meal duration, rather than eating rate, appeared to account for the extra calories consumed by obese bingers (vs non-bingers) in two previously mentioned studies.[48,49] Guss et al[43] reported no difference in eating rate between normal-weight controls, obese bingers and non-bingers, and normal-weight bulimic individuals during a single-item (ice cream) meal. However, in a multiple-item meal, subjects with bulimia and obese subjects without BED ate at a faster rate by weight than the non-obese controls or the subjects with BED.

Prior to laboratory studies, data on specific food choices during binge episodes were also limited to self-report and anecdotal information. Marcus and Wing[22] found that obese bingers, like normal-weight bulimics, preferred high-calorie, easily ingested foods. Such foods were usually high in fat, sugar, and/or salt and representative of those that the subjects chose to exclude from their reducing diets (i.e., sweets, snack foods, pastries, cookies). While Goldfein et al[49] reported no difference in the macronutrient composition of food intake between obese bingers and non-bingers during a multiple-item binge meal in the laboratory, Yanovski et al[48] reported intake of a significantly greater percentage of calories from fat, and less from protein, in obese bingers under similar conditions. Using self-reported food intake data, Yanovski and Sebring[21] reported a greater percentage of calories from both fat and fiber (grams/100 kcal of food) in obese women with and without BED on binge vs non-binge days. In comparison, using dietary recall and food records, Rossiter et al[47] reported that non-purging bulimics consumed significantly more calories, less protein, and less fiber on binge days vs non-binge days.

BINGE EATING TREATMENT OF OBESE PERSONS: PAST, PRESENT, AND FUTURE

Much of the controversy surrounding the treatment of obese binge eaters has revolved around whether weight loss, or extinction of the binge eating behavior, should take priority. The past assumptions that either weight loss or behavioral programs alone could provide adequate treatment for this population have met with disappointing results. Ideally, treatment programs for obese bingers should incorporate a nutritionally sound weight loss plan with a behavioral component focused specifically on cognitions and actions associated with binge eating. As more controlled drug studies are reported, perhaps the specific effects of various types of antidepressants, appetite suppressants, and thermogenic agents on binge eating will be clarified. A review of past and present treatment modalities that focus on weight loss and/or binge behavior are discussed below and presented in Table 4–2.[25]

Behavioral Treatment

The origins of "standard" behavioral treatment were built on the premise that manipulation of one's environment (rather than examination of issues that lead to specific behaviors) should have the greatest impact on future behavioral changes.[50] Early techniques directed at control of eating behavior and weight often included self-monitoring of calories, stimulus control and food substitution, and exercise. A number of reports have pointed out the inadequacy of such a general behavioral approach in the treatment of binge eaters.[51,52] In 1976, Wilson[51] astutely pointed out that individuals who engage in binge eating often exhibit extremely

Table 4–2 Response of Obese Binge and Non-Binge Eaters to Weight Loss Treatment

Author	Treatment, Weeks (diet/program)	Type of Criteria	Pre-Rx Wt (kg)		Number (F/M)		Drop Outs During Program		Weight Loss kg (% total body weight)		Follow-up kg Regained (% of lost wt regained)		Number in Follow-up/ Number Started	
			BE	NBE	BE	NBE	BE	NBE	BE	NBE	BE	NBE	BE	NBE
Yanovski et al, 1993	VLCD + BT 12/26	BED;[1] BES[2]	114.3	104.5	21F	17F	2 (10%)	0 (0)	19.6 (18%)	21.3 (21%)	3 months[3] 3.7 (19%) / 12 months[3] 8.5 (42%)	3 months 2.5 (13%) / 12 months 10.4 (51%)	3 months 20/21 / 12 months 16/21	3 months 17/17 / 12 months 17/17
LaPorte, 1992	VLCD + BT 10/10	BES	108.1	109.0	19F 6M	15F 9M	5F 3M (32%)	1F 3M (17%)	18.7 (17%)	20.2 (19%)	N/A	N/A	N/A	N/A
Wadden et al, 1992	VLCD + BT 12/26	Binge eaters (BE) episodic overeaters (EO)[4]	BE: 97.8 EO: 99.0	101.6	BE: 29F EO: 26F	180F	BE: 14 (47%) EO[5] 15 (58%)	68 (37%)	BE: 21.5 (22%) EO: 19.4 (20%)	21.7 (21%)	Not reported[6]	Not reported	12 months 7/29 BE 6/26 EO	12 months 73/180
de Zwaan et al, 1992	CBT vs DM ± fluvoxamine[7]	Self-report + clinical interview[8]	35.8[9] kg/m2	36.7 kg/m2	22F	44F	7 (32%)	9 (21%)	6.1	5.6	12 months 4.6 kg (76%)	12 months 1.6 kg (28%)	N/A	N/A
Marcus et al, 1990[10]	BT ± fluoxetine 52/52	DSM-III[11]	110.1	94.8	20F 2M	22F 2M	13 (59%)	11 (48%)	Fluox: 3.9 (4%) Placebo +0.25 kg (0%)	Fluox: 11.5 (12%) Placebo +0.27 (0%)	3–6 months Fluox[12] +6.6 (>100%) Placebo +0.73 (>100%)	3–6 months Fluox[12] +4.4 (38%) Placebo –1.4 (>100% addnl loss)	3–6 months 7/22	3–6 months 8/23

continues

Table 4–2 continued

Author	Treatment, Weeks (diet/program)	Type of Criteria	Pre-Rx Wt (kg)		Number (F/M)		Drop Outs During Program		Weight Loss kg (% total body weight)		Follow-up kg Regained (% of lost wt regained)		Number in Follow-up/ Number Started	
			BE	NBE	BE	NBE	BE	NBE	BE	NBE	BE	NBE	BE	NBE
Marcus et al, 1988	BT[13] 10/10	DSM-III	84.2	81.2	35F	33F	9[14] (26%)	3 (9%)	4.7 (5%)	5.2 (6%)	6 months 2.8 kg (60%)[15] 12 months 3 kg (65%)	6 months 0.5 kg (10%) 12 months 2.6 kg (50%)	6 month 26/35 12 month 26/35	6 month 30/33; 12 month 30/33
Keefe et al, 1984[16]	BT 9/9	DSM-III	94.4	86	23 ?M/F	21 ?M/F	16		1.9[17] (2%)	4.4 (5%)	6 months −1.1 kg (60% addnl loss)	6 months −1.1 kg (30% addnl loss)	N/A	N/A

Note: BE = binge eater, NBE = non-binge eater, VLCD = very-low-calorie diet, BT = behavioral therapy, CBT = cognitive behavioral therapy, DM = dietary management. [1]BED = preliminary DSM-IV criteria for binge eating disorder as assessed by the QEWP. [2]BES = binge eating scale (26). [3]Regain calculated for the 16/21 BED (+) subjects completing all follow-up visits. [4]BE defined by DSM-III-R criteria for bulimia nervosa with omission of purging, episodic overeaters defined by frequent episodes of overeating without subjective loss of control. [5]EO were significantly more likely to drop out of treatment following refeeding than BE and NBE, p < 0.003. [6]Overall weight regain was 8.8 kg at one year; however, separate figures were not reported for BE, EO, and NBE. [7]This was a double-blind placebo controlled study evaluating effectiveness of cognitive behavioral therapy (CBT) vs standard dietary management without behavior therapy (DM) and fluvoxamine vs placebo. No differences in weight loss outcome measures were found as a function of treatment type. [8]Self-report of moderate to severe binge eating on questionnaire +/– criteria for bulimia nervosa without fulfilling purging or frequency criteria. [9]Weight in kg not reported. BMI given. [10]Some of these data are previously unpublished. [11]DSM-III criteria for bulimia do not require compensatory purging. [12]Refers to group that was on active drug during the study. All medications were stopped at study endpoint. [13]BT was modified or standard. No differences of outcome measured were seen as a result of treatment type (modified vs standard therapy). [14]Binge eaters vs non-binge eaters, p < 0.07. [15]Binge eaters vs non-binge eaters, p = 0.02. [16]Study was retrospective. Only completers interviewed, therefore drop-out and follow-up rate cannot be calculated. [17]p < 0.05, binge eaters vs non-binge eaters.

Source: Reprinted with permission from S.J. Yanovski, Binge Eating Disorder: Current Knowledge and Future Directions, *Obesity Research*, Vol. 1, No. 4, p. 314, © 1993.

controlled and appropriate eating behavior during non-binge periods. Subsequently, Loro and Orleans[7] described the need for a highly individualized behavioral approach to treating obese bingers, whereby specific triggers and consequences of binge eating episodes must be considered (Table 4–3). Keefe et al[8] reported that obese bingers experienced less weight loss following nine weeks of "standard" behavioral treatment, and at six-month follow-up, than obese non-bingers. More recently, Marcus et al[39] compared the weight loss results of obese female bingers and non-bingers randomly assigned to either standard or modified behavioral weight control programs. Standard treatment emphasized self-monitoring of food intake, stimulus control techniques, self-reinforcement, and goal setting. The modified program also included binge-oriented behavioral strategies such as a structured meal plan, the use of exercise as a binge alternative, and cognitive training to counteract negative thoughts about dieting and binge eating. Unfortunately, binge eaters in both groups had a significantly higher drop-out rate, and regained their weight significantly more quickly than non-bingers. Thus, to date, the use of standard or modified behavioral treatment alone has had limited clinical utility in the treatment of obese binge eaters.

Weight Loss Treatment

Early findings by Gormally et al[52] suggested a relationship between obese bingers who weight cycled, and poor long-term weight control. They later proposed that obese bingers might require calorically liberal weight loss programs, which would promote a greater likelihood of compliancy than very-low-calorie diets (VLCDs).[6] However, since subsequent data has failed to confirm that dietary restriction exacerbates binge behavior in obese bingers,[21,26] studies on weight loss in obese bingers typically employ the use of VLCDs, usually in combination with some type of behavioral therapy.[46,53] LaPorte[53] reported no significant differences in weight loss, dietary adherence, or drop-out rate between obese bingers and non-bingers enrolled in a 10-week VLCD program, but did note a trend toward a higher drop-out rate among bingers. No follow-up data were reported for this group. Wadden et al[46] described similar results for three groups of obese women (bingers, episodic overeaters, and non-bingers) participating in a 26-week VLCD program. There were no significant differences in weight loss either during the program or at one-year follow-up. Interestingly, episodic overeaters (who report binge eating without loss of control) were significantly more likely to drop out of treatment during the last six weeks of the study than subjects in either of the other groups. Yanovski et al[21] also compared the responses of obese bingers and non-bingers enrolled in a 12-week, 800 calorie per day weight loss program. They found no difference in mean weight loss at the end of treatment, but reported that bingers lost significantly less weight at a particular point in treatment than the

Table 4–3 Antecedents and Consequences of Binge Eating with Suggested Behavioral Treatment Approaches

Results of Functional Analysis—Antecedents	Suggested Treatment Approaches—Antecedent Control
Anxiety related to external stress and deficient coping skills	Anxiety management (Suinn, 1977); Progressive muscle relaxation (Goldfried & Davidson, 1976)
Recurrent interpersonal conflicts related to deficient assertion and interpersonal problem-solving skills	Assertion and interpersonal problem-solving training (Bower & Bower, 1976); Operant treatment for marital discord (Weiss, Hops, & Patterson, 1973)
Irrational thinking, cognitive distortions, and self-critical thinking leading to negative feeling states	Rational emotive therapy (Ellis, 1962); Cognitive therapy (Beck, 1976); Cognitive ecology (Mahoney & Mahoney, 1976)
Obsessions and preoccupations with thoughts about food	Delay therapy (Meyer, 1973); Thought stopping (Cautela, 1969)
Frustration and disappointment from unrealistic weight loss goals and expectations	Realistic goal setting (Jeffrey & Katz, 1977; Stuart & Davis, 1972)
Boredom resulting from unstructured time	Exercise and activity counseling to structure free time (Meyer & Henderson, 1974; Stuart, 1978)
High access to privacy and preferred binging settings	Restrict privacy and access to preferred settings
Hunger related to overly strict dieting and exhaustion from strenuous exercise	Eliminate strict diets and extreme approaches to exercise by shaping adaptive and sensible eating and activity habits (Jeffrey & Katz, 1977; Mahoney & Mahoney, 1976; Stuart & Davis, 1972)
Consequences	*Consequence Control*
Positive thoughts and feelings related to anticipating and ingesting preferred foods	Aversive conditioning (Morganstern, 1973; Wijesinghe, 1973); Cognitive therapy (Beck, 1976)
Low immediate response costs of binge eating	Raise immediate response costs of gaining access to preferred foods through environmental control (Stuart & Davis) and contingency contracting (Mann, 1972; Reznick & Balch, 1977)

continues

Table 4–3 continued

Results of Functional Analysis— Consequences	Suggested Treatment Approaches— Consequence Control
Delayed negative psychological consequences of binge eating	Replace self-critical and self-punishing statements with positive problem-solving statements (Jeffrey & Katz, 1977; Mahoney & Mahoney, 1976); Reframe binging behavior as a useful learning experience (Watzlawick & Weakland, & Fisch, 1974)
Relief from stress, anxiety, hunger, and boredom	See Antecedent Control section
Positive (even inadvertent) social reinforcement and attention	Reprogram social and family environment using contingency contracting and spouse involvement (Jeffrey & Katz, 1977; Mann, 1972; Saccone & Israel, 1978)
Rebellion against weight reduction regimen, diet, or external authority	Counter-control strategies (Davison) including paradoxical injunctions (Watzlawick, Beavin, & Jackson, 1967), paradoxical intentions (Ascher & Efran, 1978; Frankl, 1975), behavioral prescriptions and directives (Haley, 1976), and reframing (Watzlawick & Weakland, & Fisch, 1974)

Source: Reprinted from A.D. Loro and C.S. Orleans, Binge Eating in Obesity: Preliminary Findings and Guidelines for Behavioral Analysis and Treatment, Copyright 1981, Pages No. 155–166, with kind permission from Elsevier Science Ltd, The Boulevard, Langford Lane, Kidlington OX5 1GB, UK.

non-bingers. They also noted that dietary lapses reported by bingers during the VLCD and the refeeding period were significantly larger than those reported by non-bingers. But, because bingers were far more accurate in reporting food intake than non-bingers in this study, the validity of this finding is not clear. While mean weight regain was similar at 12 months post-treatment, 25% of obese bingers had apparently regained more than half of their lost weight by the third post-treatment month. At one-year post-treatment, 25% to 35% of the bingers either refused or were lost to follow-up. All non-bingers remained available and compliant in terms of follow-up. In summary, these studies suggest that obese bingers may be more prone to (1) drop out of treatment prematurely, (2) refuse long-term follow-up, and (3) regain lost weight more rapidly than non-bingers. Nonetheless, the nonsignificant differences in weight change between groups in most of these short-term studies suggest that both obese bingers and non-bingers regularly engage in eating behaviors that promote chronic caloric excess. As suggested earlier, obese bingers appear better able to confront certain aspects of their obesity-sustaining behavior than non-bingers, "diet-resistant" individuals, or episodic overeaters. The latter groups often deny or grossly underestimate average caloric intake, complain of a chronic inability to lose weight, and/or deny abnormalities in their eating behavior.[18,21,46] These differences should be considered when discussing treatment options.

Cognitive Behavioral Therapy

Cognitive-behavioral therapy (CBT) is a form of treatment that seeks to extinguish deviant or harmful behavior by addressing its underlying psychopathology. In the recent past CBT has been effective in eliminating the binge/purge cycle typically seen in bulimia nervosa,[54] and has since been adapted for use with non-purging obese bingers.[55,56] The focus of CBT in this population is elimination of binge eating behavior, and not weight loss. Thus, success is measured in terms of a reduction in thoughts and actions associated with binge episodes. Since weight loss is not an absolute response to this type of treatment, CBT alone would be inappropriate for individuals requiring emergent weight loss for medical reasons. For obese bingers, CBT often combines techniques of standard behavioral treatment with techniques that focus on identifying and altering dysfunctional cognitions, attitudes, and beliefs, which may trigger and perpetuate binging behavior. Based on self-report data, Telch et al[55] reported a reduction in frequency of binge episodes in a group of obese subjects shortly after completion of CBT. Recently, Smith et al[56] described a significant reduction in the number of binge days reported by obese bingers from pre- to post-treatment with CBT. In this study, the EDE, administered to subjects pre- and post-treatment, confirmed that reduced binging was accompanied by a marked reduction in psychopathology. Depression, assessed by the BDI, also decreased following CBT. Mean weight loss during this 18-week period was minimal, but tended to occur in individuals with the most significant reductions in binge behavior. While reduced binge frequency defines successful CBT, it is still surprising that significant weight loss is not routinely observed. Future studies should consider the type of caloric compensation that occurs following CBT such that obese bingers often exhibit minimal weight loss.

Pharmacotherapy

Pharmacotherapy specific for binge eating behavior has considered the use of agents that alter mood and/or neuroendocrine factors involved in appetite regulation (i.e., neurotransmitters, neuropeptides, and hormones). Certain antidepressants and opiate antagonists have shown promising results in reducing binge frequency in normal-weight bulimic individuals[57,58] and offer potential use for obese bingers. Weight loss, an unanticipated side effect of a certain class of antidepressants (serotonin reuptake inhibitors) has made their use particularly promising for obese binge eaters. Marcus et al[59] compared weight loss results in obese female binge and non-binge eaters who received either fluoxetine (a bicyclic antidepressant) plus behavior modification (BM) or placebo plus BM, over a 52-week period. Regardless of prior binge behavior, patients treated with fluoxetine plus BM lost significantly more weight than those treated with placebo plus BM. While weight loss didn't differ significantly within the drug treatment group, a trend for bingers to have lost less weight than non-bingers by study week 52 (3.9 vs 11.5 kg) was observed. Thus, the utility of fluoxetine in future obesity treatment does not appear to be specific to reducing binge behavior. In an eight-week placebo controlled double-blind study, Alger et al[60] compared the effects of placebo, naltrexone (an opiate antagonist), and imipramine (a tricyclic antidepressant) on binge eating behavior in both normal-weight females with bulimia and obese females who binged. Interestingly, they noted a significant reduction in binge duration among normal-weight bulimic women treated with naltrexone and obese women who binge treated with imipramine. They also reported a reduction in binge frequency for obese bingers in both drug groups, but this drop did not differ significantly from that observed in the obese placebo group. The authors made the point that no dietary intervention was provided to any of the study groups, yet it is still surprising that despite reported reductions in both binge duration and frequency in the obese women, no body weight change was observed. This again suggests either inaccurate reporting by the subjects, or compensatory caloric consumption that maintained body weight. De Zwaan et al[24] compared weight loss response to several interventions: (1) CBT plus fluvoxamine, (2) CBT plus placebo, (3) dietary management (DM) plus fluvoxamine, and (4) DM plus placebo, in emotionally disturbed obese female bingers and non-bingers recruited from an outpatient psychiatry clinic. No difference was reported in amount of weight lost between binge and non-binge eaters either at the end of the study, or at one-year follow-up. However, binge eaters regained three times more weight than non-bingers (4.6 vs 1.5 kg) during the first post-treatment year. Thus, this study provided no evidence that weight loss was influenced by treatment condition or prior binge status in obese female bingers and non-bingers with prior histories of "emotional problems." Pondimin (an anorectic agent) and Ionamin (a sympathomimetic amine) are common drug combinations used in the treatment of general obesity. Thorough evaluation of this combination should provide insight into future drug management of binge eating among obese persons.

NIGHT-EATING AND OBESITY: HISTORY, DEFINITION, DIAGNOSTIC CRITERIA, AND PREVALENCE

Anecdotal reports of a "tendency for obese individuals to consume the majority of their food from late in the evening into the early hours of the morning" are found in some of the earliest obesity treatment literature.[61–64] However, it wasn't until 1955 that Stunkard et al[19] attempted to fully characterize a pattern of "night-eating" among the obese in terms of criteria, etiology, and obesity-related implications. Stunkard encountered repeated reports of this particular eating pattern from a group of morbidly obese females seeking weight control treatment in an obesity clinic, and went on to establish criteria specific to this condition. The criteria included (1) nocturnal hyperphagia, or consumption of at least 25% of total daily calories during the period following the evening meal; (2) insomnia or sleeplessness three or more times per week; and (3) morning anorexia, defined as negligible (i.e., juice or coffee) or no intake at the traditional breakfast time.[19] Not surprisingly, Stunkard's subjects lost significant weight as hospital inpatients, when nighttime food intake was involuntarily restricted, but quickly regained weight after discharge, when night-eating behavior resumed.

While Stunkard proposed both physiological (e.g., insulin-induced) and psychological etiologies for this eating pattern,[19] the past 40 years have failed to provide data to either support or refute such possibilities. In a subsequent paper, Stunkard[1] described both similarities and differences that he observed between obese binge eaters and night-eaters requiring weight control treatment (Table 4–1). Similarities included manifestation of both binge eating and night-eating during periods of life stress, and a decline in both behaviors with alleviation of stress. He noted that the onset of binge eating usually occurred in response to a specific and highly personal precipitating event (e.g., unresolved anger at a spouse), and that intense physical discomfort and self-condemnation typically followed eating binges. On the other hand, he described night-eating as more time dependent, or periodic, than binge eating, less related to a specific identifiable trigger, and rarely associated with the self-reprisal and guilt reported following binge eating. (In clinical practice, the actual distinction between obese bingers and night-eaters may not be as clear. Personal interviews by this author found many obese night-eaters who express great confusion, distress, and hopelessness over their inability to maintain the dietary self-control, which they exhibit during the day, after nightfall.)

The most recent definition of the nocturnal eating (drinking) syndrome published by the American Sleep Disorders Association (ASDA)[65] describes a condition characterized by recurrent awakenings during the sleep period and an inability to return to sleep without eating or drinking. Accordingly, the minimal diagnostic criteria for this syndrome include (1) frequent and recurrent awakenings to eat or drink and (2) normal sleep onset following the ingestion of the desired food or drink (Exhibit 4–4).[65(p103)] With limited regard for Stunkard's early

Exhibit 4–4 Diagnostic Criteria for Nocturnal Eating (Drinking) Syndrome (780.52–8)

A. A complaint of difficulty maintaining sleep.*
B. Frequent and recurrent awakenings to eat or drink.*
C. Sleep onset is normal following ingestion of the desired food or drink.*
D. Polysomnographic monitoring demonstrates an increase in the number or duration of awakenings.*
E. No evidence of psychiatric or medical disorder to account for the complaint (e.g., hypoglycemia, bulimia).
F. Absence of any other sleep disorder producing difficulty maintaining sleep.

Note: If the disorder is predominantly one of eating at night, then state and code the disorder as nocturnal eating syndrome; if predominantly one of drinking at night, nocturnal drinking syndrome.
*Polysomnographic feature: normal major sleep period except for increased number of awakenings.
Courtesy of the American Sleep Disorders Association, 1990, Rochester, Minnesota.

---

work[1,19] the ASDA further describes this eating pattern as typically occurring in infants and children, and as relatively rare in adults. Without proposing a specific etiology for this behavior, they do suggest that once learned, the awakenings to eat may continue even when the underlying cause is treated. In light of more recent literature on adult night-eating and sleep-eating, modification of the nosology of the nocturnal eating (drinking) syndrome is presently being considered.[66]

Prevalence

Not surprisingly, Stunkard[1] provided the earliest prevalence data on night-eating in obese adults. Of 40 adults in a special study clinic for severe obesity during a six-year period, incidence of the night-eating syndrome was approximately 65%. Incidence of night-eating dropped to 12% in a study based on questionnaire responses of 100 randomly selected obese patients in the general nutrition clinic of the same hospital. Night-eating was not reported at all (0% incidence) in a group of 38 normal-weight control subjects. Although these early data were derived from a biased sample of "diet-resistant" morbidly obese individuals referred to a special clinic, the presence of an eating behavior that is potentially weight dependent is indicated, and perhaps more commonly observed in a subset of extremely obese individuals. Since then, the ASDA has suggested that an estimated 5% of the population aged six months to three years may suffer from the nocturnal eating (drinking) syndrome, with a marked reduction noted after weaning.[65] They were, however, unable to provide any prevalence data with regard to adults. Recently,

Aronoff et al[67] have reported an incidence of the night-eating syndrome and/or the nocturnal eating (drinking) syndrome of 49% in 110 obese individuals seeking treatment for either weight control or sleep disturbances. This prevalence data is strikingly different from that recently reported by others. Spaggiari et al,[68] for example, reported that obese night-eaters represented less than 5% of outpatients referred to their sleep disorders center over an 18-month period. Winkelman et al[69] described an incidence of less than 1% in a group of 133 obese subjects presenting to an eating disorders clinic for weight control treatment. Schenck et al[70] similarly reported sleep-related eating (different from night-eating in that subjects are asleep during eating episodes) in only 0.5% of all adult referrals to their sleep disorders clinic over a five-year period.

These prevalence differences become clearer when one considers, as Stunkard[1] did, the populations from which these samples were derived. In the study by Aronoff et al,[67] most of the subjects were affiliated with the hospital obesity research center and tended to have extremely high body weights. The prevalence data from both Spaggiari et al[68] and Schenck et al[70,71] were derived from individuals of all body weights seeking treatment for a variety of sleep-related conditions. The mean body mass index (BMI) in their samples of adult night-eaters and sleep-eaters was significantly lower than that reported by Aronoff et al (28 and 27 vs 55). Winkelman's data,[69] derived from subjects seeking treatment for various eating disorders, included normal-weight, severely underweight, and overweight individuals. While BMI data were not provided, the mean BMI of their sample was most likely also significantly lower than that of the obese night-eaters previously or recently described.[1,19,67]

More than 90% of Stunkard's original sample of obese night-eaters were female,[1,19] whereas 76% of those described by Aronoff et al[67] were male. This difference may be due in part to the fact that 40 years ago men were less likely to seek treatment for weight control than women. If we consider the likelihood that males still wait until they are at higher weights and are often sicker than females before seeking treatment, and that night-eating may be positively correlated with weight,[67] it is not surprising that in an extremely obese population, males would represent a larger proportion of night-eaters. While 60% of the adult night-eaters described by Spaggiari et al[68] were male, their sample size was quite small (n = 10). Sixty-six percent of Schenck's sample of overweight sleep-eaters were female,[70,71] again suggesting that in women (more than men), a 10 to 15 kg weight gain might be a major impetus for seeking treatment.

MEDICAL CONDITIONS ASSOCIATED WITH NIGHT-EATING

Obstructive sleep apnea (OSA), characterized by impeded airflow and respiratory pauses during sleep, and Pickwickian syndrome (PS), characterized by hypoventilation, arterial oxygen desaturation, and carbon dioxide retention, are serious medical conditions that have been associated with obesity.[72-74] While a clear link between onset of these conditions and establishment of a night-eating pattern has not been reported, all appear to manifest at or above individual threshold weights,[75] and to be associated with disrupted sleep patterns. Skillful interviewing and appropriate testing can help ascertain whether an obese night-eater has acquired this eating pattern as a result of physiological sleep disruption, or, whether pre-existing night-eating behavior, resulting in weight gain, has contributed to the onset of OSA and/or PS, and further sleep fragmentation. While resolution of OSA and PS have been observed with even moderate weight loss, it is unclear whether concurrent night-eating also diminishes and contributes to further weight loss. Nocturia, often reported by obese individuals on large doses of diuretics, or with poorly controlled diabetes, has also been considered as a potential cause of nighttime awakening, which can result in night-eating. However, in a recent case study, neither OSA nor nocturia could account for the awakening and subsequent eating episodes exhibited by an obese night-eater in a laboratory setting.[20] Thus, to date, data to substantiate a physiological basis for night-eating are not available. High levels of hunger and disinhibition, like those observed in obese bingers on VLCDs, remain as the most likely contributors to night-eating behavior. See Figure 4–1.

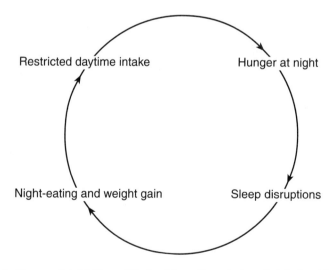

Figure 4–1 Hunger, disinhibition of dieting (sleep disruption), and nighttime binge eating. *Source:* Reprinted with permission from N.J. Aronoff et al., The Relationship Between Daytime and Nighttime Food Intake in an Obese Night-Eater, *Obesity Research,* Vol. 2, No. 2, p. 150, © 1994.

CLINICAL CHARACTERISTICS OF OBESE NIGHT-EATERS

Current literature has identified a number of distinct groups of individuals with sleep-related eating disorders (SREDs). Along with obese night-eaters, overweight night-eaters, normal-weight and overweight sleep-eaters, and normal-weight bulimic night-bingers have been described.[1,19,20,65,67–71,75–80] For the purpose of this section, characteristics of obese night-eaters and sleep-eaters will be compared.

Sleep-eaters of the type described by Schenck et al[70,71] generally report moderate, but distressing, weight gain in response to eating that occurs secondary to a primary sleep disorder. They also tend to report unremarkable weight histories prior to the onset of sleep-eating, and often unsuccessfully attempt to restrict daytime food intake to compensate for the unknown calories consumed during various sleep states. Treatment of the underlying sleep disorder in this group frequently results in the disappearance of the sleep-eating behavior and a return to usual weight. Conversely, obese night-eaters, like binge eaters, tend to report early onset of obesity (i.e., in childhood or adolescence) and multiple failed attempts at weight loss. They also frequently report large "stress-induced" weight gains, and subsequent exacerbation of both medical and sleep conditions, which drive them to seek treatment. The nocturnal hyperphagia typical of this eating pattern can occur throughout the period between dinner and bedtime, and/or during one or more nightly awakenings. In either case, excessive amounts of calories are consumed during night-eating episodes. While age of onset of night-eating is quite variable, anecdotal patient reports have linked the establishment of this eating pattern to specific traumatic childhood events. One overweight patient, for example, recalled that as a child she was awakened to go to the bathroom two to three hours after being put to sleep so she would not wet her bed. When bedwetting was no longer a problem, she would still awaken two to three hours after going to bed and go to the kitchen for a high-calorie snack. Another obese patient was reportedly fed excessive amounts of food late at night in an attempt by his mother to keep him awake until her abusive husband, whom she feared, returned home from working the late shift at his job. Subsequently, this individual also found it quite difficult to break a destructive sleep/meal pattern established in early childhood. Unlike sleep-eaters who usually learn of their behavior from family members, or from the mess in the kitchen on mornings following a sleep-eating bout, night-eaters report being awake. Limited polysomnographic data have confirmed this to be true.[20]

Calorie/Food Intake of Obese Night-Eaters

Since obese night-eaters, unlike sleep-eaters, are awake during their nighttime eating episodes, it might follow that they are more aware of their nocturnal food consumption. Unfortunately, an unwillingness to self-report this secretive behavior (usually related to humiliation about the quantities and types of food they consume), compounded by a lack of awareness by health professionals that such an eating pattern exists, has resulted in a paucity of food intake data for this group.

While the Stunkard criteria[19] suggest an intake of at least 25% of total daily calories after the evening meal as indicative of night-eating, it seems likely that consumption of more than 40% might be more accurate. An unpublished analysis of the weekly food records of an obese night-eater revealed an average intake of approximately 1500 calories from lunch and dinner meals combined, with approximately 30% of calories from fat. A separate analysis of food consumed from approximately 7 PM to 11 PM revealed an average consumption of another 1700 calories (53% of total daily intake), 50% of which were from fat. The high-fat sweets and salty snacks reportedly consumed after dinner are similar to those reportedly consumed by obese and bulimic individuals during binge episodes.[22,48] Not surprisingly, when this patient modified (i.e., to low-fat choices), reduced, or eliminated her PM snacks, weight loss followed.

In an attempt to determine the relationship between daytime and nighttime food intake in this population, Aronoff et al[20] manipulated daytime intake and monitored nighttime intake of an obese night-eater (D.L.) in a laboratory setting. From self-report data, D.L. reported an average daytime intake at lunch and dinner of approximately 1286 kcal, and a nighttime intake of 1036 kcal (45% of total daily calories), mostly from sandwiches containing cheese, cold cuts, and mayonnaise. In the laboratory, when D.L. was provided with a daytime intake of 600 kcal, nighttime intake increased to 3004 kcal (83% of total daily calories). When daytime intake was increased to 1800 kcal, nighttime intake decreased to 2350 kcal (57% of total daily calories). Thus, while caloric compensation was not perfect, laboratory data revealed a negative correlation between daytime and nighttime food intake.

METABOLIC CONSEQUENCES OF NIGHT-EATING (THE OBESITY PERPETUATION THEORY)

While night binging has been reported in both underweight individuals with anorexia nervosa and normal-weight individuals with and without bulimia,[77–80] negative metabolic consequences potentially associated with this eating pattern may be related to situations of excess energy storage. Unfortunately, few recent studies have directly addressed the impact of mealtime and frequency on metabolism and body weight in overweight humans.[20,81–86] In terms of an animal model, obese night-eaters tend to alter their food intake in a fashion highly analogous to that observed in genetically obese Zucker rats (*fa/fa*). For example, both tend to consume the majority of excess energy at a time of day when their leaner counterparts are either asleep (i.e., light phase for rats and dark phase for humans) or consuming very limited amounts of food. Both groups also tend to exhibit a reduction in meal frequency, an increase in meal size, and longer between-meal intervals than their lean counterparts.[87] An early animal study addressed the effect of reduced meal frequency on body composition. Cohn and Joseph[88] found that animals who received forced bolus feedings one or two times per day weighed the same, but were significantly fatter than controls fed an equal amount of calories ad libitum throughout the day. Sensi and Capani[84] reported no difference in weight loss between two groups of obese patients receiving either one morning or one evening hypocaloric (684 kcal) meal/day. Bellisle et al[85] have described an inverse relationship between meal distribution and body weight in humans. Others have described the impact of meal time, meal size, meal frequency, and behavior modification in promoting effective weight loss.[83,86]

The lipogenic-lipolytic cycle of fuel storage and utilization described for both rats[89] and humans[90] would suggest that excessive energy intake at a time of day when energy expenditure is generally less than intake (i.e., daytime for rats and nighttime for humans) might disrupt the cycle in such a way that both obesity and fatness are perpetuated. Thus, meal times, meal frequency, and meal size (or energy content) all appear to have metabolic implications in terms of successful treatment of obesity.

STRATEGIES FOR MANAGING BINGE NIGHT-EATING OF OBESE PATIENTS

Behavioral and Dietary Treatment

Just as food intake data are limited, so are reports of behavioral or dietary treatment of night-eating. Coates[76] reported the need to totally eliminate access to food at night (i.e., locking refrigerators, pantries, etc.) as the only successful means of alleviating night-eating in an adult male patient. In 1989, Williamson et al[79] used a contingency management program to treat nocturnal binge eating and rumination in a female with bulimia nervosa. The subject of this report was rewarded with controlled access to her beloved jewelry collection (which she had turned over to her therapist at treatment onset) following nights when she refrained from nighttime binge eating and rumination. At the same time, this patient was enrolled in a cognitive behavioral group for bulimia. While nighttime binge eating and rumination resolved over time, it is not clear which treatment contributed most to this patient's recovery. Aronoff et al[20] reported the use of behavior modification related to both dietary and sleep habits in successful treatment of an obese male night-eater (D.L.). In an attempt to reduce daily calorie consumption and improve both quality and duration of his sleep, D.L. was encouraged to eat three balanced 500 kcal meals/day, to consume only fat-free snacks after dinner, to avoid caffeinated beverages after lunchtime, and to avoid unplanned naps throughout the day. While D.L. still reports occasional nighttime awakenings, especially in times of stress, he has lost more than 40 kg since he confronted and sought treatment for his night-eating. Less successful long-term results are reported for a female night-eater who self-reported an average post-dinner intake of 1700 kcal, of which at least 50% of kcal were from fat. Despite significant weight loss during a period of a few weeks when she replaced nighttime snacks of ice cream, nuts, potato chips, candy bars, and pastries with cold cereal, popsicles, licorice, and gummy candy, a return to high-fat choices has prevented further weight loss. Insufficient funds to continue weekly psychotherapy sessions probably contributed to this patient's difficulty adhering to nighttime dietary recommendations.

Treatment of Sleep Disorders and Medical Conditions Associated with Night-Eating

Night-eating was previously suggested to be an indirect cause or an unforeseen effect of certain obesity-induced sleep disorders (i.e., OSA, PS). If so, the beneficial effect of identification and treatment of one nighttime condition on another must be considered. For example, Eveloff and Millman[75] reported on a male patient with obesity and OSA, both secondary to sleep-related eating. Subsequent incarceration in prison, with involuntary nighttime food restriction, led to weight loss and significant clinical improvement of OSA. Unfortunately, release from prison resulted in a return to night-eating, weight gain, and recurrence of OSA symptomology. There are little or no data to support the contention that successful treatment of a sleep-related respiratory disturbance in a documented night-eater would result in extinction of the night-eating behavior. Yet, it would make sense that improved sleep consolidation and quality would result in less nighttime awakenings during which one could exhibit nocturnal eating.

While weight loss remains the primary recommendation for treatment of both OSA and PS, it is generally the most difficult to achieve. The nightly use of nasal continuous or "as needed" positive airway pressure devices (CPAP or Bi-PAP) have been effective in the treatment of both OSA and PS. Patients often report experiencing both "a good night's sleep" and "dreaming" for the first time in many years, following the proper implementation of either device. Decreased daytime hypersomnolence, hypertension, and improved cardiovascular, psychological, and cognitive functioning have been reported with long-term use.[74] The latter two improvements can often enhance cooperation with concurrent weight control treatment. Other treatments for sleep apnea including tongue-retaining devices (TRDs) and uvulopalato- or nasal reconstructive surgery (to improve nasal or upper airway airflow) have met mixed success.

For obese night-eaters who report nocturnal awakenings to urinate (nocturia), and a consequent need to eat or drink in order to resume sleep, a number of treatment strategies can be tried. If the nocturia is also associated with daytime poly-uria, polydipsia, or other signs of diabetes mellitus, this condition should be ruled out or treated. Nocturia is also prevalent in ambulatory obese individuals who opt to take prescribed diuretics (for edema, congestive heart failure, etc.) in one large nighttime dose when they are home, rather than over the course of a day, when access to a suitable bathroom may be limited. This behavior can result in multiple nightly awakenings to urinate, and subsequent eating bouts. The value of an unin-terrupted night's sleep must be discussed with these patients and strategies planned for taking daytime diuretic medications as well as for urination in the morning and afternoon. Fluid restriction, especially late in the evening, should also be considered in this population.

Pharmacotherapy

Schenck et al[70,71] have described highly successful pharmacological treatment of the sleep-related eating observed in patients presenting to their sleep disorders center. Drug choice or combination was dependent on the primary sleep disorder with which the patient presented. For example, dopaminergic drugs (either alone or in combination with other drugs) were effective in treating sleepwalking sleep-eaters. A significant reduction in night-eating was also reported by Spaggiari et al[68] in moderately obese adult subjects receiving bedtime treatment with d-fenfluramine. Unfortunately, due to the complicated medical problems that of-ten accompany morbid obesity, use of these drugs cannot be generalized to all populations of night-eaters.

CONCLUSION

Both binge eating and night-eating represent disordered eating patterns that very likely play a role in the perpetuation of obesity. While both behaviors have been observed in severely underweight and normal-weight individuals (e.g., those with anorexia and bulimia nervosa), the potential for suffering negative health consequences is limited in the absence of caloric excess. Although the recent burst of reported prevalence data on binge eating far outnumber that on night-eating among obese persons, past and recent night-eating data suggest that it is probably as prevalent among obese individuals seeking weight control treatment as binge eating. In fact, future study of obese nighttime bingers might provide even more striking prevalence data. While degree and age of onset of obesity, gender, diet history, and "response to stress" all appear to influence the degree and frequency of binge eating and night-eating, in neither case has a specific etiology been iden-tified. It is likely that the multifaceted nature of eating behavior will preclude such a discovery. Preferred food choices during self-reported and laboratory monitored binge eating or night-eating episodes are those that are traditionally excluded when strict weight loss efforts are employed (i.e., high-fat snacks, desserts, cold cuts, etc.). For obese binge eaters, further research involving a combination of diet, CBT, and pharmacotherapy appears most promising. Collaborative research between obesity and sleep specialists could provide the most valuable treatment options for obese night-eaters. The strong likelihood that binge eating and night-eating behaviors coexist in a specific subset of obese individuals reinforces the need for highly focused and aggressive research in both areas. For the practitioner, awareness of binge eating and night-eating symptoms, and skill with techniques to screen for them are important when working with patients seeking help with weight-related conditions.[91] Because these disorders occur in persons of normal weight and of severe overweight who are struggling with weight and food, all health professionals should take a proactive role in identifying and helping patients plan day-to-day strategies to cope with these food and weight disorders.

REFERENCES

1. Stunkard AJ. Eating patterns and obesity. *Psychiatric Quarterly.* 1959;33:284–295.
2. Stunkard AJ. A history of binge eating. In: Fairburn CG, Wilson GT, eds. *Binge Eating: Nature, Assessment, and Treatment.* New York: Guilford Press; 1993:15–34.
3. Morris W, ed. *The American Heritage Dictionary of the English Language.* New York: American Heritage Publishing Co and Houghton Mifflin Co; 1969.
4. Russell G. Bulimia nervosa: an ominous variant of anorexia nervosa. *Psych Med.* 1979;9:429–448.
5. American Psychiatric Association. *Diagnostic and Statistical Manual of Mental Disorders.* 3rd ed. Washington, DC: American Psychiatric Association; 1980.
6. Gormally J, Black S, Daston S, Rardin D. The assessment of binge eating severity among obese persons. *Addict Behav.* 1982;7:47–55.
7. Loro AD, Orleans CS. Binge eating in obesity: preliminary findings and guidelines for behavioral analysis and treatment. *Addict Behav.* 1981;6:155–166.
8. Keefe PH, Wyshogrod D, Weinberger E, Agras WS. Binge eating and outcome of behavioral treatment of obesity: a preliminary report. *Behav Res Ther.* 1984;22:319–321.
9. Marcus MD, Wing RR, Lamparski DM. Binge eating and dietary restraint in obese patients. *Addict Behav.* 1985;10:163–168.
10. Spitzer RL, Devlin MJ, Walsh BT, et al. Binge eating disorder: a multisite field trial of the diagnostic criteria. *Int J Eating Dis.* 1992;11:191–203.
11. Spitzer RL, Yanovski S, Wadden T, et al. Binge eating disorder: its further validation in a multisite study. *Int J Eating Dis.* 1993;13:137–153.
12. American Psychiatric Association. *Diagnostic and Statistical Manual of Mental Disorders.* 3rd ed., rev. Washington, DC: American Psychiatric Association; 1987.
13. Wilson GT, Walsh BT. Eating disorders in the DSM-IV. *J Abn Psych.* 1991;100:362–365.

14. Walsh BT. Diagnostic criteria for eating disorders in DSM-IV: Work in progress. *Int J Eating Dis.* 1992;11:301–304.

15. American Psychiatric Association. *Diagnostic and Statistical Manual of Mental Disorders.* 4th ed. Washington, DC: American Psychiatric Association; 1994.

16. Lansky D, Brownell KD. Estimates of food quantity and calories: errors in self-report among obese patients. *Am J Clin Nutr.* 1982;35:727–732.

17. Bandini LG, Schoeller DA, Cyr HN, Dietz WH. Validity of reported energy intake in obese and nonobese adolescents. *Am J Clin Nutr.* 1990;52:421–425.

18. Lichtman SW, Pisarska K, Berman ER, et al. Discrepancy between self-reported and actual caloric intake and exercise in obese subjects. *N Engl J Med.* 1992;327:1893–1898.

19. Stunkard AJ, Grace WJ, Wolff HG. The night-eating syndrome: a pattern of food intake among certain obese patients. *Am J Med.* 1955;19:78–86.

20. Aronoff NJ, Geliebter A, Hashim SA, Zammit GK. The relationship between daytime and night-time food intake in an obese night-eater. *Obes Res.* 1994;2:145–151.

21. Yanovski SZ, Sebring NG. Recorded food intake of obese women with binge eating disorder before and after weight loss. *Int J Eating Dis.* 1994;15:135–150.

22. Marcus MD, Wing RR. Binge eating among the obese. *Ann Behav Med.* 1987;9:23–27.

23. Lowe MR, Caputo GC. Binge eating in obesity: toward the specification of predictors. *Int J Eating Dis.* 1991;10:49–55.

24. de Zwaan M, Nutzinger DO, Schoenbeck G. Binge eating in overweight women. *Compr Psychiatry.* 1992;33:256–261.

25. Yanovski SZ. Binge eating disorder: current knowledge and future directions. *Obes Res.* 1993;1:306–324.

26. Wilson GT, Nonas CA, Rosenblum GD. Assessment of binge-eating in obese persons. *Int J Eating Dis.* 1993;13:25–33.

27. Hawkins RC II, Clement PF. Development of a self-report measure of binge eating tendencies. *Addict Behav.* 1980;5:219–226.

28. Stunkard AJ. "Restrained eating": what it is and a new scale to measure it. In: Cioffi LA, ed. *The Body Weight Regulatory System: Normal and Disturbed Mechanisms.* New York: Raven Press; 1981:243–251.

29. Herman CP, Mack D. Restrained and unrestrained eating. *J Personality.* 1975;43:647–660.

30. Stunkard AJ, Messick S. The three-factor eating questionnaire to measure dietary restraint, disinhibition and hunger. *J Psychosom Res.* 1985;29:71–83.

31. Pudel VE, Metzdorff M, Oetting MX. Zur persoehnlichkeit adipoeser in psychologischen tests unter beruecksichtigung latent fettsuechtiger. *Z Psychosom Med Psychoanalyse.* 1975;21:345–350.

32. Cooper Z, Fairburn CG. The eating disorders examination: a semi-structured interview for the assessment of the specific psychopathology of eating disorders. *Int J Eating Dis.* 1987;6:1–8.

33. Beck AT, Ward CH, Mendelson M, Mock JE, et al. An inventory for measuring depression. *Arch Gen Psych.* 1961;4:561–571.

34. Derogatis LR, Melisaratos N. The brief symptom inventory: an introductory report. *Psychol Med.* 1983;13:595–605.

35. Marcus MD, Smith D, Santelli R, Kaye W. Characterization of eating disordered behavior in obese binge eaters. *Int J Eating Dis.* 1992;12:249–255.

36. Kolotkin RL, Revis ES, Kirkley BG, Janick L. Binge eating in obesity: associated MMPI characteristics. *J Consult Clin Psychol.* 1987;55:872–876.

37. Telch CF, Agras WS, Rossiter EM. Binge eating increases with increasing adiposity. *Int J Eating Dis.* 1988;7:115–119.

38. Lingswiler WM, Crowther JH, Stephens MAP. Emotional reactivity and eating in binge eating and obesity. *J Behav Med.* 1987;10:287–298.

39. Marcus MD, Wing RR, Hopkins J. Obese binge eaters: affect, cognitions, and response to behavioral weight control. *J Consult Clin Psychol.* 1988;56:433–439.

40. Marcus MD, Wing RR, Ewing L, Kern E, et al. Psychiatric disorders among obese binge eaters. *Int J Eating Dis.* 1990;9:69–77.

41. Kanter RA, Williams BE, Cummings C. Personal and parental alcohol abuse and victimization in obese binge eaters and non-bingeing obese. *Addict Behav.* 1993;17:439–445.

42. Herman CP, Polivy J. Restrained eating. In: Stunkard AJ, ed. *Obesity.* Philadelphia: WB Saunders; 1980.

43. Guss JL, Kissileff HR, Walsh BT, Devlin MJ. Binge eating behavior in patients with eating disorders. *Obes Res.* 1994;2:355–363.

44. Rossiter EM, Wilson GT, Goldstein L. Bulimia nervosa and dietary restraint. *Behav Res Ther.* 1989;27:465–468.

45. Beglin SJ, Fairburn CG. What is meant by the term "binge"? *Am J Psychiatry.* 1992;149:123–124.

46. Wadden TA, Foster GD, Letizia KA. Response of obese binge eaters to treatment by behavioral therapy combined with very low calorie diet. *J Consult Clin Psychol.* 1992;60:808–811.

47. Rossiter EM, Agras WS, Telch CF, Bruce B. The eating patterns of non-purging bulimic subjects. *Int J Eating Dis.* 1992;11:111–120.

48. Yanovski SZ, Leet M, Yanovski JA, et al. Food intake and selection of obese women with binge eating disorder. *Am J Clin Nutr.* 1992;56:975–980.

49. Goldfein JA, Walsh BT, LaChaussee JL, et al. Eating behavior in binge eating disorder. *Int J Eating Dis.* 1993:13.

50. Stuart RB, Davis B. *Slim Chance in a Fat World: Behavioral Control of Obesity.* Champaign, IL: Research Press; 1972.

51. Wilson GT. Obesity, binge eating and behavior therapy: some clinical observations. *Behav Ther.* 1976;7:700–701.

52. Gormally J, Rardin D, Black S. Correlates of successful response to a behavioral weight control clinic. *J Counsel Psychol.* 1980;27:179–191.

53. LaPorte DJ. Treatment response in obese binge eaters: preliminary results using a very low calorie diet (VLCD) and behavior therapy. *Addict Behav.* 1992;17:247–257.

54. Fairburn CG, Jones R, Peveler RC, Carr SJ, et al. Three psychological treatments for bulimia nervosa: a comparative trial. *Arch Gen Psych.* 1991;48:463–469.

55. Telch CF, Agras WS, Rossiter EM, et al. Group cognitive-behavioral treatment for the non-purging bulimic: an initial evaluation. *J Consult Clin Psychol.* 1990;58:629–635.

56. Smith D, Marcus MD, Kaye W. Cognitive-behavioral treatment of obese binge eaters. *Int J Eating Dis.* 1992;12:257–262.

57. Pope HG, Hudson JI, Jonas JM, Yurgelun-Todd D. Bulimia treated with imipramine: a placebo-controlled double-blind study. *Am J Psychiatry.* 1983;140:554–558.

58. Freeman CPL, Hampson M. Fluoxetine as a treatment for bulimia nervosa. *Int J Obes.* 1987;11:171–177.

59. Marcus MD, Wing RR, Ewing L, et al. A double-blind, placebo-controlled trial of fluoxetine plus behavior modification in the treatment of obese binge-eaters and non-binge-eaters. *Am J Psychiatry.* 1990;147:876–881.

60. Alger SA, Schwalberg MD, Bigaouette JM, et al. Effect of a tricyclic antidepressant and opiate antagonist on binge-eating behavior in normoweight bulimic and obese, binge-eating subjects. *Am J Clin Nutr.* 1991;53:865–871.

61. Lesses MF, Myerson A. Human autonomic pharmacology XVI. Benzedrine sulfate as an aid in the treatment of obesity. *N Engl J Med.* 1938;218:119–124.

62. Trulson M, Walsh ED, Caso EK. A study of obese patients in a nutrition clinic. *J Am Diet Assoc.* 1947;23:1941–1946.

63. Beaudoin R, Mayer J. Food intakes of obese and nonobese women. *J Am Diet Assoc.* 1953;29:29–33.

64. Dole VP, Schwartz IL, Thaysen JH, et al. Treatment of obesity with a low protein calorically unrestricted diet. *Am J Clin Nutr.* 1954;2:381–390.

65. Diagnostic Classification Steering Committee, Thorpy MJ, Chair. *International Classification of Sleep Disorders: Diagnostic and Coding Manual.* Rochester, MN: American Sleep Disorders Association; 1990:101–104.

66. Schenck CH, Zammit GK, Winkelman JW, et al. A proposed data-based revision of the diagnostic category "nocturnal eating (drinking) syndrome" contained in the international classification of sleep disorders. Presented at the Ninth Annual Meeting of the American Sleep Disorders Association; Nashville, TN, June 1995.

67. Aronoff NJ, Zammit GK, Urioste R. The incidence of night-eating in an obese adult population. Presented at the Eighth Annual Meeting of the American Sleep Disorders Association, Boston, MA, June 6, 1994.

68. Spaggiari MC, Granella F, Parrino L, et al. Nocturnal eating syndrome in adults. *Sleep.* 1994;17:339–344.

69. Winkelman J, Herzog D, Atala K, et al. Epidemiology of sleep-related eating disorder in psychiatric and non-psychiatric populations. *Sleep Res.* 1994;23:345.

70. Schenck CH, Hurwitz TD, Bundlie SR, Mahowald MW. Sleep-related eating disorders: polysomnographic correlates of a heterogeneous syndrome distinct from daytime eating disorders. *Sleep.* 1991;14:419–431.

71. Schenck CH, Hurwitz TD, O'Connor KA, Mahowald MW. Additional categories of sleep-related eating disorders and the current status of treatment. *Sleep.* 1993;16:457–466.

72. Hartman EM, Wynne JW, Block AJ. The effect of weight loss on sleep-disordered breathing and oxygen desaturation on morbidly obese men. *Chest.* 1982;82:291–294.

73. Sanders MH, Gruendl CA, Rogers RM. Patient compliance with nasal CPAP therapy for sleep apnea. *Chest.* 1986;90:330–333.

74. Zammit GK. Sleep disorders associated with obesity. Charles Press. In press.

75. Eveloff SE, Millman RP. Sleep-related eating disorder as a cause of obstructive sleep apnea. *Chest.* 1993;104:629–630.

76. Coates TJ. Successive self-management strategies toward coping with night eating. *J Behav Ther Exp Psychiatry.* 1978;9:181–183.

77. Guirguis WR. Sleepwalking as a symptom of bulimia. *Br Med J.* 1986;293:587–588.

78. Oswald IO, Adam K. Rhythmic raiding of refrigerator related to rapid eye movement sleep. *Br Med J.* 1986;292:589.

79. Williamson DA, Lawson OD, Bennett SM, Hinz L. Behavioral treatment of night bingeing and rumination in an adult case of bulimia nervosa. *J Behav Ther Exp Psychiatry.* 1989;20:73–77.

80. McSherry J, Asham G. Bulimia and sleep disturbances. *J Fam Pract.* 1990;30:102–103.

81. Fabry P, Fodor J, Hejl Z, et al. The frequency of meals: its relation to overweight, hypercholesterolemia, and decreased glucose tolerance. *Lancet.* 1964;1:614–615.

82. Adams CE, Morgan KJ. Periodicity of eating: implications for human food consumption. *Nutr Res.* 1981;1:525–550.

83. Armstrong S, Shahbaz C, Singer S. Inclusion of meal-reversal in a behavior modification program for obesity. *Appetite.* 1981;2:1–5.

84. Sensi S, Capani F. Chronobiological aspects of weight loss in obesity: effects of different meal timing regimens. *Chronobiology Int.* 1987;4:251–261.

85. Bellisle F, Rolland-Cachera M-F, Deheeger M, Guilloud-Bataille M. Obesity and food intake in children: evidence for a role of metabolic and/or behavioral daily rhythms. *Appetite.* 1988;11:111–118.

86. Schlundt DG, Hill JO, Sbrocco T, et al. The role of breakfast in the treatment of obesity: a randomized clinical trial. *Am J Clin Nutr.* 1992;55:645–651.

87. Becker EE, Grinker JA. Meal patterns in the genetically obese Zucker rat. *Physiol Behav.* 1977;18:685–692.

88. Cohn C, Joseph D. Changes in body composition attendant on force feeding. *Am J Physiol.* 1959:965–968.

89. LeMagnen J, Devos M, Gaudilliere J-P, et al. Role of a lipostatic mechanism in regulation by feeding of energy balance in rats. *J Comp Physiol Psychol.* 1973;84:1–23.

90. Armstrong S. A chronometric approach to the study of feeding behavior. *Neuro Biobehav Rev.* 1980;4:27–53.

91. Bruce B, Wilfley D. Binge eating among the overweight population: a serious and prevalent problem. *J Am Diet Assoc.* 1996;96:58–61.

CHAPTER 5

Trends in Prevalence of Overweight in the United States and Other Countries

Sharron Dalton

TRENDS IN THE PREVALENCE OF OVERWEIGHT

Media coverage of the average American's body weight was extensive in the summer of 1994. The newly released data on prevalence of overweight in the United States showed a dramatic increase in the 1980s decade. Adult Americans had gained an average of just over 8 lbs according to data from the 1980 and the 1991 surveys of the National Health and Nutrition Examination Studies (NHANES).[1] The 8-lb weight gain translated into an increase in overweight prevalence of 8%, from 25% to 33% of the U.S. population. This increase in overweight from one out of four to one out of three Americans was attributed to a plentiful, very palatable, and energy-dense food supply, an increased consumption of alcohol, and decreased caloric expenditure.[2] One headline read, "America the Bountiful," and, in smaller print, blamed the problem on "gluttony and sloth."[3] A rather more blunt headline reporting a similar weight increase in the United Kingdom[4] read "Britain's Obesity Caused by Sloth More Than Greed."[5] Whatever the reason, the evidence is mounting. Prevalence of overweight is increasing worldwide and the United States is in the lead.[6,7]

Prevalence reports of overweight and obesity require particular attention to the labels or definitions assigned to the categories of weight distribution. (See Chapter 1 regarding definitions of overweight and obesity.) The distribution of weight in the United States using NHANES 1988–1991 data is described according to body mass index (BMI) categories in the 1995 Institute of Medicine (IOM) report on weight (see Figure 5–1). Some of the difficulties of definition regarding cutoff points and categorical descriptors are illustrated here. The IOM report notes that the prevalence of overweight and obesity is of "epidemic proportions," but points out in reference to Figure 5–1 that "the gradation indicates that most individuals are not obese, and most obese persons are not severely so."[8(pp50–51)] This statement

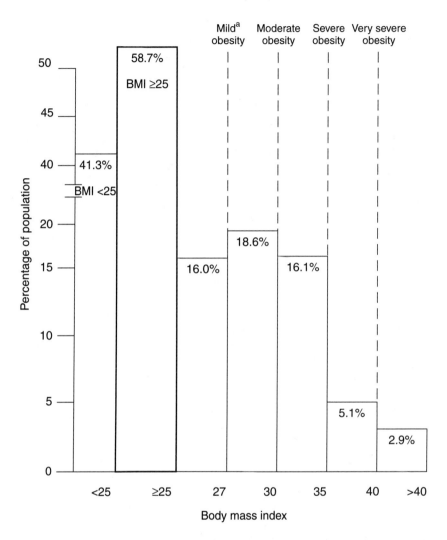

^aThe various descriptors of the degree of obesity apply to individuals aged 35 and older and are associated with particular BMIs (mild obesity at a BMI of approximately 27, moderate obesity at 30, severe obesity at 35, and very severe obesity at approximately 40 or more).

Figure 5–1 The spectrum of weight in the United States (1988–1991). *Source:* Adapted with permission from *Weighing the Options: Criteria For Evaluating Weight Management Programs.* Copyright 1995 by the National Academy of Sciences. Courtesy of the National Academy Press, Washington, D.C.

is correct according to the definition of mild and moderate obesity by using the designated cutoff points of body mass index (BMI) as ≥ 27.3 for women and ≥ 27.8 for men. If, however, the World Health Organization (WHO) criterion of obesity as a BMI ≥ 25[9] is applied to this data, the prevalence of obesity in the United States would be 58.7%. We would then describe the incidence of obesity in the United States as greater than one out of two persons, rather than one out of three persons.

Comparison of the 1988–1991 NHANES III data for adults with the three earlier surveys indicate dramatic increases in the prevalence of overweight in the United States (Table 5–1). The jump between the third and fourth surveys is striking, particularly for white men and women. Overall and within race and sex groups, the age-adjusted prevalence of overweight was significantly higher in the 1988–1991 survey than in the previous three surveys. The trend in weight increase by age occurred in all age groups and was greatest for men and women 50 to 59 years. The highest prevalence of overweight by age group was 52% for women 50 to 59 years. While the rate of increase was greater for white men and women, prevalence of overweight in 1988–1991 was greatest among black women (49.2%) and Mexican American women (48.1%). The increase in BMI of Mexican American men between the 1984 Hispanic NHANES and 1991 was from 31% to 40% and among Mexican American women from 41.5% to 48%.[1] Figure 5–2 presents the prevalence trends of overweight among adult Americans according to race and sex.

Figures 5–3 and 5–4 show trends similar to adults for children 6 to 11 years and 12 to 17 years from NHANES data.[10] The prevalence of overweight was 22% for children and adolescents of all race-ethnic groups combined according to data collected between 1988–1991. Overweight was defined as the weight at the 85th percentile of BMI according to 1970 data. Among girls in both age groups, non-Hispanic blacks had the highest prevalence of overweight and non-Hispanic whites had the lowest prevalence. For boys 6 to 11 years, non-Hispanic whites had the lowest prevalence of overweight; for boys 12 to 17 years, non-Hispanic blacks had the lowest prevalence. Similar to adults, increase in overweight prevalence observed among children since 1965 occurred mainly between 1980 and 1991.

Increasing obesity is a global trend. For example, according to nationwide data in the United Kingdom between 1980 and 1993, the mean BMI for men increased from 24.3 to 25.9, about one and a half BMI units, and for women from 23.9 to 25.7, nearly two BMI units.[11] During the same period of time in the United States, the BMI increased less than one BMI unit for men and just over one BMI unit for women. Although the baseline weight of men and women in the United Kingdom was less than that of men and women in the United States in 1980, both men and women have increased at a greater rate than their counterparts in the United States.

Using the World Health Organization classification for obesity (BMI ≥ 25) rather than for overweight (BMI ≥ 25), Epstein and Higgins[12] compared international prevalence of obesity in different populations from various studies.[13–17] Obesity is defined

Table 5–1 Age-Adjusted and Age-Specific Mean Body Mass Index (BMI), U.S. Population 20 through 74 Years of Age*

Population Group	Mean BMI by Study				Prevalence (%)	
	NHES (1960–1962)[†]	NHANES I (1971–1974)	NHANES II (1976–1980)	NHANES III Phase I (1988–1991)	1976–1980	1988–1991
Age 20–74 yr	24.8	25.2	25.3	26.3	25.4	33.3
Race/sex						
White						
Men	25.1	25.6	25.5	26.3	24.2	32.0
Women	24.4	24.6	24.8	26.1	24.4	33.5
Black						
Men	24.8	25.7	25.5	26.6	26.2	31.8
Women	26.8	27.3	27.5	28.3	44.5	49.2
Sex/age, yr						
Men 20–74	25.0	25.5	25.5	26.3	24.1	31.7
20–29	24.3	24.5	24.3	24.9	15.1	20.2
30–39	25.2	26.1	25.6	26.1	24.4	27.4
40–49	25.6	26.2	26.4	27.3	32.4	37.0
50–59	25.6	26.0	26.2	27.6	28.2	42.1
60–74	24.9	25.4	25.7	26.9	26.8	40.9
Women 20–74	24.7	24.9	25.1	26.3	26.5	34.9
20–29	22.2	23.0	23.2	24.1	14.7	20.2
30–39	24.1	24.7	24.9	26.4	23.8	34.3
40–49	25.2	25.7	25.7	26.7	29.0	37.6
50–59	26.4	26.2	26.5	28.5	36.5	52.0
60–74	27.2	26.5	26.5	27.2	37.3	41.3

*Pregnant women excluded. NHES indicates National Health Examination Survey; NHANES, National Health and Nutrition Examination Survey.
[†]A total of 0.9 kg was subtracted from measured weight to adjust for weight of clothing.
Source: Reprinted with permission from the *Journal of the American Medical Association,* Vol. 272, pp. 205–211, Copyright 1994, American Medical Association.

as a BMI of 30 and over by age group in Table 5–2. The data were drawn from eight industrialized and six developing countries reported in 1987–1988. The prevalence of obesity appears higher in the industrialized countries with a tendency to be higher among women than men. The women in Costa Rica and Nicaragua, however, also have a comparatively high incidence of obesity.

Table 5–3 presents mean BMI data, age and sex adjusted, from the Intersalt Cooperative Research Group[18] an international initiative to study health risk. Also

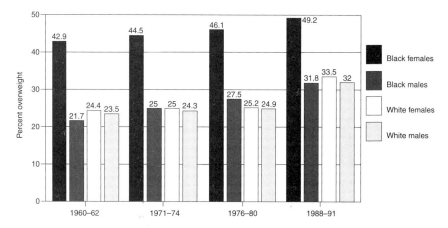

Figure 5–2 Prevalence of overweight Americans age 20–74 years. Overweight is defined as a body mass index greater than or equal to 27.8 kg/m² and 27.3 kg/m² for males and females, respectively. *Source:* Data from R.J. Kuczmarski et al., Increasing Prevalence of Overweight Among U.S. Adults, *Journal of the American Medical Association,* Vol. 272, pp. 205–211, © 1994, the American Medical Association.

presented in Table 5–3 are data on BMI at the 90th percentile from the World Health Organization (WHO) MONICA study,[19] which included comprehensive data from 38 European Centers participating in this health monitoring project.

The European data reported that the 90th percentile was about 31 BMI in men and 33 in women, indicating that the prevalence of obesity in adults is considerably higher than 10%. Had the 15th percentile cutoff point been applied, the prevalence would be much greater. Very high body mass indexes among the women from Eastern and Southern European countries are notable. The heaviest men and women are to be found in places as far apart as Lithuania and Malta. The differences among various populations are much greater overall among women than among men. Although markedly low BMI values are notable in China and India, obesity is an emerging problem in developing countries in tandem with the continuing problem of undernutrition. Urbanization, new eating habits, and pockets of affluence are important influences.

Results reported in 1995 from an international study of hypertension and obesity among persons of West African heritage living in six societies at different stages of social, economic, and technological development demonstrated weight differences related to "nurture" rather than "nature." The International Collaborative Study on Hypertension in Blacks (ICSHB)[20] defined overweight as >27.8 for men and >27.3 for women. The prevalence of overweight increased sharply from rural Africa to urban United States with significantly more prevalence among

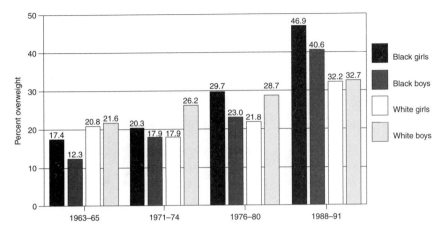

Figure 5–3 Prevalence of overweight Americans age 6–11 years. Based on sex- and age-specific percentile cutoffs for triceps skinfold data for children from the National Health and Nutrition Examination Surveys II and III. Children with triceps skinfolds greater than or equal to those of children of the same age and sex in the 85th percentile are considered overweight. *Source:* Data from R.P. Troiano et al., Overweight Prevalence and Trends for Children and Adolescents: The National Health and Nutrition Examination Surveys, 1963 to 1991, *Archives of Pediatrics and Adolescent Medicine,* Vol. 149, pp. 1085–1091, © 1995.

women than men. The age-adjusted prevalence rates for overweight ranged from a low of 7.4% among urban Nigerian males to 63.2% for the African American women. Nearly 60% of African American women 25 to 34 years were overweight in striking contrast to 14.8% of urban Nigerian women of the same age group. This multinational study clearly shows the potent impact of environmental factors on the distribution and level of obesity among persons with similar racial heritage.

SOURCES OF DATA ON PREVALENCE OF OVERWEIGHT

The procedures used to collect data on weight for height include physical measurement and self-reported surveys. The NHANES is a nationally representative cross-sectional survey with an in-person interview and a medical examination, including measurement of height and weight.[21] Between 6000 and 13,000 adults aged 20 through 74 years were examined in each of four separate national surveys from 1960 to 1991. Between 3000 and 14,000 youths aged 6 through 17 years were examined in five separate national surveys from 1963 to 1991.[1]

As described in Chapter 1, in order to compare data over time, the NHANES defined overweight as a BMI value ≥27.8 for men and ≥27.3 for women. These are sex-specific values of BMI at the 85th percentile from NHANES II and represent approximately 124% of desirable weight for men and 120% of desirable weight

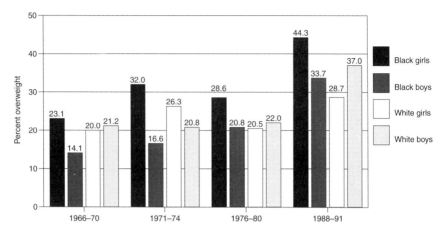

Figure 5–4 Prevalence of overweight Americans age 12–17 years. Based on sex- and age-specific percentile cutoffs for triceps skinfold data from the National Health and Nutrition Examination Surveys II and III. Children with triceps skinfolds greater than or equal to those of children of the same age and sex in the 85th percentile are considered overweight. *Source:* Data from R.P. Troiano et al., Overweight Prevalence and Trends for Children and Adolescents: The National Health and Nutrition Examination Surveys, 1963 to 1991, *Archives of Pediatrics and Adolescent Medicine,* Vol. 149, pp. 1085–1091, © 1995.

for women defined as the midpoint of the range of weights for a medium frame from the 1983 Metropolitan Height and Weight tables. Weights and heights are measured according to standardized procedures by trained staff. The Hispanic Health and Nutrition Examination Survey (HHANES) was conducted between 1982 and 1984, the first large-scale assessment of the health and nutritional status of the U.S. Hispanic population of Mexican Americans, Puerto Rican, and Cuban subgroups.[22] NHANES III (1988–1991) included an oversampling of the Hispanic population, the second largest minority group and among the fastest growing in the United States.

The U.S. Department of Agriculture (USDA) Continuing Survey of Food Intakes by Individuals (CSFII) age 20 and older publishes self-reported heights and weights. Among adults 20 years and older, about one in three (31%) reported themselves to be overweight according to 1996 data.[23] In contrast to NHANES data, the CSFII reported that the highest percent of overweight men (38.7%) were those 40 to 49 years old; the highest percent of overweight women (38.9%) were those 60 to 69 years old. NHANES III reported the 50- to 59-year decade as that of the highest overweight prevalence for white men and women. One might ask if the differences reflect self-reported vs measured weight for height. The criterion used was the same as NHANES III.

Table 5–2 Prevalence of Obesity (BMI ≥30): International Comparisons

Country	Age (yr)	Prevalence (%)		Reference
		Men	Women	
Finland	20–29	3.0	3.0	Rissanen et al[13]
	30–39	7.3	6.8	
	40–49	9.8	17.9	
	50–59	12.2	30.2	
	60–69	14.0	26.2	
	70+	13.3	33.1	
	20+	10	18	
Netherlands	20–34	1.9	2.0	Gurney and Gorstein[14]
	35–49	4.2	5.0	
	50–64	5.4	10.3	
United Kingdom	20–24	3	5	Millar and Stephens[15]
	25–34	6	6	
	35–44	8	8	
	45–54	8	12	
	55–64	9	14	
	20–64	8	9	
Italy	15–44	4.8	3.9	Gurney and Gorstein[14]
	45–64	9.9	11.1	
United States	20–24	7	7	Millar and Stephens[15]
	25–34	10	12	
	35–44	12	16	
	45–54	16	18	
	55–64	14	21	
	20–64	12	15	
Canada	25–34	6	4	Millar and Stephens[15]
	35–44	11	8	
	45–54	12	14	
	55–64	14	13	
	25–64	9	8	
Australia	25–34	4.0	5.7	Gurney and Gorstein[14]
	35–44	6.2	7.5	
	45–54	10.2	11.0	
	55–64	9.6	12.5	
	25–64	7	7	Bray[16]

continues

Table 5–2 continued

Country	Age (yr)	Prevalence (%) Men	Prevalence (%) Women	Reference
South Africa	15–24	3.6	4.6	Jooste et al[17]
	25–34	13.2	10.5	
	35–44	14.3	15.6	
	45–54	20.9	23.8	
	55–64	19.8	31.7	
	15–64	14.7	18.0	
Costa Rica	40–45	5.7	14.4	Gurney and Gorstein[14]
El Salvador	40–45	0.0	1.5	
Guatemala	40–45	0.0	5.6	
Honduras	40–45	2.8	6.0	
Nicaragua	40–45	3.1	16.4	
Panama	40–45	2.3	1.7	

Source: Reprinted with permission from F.H. Epstein and M. Higgins, Epidemiology of Obesity, In *Obesity,* P. Bjorntorp and B.N. Brodoff, eds., p. 332, © 1992, Lippincott–Raven Publishers.

Data regarding prevalence of height and weight are also self-reported in the U.S. National Health Interview Survey (NHIS) and the Prevention Behavioral Risk Factor Surveillance System (BRFSS) conducted by the Centers for Disease Control.[24] These interview surveys examine which groups of people feel that they are overweight, what methods they think are most effective in weight reduction, and how their weight has changed between surveys.

International data is not uniformly available, but a growing number of collaborative health studies are reporting weight data in addition to other factors under study. The WHO MONICA study[19] is the most comprehensive data on the prevalence of obesity in Europe. The majority of these data were collected between 1983 and 1986. Because of migration among countries, the samples are not necessarily representative of the countries in which they are located. Canadian[25] and U.K. data[11] are collected in national surveys of representative samples and reported in government publications.

A 1993 international workshop organized by the National Task Force on Prevention and Treatment of Obesity and a U.S.-Japanese initiative reported prevalence of obesity from several international studies and focused attention on the changing patterns of obesity among differing populations and the changing dietary patterns now recognized as a contributing risk factor for a number of chronic diseases.[26]

Table 5–3 Mean Body Mass Index (BMI) and Obesity (BMI ≥90th Percentile): International Comparisons Based on the Intersalt and MONICA Projects

Area	Country	Mean BMI*	BMI at 90th Percentile Point† Men	Women
Northern Europe	Denmark	24.5	30.3	30.0
	Sweden		29.1, 30.4	29.6, 32.0
	Finland	25.4, 25.3	31.6, 31.6, 31.7	32.7, 31.4, 33.0
	Iceland	24.5	30.3	30.5
Western and Central Europe	United Kingdom	25.7, 24.8, 25.2	30.1, 30.2	32.4, 31.4
	Netherlands	24.4		
	Belgium	25.9, 24.9	30.4, 31.5	32.5, 33.6
	France		29.8, 32.5	30.2, 34.2
	Federal Republic of Germany	24.5, 24.5	30.8, 30.9, 31.3, 31.9	31.5, 32.7, 33.2, 32.1
	Switzerland		30.3, 31.8	30.8, 31.2
	Luxemburg		30.8	32.1
Southern Europe	Italy	28.0, 25.4, 25.4, 25.4	30.3, 31.3	31.5, 32.6
	Malta	26.9	32.7	36.5
	Portugal	25.8		
	Spain	25.4, 26.7	30.3	33.4
Eastern Europe	German Democratic Republic	24.9	30.9, 30.6, 31.2	32.0, 33.6, 34.2
	Hungary	26.2	30.8, 31.6	32.4, 33.8
	Poland	26.4, 26.5	31.7	34.3
	Yugoslavia		31.2	34.9
	Czechoslovakia		32.4	34.9
	USSR	25.7	30.6, 30.8, 30.4, 31.1, 30.7	34.5, 36.0, 34.3, 36.1, 36.2
North America	United States	26.4, 30.3, 28.2, 28.0, 25.1	29.9	31.8
	Canada	25.1, 25.2		
South and Central America	Argentina	25.0		
	Brazil	23.4, 21.2		
	Colombia	23.0		

continues

Table 5–3 continued

Area	Country	Mean BMI*	BMI at 90th Percentile Point†	
			Men	Women
	Mexico	24.4		
	Trinidad	28.2		
Asian-	India	20.1, 23.7		
Pacific area	Japan	21.6, 22.5, 23.1		
	Hawaii	31.2		
	Taiwan	23.1		
	South Korea	22.2		
	Papua, New Guinea	21.7		
	People's Republic of China	22.8, 21.3, 23.8	27.6	29.5
	New Zealand		29.5	29.9
	Australia		29.8, 30.8	30.0, 31.5
Africa	Kenya	20.8		
	Zimbabwe	26.1		

Note: Multiple values within a country refer to different cities.
*Mean BMI refers to age-adjusted values of men and women age 30–59 years (INTERSALT data).[18]
†The 90th percentile points refer to men and women age 35–64 years (MONICA data).[19]
Source: Reprinted with permission from F.H. Epstein and M. Higgins, Epidemiology of Obesity, In *Obesity*, P. Bjorntorp and B.N. Brodoff, eds., p. 334, © 1992, Lippincott–Raven Publishers.

TRENDS IN WEIGHT CHANGE AND PERCEPTION OF OVERWEIGHT AND UNDERWEIGHT

Compared to a cohort of individuals followed over time, cross-sectional data of representative samples, such as NHANES, may reflect immigration, emigration, and variation in mortality rates, although the effect of these factors is likely to be small. Also, estimates from such a series of cross-sectional surveys do not show the proportions of individuals who became overweight, remained overweight, or lost weight, but rather indicate the net effects of these individual changes in weight. Therefore, cross-sectional data at different time points does not describe weight change patterns as well as longitudinal data.

A national sample weighed at two points 10 years apart showed that the incidence of major weight gain (defined as an increase of five or more BMI units) was highest in those 25 to 34 years old and then decreased with age.[27] The pattern was the same for men and women, but the incidence of major weight gain was approximately twice as high among women within all age groups compared to men. Compared to white women, black women 35 to 44 years old gained more weight on average, were more likely to have experienced a major weight gain, and were more likely to become overweight. Using the same data to estimate the 10-year risk of becoming overweight, those who were 35 to 44 years old had the highest risk of becoming overweight (men 16% and women 13.5%). This estimate did not include risk of becoming severely overweight.[28]

Self-perception of being overweight was examined in NHANES III and compared with measured BMI.[29] Overweight females were more likely than overweight males in all age categories to think of themselves as overweight. Among females 20 to 39 years of age who were overweight, 97% of whites, 91% of blacks, and 87% of Mexican Americans thought of themselves as overweight. Among 40- to 59-year-old females the percentages in each of the racial groups were similar. Over 80% of white males and over 70% of black and Mexican American males who were overweight perceived themselves overweight.

Among all racial groups, females who were not overweight but thought of themselves as being overweight were greater than men. Among white females, 51% of women 20 to 39 years old, 60% of those 40 to 59 years old, and 39% over 60 years old who were not overweight thought that they were overweight. Percentages were lower (41% to 46%) for non-Hispanic black and Mexican American females. About half the percentages of males compared to females in all age and racial categories who were not overweight perceived that they were overweight. The trends are similar from the NHIS data, suggesting that recognition of overweight may not be as great a problem as misrecognition of underweight among those who are underweight or misrecognition of overweight among those whose weight is normal. This misrecognition of weight status appears to be more common among females than males and among younger than older people.

ATTEMPTS TO CONTROL WEIGHT

On average, 30% of males and 53% of females reported that they tried to lose weight in the past 12 months in the NHANES III 1988–1991 survey.[29] In every age group, a higher percentage of white females reported trying to lose weight than males or black or Mexican American females. Higher percentages of overweight males and females reported that they were currently trying to lose weight than people in other weight categories. Of those in an acceptable weight category, over 40% of white women between 20 and 60 years old reported trying to lose weight compared to about 30% of black women. Overall, more females than males reported that they were currently trying to lose weight regardless of their weight status.

Weight loss practices reported to be used by more than 70% of males and females 18 years and older among all racial groups was dieting and/or exercise.

Females were more likely than males to use over-the-counter products, meal replacements, and vitamin supplements for weight loss and to participate in organized weight loss programs. Use of fasting, laxatives, body wraps, vomiting, and surgery was reported by small percentages of the population. Among adolescents 12 to 15 years old, 19% reported that they were currently trying to lose weight, compared with 26% of adolescents 16 to 19 years old. Among overweight adolescents 12 to 15 and 16 to 19 years old, 44% and 56%, respectively, reported that they were making an effort to lose weight. The relatively high number (15% to 20%) of acceptable-weight adolescents 12 to 19 years old who reported trying to lose weight are of concern.

THE HEALTHY PEOPLE 2000 INITIATIVE OF THE U.S. DEPARTMENT OF HEALTH AND HUMAN SERVICES[30,31]

Healthy People 2000 is a Public Health Service government initiative that set objectives to be achieved by the year 2000, addressing improvements in health status, risk reduction, public and professional awareness of prevention, health services and protective measures, and surveillance methods. Body weight is included in two of the priority areas, nutrition and physical activity and fitness. Baseline data for weight against which progress is measured was prevalence of overweight according to NHANES II 1976–1980 data. Baseline for physical activity was 1985 survey data.

The 1995 midcourse review of progress toward the objectives reported the status of each objective in terms of percentage of target achieved. Of the 13 nutrition objectives for which tracking data was available, three addressed weight and three addressed reduced-fat and reduced-calorie foods. Two of the weight objectives had moved in the wrong direction. Overweight prevalence percent of target achieved was *minus* 133% and weight loss practices among overweight was *minus* 50%. Figures 5–5 and 5–6 illustrate the trend in weight change in comparison to the 2000 year target.

Availability of reduced-fat processed foods had exceeded (125%) the target. Worksite nutrition/weight management programs had achieved 43% of the target and low-fat, low-calorie restaurant food choices had achieved nearly 25% of the target in 1995. Although progress was made toward labeling food with portion sizes that are customarily consumed, the report stated that in order to reverse the overweight trends, actions are needed to help people reduce their fat consumption, increase their fruit and vegetable intake, and pursue more physical activity. The most alarming trend in the status of physical activity and fitness is that progress toward achieving daily school physical education in grades 9 through 12 had reversed by 100% and the target of providing quality school physical education had reversed by 600%. The report emphatically states clearly that one of the most important public health challenges is moving our society from a sedentary one to a

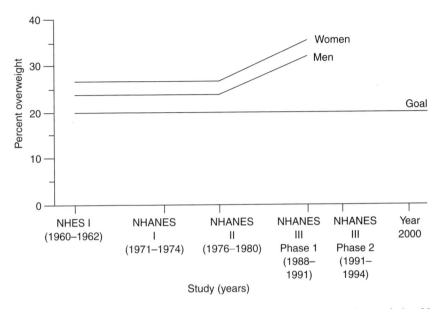

Figure 5–5 Trends in age-adjusted prevalence of overweight for the U.S. population 20 through 74 years of age, compared with the year 2000 health objective for overweight. NHES indicates National Health Examination Survey; NHANES, National Health and Nutrition Examination Survey. *Source:* Reprinted with permission from the *Journal of the American Medical Association,* Vol. 272, pp. 205–211, Copyright 1994, American Medical Association.

more physically active one. Also clear is that providing and consuming fat-reduced foods does not reduce total food consumption. As the percent of calories consumed as fat decreased, body weight increased.

TRENDS IN FACTORS RELATED TO OVERWEIGHT

What are the prospects for slowing the trend of increasing overweight or of achieving a healthy body weight in the future? Predictions regarding the future body weight of individuals necessarily focus on environmental factors related to weight change such as energy intake and energy expenditure rather than regulatory mechanisms largely affected by genetics because understanding of these mechanisms and related medical or pharmaceutical interventions has not kept pace with the rate of increase in body weight. Forecasts about body weight trends are based on studies of excess use of food and drink and paucity of physical activity.

Trends in transportation and leisure activities as well as change in dietary patterns may explain increase in body weight among developed countries and are of

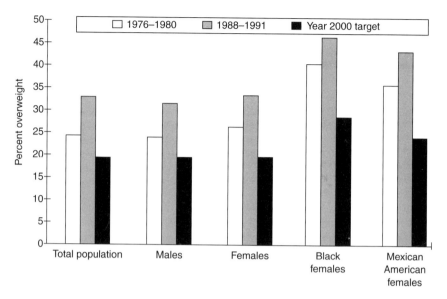

Figure 5–6 Prevalence of overweight Americans age 20–74 years compared to target health goals for weight. Data are from the National Health and Nutrition Examination Surveys (NHANES) II (1976–1980) and III Phase I (1988–1991), conducted by the National Center for Health Statistics, and target goals are from *Healthy People 2000* (DHHS, 1991). *Source:* Adapted with permission from *Weighing the Options: Criteria for Evaluating Weight Management Program,* p. 52, © 1995, National Academy Press.

growing relevance to the worldwide increase in prevalence of overweight. These trends are in addition to the factors frequently studied as affecting increased body weight in developing countries, which are reduction in infectious disease, consequences of rapid economic development such as urbanization, changes in time allocation patterns and roles of women, mechanization, and intense advertising aimed at creating a desire for a "Western" diet with larger consumption of animal and high-fat foods.[32]

During the 1980s decade of dramatic increase in average body weight in the United States, the overall mean energy intake increased among adolescents and adults by approximately 100 to 300 calories.[33] Increases in energy intake ranged from 1% to 13% in males 12 years and older and 14% to 17% in females 16 years and over across age groups between 1978–1991. In terms of calorie consumption as people grow older, the average daily energy consumption of women decreased about 100 calories for each 10-year increase in age from 1957 calories (20 to 29 years) to 1629 calories (50 to 59 years). Men decreased from an average of 3025 calories (20 to 29 years) to 2341 calories (50 to 59 years), nearly 200 calories less each decade increase in age. Yet, in spite of calorie decrease, the 50- to 59-year age group of both men and women increased in body weight at a greater rate than any other age or race group.

Although caloric intake does not predict obesity very well, the increased trend in weight is clearly related to an overall increase in calorie consumption. However, an analysis of diet, activity, and social class trends in Britain suggest that the prevalence of obesity has doubled in the 1980s decade because of modern inactive lifestyles as a more dominant factor than diet.[4] As shown in Figure 5–7 the average energy and fat intake in Britain has declined substantially as obesity rates have escalated. The implication is that levels of physical activity, and hence energy needs, have declined even faster. Greater use of cars, rather than walking, and television viewing are two major factors suggested in Figure 5–7 to explain the change in energy expenditure. These indicate "that the primary causes of the problem lie in environmental or behavioral changes affecting large sections of the

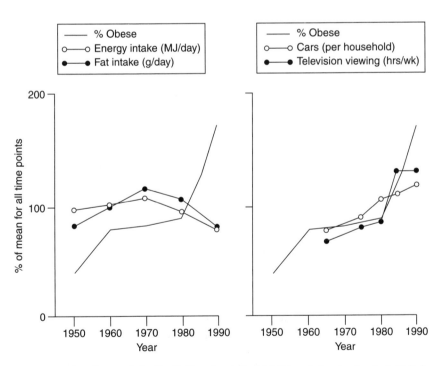

Figure 5–7 Secular trends in diet (left) and activity (right) in relation to obesity in Britain. *Source:* Prentice AM, Jebb SA. *BMJ* 1995;311:437–439. *Source:* Reprinted with permission from A.M. Prentice and S.A. Jebb, Obesity in Britain: Gluttony or Sloth?, *British Medical Journal,* Vol. 311, pp. 437–439, © 1995, BMJ Publishing Group.

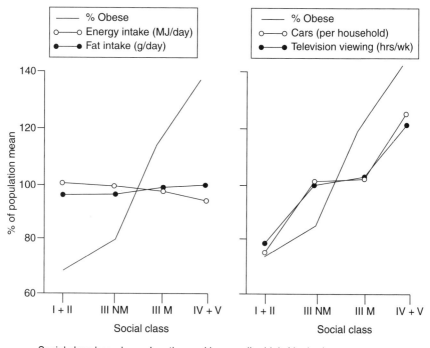

Social class based on education and income (I = high; V = low).

Figure 5–8 Social class trends in diet (left) and activity (right) in relation to obesity in Britain. *Source:* Prentice AM, Jebb SA. *BMJ* 1995;311:437–439. *Source:* Reprinted with permission from A.M. Prentice and S.A. Jebb, Obesity in Britain: Gluttony or Sloth?, *British Medical Journal,* Vol. 311, pp. 437–439, © 1995, BMJ Publishing Group.

population because the escalating rates of obesity are occurring in a relatively constant gene pool and hence against a constant metabolic background."[4(p437)]

Figure 5–8 shows that the same markers of inactivity describe the strong social class trend for obesity rather than a dietary explanation. The paradox of increasing obesity in the face of decreasing food intake is explained as an energy expenditure decline greater than energy intake, thus leading to an overconsumption of energy relative to a greatly reduced requirement.

A large prospective study of 12,000 Finnish adults over five years identified low levels of physical activity as a more important risk factor for excess weight gain than any aspects of the usual diet.[34] The conclusions reached in the United Kingdom and Finland may well apply to the United States. The 1996 Report of the Surgeon General, *Physical Activity and Health,* states that "despite common knowledge that exercise is healthful, more than 60 percent of American adults are not regularly active, and 25 percent of the adult population are not active at all."[35(p5)]

These analyses suggest a strong note of caution to the simple assumption that overweight and obesity are largely a matter of greed or gluttony, encouraged by a very palatable diet persuasively advertised and widely available at reasonable cost compared to income. During the dynamic phase of weight gain, food consumption of obese people must be excessive. But low activity levels must surely play a major role in the astonishing prevalence and increasing rate of obesity.

REFERENCES

1. Kuczmarski RJ, Flegal KM, Campbell SM, Johnson CL. Increasing prevalence of overweight among US adults. *JAMA.* 1994;272:205–211.

2. PiSunyar X. The fattening of America. *JAMA.* 1994;272:283.

3. Anonymous. America the bountiful. *New York Times.* 1994;July 19:A18.

4. Prentice AM, Jebb SA. Obesity in Britain: gluttony or sloth? *Br Med J.* 1995;311:437–439.

5. Hawkes N. Britain's obesity caused by sloth more than greed. *The Times of London.* 1995;Aug 11:5.

6. World Health Organization. Diet, nutrition, and the prevention of chronic diseases. Report of a WHO Study Group. Geneva: WHO Technical Report 797; 1990.

7. Bray GA. Etiology and prevalence of obesity. In Bouchard C, ed. *The Genetics of Obesity.* Boca Raton, FL: CRC Press; 1994:17–33.25.

8. Institute of Medicine. *Weighing the Options: Criteria for Evaluating Weight Management Programs.* Washington, DC: National Academy Press; 1995.

9. World Health Organization. Physical Status: The Use and Interpretation of Anthropometry: Report of a WHO Expert Committee. Geneva: WHO Technical Report 854; 1995.

10. Troiano RP, Flegal KM, Kuczmarski RJ, Campbell SM, Johnson CL. Overweight prevalence and trends for children and adolescents: the National Health and Nutrition Examination Surveys, 1963 to 1991. *Arch Pediatr Adolesc Med.* 1995;149:1085–1091.

11. Bennett N, Dodd T, Flatley J, Freeth S, Bolling K. Health Survey for England 1993. Series HS no 3. London: HMSO; 1995.

12. Epstein FH, Higgins M. Epidemiology of obesity. In: Bjorntorp P, Brodoff BN, eds. *Obesity.* Philadelphia: JB Lippincott Co; 1992:330–342.

13. Rissanen A, Heliovaara M, Aromaa A. Overweight and anthropometric changes in adulthood: a prospective study of 17000 Finns. *Int J Obes.* 1988;12:391–401.

14. Gurney M, Gorstein J. The global prevalence of obesity: an initial overview of available data. *World Health Stat Q.* 1988;41:251–260.

15. Millar WJ, Stephens T. The prevalence of overweight and obesity in Britain, Canada, and the Unied States. *Am J Public Health.* 1987;77:38–45.

16. Bray GA. Overweight is risking fat: definition, classification, prevalence, and risks. *Ann NY Acad Sci.* 1987;14–20.

17. Jooste Pl, Steenkamp JH, Benade AJS. Prevalence of overweight and obesity and its relation to coronary heart disease in the CORIS study. *S Afr Med J.* 1988;74:101–109.

18. Intersalt Cooperative Research Group. Intersalt: an international study of electrolyte excretion and blood pressure. Results for 25 hour urinary sodium and potassium excretion. *Br Med J.* 1988;297:319–328.

19. World Health Organization. MONICA Project: risk factors. *Int J Epidemiol.* 1989;18(suppl): S46–S55.

20. Rotini CN, Cooper RS, Ataman SL, et al. Distribution of anthropometric variables and the prevalence of obesity in populations of West African origin: The International Collaborative Study on Hypertension in Blacks (ICSHIB). *Obes Res.* 1994;3(suppl 2):95s–106s.

21. National Center for Health Statistics. Plan and Operation of the Third National Health and Nutrition Examination Survey, 1988–94. Vital and Health Statistics Series 1, No. 32. Hyattsville, MD: NCHS; 1987.

22. Centers for Disease Control. Prevalence of overweight for Hispanics—United States, 1982–1984. *JAMA.* 1990;263:631–632.

23. Cleveland LE, Goldman JD, Borrud LG. Data Tables: Results from USDA's Continuing Survey of Food Intakes by Individuals and 1994 Diet and Health Knowledge Survey. Agricultural Research Service. Riverdale, MD: US Dept of Agriculture; 1996.

24. Interagency Board for Nutrition Monitoring and Related Research (IBNMRR). Wright J, ed. Nutrition Monitoring in the United States: The Directory of Federal and State Nutrition Monitoring Activities. Hyattsville, MD: DHHS Pub No. (PHS)92-1255-1; 1994.

25. Health and Welfare Canada. *Promoting Healthy Weights in Canada.* Minister of Supply and Services; 1988.

26. Hubbard VS, ed. Prevention of obesity: populations at risk, etiologic factors and intervention strategies. *Obes Res.* 1995;3(suppl 2):75s–306s.

27. Williamson DF, Kahn HS, Remington PL, Anda RF. The 10-year incidence of overweight and major weight gain in US adults. *Arch Intern Med.* 1994;150:665–672.

28. Williamson DF, Pamuk ER. The association between weight loss and increased longevity: a review of the evidence. *Ann Intern Med.* 1993;119:731–736.

29. Federation of American Societies for Experimental Biology, Life Sciences Research Office. Prepared for the Interagency Board for Nutrition Monitoring and Related Research. Third Report on Nutrition Monitoring in the United States: Volume 1. Washington, DC: US GPO; 1995.

30. US Department of Health and Human Services. Public Health Service. Healthy People 2000, National Health Promotion and Disease Prevention Objectives. Washington, DC: DHHS publication (PHS)88-50210; 1990.

31. US Department of Health and Human Services. Public Health Service. Healthy People 2000. Midcourse Review and 1995 Revisions. Washington, DC: DHHS; 1996.

32. Popkin FM, Paeratakul S, Zhai F, Keyou G. A review of dietary and environmental correlates of obesity with emphasis on developing countries. *Obes Res.* 1995;3:145S–153S.

33. McDowell MA, Briefel RR, Alaimo K , et al. Energy and macronutrient intakes of persons ages 2 months and over in the United States: Third National Health and Nutrition Examination Survey, Phase 1, 1988–91. National Center for Health Statistics: Advance Data. Washington, DC: DHHS Publ 255 (PHS) 95-1250; 1994.

34. Rissanen AM, Heliovaara M, Knekt P, Reunanen A, Aromaa A. Determinants of weight gain and overweight in adult Finns. *Eur J Clin Nutr.* 1991;45:419–430.

35. US Department of Health and Human Services. *Physical Activity and Health: A Report of the Surgeon General.* Atlanta, GA: USDHHS, Centers for Disease Control and Prevention, National Center for Chronic Disease Prevention and Health Promotion; 1996.

CHAPTER 6

Genetic Factors and Body Weight Regulation*

Claude Bouchard

INTRODUCTION

The prevalence of overweight and obesity in industrialized nations is strikingly high. This is recognized by all health authorities irrespective of political regime and national wealth. In the United States, it has been estimated that obesity is responsible for about 5% of total health care costs.[1] In 1986, obesity was responsible for about $40 billion of the total health costs, primarily because of the adverse effects of obesity on diabetes, cardiovascular diseases, gallbladder disease, hypertension, and cancer.

Excess body weight is perceived as a problem by a great number of adults. Based on four U.S. surveys summarized recently by the National Institutes of Health Technology Assessment Conference Panel,[2] about 33% of adult women and 20% of adult men are currently trying to lose weight. In addition, about 25% of each sex are trying to maintain their present weight. Among those trying to lose weight, the time spent on a weight loss regimen during the previous year averaged about six months. The same surveys also indicated that diet and exercise were the most common methods used when adults attempted to lose weight, each with a frequency ranging from about 60% to 80%. The Conference Panel also estimated that Americans were spending about $30 billion a year on weight loss products and services.

With recent advances in human genetics and molecular biology, scientists studying the causes of human obesity have become more optimistic about identifying the genes that predispose one to obesity. The growing understanding of the human genome, the high degree of homology between humans and common laboratory mammal models for a large number of genes and chromosomal regions, and the availability of a variety of technologies and tools to study and manipulate DNA in the laboratory are among the most important reasons for the present level

---

Source: Copyright © 1997, Claude Bouchard.

of hope in the obesity research community. The genes associated with an increased susceptibility to weight gain and obesity will eventually be identified and characterized. However, the difficulties to be overcome should not be underestimated. Weight control practitioners still have a long way to go, as human obesity is not a simple entity.

THE PHENOTYPES

Interest in the genetics of human obesity has increased considerably during the last decade, partly because of the realization that some forms of obesity were associated with high risks for various morbid conditions and a higher mortality rate. Obesity cannot be seen as a homogeneous phenotype. Four different types of human obesity can be recognized.[3,4] This does not refer to the heterogeneity of the clinical manifestations of obesity or their determinants but only to the phenotype of body fat itself (Exhibit 6–1). The first type is characterized by excess total body fat without any particular concentration of fat in a given area of the body. The second type is defined as excess subcutaneous fat on the trunk, particularly in the abdominal area (android or male type of obesity). The third is characterized by an excessive amount of fat in the abdominal visceral area (abdominal visceral obesity). The last type is defined as gluteofemoral obesity and is observed primarily in women (gynoid obesity). Thus, excess fat can be stored primarily in the truncal-abdominal area or in the gluteal and femoral area. This implies that a given body fat content of, for example, 30% or 50 kg, may exhibit different anatomical distribution characteristics in different people.

These types of obesity are not fully independent of one another as shown by the data in Figure 6–1. The level of covariation among the body fat phenotypes ranges from about 30% to 50%. One implication of this is that studies designed to inves-

---

Exhibit 6–1 Types of Obesity Phenotypes in a Health Perspective

TYPE I OBESITY:	Excess body mass or percent fat
TYPE II OBESITY:	Excess subcutaneous truncal-abdominal fat (android)
TYPE III OBESITY:	Excess abdominal visceral fat
TYPE IV OBESITY:	Excess gluteofemoral fat (gynoid)

Source: C. Bouchard, Variation in Human Body Fat: The Contribution of the Genotype, In G. Bray, D. Ricquier, and B. Speigelman, eds., *Obesity: Towards a Molecular Approach,* Copyright © 1990, Alan R. Liss. Reprinted by permission of Wiley-Liss, Inc., a subsidiary of John Wiley & Sons, Inc.

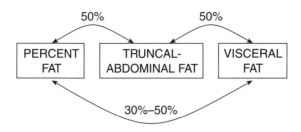

Figure 6–1 Common variance between three body fat phenotypes. Fat mass estimated from underwater weighing; truncal-abdominal fat assessed from skinfolds or CT scans; abdominal visceral fat estimated by CT scan at the L4-L5 vertebrae. *Source:* Reprinted with permission from *The Genetics of Obesity.* Copyright CRC Press, Boca Raton, Florida, © 1994.

tigate the causes of individual differences in the various body fat phenotypes, including genetic causes, should control for these levels of covariation.

The correlation between the body mass index (BMI) and total body fat or percent body fat is reasonable in large and heterogeneous samples. The predictive value of the BMI is much less impressive in a given individual when the BMI is below 30 kg/m² or so. The common variance between BMI and percent body fat derived from underwater weighing in large samples of adult men and women, 35 to 54 years of age, attains only about 40% (Table 6–1). At the extremes of body fat content distribution, BMI is more closely associated with percent body fat. The common variance may reach 60% or more. This is not entirely satisfactory as genetic studies deal with individual differences in the phenotype of interest and to be successful, the phenotype of complex multifactorial traits must be measured with a reasonable degree of precision. Thus, the BMI is an indicator of heaviness and only indirectly of body fat.[5,6] Any estimate of the genetic effect on BMI is

Table 6–1 Common Variance ($r^2 \times 100$) Between BMI and Body Composition in Adults, 35 to 54 Years of Age

	BMI in 342 Males	BMI in 356 Females
Percent fat	41	40
Fat-free mass	37	25
Sum 6 skinfolds	58	67
Trunk/limb skinfolds	10	8

Note: Percent fat and fat-free mass were derived from underwater weighing assessment of body density.

Source: Reprinted with permission from C. Bouchard, Human Obesities: Chaos or Determinism?, in *Obesity in Europe 91, Proceedings of the 3rd European Congress on Obesity,* G. Ailhaud et al., eds, © 1991, John Libbey & Company Ltd.

influenced in unknown proportions by the contribution of the genotype to fat mass, muscle mass, skeletal mass, and other components. Nevertheless, the BMI is worth considering because of its clinical use.

The same point can be made for regional fat distribution phenotypes. Thus the correlation between waist-to-hip circumference ratio (WHR) and abdominal visceral fat is positive and generally significant in various populations, but the association is characterized by a wide scatter of scores. In a study of 51 adult obese women, the correlation between WHR and abdominal visceral fat assessed by computed tomography (CT) reached 0.55.[7] For a WHR of about 0.80, visceral fat area at the L4-L5 level ranged from about 50 cm^2 to approximately 200 cm^2. Although the covariation between total body fat and abdominal visceral fat is statistically significant, the relationship is also characterized by a high degree of heterogeneity. As shown in Table 6–2, when BMI and percent body fat are constrained to narrow ranges, there is generally a threefold range for the amount of CT-assessed abdominal visceral fat in adult males. Thus, in 16 men with BMI values of 30 or 31 and a percentage of body fat ranging from 30 to 33, mean abdominal visceral fat was 153 cm^2 with a range from 77 to 261 cm^2. The same lack of coupling between BMI, percent body fat, and abdominal visceral fat was observed in adult women.[8]

These data suggest that even though it may be useful to use the BMI or a prediction of abdominal visceral fat in clinical settings, in field work or large population surveys, the practice is not recommended in the context of scientific and clinical research designed to understand the causes and metabolic consequences of variation in body fat content or in fat topography.

Because of the many causes and manifestations of body fat, one should use the term "obesities" rather than "obesity." The situation is complex as the phenotypes are not of the simple Mendelian kind. Segregation of the genes is not readily per-

Table 6–2 Variation in Amount of Abdominal Visceral Fat Measured by CT Scan at L4-L5 for Given BMI and Percent Body Fat Classes in Adult Males

		% Fat	Visceral Fat in cm^2		
N	BMI	(range)	Mean	Min	Max
15	21–22	14–18	58	31	84
19	24–25	19–24	89	50	140
18	27–28	25–29	133	63	199
16	30–31	30–33	153	77	261

Note: Percent fat derived from underwater weighing.

Source: Reprinted with permission from C. Bouchard, J.P. Despres, and P. Mauriege, Genetic and Nongenetic Determinants of Regional Fat Distribution, *Endocrine Reviews*, Vol. 14, pp. 72–93, 1993, © The Endocrine Society.

ceived and whatever the influence of the genotype on etiology, it is generally attenuated or exacerbated by nongenetic factors. In other words, variation in human body fat is caused by a complex network of genetic, nutritional, metabolic, energy expenditure, psychological, and social variables.

GENETIC EPIDEMIOLOGY OF BODY MASS AND BODY FAT

Attempts to define the genetic basis of obesity probably began in the 1920s with Davenport's study of body build and its inheritance.[9] Before the 1970s, a number of papers were published on the topic, based on weight-for-height data. For the past 15 years or so, a number of reports discussing the level of heritability and the segregation pattern of body mass for stature and other indicators of obesity have been published.

Seventy years after Davenport's paper,[9] what have researchers learned from genetic epidemiology? First, the estimates of heritability are quite heterogeneous (Table 6–3). However, a trend in the degree of heritability is apparent[10]: estimates based on twin studies are the highest (as high as 80% and more of the phenotype variance), while those derived from adoption studies are the lowest, ranging from ~10% to 30%. Heritability values computed from nuclear-family data fall between these extremes. When several types of relatives are used in the same analyses, heritability estimates generally range from 25% to 40% of the age- and gender-adjusted phenotype variance. There is no clear evidence for a specific maternal or paternal effect, and the common familial environmental effect is marginal.[10]

Second, several studies based on familial data have considered the hypothesis that a single major gene for high body mass was segregating. Table 6–4 presents

Table 6–3 Heritability Levels for Human BMI/Body Fat from Vairous Types of Studies

Type of study	Heritability/ Transmission (%)	Maternal/ Paternal	Familial Environment
Nuclear families	30–50	No	Minor
Adoption studies	10–30	Mixed results	Minor
Twin studies	50–80	No	No
Combined strategies	25–40	No	Minor

Source: Adapted with permission from C. Bouchard, Genetics of Obesity: Overview and Research Directions, In *The Genetics of Obesity,* C. Bouchard, ed., pp. 223–233. Copyright CRC Press, Boca Raton, Florida, © 1994.

Table 6–4 Overview of Segregation Analysis Results for BMI/Obesity Phenotypes

Multifactorial Transmission (%)	Major Effect	Major Gene	Gene Frequency	Studies
41	Yes, 20%	Yes	0.25	Province et al, 1990
34	Yes	Yes	0.21	Price et al, 1990
42	Yes, 35%	Yes	0.25	Moll et al, 1991
39	Yes	No	Non-Mendelian	Tiert et al, 1992[a]
42	Yes, 20%	No	Non-Mendelian	Rice et al, 1993
Yes	Yes	Age and sex related	0.22	Boercki, 1993
25	Yes, 45%	Yes	0.30	Rice et al, 1993[b]

[a]Weight adjusted for height.
[b]Percent body fat.

some of these studies.[10] If one considers only the studies that have used body mass adjusted for height in one way or another, several have found evidence for a major effect, compatible with a major gene (Mendelian transmission). However, some studies did not find support for a major gene and other reports could not find Mendelian transmission unless age and/or gender variations in the major gene were taken into account. From this small body of data, it appears that a major recessive gene accounts for ~20% to 25% of the variance; with age-associated effects, a gene frequency of ~0.2.

Third, from some epidemiological studies, it can be estimated that about 25% to 30% of cases of obese individuals have normal-weight parents, despite the fact that the risk of becoming obese is much higher if the affected individual has obese parents. Indeed, families with one or two morbidly obese parents have two to three times the risk of having an obese adult offspring, compared with families in which neither parent is morbidly obese. Moreover, obese individuals tend to be much heavier than those of the previous generation, and the prevalence of obesity is clearly increasing from generation to generation.[11]

GENETIC EPIDEMIOLOGY OF FAT TOPOGRAPHY

Regional fat distribution has been shown to be an important determinant of the relationship between obesity and health and an independent risk factor for various morbid conditions, like cardiovascular diseases or non–insulin-dependent diabetes. See Bouchard et al[12] for a review of the genetics of fat topography phenotypes.

Truncal-Abdominal Subcutaneous Fat

Upper body obesity is more prevalent in males than in females and it increases in frequency with age in males and after menopause in females. It is moderately correlated with total body fat and appears to be more prevalent in individuals habitually exposed to stress. In females, it is also associated with levels of plasma androgens and cortisol. In addition, the activity of abdominal adipose tissue lipoprotein lipase is elevated with higher levels of truncal-abdominal fat.[13]

Evidence for familial resemblance in body fat distribution has been reported.[14] Based on skinfold measurements obtained in 173 monozygotic and 178 dizygotic pairs of male twins, Selby et al[15] concluded that there was a significant genetic influence on central deposition of body fat. Using data from the Canada Fitness Survey and the strategy of path analysis, Pérusse et al[16] showed that the transmissible effect across generations reached about 40% for trunk skinfolds (sum of subscapular and suprailiac skinfolds), limb skinfolds (sum of biceps, triceps, and medial calf skinfolds), and the trunk-to-limb skinfold ratio and 28% for the waist-to-hip ratio.

The biological and cultural components of transmission of regional fat distribution were further assessed with data from the Quebec Family Study.[17] Two indicators of regional fat distribution were considered. The trunk-to-limb skinfold ratio and the subcutaneous fat-to-fat mass ratio were obtained by dividing the sum of the six skinfolds by fat mass derived from body density measurements. Genetic effects of 25% to 30% were observed. When the influence of total body fat was taken into account, the profile of subcutaneous fat deposition was found to be characterized by higher heritability estimates reaching about 40% to 50% of the residual variance.[3,18] These results imply that for a given level of fatness, some individuals store more fat on the trunk or abdominal area than others.

Results from two studies suggest the influence of major genes for regional fat distribution phenotypes. In one study, Hasstedt et al[19] reported a major gene effect explaining 42% of the variance in a relative fat pattern index defined as the ratio of the subscapular skinfold to the sum of the subscapular and suprailiac skinfold thicknesses. Recent results from the Quebec Family Study suggest major gene effects for the trunk-to-extremity skinfold ratio, adjusted for total fat mass, accounting for about 35% of the phenotypic variance.[20]

Abdominal Visceral Fat

Researchers know less about the causes of individual differences in abdominal visceral fat level than the causes of differences in other body fat depots. Visceral fat increases with age, in both genders, in lean as well as obese individuals.[21] Males have on the average more visceral fat than females and obese have more than lean persons. However, the level of visceral fat is only moderately correlated with total body fat, with a common variance level ranging from about 30% to 50%. In women, high plasma androgen and cortisol concentrations are commonly seen with augmented amounts of visceral fat. In addition, high lipoprotein lipase and lipolytic activities in the visceral adipose depot are observed, but we do not know if these characteristics are causes or effects of visceral obesity. Data from the Quebec Family Study indicate that significant familial aggregation is observed for level of abdominal visceral fat beyond that seen for total body fat. The study suggests that the heritability of abdominal visceral fat with proper control for total body fat reaches about 56% of the phenotype variance.[22]

Further indication that genotype may be an important determinant of subcutaneous fat distribution and abdominal visceral fat phenotypes comes from an overfeeding experiment with identical twins[4] and a negative energy balance study also with pairs of identical twins.[23] The overfeeding experiment revealed about six times more variance between pairs than within pairs for the increases with overfeeding in subcutaneous fat distribution and in CT-assessed abdominal visceral fat after controlling for gains in total fat. Significant intrapair resemblance was also obtained in the negative energy balance experiment for the loss of abdominal visceral fat.

EXPERIMENTAL OVERFEEDING

Some individuals are recognized to be prone to excessive accumulation of fat, and for whom losing weight is a continuous battle, while others seem relatively protected against fat accumulation. We have recently tried to test whether such differences could be accounted for by inherited differences. We asked whether there were differences in the sensitivity of individuals to gain fat when chronically exposed to positive energy balance and whether such differences were dependent or independent of the genotype. If the answer to these questions was affirmative then one would have to conclude that there was a significant genotype-energy balance interaction effect. The results from two experiments suggested that such an effect was likely to exist for body weight, body fat, fat distribution, metabolic rates, and several aspects of carbohydrate and lipid metabolism.

The Short-Term Experiment

In the first study, six pairs of male MZ twins were exposed to a 1000 kcal per day energy intake surplus for a period of 22 consecutive days.[24,25] Individual differences in body weight, fat mass, subcutaneous fat, and site of fat deposition gains were observed with this short-term overfeeding protocol but these differences were not randomly distributed. Indeed, significant intrapair resemblance was observed for changes in most body composition and fat distribution variables despite the fact that the treatment was of short duration and that the changes induced by the treatment were not large. The intrapair resemblance in the response to overfeeding, as assessed by the intraclass coefficient computed with the individual changes, reached 0.88 for total fat mass and 0.76 for fat-free mass. Subjects gained body weight and body fat but there was a nonsignificant 7% increase in resting metabolic rate.[26]

The Long-Term Experiment

Twelve pairs of male MZ twins ate a 1000 kcal per day caloric surplus, six days a week, during a period of 100 days.[4] Significant increases in body weight and fat mass were observed after the period of overfeeding. Data showed that there were considerable interindividual differences in the adaptation to excess calories and that the variation observed was not randomly distributed, as indicated by the significant within-pair resemblance in response. For instance, there was at least three times more variance in response between pairs than within pairs for the gains in body weight, fat mass, and fat-free mass (Table 6–5 and Figure 6–2). These data, and those of the study testing response to short-term overfeeding,[24,25] demonstrate that some individuals are more at risk than others to gain fat when energy intake surplus is set at the same

Table 6–5 Effects of 100-Day Overfeeding Treatment and Intrapair Resemblance in the Absolute Response

Variable	Before Overfeeding $(X \pm sd)$	After Overfeeding $(X \pm sd)$	Within-Pair Resemblance F Ratio	Within-Pair Resemblance Intraclass
Body weight (kg)	60.3 ± 8.0	68.4 ± 8.2**	3.43*	0.55*
Body mass index (kg/m)	19.7 ± 2.0	22.4 ± 2.0**	2.85*	0.48*
Percent fat	11.3 ± 5.0	17.8 ± 5.7**	2.92*	0.49*
Fat mass (kg)	6.9 ± 3.5	12.3 ± 4.5**	3.00*	0.50*
Fat-free mass (kg)	53.4 ± 6.6	56.1 ± 6.7*	2.34	0.40
Fat mass/fat-free mass	0.13 ± 0.06	0.22 ± 0.08**	3.30*	0.53*
Subcutaneous fat (mm)	75.9 ± 21.2	129.4 ± 32.9**	2.77*	0.47*
Body energy (MJ)	497 ± 12	719 ± 176**	3.12*	0.51*

*P < 0.05; **P < 0.0001.

Note: Statistical significance was established from a two-way analysis of variance for repeated measures on one factor (time). F ratio of between-pairs over within-pairs variances. Intraclass coefficient is used to assess the within-pair resemblance in response to the treatment.

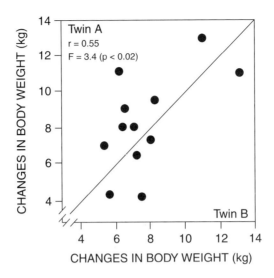

Figure 6–2 Changes in body weight in response to a 100-day overfeeding protocol in 12 pairs of young adult male identical twins. *Source:* Reprinted by permission of *The New England Journal of Medicine,* C. Bouchard et al., Volume 322, p. 1479, 1990. Copyright 1990. *Massachusetts Medical Society.* All rights reserved.

level for everyone and when all subjects are confined to a sedentary lifestyle. The within-identical-twin-pair response to the standardized caloric surplus suggests that the amount of fat stored is likely influenced by the genotype.

At the beginning of the overfeeding treatment, almost all the daily caloric surplus was recovered as body energy gain, but the proportion decreased to 60% at the end of the 100-day protocol.[27] The weight gain pattern followed an exponential course with a half-duration of about 86 days. We estimate that the weight gain attained in the experiment reached about 55% of the maximal weight gain that would be expected if the overfeeding protocol had been continued indefinitely.[27] The mean body mass gain for the 24 subjects of the 100-day overfeeding experiment was 8.1 kg, of which 5.4 kg were fat mass and 2.7 kg were fat-free mass increases. Assuming that the energy content of body fat is about 9300 kcal per kg and that of fat-free tissue is 1020 kcal per kg, then an average of about 63% of the excess energy intake was recovered as body mass changes. This proportion is of the same order as that reported by other investigators,[28,29] i.e., between 60% and 75% of total excess energy intake. There were, however, individual differences among the 24 subjects with respect to the amount of fat and fat-free tissue gained.

Resting metabolic rate in absolute terms increased by about 10% with overfeeding. However, the increase was only marginal when it was expressed by unit of fat-free mass.[30,31] The intrapair resemblance for the changes in resting metabolic rate brought about by overfeeding was significant but it became nonsignificant when changes in body mass or body composition were taken into account. The thermic response to food, as assessed by indirect calorimetry for a period of 4 hours following the ingestion of a 1000 kcal meal of mixed composition, did not increase with overfeeding when resting metabolic rate was subtracted from postprandial energy expenditure.[30] In contrast, postprandial energy expenditure and the total energy cost of weight maintenance increased significantly but the increments were mostly due to the gain in body mass.

EXPERIMENTAL NEGATIVE ENERGY BALANCE

Seven pairs of young adult male identical twins completed a negative energy balance protocol during which they exercised on cycle ergometers twice a day, 9 out of 10 days, over a period of 93 days while being kept on a constant daily energy and nutrient intake. The mean total energy deficit caused by exercise above the estimated energy cost of body weight maintenance reached 244 MJ. Baseline energy intake was estimated over a period of 17 days preceding the negative energy balance protocol. Mean body weight loss was 5.0 kg and it was entirely accounted for by the loss of fat mass. Fat-free mass was unchanged. Body energy losses reached 191 MJ, which represented about 78% of the estimated energy deficit. Decreases in metabolic rates and in the energy expenditure of activity not associated with the cycle ergometer protocol must have occurred to explain the difference between the estimated energy deficit and the body energy losses. Subcutaneous fat loss was slightly more pronounced on the trunk than on the limbs as estimated from skinfolds, circumferences, and computed tomography. The reduction in abdominal visceral fat area was quite striking, from 81 cm^2 to 52 cm^2. At the same submaximal power output level, subjects oxidized more lipids than carbohydrates after the program as indicated by changes in the respiratory exchange ratio. Intrapair resemblance was observed for changes in body weight, fat mass, percent fat, body energy content, sum of 10 skinfolds, abdominal visceral fat, and respiratory exchange ratio during submaximal work. Even though there were large individual differences in response to the negative energy balance and exercise protocol, subjects with the same genotype were more alike in responses than subjects with different genotypes, particularly for body fat, body energy, and abdominal visceral fat changes. High lipid oxidizers and low lipid oxidizers during submaximal exercise were also seen despite the fact that all subjects had experienced the same exercise and nutritional conditions for about three months.

The main purpose of the study was to establish whether there were individual differences in response to negative energy balance solely produced by endurance exercise and to demonstrate whether these differences in response were greater between genotypes than for a given genotype. Changes in body mass, body fat, and body energy content were characterized by more heterogeneity between twin pairs than within pairs. These results are remarkably similar to those reported earlier for body mass, body fat, and body energy gains with 12 pairs of twins subjected to a 100-day overfeeding protocol.[4]

DETERMINANTS OF BODY WEIGHT REGULATION

The list of the determinants of energy balance and ultimately body weight regulation continues to grow. It is impossible here to present a detailed review of all these determinants. The focus will rather be on those for which there is evidence concerning a role of the genotype or a lack of it.

Energy Intake and Food Preference

Familial resemblance in nutrient intake has been reported in spouses as well as in parents and their children. Results from twin studies showed that monozygotic twins were more alike than dizygotic twins regarding their diets. Moreover, a genetic influence on the concentration of nutrients in the diet and on the selection of some foods, particularly with a bitter taste, was reported. These results suggest a possible role of heredity in the regulation of nutrient intake even though lifestyle and environmental factors contribute to the similarity observed within twin pairs.[32]

We have also investigated the potential role of heredity on macronutrient selection and energy intake in a group of 375 families of the Quebec Family Study. Data were available on nine different kinds of relatives by descent or by adoption. As expected, significant familial resemblance accounting for about 30% to 40% of the variance was observed for energy and macronutrient intakes. The familial resemblance noted for energy intake was largely explained by environmental conditions and lifestyle characteristics shared by family members. This was also true for familial resemblance in macronutrient intake. However, evidence was found for a relatively minor genetic effect (about 20%) in the determination of individual differences in the proportion of energy derived from lipids and carbohydrates.[32]

The observation of a potential role of heredity on macronutrient preference raises the possibility that food choice may be involved in determining the inherited susceptibility of some people to obesity. This observation is compatible with the data indicating an increased preference for lipids in obese and postobese subjects in comparison to lean controls.

Metabolic Rates

Resting metabolic rate accounts for about 70% of daily energy expenditure and is influenced by age and gender. The intraindividual variation in resting metabolic rate measurements has been estimated to be about 4% to 6%, a value that includes both the normal day-to-day fluctuation in resting metabolic rate and the technical error associated with its assessment. When resting metabolic rate is adjusted for body mass or body composition, age, and sex, the residual variance reaches about ±200 to 300 kcal per day, which represents about ±10% to 15% of the resting metabolic rate. Thus, the unexplained resting metabolic rate variance is substantial. These observations have been instrumental in the development of the hypothesis that inherited differences were associated with resting metabolic rate. Indeed, twin and family studies suggest that about 30% to 40% of the variance in resting metabolic rate could be attributed to genetic differences.[33]

The thermic effect of food is the integrated increase of energy expenditure after food ingestion. In the only study reported to date,[33] energy expenditure was recorded during four hours after a 1000 kcal carbohydrate meal in pairs of fraternal twins and identical twins as well as in parent-offspring pairs. The heritability of the thermic response to food has been estimated to be at least 30% and perhaps more. The biological significance of such a heritability level is highlighted by the fact that the standard deviation of energy expenditure over four hours in this study reached about 20 kcal and the 95% confidence intervals were within ±4% of the thermic response to the meal (mean response of about 8%).[33]

Level of Physical Activity

Studies of the genetic effect on the level of habitual physical activity or the amount of energy expended for daily physical activity are limited. Results from a few twin studies[23,38] have shown that activity level may be partly inherited. Using data obtained from a nationwide survey on physical fitness and physical activity habits in Canada, the importance of familial resemblance in leisure-time energy expenditure was considered in a total of 18,073 individuals living in thousands of households. Detailed information on frequency, duration, and intensity of activities performed on a daily, weekly, monthly, and yearly basis was obtained by questionnaire and used to compute the average daily energy expenditure (kcal expended per day per kg of body weight) for each subject of the cohort. Familial correlations of 0.28, 0.12, and 0.21 were obtained among pairs of spouses (N = 1024 pairs), parent-offspring (N = 1622), and siblings (N = 1036), respectively. These results suggest that the genetic contribution to interindividual differences in leisure-time energy expenditure is probably quite weak.[34]

Two different indicators of physical activity were also considered in the Quebec Family Study based on 1610 members of 375 families encompassing nine types of relatives by descent or adoption. Thus, habitual physical activity and exercise participation were obtained from a three-day activity record completed by each individual during two weekdays and one weekend day. Heritability reached 29% for habitual physical activity but was 0% for exercise participation.[35] These results were interpreted as an indication of inherited differences in the propensity to be spontaneously active.

More recently, the level of habitual physical activity was investigated with the Caltrac accelerometer in 100 children, 4 to 7 years of age, 99 mothers, and 92 fathers from the Framingham Children's Study. Over the course of one year, data were obtained with the mechanical device for about 10 hours per day for an average of nine days in children and eight days in fathers and mothers. When both parents were active, the children were 5.8 times as likely to be active as children of two inactive parents.[36] These results are compatible with the theory that genetically transmitted factors may predispose a child to be active or inactive.

Substrate Oxidation

One biological characteristic that is associated with the risk of becoming obese over time is the profile of carbohydrate and lipid oxidized, the high lipid oxidizer being at a reduced risk, even though the overall effect is rather small. This can be indirectly assessed using the respiratory quotient as an indicator of the relative proportion of fat or carbohydrates oxidized, provided testing conditions are carefully standardized.

There are inherited differences in the predisposition to oxidize relatively more lipids or carbohydrates as shown by twin and family studies.[33] This finding has been reinforced by the results of our long-term overfeeding study. Indeed, we found a significant within-pair resemblance (within genotype) for changes in respiratory quotient, at rest and for four hours following a mixed-meal challenge, as a result of chronic exposure to overfeeding over a period of 100 days. Similar findings were reported when identical twins were exposed to a negative energy balance protocol for 93 days.[23] These results indicate that there are individuals prone to oxidize more fat than carbohydrates even when energy intake, macronutrient composition of the diet, and level of physical activity were standardized for more than three months. The twin resemblance observed suggests that genes have something to do with this phenomenon.

Skeletal Muscle Metabolism

The ability of skeletal muscle tissue to oxidize lipid substrates is correlated with the pattern of substrates oxidized in a variety of conditions. We have investigated the biochemical characteristics of skeletal muscle from biopsy samples obtained in pairs of brothers, and pairs of fraternal and identical twins. The importance of interindividual variability in the enzyme activity profile of human skeletal muscle confirms that one may find high and low activity levels of enzyme markers involved in the catabolism of different substrates in healthy sedentary individuals of both genders. Numerous factors are undoubtedly involved in accounting for such large interindividual variations. Genetic factors appeared to be responsible for about 25% to 50% of the total phenotypic variation in the activities of the regulatory enzymes of the glycolytic and citric acid cycle pathways and in the variation of the oxidative to glycolytic activity ratio.[37]

Adipose Tissue Metabolism

Lipoprotein lipase is a key enzyme in the process leading to lipid storage in adipose tissue. Based on lipoprotein lipase activity assessments made on suprailiac adipose tissue samples in sets of fraternal and identical twins, a significant heritability level was reported. Furthermore, the acute changes in adipose tissue lipoprotein lipase activity to a prolonged and strenuous bout of exercise are characterized by a greater resemblance within identical twin pairs than in fraternal twins. Thus, twin studies tend to support the notion that inherited characteristics are involved in the regulation of adipose tissue lipoprotein lipase activity.[38,39]

Mobilization of lipids from the adipose tissue stores of the body depends on the metabolic process known as lipolysis. Data on the genetic effects on adipose tissue lipolysis are equivocal. In one twin study, significant heritability levels for submaximal and maximal epinephrine-stimulated suprailiac adipose cell lipolysis were reported.[40] These results were confirmed for isolated fat cells from the abdominal depot but not from the femoral site in a subsequent study performed with parents and their children as well as with twins. On the other hand, studies on identical twins subjected to chronic exercise or chronic overfeeding for short (22 days) and long (100 days) periods indicate that the genotype is involved, to a large extent, in the regulation of the abdominal adipocyte lipolytic response.[41]

Nutrient Partitioning

Nutrient partitioning can be defined in terms of the pattern of deposition of the ingested energy in the form of fat (lipid) or lean (protein) tissue. In adult human beings, the prime metabolic fate of the ingested energy is to sustain adenosine triphosphate (ATP) synthesis for the maintenance of cells, tissues, and a variety of essential functions. Most of the dietary energy is used to meet these needs, particularly in mature individuals. By some estimates, about 99% of food energy serves for maintenance in the broad sense.

When basic maintenance needs have been met, excess dietary energy can be used to support the metabolic processes leading to protein synthesis or fat deposition. Thus, nutrient partitioning becomes an even more important metabolic property when nutrients are ingested in excess of maintenance dietary calorie needs. Nutrient partitioning in animal husbandry has been shown to be a trait that can be altered by a variety of factors, including diet and variation in energy expenditure. It is also influenced by genetic differences.

A nutrient partitioning phenotype resulting in greater protein deposition should result in a decrease in energy efficiency of energy storage in comparison to a nutrient partitioning profile favoring lipid accretion. These considerations are of considerable importance for the understanding of the etiology of excess body fat content in humans. A nutrient partitioning profile favoring lipid accretion over protein deposition is likely to contribute to a chronic state of positive energy balance for two main reasons. First, because of the higher energy efficiency of energy storage in the form of lipid deposition. Second, because when nutrient partitioning favors lipid accretion, fat-free mass is likely to progressively contribute a decreasing proportion of total body mass. In turn, resting metabolic rate will not increase at the same rate as body mass does, thus setting the stage for a state of chronic positive energy balance.

From the animal literature, we know that there are strain differences in nutrient partitioning characteristics, an indication that genes are an important determinant of the phenotype. The genetic epidemiology of the nutrient partitioning phenotype has not been considered to any extent in humans. Only one report has dealt with the heritability of nutrient partitioning characteristics and it is based on data from the Quebec Family Study. A total transmission effect of about 50% was found with a genetic transmission of approximately 20% after adjustment for the proper concomitants.[42]

SINGLE GENE EFFECTS

Association and Linkage Studies

The investigation of the association between DNA sequence variation at specific genes and obesity phenotypes has just begun. One report dealt with the A, B, and C loci of the human leukocyte antigen (HLA) system and their relations with several phenotypes of body fat content and regional fat distribution.[43] The analyses were performed on 348 adult males, 357 adult females, 468 boys and male adolescents, and 405 girls and female adolescents. No consistent pattern of association emerged for any of the phenotypes. The hypothesis that allelic variation at the class 1 loci of the HLA system (chromosomal assignment: 6p21.3) was associated with the body mass index (BMI) could not be confirmed. Thus far, no association has been found between BMI and molecular markers of the glucose transporter-1 (Glut-1) (1p35-31.3),[44] glucose transporter-4 (Glut-4) (17p13),[45] insulin (11p15.5),[45] insulin receptor (19p13.3),[45] and glucocorticoid receptor (5q31-32)[46] genes. Associations between obesity or body fat levels with apolipoprotein B (2p24-23),[47,48] red blood cell acid phosphatase (2p25),[49] low-density lipoprotein receptor (19p13.2),[50] apolipoprotein D (3q27-qter),[51] and dopamine D_2 receptor (11q23.1)[52] have been suggested.

In our laboratory, the relationship between allelic variation at the alpha 1 (1p13), alpha 2 (1q21-23), and beta (1q21-25) genes of the Na,K-ATPase, and percentage body fat, resting metabolic rate, and respiratory quotient was investigated.[53] There was a consistent trend for the percentage of body fat to be related to the restriction fragment length polymorphism (RFLP) generated in exons 21-22 of the alpha 2 gene in both males and females. The association between DNA sequence variation in the brown adipose tissue uncoupling protein (4q28-31) gene and body fat content was examined.[54] DNA samples were digested with nine restriction enzymes, but only BclI generated a RFLP with a 4.5 kb fragment (frequency = 0.72) and a 8.3 kb fragment (frequency = 0.28). Those who gained more than 7% body fat over 12 years were more frequently carriers of the 8.3 kb minor allele (62%) than those who gained less percent body fat (32%).

An association study dealing with the relationship between a RFLP generated by BglII in the 3 beta-hydroxysteroid dehydrogenase locus (1p13.1) and body fat content and regional adipose tissue distribution phenotypes was also completed.[55] Significant relationships were observed between genotypes for 11-year changes in the sum of six skinfolds, abdominal skinfold and abdominal skinfold, adjusted for the sum of six skinfolds at entry in the study. The relationships were observed in women who happened to gain considerably more fat than men over the 11-year span. Oppert et al[56] have observed that a DraI polymorphic restriction site in the alpha-2 adrenoceptor gene (10q24-26) was associated and linked with subcutaneous upper body fat in women, independently of the overall level of fatness. However, no relationship was found between a BanI beta-2 adrenoceptor RFLP (5q31-32) and a variety of obesity-related phenotypes.[56]

The data on linkage between obesity phenotypes and candidate genes or other molecular markers are even less abundant. Regions of the genome in which "obesity genes" potentially reside were explored in the Quebec Family Study using sib-pair linkage analysis.[57] Three consistent patterns of potential linkages with obesity phenotypes resulted, involving the marker loci adenosine deaminase, the Kell blood group antigen, and esterase D, which identify chromosomal regions 20q12-13.1, 7q33, and 13q14.1-14.2, respectively. The region 20q13 is also within the equivalent of the yellow (*agouti* locus) mouse model of obesity, while KEL is in the proximity of the equivalent of the mouse *ob* gene.

The sib-pair linkage approach was used by Dériaz et al[53] in their study of the genes of the Na,K-ATPase. They reported that the polymorphic markers did not reveal any evidence for linkage with percentage body fat. However, the respiratory quotient appeared to be linked to the beta gene MspI and PvuII haplotype (p = 0.008). The beta locus is located on 1q. Oppert et al[54] also used the sib-pair linkage approach to test whether there was any evidence of potential linkage between the

BclI polymorphic site of the uncoupling protein gene and body fat. Their results were consistently negative. Similarly, no evidence of linkage was reported between DraI alpha-2 and BanI beta-2 adrenoceptor gene RFLPs and a variety of body fat measures.[56]

Single Gene Mouse Models

The limited number of molecular marker studies suggest that there will probably be several genes associated and/or linked with human obesity. In addition, other important loci may also be involved. For example, five mouse mutations causing obesity are encoded on five different mouse chromosomes. These mouse obesity genes are in coding regions that have human homologous equivalents. These human homologous regions are also located on five different human chromosomes.[58]

Table 6–6 lists the mouse chromosomes encoding the defective genes and the probable human homologous regions. Two of these mouse genes have been cloned. The *agouti* locus on mouse chromosome 2 regulates coat color pigmentation. Several dominant alleles at the *agouti* locus (A^y, A^{vy}, etc.) shift the relative amounts of black (eumelanin) and yellow (phaeomelanin) pigment in the hairs of the animal pelage and cause a predominantly yellow coat color.[59,60] Pleiotropic effects of the dominant *agouti* mutations include obesity and increased susceptibility to diabetes. The *agouti* gene has been cloned,[61] and encodes a 131 amino acid protein. The gene is normally expressed predominantly in neonatal skin.[61] The dominant yellow (A^y) mutation is associated with overexpression of the gene in most tissues of the adult mouse.[59,61] The mouse *agouti* has a human homolog, which maps on 20q11.2,[60] and the coding region of the human gene is 85% identical to the mouse gene.[60] The overexpression of the *agouti* protein appears to inter-

---

Table 6–6 Possible Synteny Between Mouse Obesity Genes and Human Chromosome Regions

Locus	Transmission	Mouse Chromosome	Human Homologous Region
Diabetes (db)	Recessive	4	1p31-pter
Obese (ob)	Recessive	6	7q31
Tubby (tub)	Recessive	7	11p15.1
Fat (fat)	Recessive	8	16q22-24
Yellow (A^y)	Dominant	2	20q13

Source: Reprinted with permission from J.M. Friedman et al., *Mammalian Genome,* Vol. 1, pp. 130–144, © 1991, Springer-Verlag New York, Inc.

fere with the binding of the α-melanocyte-stimulating hormone (α-MSH) to its receptor in the hair follicle, thus blocking the activation of adenyl cyclase.[62]

The mouse *ob* gene has also been cloned, and encodes a 4.5-kb adipose tissue mRNA with a 167 amino acid open reading frame. The predicted amino acid sequence is 84% identical between human and mouse and has some features of a secreted protein.[63] The *ob* gene human equivalent is on 7q31. A nonsense mutation in codon 105 of the mouse gene has been observed in the severely obese *ob/ob* mouse line, and it expresses a 20-fold increase in adipose tissue *ob* mRNA, while a second *ob* mutant strain does not exhibit any evidence for the expression of the gene.[63]

Interestingly, the *fa* mutation, which arose in the Zucker rat strain maps to rat chromosome 5, and both the rat *fa* and the mouse *db* mutations are apparently in homologous genes.[64] The *fa/fa* rats become obese early in life and exhibit many of the physiological features observed in the *db/db* mice.

The Quantitative Trait Locus Approach

Using the quantitative trait locus (QTL) mapping approach with locus of determination (LOD) scores, new mouse genes for polygenic obesity have recently been identified (Table 6–7). Fisler et al[65] obtained a backcross between the strains *Mus Spretus* and C57BL/6J, which they called the BSB mouse. BSB exhibits a wide range of carcass lipid, from 1% to 50% and more. On the basis of the QTL approach with a large number of markers, Warden et al[66] reported that a locus (MOB-1) on BSB chromosome 7 determines the lipid content of the carcass (LOD score of 3.8). Mouse chromosome 7 is also known to encode the *tubby* gene. Although the BSB MOB-1 locus seems to be different from *tubby*, further characterization is required before a definitive conclusion can be reached. A second locus (MOB-2), on chromosome 6, affected only subcutaneous fat pads (LOD = 2.8). A third locus (MOB-3), encoded on chromosome 12, was linked to percentage of lipid in the carcass (LOD = 4.8) while MOB-4 (chromosome 15) was linked primarily to mesenteric fat (LOD = 3.8).[67] Syntenic regions with these four mouse QTLs are on human chromosomes: 10, 11, and 16; 7; 14; and 5, respectively (Table 6–7).

A mouse polygenic model of differential susceptibility to dietary fat has been developed by crossing a dietary-lipid-sensitive strain (AKR/J) with a resistant strain (SWR/J). After 12 weeks of feeding on a high-fat diet, the AKR/J strain had approximately six-fold higher carcass fat than the SWR/J strain. F2 animals and backcross data were used and, to date, three QTLs have been identified. Do1 (chromosome 4), Do2 (chromosome 9), and Do3 (chromosome 15) are linked to the level of adiposity and, in the case of Do2, also to mesenteric fat (47% of the variance).[68,69] Although regions of homology in the human genome have not been described, it appears likely that syntenic areas can be found on human chromosome 1p36-32 and 9pter-q32 for Do1, 3p21 for Do2, and 5p14-12 for Do3.

Table 6–7 QTL Loci Linked to Body Fat with Corresponding Regions of the Human Genome

Laboratory	Mouse Cross	Mouse Chromosome	Human Homologous Region
Warden et al.		6	7
	C57BL/6J		
	X	7	10, 11 and 16
	Mus Spretus	12	14
		15	5
West et al.	AKR/J	4	1p36-32 and
	X		9pter-q32
	SWR/J	9	3p21
		15	5p14-12

Source: Reproduced from *The Journal of Clinical Investigation,* 1994, Vol. 94, pp. 1410–1416 by copyright permission of The American Society for Clinical Investigation.

Transgenic Mouse Models

Results from transgenic mouse models also reveal that dysfunction in the expression of certain genes can cause obesity. A transgenic mouse with impaired corticosteroid receptor function was created by a partial knockout of the type II glucocorticoid receptor with an antisense RNA transgene.[70] The transgenic animals had increased fat deposition with a body mass that was twice as high as control animals by six months of age. This was observed despite the fact that the transgenic animals ate ~15 % less than the normal mice. It has also been reported that a transgenic mouse that expresses Glut-4 constitutively in the adipose tissue becomes quite fat, with only a moderate elevation in body mass.[71] In this latter case, nutrient partitioning appears to be altered to favor fat deposition.

CONCLUSION

Excessive body fat content is a complex multifactorial trait evolving under the interactive influences of dozens of factors from the social, behavioral, physiological, metabolic, cellular, and molecular domains. Segregation of the genes is not easily detected in familial or pedigree studies and whatever the influence of the genotype on the etiology, it is generally attenuated or exacerbated by nongenetic factors.

Efforts to understand the genetic basis of such traits can be successful only if they are based on an appropriate conceptual framework, adequate phenotype and intermediate phenotype measurements, proper samples of unrelated persons and nuclear families or extended pedigrees, and extensive candidate gene typing and other molecular markers. In this context, the distinction between "necessary" genes and "susceptibility" genes is particularly relevant. For instance, in the case of obesity, there are several examples of necessary loci resulting in excess body mass or body fat for height, that is, carriers of the deficient alleles have the disease (e.g., Prader Willi). However, they represent only a small fraction of the obese population.

A susceptibility gene is defined as one that increases susceptibility or risk for the disease but that is not necessary for disease expression. An allele at a susceptibility gene may make it more likely that the carrier will become affected, but the presence of that allele is not sufficient by itself to explain the occurrence of the disease. It merely lowers the threshold for a person to develop the disease.

In addition, it is likely that body fat content is also modulated over the lifetime of a person by a variety of gene-environment interaction effects. These effects result from the fact that sensitivity to environmental exposures or lifestyle differences varies from individual to individual because of genetic differences. Among the factors of interest are dietary fat, energy intake, level of habitual physical activity, smoking, alcohol intake, and others. Moreover, even though data are lacking on the topic, it is obvious that gene-gene interaction effects need to be considered. However, little research bearing directly on this topic has been reported so far.

A schematic representation of these various genetic modalities is depicted in Figure 6–3. The figure shows that these modalities can be operative on a complex disease such as the predisposition to become obese.

Association and linkage genetic studies are now more frequently reported. Based on the current understanding of the pathophysiology of human obesity, the candidate gene approach is likely to yield useful association and linkage results. Moreover, with the advent of a comprehensive human genetic linkage map, linkage studies with a large number of markers covering most of the chromosomal

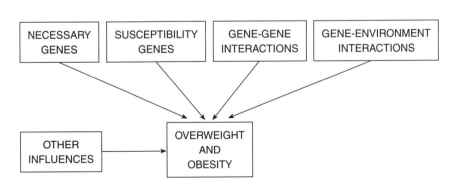

Figure 6–3 Genetic factors and causes of overweight and obesity.

length of the human genome are likely to be helpful in the identification of putative obesity genes or chromosomal regions. Recent progress in animal genetics, transfection systems, transgenic animal models, recombinant DNA technologies applied to positional cloning, and methods to identify loci contributing to quantitative traits have given a new impetus to this field.

Current research shows that a good number of genes seem to have the capacity to cause obesity or increase the likelihood of becoming obese when they are altered or dysfunctional in mammalian organisms. Even though investigation of molecular markers of obesity has barely begun, investigators have already identified about 20 genes, loci, or chromosomal regions that appear to play a role in determining obesity phenotypes. They are located on about a dozen different chromosomes. Many additional genes will surely be identified in the future such that the panel of human obesity genes, based on association, linkage, or animal models, will grow. This may reflect the cause of most human obesity cases. In other words, the susceptibility genotypes may result from allelic variations at a good number of genes.

The stage is now set for major advances in understanding the genetic and molecular basis of obesity. However, as abdominal obesity, particularly visceral obesity, is the most atherogenic, diabetogenic, and hypertensiogenic form of obesity, future studies will have to focus on these phenotypes, rather than simply on excess body mass for stature or excess body fat content. The search for susceptibility genes and the molecular variants of these genes remains a major undertaking. The task becomes even more complex when the important issues of gene-environment, gene-energy intake, gene-nutrient intake, gene-exercise, and, particularly, gene-gene interactions are considered. Investigators will need all of the human genetic, experimental genetic, and molecular biology resources to understand the genetic and molecular basis of human obesity.

REFERENCES

1. Colditz GA. Economic costs of obesity. *Am J Clin Nutr.* 1992;55:503S.
2. Technology Assessment Conference Panel. Methods for voluntary weight loss and control: Technology Assessment Conference statement. *Ann Intern Med.* 1992;116:942.
3. Bouchard C. Variation in human body fat: the contribution of the genotype. In: Bray G, Ricquier D, Spiegelman B, eds. *Obesity: Towards a Molecular Approach.* New York: Alan R Liss; 1990:17–28.
4. Bouchard C, Tremblay A, Després JP, et al. The response to long-term overfeeding in identical twins. *N Engl J Med.* 1990;322:1477–1482.
5. Bouchard, C. Human obesities: chaos or determinism? In: Ailhaud G, Guy-Grand B, Lafontan M, Ricquier C, eds. *Obesity in Europe 91. Proceedings of the Third European Congress on Obesity.* Paris: John Libbey & Company Ltd; 1992:7–14.
6. Garn SM, Leonard WR, Hawthorne VM. Three limitations of the body mass index. *Am J Clin Nutr.* 1986;44:996–997.

7. Ferland M, Després JP, Tremblay A, et al. Assessment of adipose tissue distribution by computed axial tomography in obese women: association with body density and anthropometric measurements. *Br J Nutr.* 1989;61:139–148.

8. Bouchard C. Genetics of human obesities: introductory notes. In: Bouchard C, ed. *The Genetics of Obesity.* Boca Raton, FL: CRC Press; 1994:1–15.

9. Davenport CB. *Body Build and Its Inheritance.* Washington, DC: Carnegie Institution of Washington; 1923.

10. Bouchard C. Genetics of obesity: Overview and research directions. In: Bouchard C, ed. *The Genetics of Obesity.* Boca Raton, FL: CRC Press; 1994:223–233.

11. Lissner L, Sjöström L, Bengtsson C, et al. The natural history of obesity in an obese population and associations with metabolic aberrations. *Int J Obes.* 1994;18:441–447.

12. Bouchard C, Després JP, Mauriège P. Genetic and nongenetic determinants of regional fat distribution. *Endocr Rev.* 1993;14:72–93.

13. Bouchard C, Després JP, Mauriège P, et al. The genes in the constellation of determinants of regional fat distribution. *Int J Obes.* 1991;15:9–18.

14. Donahue RP, Prineas RJ, Gomez O, Hong CP. Familial resemblance of body fat distribution: the Minneapolis children's blood pressure study. *Int J Obes.* 1992;16:161–167.

15. Selby JV, Newman B, Quesenberry CP Jr, et al. Evidence of genetic influence on central body fat in middle-aged twins. *Hum Biol.* 1989;61:179–193.

16. Pérusse L, Leblanc C, Bouchard C. Inter-generation transmission of physical fitness in the Canadian population. *Can J Sport Sci.* 1988;13:8–14.

17. Bouchard C, Pérusse L, Leblanc C, et al. Inheritance of the amount and distribution of human body fat. *Int J Obes.* 1988;12:205–215.

18. Bouchard C. Inheritance of human fat distribution. In: Bouchard C, Johnson FE, eds. *Fat Distribution During Growth and Later Health Outcomes.* New York: Alan R. Liss; 1988:103–125.

19. Hasstedt SJ, Ramirez ME, Kuida H, Williams RR. Recessive inheritance of a relative fat pattern. *Am J Hum Genet.* 1989;45:917–925.

20. Borecki IB, Rice T, Pérusse L, Bouchard C, Rao DC. Major gene influence on the propensity to store fat in trunk versus extremity depots: evidence from the Quebec Family Study. *Obes Res.* 1995;3:15–22.

21. Enzi G, Gasparo M, Biondetti PR, et al. Subcutaneous and visceral fat distribution according to sex, age, and overweight, evaluated by computed tomography. *Am J Clin Nutr.* 1986;44:739–746.

22. Pérusse L, Després JP, Lemieux S, et al. Familial aggregation of abdominal visceral fat level: results from the Quebec Family Study. *Metabolism.* Pending revision.

23. Bouchard C, Tremblay A, Després JP, et al. The response to exercise with constant energy intake in identical twins. *Obes Res.* 1994;2:400–410.

24. Poehlman ET, Tremblay A, Després JP, et al. Genotype-controlled changes in body composition and fat morphology following overfeeding in twins. *Am J Clin Nutr.* 1986;43:723.

25. Bouchard C, Tremblay A, Després JP, et al. Sensitivity to overfeeding: the Quebec experiment with identical twins. *Prog Food Nutr Sc.* 1988;12:45–72.

26. Poehlman ET, Després JP, Marcotte M, et al. Genotype dependency of adaptation in adipose tissue metabolism after short-term overfeeding. *Am J Physiol.* 1986;250:E480–E485.

27. Dériaz O, Tremblay A, Bouchard C. Non linear weight gain with long-term overfeeding in man. *Obes Res.* 1993;1:179–185.

28. Norgan NG, Durnin JVGA. The effect of 6 weeks of overfeeding on the body weight, body composition, and energy metabolism of young men. *Am J Clin Nutr.* 1980;33:978–988.

29. Ravussin E, Schutz Y, Acheson KJ, et al. Short-term, mixed-diet overfeeding in man: no evidence for 'luxuskonsumption'. *Am J Physiol.* 1985;249:E470–E477.

30. Tremblay A, Després JP, Thériault G, Fournier G, Bouchard C. Overfeeding and energy expenditure in humans. *Am J Clin Nutr.* 1992;56:857–862.

31. Dériaz O, Fournier G, Tremblay A, Després JP, Bouchard C. Lean-body mass composition and resting energy expenditure before and after long-term overfeeding. *Am J Clin Nutr.* 1992;56:840–847.

32. Pérusse L, Tremblay A, Leblanc C, et al. Familial resemblance in energy intake: contribution of genetic and environmental factors. *Am J Clin Nutr.* 1988;47:629–635.

33. Bouchard C, Tremblay A, Nadeau A, et al. Genetic effect in resting and exercise metabolic rates. *Metabolism.* 1989;38:364–370.

34. Pérusse L, Leblanc C, Bouchard C. Familial resemblance in lifestyle components: results from the Canada Fitness Survey. *Can J Pub Health.* 1988;17:187–219.

35. Pérusse L, Tremblay A, Leblanc C, Bouchard C. Genetic and environmental influences on level of habitual physical activity and exercise participation. *Am J Epidemiol.* 1989;129:1012–1022.

36. Moore LL, Lombardi DA, White MJ, Campbell JL. Influence of parents' physical activity levels on young children. *J Pediatr.* 1991;118:215–219.

37. Bouchard C, Simoneau JA, Lortie G, et al. Genetic effects in human skeletal muscle fiber type distribution and enzyme activities. *Can J Physiol & Pharmacol.* 1986;64:1245–1251.

38. Savard R, Bouchard C. Genetic effects in the response of adipose tissue lipoprotein lipase activity to prolonged exercise: a twin study. *Int J Obes.* 1990;14:771–777.

39. Savard R, Després JP, Marcotte M, et al. Acute effects of endurance exercise on human adipose tissue metabolism. *Metabolism.* 1987;36:480–485.

40. Bouchard C. Inheritance of fat distribution and adipose tissue metabolism. In: Vague J, Björntorp P, Guy-Grand B, Rebuffé-Scrive M, Vague P, eds. *Metabolic Complications of Human Obesities.* Amsterdam: Elsevier Science Publishers; 1985:87–96.

41. Mauriège P, Després JP, Marcotte M, et al. Adipose tissue lipolysis after long-term overfeeding in identical twins. *Int J Obes.* 1992;16:219–225.

42. Bouchard C, Tremblay A, Després JP, Dériaz O, Dionne FT. The genetics of body energy content and energy balance: an overview. In: Bray GA, Ryan DH, eds. *The Science of Food Regulation: Food Intake, Taste, Nutrient Partitioning and Energy Expenditure.* Baton Rouge, LA: Louisiana State University Press; 1992:3–21.

43. Bouchard C, Pérusse L, Rivest J, et al. HLA system, body fat and fat distribution in children and adults. *Int J Obes.* 1985;9:411–422.

44. Weaver JU, Kopelman PG, Hitman GA. Glucose transporter (Glut 1) as a possible candidate gene for obesity. In: Ailhaud G, Guy-Grand B, Lafontan M, Ricquier C, eds. *Obesity in Europe 91. Proceedings of the Third European Congress on Obesity.* London: John Libbey; 1992:89–93.

45. Weaver JU, Kopelman PG, Hitman GA. Central obesity and hyperinsulinaemia in women are associated with polymorphism in the 5' flanking region of the human insulin gene. *Eur J Clin Invest.* 1992;22:265–270.

46. Weaver JU, Hitman GA, Kopelman PG. An association between a BcII restriction fragment length polymorphism of the glucocorticoid receptor locus and hyperinsulinaemia in obese women. *J Mol Endocrinol.* 1992;9:295–300.

47. Rajput-Williams J, Wallis SC, Yarnell J, et al. Variation of apolipoprotein-β gene is associated with obesity, high blood cholesterol levels, and increased risk of coronary heart disease. *Lancet.* 1988;2:1442–1446.

48. Saha N, Tay JSH, Heng CK, Humphries SE. DNA polymorphisms of the apolipoprotein B gene are associated with obesity and serum lipids in healthy Indians in Singapore. *Clin Genet.* 1993;44:113–120.

49. Lucarini N, Finocchi G, Gloria-Bottini F, Macioce M, et al. A possible genetic component of obesity in childhood. Observations on acid phosphatase polymorphism. *Experientia.* 1990;46:90–91.

50. Zee RYL, Griffiths LR, Morris BJ. Marked association of a RFLP for the low density lipoprotein receptor gene with obesity in essential hypertensives. *Biochem Biophys Res Commun.* 1992;189:965–971.

51. Vijayaraghavan S, Hitman GA, Kopelman PG. Apolipoprotein D polymorphism: a genetic marker for obesity and hyperinsulinemia. *J Clin Endocrinol Metab.* 1994;79:568–570.

52. Comings DE, Flanagan SD, Dietz G, et al. The dopamine D_2 receptor (DRD2) as a major gene in obesity and height. *Biochem Med Metab Biol.* 1993;50:176–185.

53. Dériaz O, Dionne FT, Pérusse L, et al. DNA variation in the genes of the Na,K-adenosine triphosphatase and its relation with resting metabolic rate, respiratory quotient, and body fat. *J Clin Invest.* 1994;93:838–843.

54. Oppert JM, Vohl MC, Chagnon M, et al. DNA polymorphism in the uncoupling protein (UCP) gene and human body fat. *Int J Obes.* 1994;18:526–531.

55. Vohl MC, Dionne FT, Pérusse L, et al. Relation between BglII polymorphism in 3β-hydroxysteroid dehydrogenase gene and adipose tissue distribution in humans. *Obes Res.* 1994;2:444–449.

56. Oppert JM, Tourville J, Chagnon M, et al. DNA polymorphisms in the α_2- and β_2-adrenoceptor genes and regional fat distribution in humans: association and linkage studies. *Obes Res.* 1995;3:249–255.

57. Borecki IC, Rice T, Pérusse L, Bouchard C, Rao DC. An exploratory investigation of genetic linkage with body composition and fatness phenotypes: the Quebec Family Study. *Obes Res.* 1994;2:213–219.

58. Friedman JM, Leibel RL, Bahary N. Molecular mapping of obesity genes. *Mam Gen.* 1991;1:130–144.

59. Yen TT, Gille AM, Frigeri LG, Barsh GS, Wolff GL. Obesity, diabetes, and neoplasia in yellow A^vy/- mice: ectopic expression of the *agouti* gene. *FASEB J.* 1994;8:479–488.

60. Kwon HY, Bultman SJ, Löffler C, et al. Molecular structure and chromosomal mapping of the human homolog of the *agouti* gene. *Proc Natl Acad Sci.* 1994;91:9760–9764.

61. Bultman SJ, Michaud EJ, Woychik RP. Molecular characterization of the mouse *agouti* locus. *Cell.* 1992;71:1195–1204.

62. Lu D, Willard D, Patel IR, et al. *Agouti* protein is an antagonist of the melanocyte-stimulating-hormone receptor. *Nature.* 1994;371:799–802.

63. Zhang Y, Proenca R, Maffei M, et al. Positional cloning of the mouse obese gene and its human homologue. *Nature.* 1994;372:425–432.

64. Truett GE, Bahary N, Friedman JM, Leibel RL. Rat obesity gene fatty (*fa*) maps to chromosome 5: evidence for homology with the mouse gene diabetes. *Proc Natl Acad Sci USA.* 1991;88:7806–7809.

65. Fisler JS, Warden CH, Pace MJ, Lusis AJ. A new mouse model of multigenic obesity. *Obes Res.* 1993;1:271–280.

66. Warden CH, Fisler JS, Pace MJ, Svenson KL, Lusis AJ. Coincidence of genetic loci for plasma cholesterol levels and obesity in a multifactorial mouse model. *J Clin Invest.* 1993;92:773–779.

67. Warden CH, Fisler JS, Shoemaker SM, Wen PZ. Identification of four chromosomal loci determining obesity in a multifactorial mouse model. *J Clin Invest.* 1995;95:1545–1552.

68. West DB, Waguespack J, York B, Goudey-Lefevre J, Price RA. Genetics of dietary obesity in AKR/J x SWR/J mice: segregation of the trait and identification of a linked locus on chromosome 4. *Mamm Genome*. 1994;5:546–552.

69. West DB, Goudey-Lefevre J, York B, Truett GE. Dietary obesity linked to genetic loci on chromosomes 9 and 15 in a polygenic mouse model. *J Clin Invest*. 1994;94:1410–1416.

70. Pépin MC, Pothier F, Barden N. Impaired type II glucocorticoid-receptor function in mice bearing antisense RNA transgene. *Nature*. 1992;235:725–728.

71. Shepherd PR, Gnudi L, Tozzo E, Yang H, Leach F, Kahn BB. Enhanced glucose disposal and obesity in transgenic mice overexpressing Glut-4 selectively in fat. *J Biol Chem*. 1993;268:22243–22246.

CHAPTER 7

Mechanisms of Appetite and Body Weight Regulation

Joseph R. Vasselli
Carol A. Maggio

BASIC CONCEPTS

Perhaps the most basic question asked by investigators in considering the excess of body fat that defines the obese condition is: What kind of disturbance of energy balance permits obesity to develop? This chapter addresses this question, although final answers remain speculative.

The nature of body weight regulation is discussed assuming that setpoints exist for individuals at various weights. A regulatory model illustrates how alterations in the short-term control component or the long-term monitoring component modulate food intake and body weight. These regulatory systems include the brain and its neurotransmitters, the gut and its peptides, the liver and its metabolic processes, the adipose tissue and its secreted proteins such as leptin, and finally, the endocrine hormones. The brain is described as an integrator of feeding stimulation and satiety signals; the proposed neural, endocrine, and metabolic mechanisms in each of the related systems is then presented. Finally, the possibility of manipulating this complex system is considered, given its strong compensatory characteristic of responding more vigorously to weight loss than to gradual weight gain. The question and implications of alternating the setpoint with pharmaceutical agents concludes the chapter.

Energy Balance and the Setpoint

A logical starting point for an analysis of weight regulation is the energy balance equation, which, simply stated, is

$$\text{Change in energy stores} = \text{Energy intake} - \text{Energy expenditure}$$

If body weight represents the energy stores to be balanced by energy intake, then the equation implies that body weight will be maintained at a stable value when the level of energy intake equals the level of energy expenditure. Of course, obesity will develop in a person when energy intake consistently exceeds energy expenditure.[1] This simple principle can lead to some complex questions.

First, the question immediately arises as to whether a regulatory system exists in the mature organism that is designed to maintain body weight at some fixed level. In fact, a good deal of empirical data demonstrates that the body weights of animals and humans will actively be defended following experimental manipulations.[2] Accordingly, the assumption of an active regulatory system for body weight operating around a fixed value, or "setpoint,"[3] has become the basis for many analyses of potential disorders that may lead to obesity,[4,5] and is the focus of a good deal of human and animal research attempting to demonstrate body weight regulatory mechanisms.[6,7] The hypothesis of a body weight setpoint with an active regulatory system implies, of course, that under constant environmental conditions, people will maintain their weights within relatively narrow limits. The great diversity of human body weight, however, and the significant weight changes seen in many people during adulthood suggest that if setpoints exist, they do so over a wide range. Moreover, consistent with a setpoint hypothesis, it is unnecessary to assume that obesity is the result of a regulatory disorder. One need assume only that body weight setpoints exist and are maintained at higher levels in obese individuals.

Second, if a disorder of the mechanism controlling body weight is assumed, then the question arises as to how the disorder is expressed. In terms of the energy balance equation, an imbalance leading to excess caloric storage can be created by increased caloric intake in the face of normal levels of energy expenditure,[8] unchanged caloric intake with reduced energy expenditure,[9] or a combination of these factors. One can quickly see that overeating, metabolic rate changes, changes in the level of exercise, and interactions among these factors can all contribute to excess weight gain. Finally, although significant progress has been made in identifying the genetic bases of several types of animal obesity (see discussion below), the genetic factors leading to human obesity have yet to be determined.

What Is Disordered in Obesity?

Earlier hypotheses on the disorders leading to obesity were relatively simple in approach. Overeating, viewed as a sustained imbalance on the input side of the energy equation, was the primary cause suggested by early observers.[10] Accordingly, attention was initially focused on identifying potential excesses in the feeding behavior of the obese, and their psychologic basis. While it is clear that some obese individuals overeat,[11] evidence that the obese consistently overeat, relative to metabolic mass, or reliably show enhanced preferences for palatable food items relative to lean individuals,[12] is not convincing. Thus, while it is true that surplus energy will lead to the deposition of excess body fat, it is unclear that many obese people become so simply by means of caloric overconsumption. Newer behavioral notions stress motivational factors that prompt the obese to overeat under special circumstances.[13] See Chapter 17 on emotional eating and Chapter 4 on binge eating and night-eating.

Similarly, consistent with a focus on feeding behavior, early analyses of biologic factors in obesity focused on the potential neural bases of overeating in the obese. The widely held hypothesis that an imbalance between two hypothalamic brain "centers" reciprocally controlling hunger and satiety may underlie overeating and obesity[14] is now seen as an oversimplification. Obesity stemming from endocrine disorders was identified by early investigators, but is recognized as a relatively rare condition.[15] Finally, although inactivity clearly is correlated with obesity, the view that excess body fat is the result of chronically decreased exercise may be applicable only to some obese individuals.[16]

Newer approaches to the causes of obesity stress that it is not a unitary disorder, but may involve alterations in one or more of the body's regulatory systems, potentially with a genetic basis. These regulatory systems include the brain and its neurotransmitters, the gut and its peptides, the liver and its metabolic processes, the adipose tissue and its secreted proteins, and endocrine hormones. Thus, quite discrete disorders may underlie various types of obesity. To facilitate an analysis of these factors and their interactions, this chapter will first consider the components of a simplified appetite–body weight regulatory system. The terms "appetite" and "hunger," usually distinguished from each other in terms of external vs internal initiating stimuli,[17] are used interchangeably in the following discussion.

A SIMPLIFIED REGULATORY MODEL

In considering the structure of hypothetical appetite and body weight regulatory systems, workers in the area classically have inferred the existence of two regulatory components: a *short-term* component that controls the onset and cessation of feeding on a meal-related basis, and a *long-term* component that monitors body nutrient depletion and repletion over extended periods.[18,19] In theory, these two components will modulate intake such that body weight is maintained, with some fluctuations, within a relatively narrow range. The two components, although having distinct mechanisms, may be assumed to interact in an additive way in performing regulatory corrections of body weight. Specifically, the potency of short-term satiety signals may be decreased or enhanced in accord with long-term regulatory influences reflecting the nutrient state of the organism.[20] See Figure 7–1.

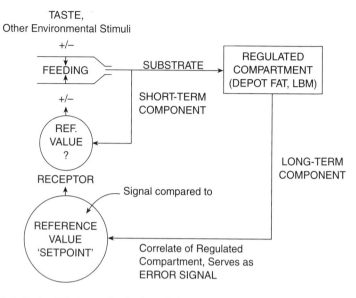

Figure 7–1 A simplified appetite–body weight regulation model.

As indicated in Figure 7–1, feeding stimulated by both internal and external factors provides energy substrate to the body, the unused portion of which is stored primarily in depot fat. The body's fat mass is presumed to be the regulated compartment, since moderate fluctuations of adult body weight consist mainly of alterations of body fat. Extreme weight reductions, however, may result in the involvement of lean body mass as a regulated entity as well. The regulated compartment generates neuronal or endocrine factors that are reliable correlates of its size and which serve as error signals to a receptor having a reference value, or setpoint, for such signals. After comparison of the error signal with the reference value, presumably in the brain, the receptor initiates signals that ultimately provide stimulatory or inhibitory influences on the feeding mechanism. This is the long-term regulatory component of the system.

Signals controlling meal intake presumably arise from the gut, where newly introduced substrate is first sensed. These signals activate a short-term regulatory component operating within a much more limited time frame, which may also use error signals and a reference value such as monitoring gut nutrient levels during a meal. However, for some types of gastrointestinal stimulation, the passive accumulation of purely negative feedback signals, such as distension from increasing stomach volume, may suffice to inhibit feeding. In this model, long-term and short-term feeding influences can summate or cancel each other, in accordance with the state of the gut and body fat stores. Their effects are integrated and expressed by the final common pathway, the feeding mechanism of the brain itself. Although the feeding response may be stimulated by external factors such as taste, temperature, and even psychological events, the effects of feeding initiated in this way ultimately will be reflected in the body's regulatory system.

It should be noted that an *active* regulatory system for body weight need not be assumed. Increasing or decreasing levels of feedback inhibition, in the absence of a reference value (setpoint), can account for weight stability as long as feeding stimulatory influences remain constant.[21] This represents a *passive* body weight control system, through which body weight levels ultimately reflect, rather than resist, environmental feeding influences. In this discussion, an *active* body weight regulatory system is assumed.

PHYSIOLOGIC MECHANISMS INVOLVED IN REGULATION

The Brain and Its Neurotransmitters

Earlier Notions

The "dual center" theory of feeding control evolved from extensive brain lesion and stimulation work focused on two specific areas in the hypothalamus, and the potential interconnections between them. According to the theory,[22] impulses from the lateral hypothalamus (LH), or feeding center, initiate eating when incoming information signals nutrient depletion. As eating proceeds, feeding impulses are inhibited by stimulation from the ventromedial hypothalamus (VMH), or satiety center, which lies close to the brain's vascular bed and the cerebrospinal fluid (CSF), and can monitor rising nutrient levels. Support for this theory is found in the fact that destruction of the VMH by electrolytic lesion or other means leads to hyperphagia and obesity, while destruction of the LH leads to hypophagia and weight loss.[3]

The dual center theory was made considerably more powerful by the parallel development of the glucostatic hypothesis,[14] which identified the rate of glucose utilization as a potential error signal for the initiation or cessation of feeding. As a major tenet of the glucostatic hypothesis, insulin-sensitive glucoreceptors capable of monitoring glucose utilization were posited for the VMH. Such receptors would directly reflect peripheral metabolic events, and make accurate feedback control by the VMH satiety center possible. However, as further experiments either directly or indirectly tested the assumptions of the dual center theory and the glucostatic hypothesis, it became clear that these notions, although appealing in explanatory and integrative power, were inadequate to represent the complexity of the neural and metabolic events controlling feeding.[23] Although the LH and medial hypothalamic (MH) areas of the brain remain a focus of study for the regulation of feeding behavior, these locations are now seen as integrative components in a complex system of incoming and outgoing excitatory and inhibitory influences, mediated by a variety of tracts and neurotransmitters.[24]

Hypothalamic Neurotransmitter Systems

Interest is now focused on the paraventricular nucleus (PVN), located anteriorally and dorsally in the MH, as an integrator of satiety influences, and on the perifornical region of the LH (PFH), as an integrator of feeding stimulatory influences. These areas are known to respond to a host of neurotransmitters that modulate their basic effects on feeding.[25] A major satiety function for the PVN was originally demonstrated by MH lesions centered in the PVN, as well as knife cuts of a tract exiting from the PVN and descending to the medulla. These manipulations lead to hyperphagia and obesity, presumably because of the loss of feeding-inhibitory influences originating in the PVN.[26]

Two neurotransmitter systems have been especially well characterized in relation to hypothalamic feeding control areas. First, the catecholamine (CA) neurotransmitters were shown to exert reciprocal excitatory and inhibitory influences over PVN and LH-PFH function. Specifically, microinjections of norepinephrine (NE) into the PVN stimulated feeding,[27] while microinjections of NE, epinephrine, and dopamine (DA) into the PFH inhibited feeding.[28] Because these locations were identified as feeding inhibitory and feeding stimulatory, respectively, injections of these CA neurotransmitters must exert inhibitory influences over normal function in each location. Following these original observations, it became clear that CA neurotransmitters acting endogenously in these brain areas influence intake via discrete effects on the onset and cessation of feeding,[29,30] and specific influences on macronutrient appetites.[31] The significance of the CA feeding system is demonstrated by the fact that destruction of an ascending CA tract known as the ventral noradrenergic bundle, which terminates in the LH, leads to hyperphagia and obesity, presumably because of the release of the LH from CA inhibition.[32]

The regulatory effects of two more recently identified neuropeptides, neuropeptide Y (NPY) and galanin, have also been well characterized. NPY, the most potent feeding-stimulatory neurotransmitter known, is synthesized in the arcuate nucleus of the hypothalamus and transported to the medial area of the PVN.[33] In addition to its feeding-stimulatory properties,[34] NPY appears to promote peripheral anabolic processes by stimulating both insulin and corticosterone release,[35] activating lipogenic enzyme activity in white adipose tissue,[36] reducing sympathetic nervous system activity (including brown adipose tissue activity[37]), and inhibiting lipolysis.[38] Peripheral hormone levels and metabolic status in turn regulate NPY expression in the brain.[34] Thus, NPY may play a regulatory role in the maintenance of body weight.[6,39] In support of this notion, chronic microinjections of NPY into normal rats has been shown to induce hyperphagia and obesity.[40]

Galanin is concentrated in the lateral PVN, and, like NPY, stimulates feeding,[41] but many of its peripheral effects are dissimilar to those of NPY, in that specific lipogenic mechanisms are not activated.[42] There is considerable evidence that NPY and galanin differ in their appetite-stimulating effects as well, selectively enhancing carbohydrate and fat intake, respectively.[41] Thus, NPY and galanin have different neuroanatomical substrates, and distinct behavioral and physiological effects.[43]

The existence of other neurotransmitters that alter feeding when injected into the brain, however, indicates how complex the neural control of feeding may be. Serotonin and its agonists, for example, inhibit feeding at MH sites, and seem to antagonize NE-induced feeding specifically in the PVN.[44] In turn, levels of brain serotonin are dependent on dietary intake of its amino acid precursor tryptophan, and also of carbohydrates, which enhance brain tryptophan uptake via their effects on insulin release.[45] An endogenous opioid system acting through a PVN-hindbrain circuit appears to modulate NPY-induced feeding,[46] and NPY-sensitive feeding sites have been identified in the hindbrain itself.[47] In addition, both endorphins and DA have been implicated as neurotransmitters in feeding-reward systems located in the hypothalamus and forebrain.[25] Finally, a number of previously unknown hormones/neurotransmitters that may participate in the control of feeding have recently been identified in the hypothalamus, notably leptin and its receptor,[48] glucagon-like peptide-1 (GLP-1),[49] urocortin,[50] and melanocortin and its receptor.[51] It is important to emphasize that interconnections between the forebrain, hypothalamus, cranial nerve nuclei, and brainstem areas implicated in feeding control indicate that extensive integration of feeding-related information normally takes place in the brain.[25] Relatively minor alterations in this complex anatomical and neurochemical system can alter feeding behavior and, potentially, alter body weight.

Signals from the Gastrointestinal Tract

One of the earliest theories of food intake regulation considered the stomach to be the locus of feeding control and gastric contractions to be the signal for hunger.[52] This theory fell into disfavor when no systematic relation could be demonstrated between the occurrence of gastric contractions and either reports of hunger or feeding.[53] The gastrointestinal tract is once again prominent in food intake regulation, this time as a source of signals for satiety, or the cessation of feeding.

Satiety involves both meal-related inhibitory signals and intermeal inhibitory influences.[54] Meal-related satiety signals are thought to arise within the gastrointestinal tract in response to the presence of ingested nutrients. In the stomach, satiety signals may be stimulated by distension resulting from gastric filling.[55] The process of gastric emptying, which involves feedback control of the stomach by the small intestine, also appears to participate in meal-related satiety.[56] As a meal empties from the stomach, intestinal receptors, activated by food-related stimuli, influence not only further gastric emptying but also subsequent food intake.

Transmission of satiety signals from the gastrointestinal tract to the central nervous system appears to involve both neural and peptidergic mechanisms. Electrophysiological and behavioral evidence indicates that several types of receptors in the stomach and small intestine encode information about ingested nutrients.[57,58] These are largely associated with the vagus nerve and include tension receptors, which register changes in distension; osmoreceptors, which register changes in tonicity; and chemoreceptors, which are activated by specific nutrients. In addition, numerous peptides are released when food-derived stimuli contact endocrine cells in the gastrointestinal tract. Vagal afferent fibers also appear to contain receptors for many of these peptides.[58]

Administration of the brain-gut peptide cholecystokinin (CCK) has long been known to reliably reduce meal size in many species including humans.[59,60] Strong evidence for a role of endogenous CCK in satiety comes from demonstrations that highly specific CCK receptor antagonists increase feeding.[61,62] Such studies show that the satiety effect of CCK is mediated primarily through its A receptor subtype, which is located mainly in peripheral tissues such as gut, gallbladder, pancreas and afferent vagal fibers.[63] Interestingly, the recently described Otsuka Long-Evans rat strain lacks CCK-A receptors and becomes obese.[64]

Peripheral administration of bombesin and bombesin-like peptides such as gastrin-releasing peptide and neuromedin have also been shown to reduce food intake.[65] In human volunteers, intravenous infusion of a low dose of bombesin reduced intake of a test meal in the absence of untoward side effects.[66] There is some evidence that bombesin both decreases meal size and lengthens the intermeal interval.[67] Neural ablation studies suggest that bombesin exerts its initial satiety effect within the stomach.[67]

Glucagon, a peptide of pancreatic origin, also reduces short-term food intake.[68] However, to exert a feeding-inhibitory effect, glucagon must generally be administered at higher doses than other peptides such as CCK. The feeding-inhibitory effect of administered glucagon appears to originate in the liver and is conveyed to the central nervous system by the hepatic branch of the vagus nerve. The finding that administration of a highly specific antiglucagon antibody increases feeding supports a potential role for endogenous glucagon in satiety.[69]

Finally, specific inhibition of fat intake has been observed after administration of enterostatin, the activation pentapeptide of pancreatic procolipase.[70] Enterostatin is not a gut peptide per se. Rather it is produced within the intestinal lumen when trypsin cleaves the signal peptide from procolipase. It is now clear that multiple signals for satiety are generated within the gastrointestinal tract as ingested food is processed. Precisely how these signals interact to control meal intake is not yet understood.

Liver Metabolic Influences

After a meal, absorbed glucose is taken up by the liver and provides substrate for energy and for glycogen synthesis. Two early hypotheses identified glucose in the liver as a potential feeding control signal. The first posits a hepatic glucoreceptor system that provides satiety signals to the brain for the initiation and termination of meals.[71] Dependence of this system on the liver's glycogen content is indicated by the finding that hepatic infusion of glucose via the portal vein suppresses food intake in deprived animals but not in freely-feeding, presumably glycogen-replete ones. Since these effects are abolished by vagotomy, information concerning glucose availability in the liver may be conveyed via afferent fibers in the vagus nerve. The firing rate of hepatic vagal fibers has, in fact, been shown to vary as a function of the concentration of glucose in the portal blood.[72]

In an alternate "hepatostatic" theory of food intake control, hepatic glucose metabolism is proposed as the source of signals triggering satiety and initiating feeding.[73] The critical event is viewed as alterations of pyruvate level resulting from glycolysis in response to hepatic glucose uptake in the fed state (pyruvate surfeit), and liver glycogen breakdown in the fasting state (pyruvate deficit). Feeding occurs to replenish carbohydrate reserves and prevent the onset of gluconeogenesis, which is energy costly. Again, hepatic vagal fibers are identified as the relay for information to the central nervous system (CNS). In experimental preparations supporting this hypothesis, predicted effects are in fact abolished by vagotomy. Note that, in contrast to the more general role proposed for glucose in the earlier glucostatic hypothesis, these hypotheses propose a specific role for glucose and hepatic glucoreceptors in signaling hunger and satiety, in conjunction with the state of hepatic glucose metabolism.[74]

A more general theory of the liver's role in the control of feeding has resulted from observations of the interchangeability of various metabolic fuels during states of energy depletion.[75] For example, feeding in response to insulin-induced hypoglycemia can be abolished not only, as expected, by infusions of glucose, but also by the ketone beta-hydroxybutyrate and by the sugar fructose, which does not cross the blood-brain barrier but is metabolized by the liver.[76] Because all of the body's fuels ultimately are processed by the liver, the liver has been proposed as the ideal organ to monitor shifts in substrate flow occurring during energy surplus and deficit. Specifically, the theory identifies hepatic energy production from glucose metabolism and fatty acid oxidation as key in the liver energy monitoring process.[77] During fasting, for example, a decrease in the availability of intracellular adenosine triphosphate (ATP) resulting from a shift in hepatic energy production from glycolysis and glucose oxidation to fatty acid oxidation may be sensed by membrane or intracellular receptors[74,77] and transmitted via the vagus nerve to the brain, resulting in feeding stimulation. In fact, experimental blockade of both the glucose and fatty acid oxidation pathways stimulates feeding.[78,79] Thus, the liver may influence feeding via changes in hepatic intracellular fuel status.[80] Liver-based hypotheses for the control of food intake rely on the presence of an intact vagus nerve to transmit appropriate feeding signals. While the liver may play a significant role in the normal control of feeding, the occurrence of hunger and relatively intact meal patterns have been reported in many cases in vagotomized humans and animals.[81]

Adipose Tissue Mechanisms

Leptin and Other Adipose Tissue Proteins

In addition to relatively short-term feeding control mechanisms associated with the gastrointestinal tract and liver, long-term regulatory signals have been proposed to arise from the adipose tissue. The notion that the adipose tissue may regulate its own size through feedback signals to the brain that influence levels of feeding derives from early "lipostatic" hypotheses,[82,83] and from data indicating that total adipose tissue mass is restored by the body after lipectomy.[84] It was assumed that signals conveyed to the brain from adipose tissue are bloodborne, because little or no afferent innervation of white adipose tissue has been identified.[85] The search for signals that reflect total lipid stores first focused on metabolites emerging from the adipose tissue such as glycerol and free fatty acids, breakdown products of lipolysis whose concentrations in blood increase as fat cells enlarge. Conclusive evidence for the role of such metabolites in the regulation of feeding was not found, however.[86]

The notion of a long-term regulatory signal has now received strong experimental support with the discovery by molecular biological techniques of leptin, a 167 amino acid protein expressed in and secreted from the adipose tissue.[87] In the short period of time since this exciting discovery, it has been shown experimentally that circulating leptin levels are highly correlated with body fat,[88] that leptin crosses into the brain and stimulates hypothalamic leptin receptors, which in turn decrease NPY expression and release,[89] and that leptin administration decreases food intake and body weight in obese and lean mice.[90,91] Adipocyte leptin levels and release in turn appear to be an increasing function of adipocyte size.[87] Thus, a regulatory loop from the adipose tissue to brain feeding sites and back has been established, and leptin appears to be acting as an endocrine hormone. Interestingly, although obese humans have highly elevated levels of leptin,[92] they do not spontaneously reduce their caloric intake or body weight. This has given rise to the notion of "leptin resistance"[93] in the obese, i.e., loss of the adipose tissue regulatory functions of leptin, and various mechanisms of leptin resistance in obese humans and rodents are being investigated. In obese rodent models, mutations of the hypothalamic leptin receptor induce leptin resistance,[94] while in obese humans, resistance may result from impaired entry of leptin from the circulation into the brain.[95]

Other proteins with feeding-inhibitory ability also have been identified by molecular biological techniques in the adipose tissue, including the cytokines TNF-alpha[96,97] and interleukin-6 (IL-6),[98] and a complement-like protein known as adipsin.[99] Administration of TNF-alpha has been demonstrated to differentially reduce feeding in Zucker genetically obese rats.[100,101] This chapter has already cited the identification of the feeding-inhibitory neuropeptide melanocortin and its receptor, found by studies of genetically obese mice carrying the *agouti* gene.[51] Clearly, molecular biological techniques are providing not only new candidate signals, but a valuable new approach to the study of the appetite/weight regulatory process. The majority of human obesity, however, does not appear at this point to be based on either single-gene mutations identified in experimental models,[102,103] or on the genes involved in rare human obesity syndromes.[104]

Additional Adipose Tissue Regulatory Mechanisms

There is now strong evidence that an enzymatic mechanism may contribute to the maintenance of adipose tissue mass following body weight reduction. It has long been observed that basal levels of the adipose tissue fat-storing enzyme lipoprotein lipase (LPL) increase as a result of weight loss,[105,106] a process that may enhance lipid deposition in the adipose tissue at reduced body weight. The observation was also made that not only basal levels, but meal-stimulated activity of LPL increases when adipose tissue is reduced in obese women.[107] This increase seems to be triggered by insulin released in conjunction with the meal, and would therefore contribute specifically to the uptake and storage of ingested lipid following a meal. Upon weight regain, basal levels of LPL are normalized, and enhanced LPL responsiveness disappears. While it appears that insulin mediates this process, the basis for this remarkable regulatory enzymatic response is unknown.

Finally, the size and number of the body's adipocytes may participate in body weight regulation. It is now evident that the total number of fat cells in the body may readily increase under appropriate dietary stimulation.[108] Specifically, adipocytes enlarge through the process of lipid filling, and it has been proposed that as fat cells approach maximal or "peak" size, a process of adipocyte proliferation is initiated, ultimately increasing the body's total adipocyte number.[108] This proliferative process can be triggered experimentally by extended periods of overeating, particularly of high-fat diets,[109] and results in elevated body weight and body fat. The increase of total adipocyte number would be expected to exert additional feeding-stimulatory effects as the new cells begin to fill with lipid. Because mature adipocytes cannot be eliminated except by surgical means, a new permanent body weight will be attained. Indeed, the tendency for adipocytes to maintain normal cell size indicates that adipocyte proliferation may result not only in an elevation of body weight, but in the defense of that body weight through the hormonal, metabolic, and feeding mechanisms identified above. It is notable that adipocyte LPL activity remains elevated in the Zucker obese rat despite lifelong caloric restriction, which may enable the animal to maintain its enlarged fat cell size and obese body composition despite a significant reduction of adult body weight.[110]

The Role of Endocrine Hormones

Several theories of body weight regulation involve a role for the endocrine hormones, either as direct feedback signals or as modulators of neural and metabolic processes involved in feeding and energy expenditure. One prominent hypothesis in the first category identifies the level of brain insulin as the error signal for the long-term control of body weight.[111,112] Starting with the observation that circulating levels of insulin are positively correlated with the body's adipose mass,[113] the hypothesis asserts that a representative fraction of circulating insulin crosses the blood-brain barrier and accurately indicates the size of adipose stores to hypothalamic areas capable of detecting insulin. Hypothalamic centers, in turn, alter feeding stimulation in accord with intrinsic and extrinsic neural and metabolic factors, to maintain a constant level of adiposity. According to the hypothesis, increases of interstitial insulin reflecting increased adipose tissue mass are detected in the hypothalamus and signal reductions of feeding, while decreases of insulin reflecting decreased adipose tissue mass prompt increases of feeding.

Since the introduction of this hypothesis, a considerable amount of supportive data has been generated, including the identification of insulin receptors in areas of the hypothalamus known to be involved in feeding control,[111] experimental manipulations of brain insulin levels and feeding,[114,115] and the demonstration of altered insulin levels and insulin binding in the brains of Zucker obese rats.[116] Two recent observations strengthen the hypothesis by providing mediating mechanisms for the feeding-altering effects of insulin in the brain: central insulin administration downregulates NPY expression and release at hypothalamic feeding sites,[114,117] and enhances the satiety-inducing effects of CCK.[20] Thus, brain insulin appears to be acting in a fashion similar to leptin, a finding not unlikely in light of the redundancies that are characteristic of feeding control systems.

Two additional hypotheses are based on imbalances among hypothalamic, hormonal, and autonomic nervous system activity. The glucocorticoid-autonomic hypothesis is based on the observation that changes in the level of the adrenal glucocorticoids alter fat storage.[118] Thus, the development of obesity is reversed by adrenalectomy but enhanced in Cushing's disease, which is characterized by increased adrenal steroid secretion.[119] Further, elevated glucocorticoid levels reduce the release of hypothalamic corticotrophin-releasing hormone (CRF), which itself is known to inhibit feeding at PVN sites, and stimulate autonomic sympathetic nervous system (SNS) activity. Enhanced SNS activity increases energy expenditure and protects against excess weight gain. It is well documented, however, that SNS activity is reduced and therefore altered in favor of lipid deposition in many obese models.[120] Thus, glucocorticoid hormones seem to increase feeding and enhance the accumulation of body fat via central actions on CRF levels and SNS activity. The fact that NE-induced feeding in the PVN is abolished by adrenalectomy[121] supports this hypothesis. Increased CRF levels resulting from adrenalectomy would exert inhibitory effects on PVN feeding stimulation. In summary, an excessive responsiveness to glucocorticoids may characterize individuals prone to develop obesity.[118]

A similar hypothesis concerning the etiology of obesity identifies as a primary cause a dysfunction of hypothalamic activity that results in insulin hypersecretion, decreased SNS activity favoring lipid deposition, and related metabolic abnormalities such as enhanced hepatic glucose production and increased insulin resistance.[122] These two theories view obesity as a neuroendocrine disorder involving an autonomic nervous system imbalance, potentially with a genetic basis.

Finally, amylin is a newly discovered 37 amino acid polypeptide secreted along with insulin by the pancreatic islets in response to meal ingestion.[123] Amylin is similar in structure to calcitonin gene-related peptide (CGRP), which is known to reduce food intake when microinjected into the hypothalamic area of rats and mice.[124] When administered peripherally, amylin has significant feeding-inhibitory effects via reductions of meal size.[123,125] Thus amylin may be an additional endocrine satiety signal, in this case influencing meal-related satiety.

IMPLICATIONS FOR TREATMENT

Complexity of the Weight Regulatory System

It is clear that the regulation of feeding and body weight is multiply determined, with overlapping neural, endocrine, and metabolic mechanisms designed to maintain immediate (short-term) and long-term energy reserves at relatively constant levels. Obviously, these systems not only interact in complex ways, but appear to compensate for each other in the face of interventions that alter their functioning. It is this characteristic that renders attempts at appetite control and weight reduction so difficult. Complicating the problem is the fact that weight regulatory systems respond much more vigorously to weight loss than to gradual weight gain.[8] As noted above, adipocyte number and thus total body fat can increase in the adult state via a proliferative process that appears to be unopposed. Therapies for the obese are targeted at every stage of the caloric ingestion-utilization process. Behavior modification in part alters the accessibility of food items; anorectic drugs, dietary fiber, and gastric surgery presumably reduce appetite or enhance satiety; low-calorie liquid diets bypass short-term control mechanisms entirely and more directly manipulate body weight; and exercise transiently increases energy expenditure,[126] diverting or mobilizing calories from storage. It also reportedly decreases appetite, although this last claim is questionable.[127]

Most effective weight loss therapies, however, lead to compensatory adjustments such as increased hunger and caloric intake, decreased metabolic rate, an enhanced rate of lipid storage, and/or reduced exercise levels. Of the potential treatments the practitioner can offer obese patients, the ideal one would, of course, manipulate the body weight regulatory system so that equilibrium is achieved at a lower weight level. This alternative, clearly the most attractive, also seems to be the most difficult to implement.

Can the Regulatory System Be Manipulated?

Under experimental conditions, at least one type of intervention has been shown to have the ability to decrease body weight maintenance levels without increasing appetite. This is chronic administration of the anorectic agents amphetamine and fenfluramine, members of the phenylethylamine class of compounds.[128] The case for fenfluramine is considered here, because the argument for its "setpoint-like" altering effects is well documented. Studies with fenfluramine indicate that rats treated with the drug initially reduce food intake and body weight, but upon weight stabilization increase caloric intake to normal levels. Decreased body weight is maintained. Rats that are reduced in weight before drug administration show no intake reduction when treated, but maintain the reduced weight.[129] Thus the drug acts by lowering the weight maintenance level, and only secondarily by decreasing appetite, if required, to effect a lowered body weight.[130]

Initially, investigators hypothesized that the basal metabolic rate of the treated animals was increased, permitting an increase of caloric intake during treatment to pretreatment levels.[128,129] Later studies demonstrate that rather than basal metabolic rate, the energetic cost of locomotor activity[131] and the thermic effect of food[132] are increased by the drug, and that tolerance to these effects does not develop. Several additional metabolic changes induced by fenfluramine, including decreased corticosterone release, increased insulin sensitivity, and decreased triglyceride synthesis, may also contribute to weight maintenance at a reduced level.[133] Interestingly, chronic administration of nicotine to rats has similar weight-reducing effects although caloric intake returns to normal.[134]

Several points should be made concerning these findings. First, it is clear that fenfluramine alters energy expenditure in such a way as to maintain decreased body weight in the face of normal caloric intake. This effect demonstrates that the body's weight regulatory system can at least experimentally be "reset" to a lower level. However, the decrease in weight maintenance level induced by fenfluramine is only temporary. Withdrawal of the drug results in rapid regain of the lost body weight in both animals and man.[129,135] This has prompted some to suggest that the drug be used chronically in the treatment of obesity, but the safety of such a procedure is yet to be established.[136]

Currently there is great interest in the potential use of leptin as a weight-reducing agent. Successful use of this adipose tissue hormone for weight reduction depends first upon identifying leptin injection dose and delivery parameters effective in overcoming the leptin resistance characteristic of obese persons. Moreover, unlike fenfluramine, the appetite-inhibiting effect of leptin appears to be continuous; assuming that resistance to leptin does not reappear following weight loss, weight-maintenance doses of leptin will have to be carefully titrated to balance caloric intake with caloric expenditure. Also, unlike fenfluramine, it is not clear that leptin alters energy expenditure in lean or obese humans.[137] Like fenfluramine, however, cessation of treatment with leptin in rodents is followed by rapid weight regain.[138] Therefore, long-term treatment with the hormone will be required to maintain reduced body weight. The development of leptin-like agonists that can be taken orally will make this prospect much more appealing.

CONCLUSION

The framework for considering the nature of body weight regulation presented in this chapter is flexible and inclusive, updating old hypotheses, and further developing current ones by adding new information about the mechanisms and products in these regulatory systems. By using the "big picture" approach to understand the integration of the various mechanisms that affect energy balance, the practitioner is armed with a background to explain why a specific diet, drug, or other intervention does not produce the result desired by each client. At the same time, maintaining weight and preventing weight gain appear to be both understandable and practical.

ACKNOWLEDGMENT

Preparation of this chapter was supported by Obesity Research Center CORE Grant NIH P30 DK26687.

REFERENCES

1. Astrup A. Obesity and metabolic efficiency. In: *Origins and Consequences of Obesity.* Ciba Foundation Symposia 201. Chichester, England: John Wiley & Sons; 1996:159–173.
2. Bouchard C, Bray GA, eds. *Regulation of Body Weight: Biological and Behavioral Mechanisms.* Chichester, England: John Wiley & Sons; 1996.
3. Keesey RE. A set-point analysis of the regulation of body weight. In: Stunkard AJ, ed. *Obesity.* Philadelphia: WB Saunders Co; 1980:144–165.
4. Billington CJ, Levine AS. Appetite regulation: shedding new light on obesity. *Current Biology.* 1996;6:920–923.

5. Weigle DS. Appetite and the regulation of body composition. *FASEB J.* 1994;8:302–310.

6. Davies L, Marks JL. Role of hypothalamic neuropeptide Y gene expression in body weight regulation. *Am J Physiol.* 1994;266:R1687–R1691.

7. Heyman MB, Young VR, Fuss P, Tsay R, Joseph L, Roberts SB. Underfeeding and body weight regulation in normal-weight young men. *Am J Physiol.* 1992;263:R250–R257.

8. Blundell JE, King NA. Overconsumption as a cause of weight gain: behavioural-physiological interactions in the control of food intake (appetite). In: *Origins and Consequences of Obesity.* Ciba Foundation Symposia 201. Chichester, England: John Wiley & Sons; 1996:138–158.

9. Saltzman E, Roberts SB. The role of energy expenditure in energy regulation: findings from a decade of research. *Nutr Rev.* 1995;53:209–220.

10. Newburgh LH. Obesity: energy metabolism. *Physiol Rev.* 1944;24:18–31.

11. Lichtman SW, Pisarska K, Berman ER, et al. Discrepancy between self-reported and actual caloric intake and exercise in obese subjects. *N Engl J Med.* 1992;327:1893–1898.

12. Drewnowski A. Human preferences for sugar and fat. In: Fernstrom JD, Miller GD, eds. *Appetite and Body Weight Regulation: Sugar, Fat, and Macronutrient Substitutes.* Boca Raton, FL: CRC Press; 1994:137–147.

13. Faith MS, Allison DB, Geliebter A. Emotional eating and obesity. In: *Overweight and Weight Management: A Handbook for Understanding and Practice.* Gaithersburg, MD: Aspen Pub Co; 1977.

14. Mayer J, Thomas DW. Regulation of food intake and obesity. *Science.* 1967;156:328–337.

15. Kopelman PG. Hormones and obesity. *Baillieres Clin Endocrinol Metab.* 1994;8:549–575.

16. Saris WHM. Physical activity and body weight regulation. In: Bouchard C, Bray GA, eds. *Regulation of Body Weight: Biological and Behavioral Mechanisms.* Chichester, England: John Wiley & Sons; 1996:135–148.

17. Geiselman PJ, Novin D. The role of carbohydrates in appetite, hunger, and obesity. *Appetite.* 1982;3:203–223.

18. Van Itallie TB, Smith NS, Quatermain D. Short-term and long- term components in the regulation of food intake: evidence for a modulatory role of carbohydrate status. *Am J Clin Nutr.* 1977;30:742–757.

19. Levin BE, Routh VH. Role of the brain in energy balance and obesity. *Am J Physiol.* 1996;40:R491–R500.

20. Riedy CA, Chavez M, Figlewicz DP, Woods SC. Central insulin enhances sensitivity to cholecystokinin. *Physiol Behav.* 1995;58:755–760.

21. Wirtshafter D, Davis JD. Set points, settling points, and the control of body weight. *Physiol Behav.* 1977;19:75–78.

22. Stellar E. The physiology of motivation. *Psychol Rev.* 1954;61:5–22.

23. Grossman SP. Contemporary problems concerning our understanding of brain mechanisms that regulate food intake and body weight. In: Stunkard AJ, Stellar E, eds. *Eating and Its Disorders.* New York: Raven Press; 1984:5–13.

24. Hoebel BG, Hernandez L. Basic neural mechanisms of feeding and weight regulation. In: Stunkard AJ, Wadden TA, eds. *Obesity: Theory and Therapy.* 2nd ed. New York: Raven Press; 1993:43–62.

25. Leibowitz SF, Hoebel BG. Behavioral neuroscience and obesity. In Bray GA, Bouchard C, James WPT, eds. *The Handbook of Obesity.* New York: Marcel Dekker; in press.

26. Sclafani A, Kirchgessner AL. The role of the medial hypothalamus in the control of food intake: an update. In Ritter RC, Ritter S, Barnes CD, eds. *Feeding Behavior: Neural and Humoral Controls.* New York: Academic Press; 1986:27–66.

27. Leibowitz SF, Roosin P, Rosenn M. Chronic norepinephrine injection into the hypothalamic paraventricular nucleus produces hyperphagia and increased body weight in the rat. *Pharmacol Biochem Behav.* 1984;21:801–808.

28. Leibowitz SF, Brown LL. Histochemical and pharmacological analysis of catecholaminergic projections to the perifornical hypothalamus in relation to feeding inhibition. *Brain Res.* 1980;201:315–345.

29. Myers RD, McCaleb ML. Feeding: satiety signal from intestine triggers brain's noradrenergic mechanism. *Science.* 1980;209:1035–1037.

30. Stanley BG, Schwartz DH, Hernandez L, Hoebel BG, Leibowitz SF. Patterns of extracellular norepinephrine in the paraventricular hypothalamus: relationship to circadian rhythm and deprivation-induced eating behavior. *Life Sci.* 1989;45:275–282.

31. Leibowitz SF, Weiss GF, Yee F, Tretter JB. Noradrenergic innervation of the paraventricular nucleus: specific role in control of carbohydrate ingestion. *Brain Res Bull.* 1985;14:561–567.

32. Hoebel BG. Neuroscience and motivation: pathways and peptides that define motivation. In: Atkinson RC, Herrnstein RJ, Lindzey G, Luce RD, eds. *Steven's Handbook of Experimental Psychology.* 2nd ed. New York: John Wiley & Sons; 1988:547–625.

33. Bai FL, Yamano M, Shiotani Y, et al. An arcuato-paraventricular and dorsomedial hypothalamic neuropeptide Y-containing system which lacks noradrenaline in the rat. *Brain Res.* 1985;331:172–175.

34. Sahu A, Kalra SP. Neuropeptidergic regulation of feeding behavior: neuropeptide Y. *Trends Endocrinol Metab.* 1993;4:217–224.

35. Leibowitz SF. Brain neuropeptide Y: an integrator of endocrine, metabolic and behavioral processes. *Brain Res Bull.* 1991;27:333–337.

36. Billington CJ, Briggs JE, Grace M, Levine AS. Effects of intracerebroventricular injection of neuropeptide Y on energy metabolism. *Am J Physiol.* 1991;260:R321–R327.

37. Egawa M, Yoshimatsu H, Bray GA. Neuropeptide Y suppresses sympathetic activity to interscapular brown adipose tissue in rats. *Am J Physiol.* 1991;260:R328–R334.

38. Valet P, Berlan M, Beauville M, Crampes F, Montastruc JL, Lafontan M. Neuropeptide Y and peptide YY inhibit lipolysis in human and dog fat cells through a pertussis toxin-sensitive G protein. *J Clin Invest.* 1990;85:291–295.

39. Billington CJ, Briggs JE, Harker S, Grace M, Levine AS. Neuropeptide Y in hypothalamic paraventricular nucleus: a center coordinating energy metabolism. *Am J Physiol.* 1994;266:R1765–R1770.

40. Stanley BG, Kyrkouli SE, Lampert S, Leibowitz SF. Neuropeptide Y chronically injected into the hypothalamus: a powerful neurochemical inducer of hyperphagia and obesity. *Peptides.* 1986;7:1189–1192.

41. Kyrkouli SE, Stanley BG, Hutchinson R, Seirafi RD, Leibowitz SF. Peptide-amine interactions in the hypothalamic paraventricular nucleus: analysis of galanin and neuropeptide Y in relation to feeding. *Brain Res.* 1990;521:185–191.

42. Smith BK, York DA, Bray GA. Chronic cerebroventricular galanin does not induce sustained hyperphagia or obesity. *Peptides.* 1994;15:1267–1272.

43. Leibowitz SF. Brain peptides and obesity: pharmacologic treatment. *Obesity Res.* 1995;3(suppl 4):573S–589S.

44. Simansky KJ. Serotonin and the structure of satiation. In: Smith GP, Gibbs J, eds. *Satiety: Structure and Mechanisms.* London: Oxford University Press; in press.

45. Fernstrom JD. The effect of dietary macronutrients on brain serotonin formation. In: Fernstrom JD, Miller GD, eds. *Appetite and Body Weight Regulation: Sugar, Fat, and Macronutrient Substitutes.* Boca Raton, FL: CRC Press; 1994:51–62.

46. Levine AS, Billington CJ. Peptides in regulation of energy metabolism and body weight. In: Bouchard C, Bray GA, eds. *Regulation of Body Weight: Biological and Behavioral Mechanisms.* Chichester, England: John Wiley & Sons; 1996:179–191.

47. Corp ES, Melville LD, Greenberg D, Gibbs J, Smith GP. Effect of fourth ventricular neuropeptide Y and peptide YY on ingestive and other behaviors. *Am J Physiol.* 1990;259:R317–R323.

48. Schwartz MW, Seeley RJ, Campfield LA, Burn P, Baskin DG. Identification of targets of leptin action in rat hypothalamus. *J Clin Invest.* 1996;98:1101–1106.

49. Turton MD, O'Shea D, Gunn I, et al. A role for glucagon-like peptide-1 in the central regulation of feeding. *Nature.* 1995;379:69–72.

50. Spina M, Merlo-Pich E, Chan RKW, et al. Appetite-suppressing effects of urocortin, a CRF-related neuropeptide. *Science.* 1996;273:1561–1563.

51. Fan W, Boston BA, Kesterson RA, Hruby VJ, Cone RD. Role of melanocortinergic neurons in feeding and the *agouti* obesity syndrome. *Nature.* 1997;385:165–168.

52. Cannon WB, Washburn AL. An explanation of hunger. *Am J Physiol.* 1912;29:441–454.

53. Stunkard AJ, Fox S. The relationship of gastric motility and hunger: a summary of the evidence. *Psychosom Med.* 1971;33:123–134.

54. Van Itallie TB, VanderWeele DA. The phenomenon of satiety. In: Bjorntorp P, Cairella M, Howard AN, eds. *Recent Advances in Obesity Research.* London: John Libbey & Co Ltd; 1981;3:278–289.

55. Phillips RJ, Powley TL. Gastric volume rather than nutrient content inhibits food intake. *Am J Physiol.* 1996;40:R766–R779.

56. McHugh PR, Moran TH. The stomach: a conception of its dynamic role in satiety. In: Epstein AN, Sprague J, eds. *Progress in Psychobiology and Physiological Psychology.* New York: Academic Press; 1985;2:197–232.

57. Mei N. Sensory structures in the viscera. In: Ottoson D, ed. *Progress in Sensory Physiology.* Berlin: Springer-Verlag; 1983:1–42.

58. Schwartz GJ, Moran TH. CCK elicits and modulates vagal afferent activity arising from gastric and duodenal sites. *Ann NY Acad Sci.* 1994;713:121–128.

59. Smith GP, Gibbs J. Satiating effect of cholecystokinin. *Ann NY Acad Sci.* 1994;713:236–241.

60. Pi-Sunyer FX, Kissileff HR, Thornton J, Smith GP. C-terminal octapeptide of cholecystokinin decreases food intake in obese men. *Physiol Behav.* 1982;29:627–630.

61. Reidelberger RD, O'Rourke MF. Potent cholecystokinin antagonist L 364718 stimulates food intake in rats. *Am J Physiol.* 1989;257:R1512–R1518.

62. Moran TH, Ameglio PJ, Schwartz GJ, McHugh PR. Blockade of type A, not type B, CCK receptors attenuates satiety actions of exogenous and endogenous CCK. *Am J Physiol.* 1992;262:R46–R50.

63. Wank SA, Pisegna JR, De Weerth A. Cholecystokinin receptor family. Molecular cloning, structure and functional expression in rat, guinea pig, and human. In: Reeve JR, Eysselein V, Solomon TE, Go TLW, eds. *Cholecystokinin. Ann NY Acad Sci.* 1994;713:49–66.

64. Funakoshi A, Miyaska K, Shinozaki H, et al. An animal model of congenital defect of gene expression of CCK-A receptor. *Biochem Biophys Res Comm.* 1995;210:787–796.

65. Gibbs J, Smith GP. Effects of brain-gut peptides on satiety. In: Bjorntorp P, Brodoff BN, eds. *Obesity.* Philadelphia: J.B. Lippincott Company; 1992:399–410.

66. Muurahainen NE, Kissileff HR, Pi-Sunyer FX. Intravenous infusion of bombesin reduces food intake in humans. *Am J Physiol.* 1993;264:R350–R354.

67. Stuckey JA, Gibbs J, Smith GP. Neural disconnection of gut from brain blocks bombesin-induced satiety. *Peptides.* 1985;6:1249.

68. Geary N. Pancreatic glucagon signals postprandial satiety. *Neurosci Biobehav Rev.* 1990; 14:323–338.

69. Langhans W, Zieger U, Scharrer E, Geary N. Stimulation of feeding in rats by intraperitoneal injection of antibodies to glucagon. *Science.* 1982;218:894–896.

70. Erlanson-Albertsson C, Jie M, Okada S, York DA, Bray GA. Pancreatic procolipase propeptide enterostatin specifically inhibits fat intake. *Physiol Behav.* 1991;49:1191–1194.

71. Novin D, VanderWeele DA. Visceral mechanisms in feeding: there is more to regulation than the hypothalamus. In: Sprague J, Epstein AN, eds. *Progress in Psychobiology and Physiological Psychology.* New York: Academic Press; 1976:193–241.

72. Niijima A. Glucose-sensitive afferent nerve fibers in the liver and their role in food intake and blood glucose regulation. *J Auton Nerv Syst.* 1983;9:207–216.

73. Russek M. Current status of the hepatostatic theory of food intake control. *Appetite.* 1981;2:137–143.

74. Scharrer E, Lutz TA, Rossi R. Coding of metabolic information by hepatic sensors controlling food intake. In: Shimazu T, ed. *Liver Innervation.* London: John Libbey & Co; 1996:381–388.

75. Friedman MI, Stricker EM. The physiological psychology of hunger: a physiological perspective. *Psychol Rev.* 1976;83:409–431.

76. Stricker EM, Rowland N, Saller CF, Friedman MI. Homeostatis during hypoglycemia: central control of adrenal secretion and peripheral control of feeding. *Science.* 1977;196:79–81.

77. Friedman MI, Rawson NE. Fuel metabolism and appetite control. In: Fernstrom JD, Miller GD, eds. *Appetite and Body Weight Regulation: Sugar, Fat, and Macronutrient Substitutes.* Boca Raton, FL: CRC Press; 1994:63–76.

78. Tordoff MG, Rawson N, Friedman MI. 2,5-Anhydro-D-mannitol acts in liver to initiate feeding. *Am J Physiol.* 1991;261:R283–R288.

79. Langhans W, Scharrer E. Evidence for a vagally mediated satiety signal derived from hepatic fatty acid oxidation. *J Auton Nerv Syst.* 1987;18:13–18.

80. Rawson NE, Ulrich PM, Friedman MI. Fatty acid oxidation modulates the eating response to the fructose analogue 2,5-anhydro-D-mannitol. *Am J Physiol.* 1996;40:R144–R148.

81. Novin D. The integration of visceral information in the control of feeding. *J Auton Nerv Syst.* 1983;9:233–245.

82. Kennedy GC. The role of depot fat in the hypothalamic control of food intake in the rat. *Proc R Soc Lond.* 1953;140:578–592.

83. Liebelt RA, Bordelon CB, Liebelt AG. The adipose tissue system and food intake. *Prog Physiol Psych.* 1973;5:211–252.

84. Faust IM, Johnson PR, Hirsch J. Adipose tissue regeneration following lipectomy. *Science.* 1977;197:391–393.

85. Rosell S, Belfrage E. Blood circulation in adipose tissue. *Physiol Rev.* 1979;59:1078–1104.

86. Carpenter RG, Grossman SP. Plasma fat metabolites and hunger. *Physiol Behav.* 1983;30:57–63.

87. Zhang Y, Proenca R, Maffei M, Barone M, Leopold L, Friedman JM. Positional cloning of the mouse *obese* gene and its human homologue. *Nature.* 1994;372:425–432.

88. Frederich RC, Hamann A, Anderson S, Lollmann B, Lowell BB, Flier JS. Leptin levels reflect body lipid content in mice: evidence for diet-induced resistance to leptin action. *Nature Med.* 1995;1:1311–1314.

89. Stephens TW, Basinski M, Bristow PK, et al. The role of neuropeptide Y in the antiobesity action of the *obese* gene product. *Nature.* 1995;377:530–532.

90. Pelleymounter MA, Cullen MJ, Baker MB, et al. Effects of the *obese* gene product on body weight regulation in *ob/ob* mice. *Science.* 1995;269:540–543.

91. Halaas JL, Gajiwala KS, Maffei M, et al. Weight-reducing effects of the plasma protein encoded by the *obese* gene. *Science.* 1995;269:543–546.

92. Considine RV, Sinha MK, Heiman ML, et al. Serum immunoreactive-leptin concentrations in normal-weight and obese humans. *N Engl J Med.* 1996;334:292–295.

93. Hamann A, Matthaei S. Regulation of energy balance by leptin. *Exp Clin Endocrinol Diabetes.* 1996;104:293–300.

94. Chua SC, Chung WK, Chung WK, et al. Phenotypes of mouse *diabetes* and rat *fatty* due to mutations in the OB (leptin) receptor. *Science.* 1996;271:994–996.

95. Caro JF, Kolaczynski JW, Nyce MR, et al. Decreased cerebrospinal-fluid/serum leptin ratio in obesity: a possible mechanism for leptin resistance. *Lancet.* 1996;348:159–161.

96. Hotamisligil GS, Shargill NS, Spiegelman BM. Adipose expression of tumor necrosis factor-alpha: direct role in obesity-linked insulin resistance. *Science.* 1993;259:87–91.

97. Kern PA, Saghizadeh M, Ong JM, Bosch RJ, Deem R, Simsolo RB. The expression of tumor necrosis factor in human adipose tissue: regulation by obesity, weight loss, and relationship to lipoprotein lipase. *J Clin Invest.* 1995;95:2111–2119.

98. Greenberg AS, Nordan RP, McIntosh J, Calvo JC, Scow RO, Jablons D. Interleukin 6 reduces lipoprotein lipase activity in adipose tissue of mice *in vivo* and in 3T3-L1 adipocytes: a possible role for interleukin 6 in cancer cachexia. *Cancer Res.* 1992;52:4113–4116.

99. Rosen BS, Cook KS, Yaglom J, et al. Adipsin and the alternative pathway of complement in the regulation of energy balance. In: Bray GA, Ricquier D, Spiegelman BM, eds. *Obesity: Towards a Molecular Approach.* New York: Wiley-Liss; 1990:273–287.

100. Vasselli JR, Casey D. Increased responsiveness of Zucker obese rats to the feeding-inhibitory effects of systemically injected TNF-alpha. *FASEB J.* 1996;10:A823.

101. Plata-Salaman CR, Vasselli JR, Sonti G. Differential responsiveness of obese (fa/fa) and lean (Fa/Fa) Zucker rats to cytokine-induced anorexia. *Obes Res.* In press.

102. Xu W, Reed DR, Ding Y, Price RA. Absence of linkage between human obesity and the mouse agouti homologous region (20q11.2) or other markers spanning chromosome 20q. *Obes Res.* 1995;3:559–562.

103. Maffei M, Stoffel M, Barone M, et al. Absence of mutations in the human *OB* gene in obese/diabetic subjects. *Diabetes.* 1996;45:679–682.

104. Reed DR, Ding Y, Xu W, Cather C, Price RA. Human obesity does not segregate with the chromosomal regions of Prader-Willi, Bardet-Biedl, Cohen, Borjeson or Wilson-Turner syndromes. *Int J Obes.* 1995;19:599–603.

105. Schwartz RS, Brunzell JD. Increase of adipose tissue lipoprotein lipase activity after weight loss. *J Clin Invest.* 1981;67:1425–1429.

106. Kern PA, Ong JM, Saffari B, Carty J. The effects of weight loss on the activity and expression of adipose-tissue lipoprotein lipase in very obese humans. *N Engl J Med.* 1990;322:1053–1059.

107. Eckel RH, Yost TJ. Weight reduction increases adipose tissue lipoprotein lipase responsiveness in obese women. *J Clin Invest.* 1987;80:992–997.

108. Faust IM, Johnson PR, Stern JS, Hirsch J. Diet-induced adipocyte number increases in adult rats: a new model for obesity. *Am J Physiol.* 1978;235:E279–E286.

109. Hill JO, Dorton J, Sykes MN, DiGirolamo M. Reversal of dietary obesity is influenced by its duration and severity. *Int J Obes.* 1989;13:711–722.

110. Vasselli JR, Cleary MP, Jen KC, Greenwood MRC. The development of food motivated behavior in free-feeding and food-restricted Zucker fatty (fa/fa) rats. *Physiol Behav.* 1980;25:565–574.

111. Schwartz MW, Figlewicz DP, Baskin DG, Woods SC, Porte D Jr. Insulin in the brain: a hormonal regulator of energy balance. *Endocrine Rev.* 1992;13:387–414.

112. Woods SC, Chavey M, Park CR, et al. The evaluation of insulin as a metabolic signal influencing behavior via the brain. *Neurosci Biobehav Rev.* 1996;20:139–144.

113. Bagdade JD, Bierman EL, Porte D Jr. The significance of basal insulin levels in the evaluation of the insulin response to glucose in diabetic and nondiabetic subjects. *J Clin Invest.* 1967;46:1549–1557.

114. Brief DJ, Davis JD. Reduction of food intake and body weight by chronic intraventricular insulin infusion. *Brain Res Bull.* 1984;12:571–575.

115. Sipols AJ, Baskin DG, Schwartz MW. Effect of intracerebroventricular insulin infusion on diabetic hyperphagia and hypothalamic neuropeptide gene expression. *Diabetes.* 1995;44:147–151.

116. Figlewicz DP, Dorsa DM, Stein LJ, et al. Brain and liver insulin binding is decreased in Zucker rats carrying the "fa" gene. *Endocrinology.* 1985;117:1537–1543.

117. Sahu A, Dube MG, Phelps CP, Sninsky CA, Kalra PS, Kalra SP. Insulin and insulin-like growth factor II suppress neuropeptide Y release from the nerve terminals in the paraventricular nucleus: a putative hypothalamic site for energy homeostasis. *Endocrinology.* 1995;136:5718–5724.

118. York DA. Central regulation of appetite and autonomic activity by CRH, glucocorticoids and stress. *Prog Neuro Endocr Immunol.* 1992;5:153–165.

119. Bray GA. Weight homeostasis. *Ann Rev Med.* 1991;42:205–216.

120. Bray GA. Obesity, a disorder of nutrient partitioning: the MONA LISA hypothesis. *J Nutr.* 1991;121:1146–1162.

121. Leibowitz SF, Roland CR, Hor L. Noradrenergic feeding elicited via the paraventricular nucleus is dependent upon circulating corticosterone. *Physiol Behav.* 1984;32:857–864.

122. Jeanrenaud B, Halimi S, vandeWerve G. Neuro-endocrine disorders seen as triggers of the triad: obesity-insulin resistance-abnormal glucose tolerance. *Diab Metab Rev.* 1985;1:261–291.

123. Lutz TA, Del Prete E, Scharrer E. Reduction of food intake in rats by intraperitoneal injection of low doses of amylin. *Physiol Behav.* 1994;55:891–895.

124. Krahn DD, Gosnell BA, Levine AS, Morley JE. Effects of calcitonin gene-related peptide on food intake. *Peptides.* 1984;5:861–864.

125. Lutz TA, Geary N, Szabady MM, Del Prete E, Scharrer E. Amylin decreases meal size in rats. *Physiol Behav.* 1995;58:1197–1202.

126. Pi-Sunyer FX, Segal KR. Relationship of diet and exercise. In: Kinney JM, Tucker HN, eds. *Energy Metabolism: Tissue Determinants and Cellular Corollaries.* New York: Raven Press; 1992:187–210.

127. Pi-Sunyer FX, Woo R. Effect of exercise on food intake in human subjects. *Am J Clin Nutr.* 1985;42:983–990.

128. Levitsky DA, Troiano R. Metabolic consequences of fenfluramine for the control of body weight. *Am J Clin Nutr.* 1992;55:167S–172S.

129. Levitsky DA, Strupp BJ, Lupoli J. Tolerance to anorectic drugs: pharmacological or artifactual. *Pharmacol Biochem Behav.* 1981;14:661–667.

130. Stunkard AJ. Regulation of body weight and its implications for the treatment of obesity. In: Carruba MO, Blundell JE, eds. *Pharmacology of Eating Disorders: Theoretical and Clinical Developments.* New York: Raven Press; 1986:101–116.

131. Evens P, Nicholidais S. Dextrofenfluramine increases energy cost of muscular effort. *Pharmacol Biochem Behav.* 1986;24:647–655.

132. Levitsky DA, Schuster J, Stallone D, Strupp BJ. Modulation of the thermogenic effect of nutrients by fenfluramine. *Int J Obes.* 1986;10:169–173.

133. Brindley DN. Phenylethylamines and their effects on the synthesis of fatty acids, triacylglycerols and phospholipids. In: Curtis-Prior PB, ed. *Biochemical Pharmacology of Obesity.* Amsterdam: Elsevier; 1983:285–308.

134. Schwid SR, Hirvonen MD, Keesey RE. Nicotine effects on body weight: a regulatory perspective. *Am J Clin Nutr.* 1992;55:878–884.

135. Guy-Grand B. Clinical studies of dexfenfluramine: from past to future. *Obes Res.* 1995;3(suppl 4):491S–496S.

136. Munro JF, Scott C, Hodge J. Appraisal of the clinical value of serotoninergic drugs. *Am J Clin Nutr.* 1992;55:189S–192S.

137. Kennedy A, Gettys TW, Watson P, et al. The metabolic significance of leptin in humans: gender-based differences in relationship to adiposity, insulin sensitivity, and energy expenditure. *J Clin Endocrin Metab.* 1997; in press.

138. Campfield LA, Smith FJ, Guisez Y, Devos R, Burn P. Recombinant mouse OB protein: evidence for a peripheral signal linking adiposity and central neural networks. *Science.* 1995;269:546–549.

CHAPTER 8

Energy Metabolism and Thermogenesis in Human Obesity

Harvey L. Katzeff

INTRODUCTION

Over the past 15 years, there has been a resurgence of research into the metabolic basis of obesity. This renewed interest is based on new techniques for the noninvasive measurement of energy expenditure and research indicating that the regulation of body weight has a significant genetic component. Previously, investigators had questioned whether the genetic and environmental causes of weight gain could be separated, and initiated studies that included comparisons of the relative body fat of identical and fraternal twins, and adoption studies comparing the relative weight of offspring to both their biological and adoptive parents. The twin studies report that identical twins raised together or apart have approximately half the variation in body weight of fraternal twins under the same conditions.[1] The adoption studies revealed that adopted offspring were more likely to be similar in body mass index (BMI) to their biological parents than to their adoptive parents.[2,3] Body fat distribution is also under genetic control, and is possibly even more subject to genetic factors than relative fatness.[4]

Although these studies indicate that genetic as well as environmental components may be important in the predisposition to excessive weight gain in humans, they do not reveal its pathogenesis. The equation of

$$D \text{ weight} = \text{Energy intake} - \text{Energy expenditure}$$

is still the basic formula of metabolism. Thus, alterations in either regulation of energy intake (appetite) or energy expenditure or both could account for the predisposition to excessive weight gain in humans.

Researchers have recently discovered a mutation in a purported protein messenger from adipose tissue (leptin) to the satiety center in the hypothalamus of the *ob/ob* mouse, a genetic animal model of obesity.[5] This mutation prevents the protein from either binding to or activating its receptor on the cell surface of neurons that normally function to suppress appetite. This results in excessive food intake and the development of obesity. The discovery of this protein and a similar protein in humans opens new prospects for researchers in physiology and molecular biology to study the regulation of satiety and indicates that genetic abnormalities in regulation of energy intake as well as energy expenditure may exist in humans. This chapter focuses on the regulation of energy metabolism in humans and the alterations in energy expenditure, both primary and secondary, that exist in human obesity.

SUBSTRATE METABOLISM

Since humans metabolize calories constantly but ingest food only intermittently, physiologic mechanisms have developed to store calories in the postprandial period and transport those calories to the viscera during fasting. This section reviews the relationship between the oxidation and storage of carbohydrate (CHO), and fat (Figure 8–1).

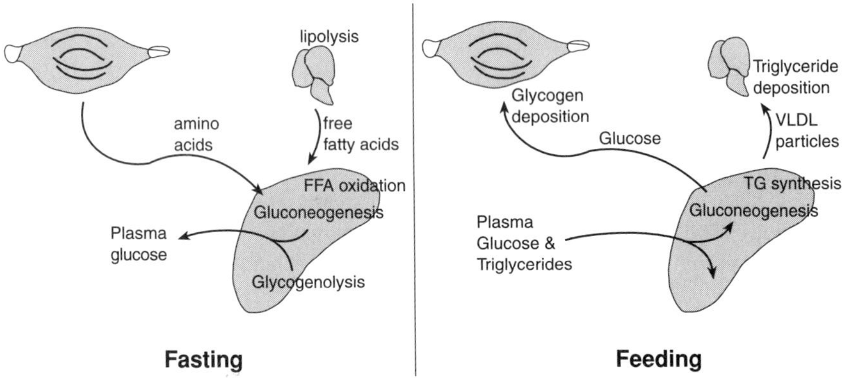

Fasting   **Feeding**

Figure 8–1 The left panel depicts the major fuel sources for hepatic glucose production during fasting. Both amino acids from muscle and free fatty acids from adipose tissue are utilized by the liver in the presence of glucagon and a decrease in insulin. The right panel depicts the transport of glucose and triglyceride synthesized in the liver to storage sites in muscle and adipose tissue. The presence of increased insulin levels are required for these processes.

Glucose

Glucose may be the most important metabolic fuel because it is the obligate fuel for oxidation by the brain. In order to maintain an adequate supply of glucose for the brain, the blood glucose level is maintained within a stable range (60 to 120 mg/dl). In the postprandial period, the major source of glucose in the blood is absorption of carbohydrates via the portal vein. This glucose load is either stored as glycogen in liver and skeletal muscle or oxidized as a fuel. However, the storage of glucose as glycogen is inefficient since 9 mg of water are required for each 1 mg of glycogen stored. Thus, the total glycogen stored in the body is only 100 gm or 400 kcal. This amount of glycogen will last through less than 24 hours of fasting if no adaptation to starvation occurs.

The liver is the major regulator of glucose metabolism. During the postprandial period, all of the ingested glucose passes through the liver via the portal vein before entering the peripheral circulation. Approximately 30% to 50% of glucose is taken up by the liver where it is converted to glycogen in response to the postprandial rise in insulin.[6] If glycogen is directly synthesized from glucose, its energy costs are approximately 5%.[6] However, recent work from Magnusson et al[7] suggests that at least a third of glycogen stores are produced from three carbon glucose precursors, which significantly increases the metabolic cost of glycogen storage.

During the postprandial rise in blood glucose, an increase in the serum insulin level is required to stimulate the necessary increase in glucose uptake in both skeletal muscle and adipose tissue. This rise in serum insulin is necessary to maintain a normal serum glucose level. Individuals who are insulin resistant have a reduced glucose uptake in skeletal muscle in response to the normal rise in serum insulin in the postprandial period. In response to this defect, insulin levels rise to elevated levels to maintain a normal glucose uptake. Although individuals can be insulin resistant in respect to cellular glucose uptake, they are not resistant to stimulatory effects of insulin on protein or triglyceride synthesis. The mechanisms for this dichotomy in insulin action are unclear but abnormalities in the postinsulin receptor second messenger system are thought to be involved.[8] Due to the selective resistance to glucose uptake only, individuals who are insulin resistant may be more efficient at storing calories as fat in the postprandial period as hypothesized and described in greater detail below.

During fasting, the only source of glucose is via its release into the circulation from the liver. This occurs when the serum insulin concentration falls and the plasma concentration of glucagon increases. In response to these hormonal changes, there is stimulation of glycogenolysis and gluconeogenesis. The source of three carbon chain precursors for gluconeogenesis are ketone bodies from fatty acid oxidation and the amino acid alanine, which is transported from skeletal muscle during protein catabolism.[9]

Obese individuals are almost invariably insulin resistant and their insulin sensitivity usually improves dramatically with weight loss.[10] In many cases, insulin resistance is secondary to obesity and may not be a causative agent. Reaven[11] has suggested that there are many individuals who are insulin resistant prior to obesity and who may be at risk for obesity, diabetes mellitus, hypertension, and hyperlipidemia, which together constitute the so-called Syndrome X or Metabolic Syndrome. Recently, studies of transgenic mice who have an increased glucose sensitivity due to an increased number of glucose transporters in muscle show lower weight gain during high-fat diets than normal rats.[12] This suggests that improvement in insulin sensitivity in muscle should be an important goal in the treatment of obesity and non–insulin-dependent diabetes mellitus. Several new classes of oral hypoglycemic agents increase glucose uptake in muscle and show promise to become useful drugs in the treatment of insulin-resistant states.

Fatty Acid Metabolism

The regulation of fatty acid metabolism is critical for long-term survival and prevention of obesity. Two schools of thought have developed in respect to central nervous system regulation of adipose tissue mass. The first is that there is no direct regulation of fat mass by the central nervous system, and that total fat mass is dependent on the energy balance of an individual. However, individuals with hypothalamic tumors, genetic disorders such as Prader Willi syndrome, and traumatic or surgical lesions of the hypothalamus reveal impaired satiety with uncontrolled eating and a resulting excessive weight gain.[13] These uncommon medical conditions confirm that there is a satiety center that can regulate energy intake. Using these findings and animal data, other researchers have theorized that there are metabolic signals from fat cells to the satiety center that have a regulatory effect on appetite. Leptin, a protein believed to be a satiety signal, may be the first of several signals derived from adipose tissue to be identified that regulate both satiety and hunger.[14]

Net fat storage in fat cells occurs only during the postprandial period and the metabolic cost of storage is dependent on the method of fatty acid storage. The most efficient form of fat storage processing (requiring ~3% of total calories being stored) is the ingestion of long-chain fatty acids that enter the blood via the lymphatic system and bypass the liver. These fatty acids are then directly stored as triglyceride in peripheral adipose tissue. Triglycerides may also be produced from medium-chain fatty acids that are elongated in the liver and then transported as lipoproteins to the adipose tissue. A third mechanism for fatty acid synthesis is the de novo synthesis of fatty acids from glucose. It is uncertain to what extent if any, de novo lipogenesis occurs because it is metabolically very expensive to convert glucose to fat. The energy required for conversion is about 20% of the calories produced as fat.[15]

Because fatty acid oxidation produces only 7 carbon dioxide (CO_2) molecules for every 10 oxygen (O_2) molecules and glucose oxidation produces 10 carbon dioxide molecules for each 10 oxygen molecules consumed, the relative ratio of carbon dioxide to oxygen in expired air (respiratory quotient) can provide an estimation of the metabolic fuel oxidized. In general, the normal response to a mixed meal is a rise in the respiratory quotient (RQ) for approximately four to six hours. This indicates a net increase in glucose oxidation that is greater than any rise in fatty acid oxidation. Thus, in the postprandial period, there is a relative sparing of fatty acid oxidation, which allows for the net storage of fat calories. This is balanced by a decline in the respiratory quotient during fasting, when there is a net increase in fatty acid oxidation and a decline in glucose oxidation.[16]

This concept that diet composition may be important in the efficiency of energy storage has been studied extensively.[16] Two specific questions have been evaluated. The first is whether increasing the fat-to-carbohydrate ratio within a weight-maintenance diet alters weight gain and the second is whether overfeeding fat vs carbohydrate produces a greater weight gain. The first question is relevant to the situation in the United States because the percentage of fat in the diet has increased from 32% to 45% in this century and is associated with a marked increase in obesity.[17] Using indirect calorimetry and the respiratory quotient, investigators have found that the percent of fat oxidation increases or decreases proportionally in response to an increase or decrease in fat content of the diet. If high-fat diets induce obesity, they probably do so by increasing the calorie content of the diet, not the efficiency of weight gain.[18,19]

The second question, whether overfeeding fat vs carbohydrate induces a greater weight gain, is also controversial and no consensus exists. Data suggest that weight gain in response to fat overfeeding may be greater than carbohydrate overfeeding since the respiratory quotient does not decline with fat overfeeding.[20,21] This indicates that carbohydrate oxidation remains the same or increases despite increased fat intake. If this is the case, then there will be a relative sparing of fat oxidation and greater fat storage compared to overfeeding with carbohydrate alone. Since most people overeat a mixed diet, it is important to note that there is also a rise in the RQ during mixed overfeeding (50% carbohydrate:35% fat:15% protein). These data suggest that there is also a sparing of fat oxidation during mixed calorie overfeeding. It has been suggested that obese individuals are more efficient than lean individuals at sparing fat oxidation in the postprandial period, but the data do not reveal any differences between lean and obese subjects.[22]

Many of the differences in glucose metabolism in lean and obese individuals can be explained by insulin resistance. The decrease in skeletal muscle glucose uptake after meals may predispose affected individuals to more efficient weight gain after a carbohydrate meal but the effect is relatively small and may account only for a small increase in body weight per year. Alterations in fat metabolism are potentially more consequential. The data suggest that during overfeeding there is a relative sparing of fat oxidation, leaving more fat available for storage. However, the data do not yet appear to implicate a primary abnormality in fat metabolism in obese individuals.

Thermogenesis

Twenty-four-hour energy expenditure is the summation of numerous cellular processes. A portion of these processes, such as the Na^+/K^+ pump are required to maintain cellular integrity, and their energy costs are probably fixed. Other metabolic processes, such as digestion, storage of ingested calories, and skeletal muscle contraction, are variable. Physiologists have attempted to separate fixed and variable rates of energy expenditure into separate components. The well known basal or resting metabolic rate (BMR or RMR) is the rate of caloric expenditure of a supine individual after an overnight fast who is performing no obvious muscle work. The energy cost of digesting, transporting, and storing ingesting calories is called the thermic effect of food (TEF) and, depending on the type and size of meal ingested, the TEF may elevate the metabolic rate for four to eight hours. The energy cost of skeletal muscle contraction, or thermic effect of exercise (TEE), is based upon the work performed and also includes an increase in cardiac output and respiratory muscle effort for breathing.

The question of whether spontaneously or experimentally obese individuals expend calories at a lower rate than lean individuals has been discussed for many decades. A fascinating hypothesis for the development of obesity was proposed by the geneticist J.V. Neel in 1962.[23] He proposed that populations that had experienced frequent famines would select out for survival individuals who are metabolically most efficient, i.e., who expend the fewest calories and store a greater proportion of ingested calories as fat. When societies industrialized and the food supply became plentiful, weight gain and the incidence of non–insulin-dependent diabetes mellitus would increase. Support for this hypothesis comes from studies of Pima Indians of the Sonora desert of Arizona. These people migrated north from Mexico and have survived the dry, harsh Arizona climate as farmers for many generations. During the 20th century, rates of obesity and non–insulin-dependent diabetes mellitus have soared dramatically to the point where over 70% of the population in the Sacaton reservation are obese and 45% of adults over 40 are diabetic, the highest observed rates in the United States.[24] Recently, the Tarahumara Indians of a remote region in northern Mexico have been studied. These people have a genetic background similar to the Pima but they still live the traditional agricultural lifestyle and eat the traditional diet. Compared to the Pima, rates of obesity and diabetes among the Tarahumara are much lower, providing further support for the importance of environment and genetics in regulation of body weight.[25]

MEASURES OF ENERGY EXPENDITURE

The classic method for measurement of energy expenditure has been indirect calorimetry. This is the measurement of the difference in the quantity of inspired and expired oxygen and carbon dioxide. It is based on the fact that all cellular metabolic processes utilize oxygen as a substrate and the oxidation of fat and carbohydrate produces between 7 and 10 moles of carbon dioxide for each 10 moles of oxygen consumed. Older studies of resting energy expenditure by indirect calorimetry suffered from inconsistent results with the use of a mouthpiece and noseplug.[26] Using more sensitive gas analyzers, a newer technique places a clear plastic or Plexiglas hood ventilated with fresh air over a subject's head, which allows more normal breathing patterns and less hyperventilation and provides more consistent data than the older methods.[26]

Another method of indirect calorimetry is the use of a respiratory chamber. Subjects stay in this sealed room for up to seven days and the oxygen and carbon dioxide content of the air entering and leaving the room is sampled continuously to provide a 24-hour measurement of energy expenditure. Experiments conducted in these rooms have been extremely useful in comparing total energy expenditure to resting or basal metabolic rates.[27]

Another new technique is the measurement of urinary excretion of a single dose of $2H218O$, which uses nonradioactive isotopes of oxygen and hydrogen as water.[28] This method measures the metabolic rate in free-living humans over longer periods of time, approximately 14 days, by measuring the rate of carbon dioxide synthesis. A correction for the average daily respiratory quotient is added, which can reduce the accuracy of the measurement by up to 14%. This technique allows measurements and comparisons to be obtained over much longer time periods than indirect calorimeters allow, and averages variations in daily 24-hour energy expenditure. It has a coefficient of variation of 3% to 5% in experienced laboratories, but cost and technical difficulties in the stable isotope measurements limit its use to the research setting.

Both the respiratory chamber and the double-labeled water methods have allowed investigators to study variability in daily energy expenditure between individuals. Interestingly, individuals of similar age, sex, and size can have a 500 kcal difference in daily energy expenditure even when they are confined to a small room. This difference is due to a marked variability in spontaneous physical movement even when "resting." The authors have named this difference the "fidget factor" and it may be an important component of energy expenditure.[29]

Resting Metabolic Rate

If the basal or resting metabolic rate (RMR) is the measurement of obligate cellular thermogenesis with as little spontaneous muscle activity as possible, then the RMR should be proportional to the metabolically active cell mass. The metabolically active cell mass has been equated to be proportional to lean body mass or fat-free mass since the adipose cell has a much lower rate of oxygen consumption than other tissue. Numerous studies have attempted to measure the relationship between body composition and energy expenditure.[30–32] Ravussin et al[32] measured resting energy expenditure and assessed body composition by underwater weight on 249 nondiabetic individuals and reported that the resting energy expenditure was directly correlated to fat-free mass with an r2 of 0.82, indicating that 82% of the variation in resting energy expenditure was accounted for by fat-free mass. This relationship held for both men and women and lean and obese volunteers.

One explanation for the variability in resting energy expenditure is that in addition to fat-free mass, other factors such as thyroid hormone levels, sympathetic nervous system activity, and caloric intake may be important regulators of metabolic rate.[33] These factors also increase during periods of overfeeding and decrease during caloric restriction.[34,35] The portion of resting or basal metabolic rate that is dependent on these factors has been called adaptive thermogenesis. If differences exist in the basal metabolic rate (BMR) or resting metabolic rate (RMR) of obese and lean individuals, alterations in adaptive thermogenesis may be the reason (Figure 8–2).[22,36,39]

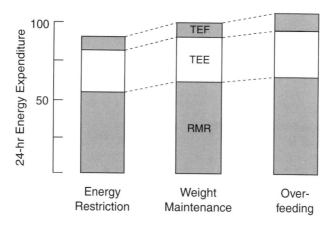

Figure 8–2 The relative change in 24-hour energy expenditure in response to over- and underfeeding. The components are RMR (resting metabolic rate), TEE (thermic effect of exercise), and TEF (thermic effect of food). There are alterations in RMR in response to dietary changes, which are out of proportion to dietary-induced changes in lean body mass. The TEF is proportional to the level of caloric intake.

The role of thyroid hormones in the regulation of resting metabolic rate has been recognized for many years but the actual cellular thermogenic processes governed by thyroid hormones are still a matter of debate and beyond the scope of this chapter. However, the serum level of triiodothyronine (T3) is increased during overfeeding and decreased during calorie restriction in both lean and obese individuals.[34] Evidence indicates that the nutritional rise and fall of this hormone is responsible for a portion of the rise and fall in RMR during over- and undernutrition.[36] There does not appear to be any significant abnormality in the nonthyroidal synthesis of T3 in obese volunteers.[36] The sympathetic nervous system is also an important regulator of RMR. Studies in both humans and rodents reveal that the central nervous system increases or decreases the rate of release of norepinephrine in response to alterations in the level of caloric intake.[37]

For many years, researchers have asked whether obese individuals have a reduced resting or basal metabolic rate. The answer is complex for several reasons. What is the appropriate metabolic yardstick to compare lean and obese individuals of the same height, age, and sex? If no yardstick is used then most studies show that the weight-stable obese individual has a greater absolute metabolic rate when compared to an average-weight individual of the same height, age, and sex.[38] When the metabolic rate is divided by fat-free mass these differences disappear and lean and obese individuals appear to have similar relative metabolic rates.[39] However, this approach does not completely answer the question since the metabolic rates of obese individuals were not measured prior to their weight gain.

In longitudinal studies of weight gain and the resting metabolic rate of Pima Indians, those subjects whose resting metabolic rates were initially lower than normal experienced weight gain and a resultant increase in RMR.[40] It is possible that in these individuals, weight gain was a response to a low RMR, a response to raise the RMR to "normal." The Vermont studies of experimental obesity are further evidence that spontaneously obese individuals may be different in respect to their energy expenditure. In the early 1970s, prisoners in Vermont participated in a series of overfeeding experiments designed to increase body weight by 20% or greater. The daily calorie intake to produce this weight gain was extremely variable (4000 to 9000 kcal/day) but more interestingly, the calorie requirement to maintain the excess weight was 2700 kcal/m2/day, which was markedly greater than that of the spontaneously obese or normal population (1800 kcal/m2/day).[41] These studies provide important evidence that spontaneously obese individuals may use their weight gain to increase their daily energy expenditure and maintain a new stable body weight. They also suggest that spontaneously lean individuals may have an adaptive mechanism to prevent excessive weight gain by dramatically increasing daily energy expenditure.

The results of a recent study at Rockefeller University are further evidence that obese individuals use excessive weight gain to maintain a normal daily energy expenditure.[42] Investigators measured the metabolic rates of spontaneously obese individuals before and after they had lost 20% of their body weight. At the reduced weight, 24-hour daily energy expenditure was approximately 300 kcal/day less than expected, suggesting that at lower body weights, obese individuals have a decreased daily energy expenditure.

These studies suggest that during periods of weight stability, the resting metabolic rates of obese individuals are similar to those of lean individuals. However, when compared to lean individuals experimentally made obese, or obese individuals who are calorie-restricted to lose weight, spontaneously obese individuals appear to have lower daily energy expenditures.

Thermic Effect of Food

The thermic effect of food (TEF) is an elevation in metabolic rate in response to food intake. It is usually described as a percentage of the absolute increase in calories over the caloric content of the test meal. The duration of the TEF is dependent on both the size and dietary composition of the meal and was originally thought to be secondary only to protein intake. The cost of digesting and metabolizing protein is approximately 25% of its energy content, whereas carbohydrate and fat are approximately 10% and 3%, respectively. The TEF of a mixed meal is approximately 8%.[43] Although the TEF is a relatively small component of the total daily energy expenditure, a 1% decrease in the TEF would be equivalent to 9125 kcal per year in a sedentary 70 kg person. This could lead to a gain in weight of 1 kg of fat if no other adaptation in energy expenditure occurred. Since the metabolic cost of storing fat is lower than the metabolic cost of storing carbohydrate, a change in the dietary composition from a high-carbohydrate diet to a high-fat diet without a change in the total caloric intake could decrease the TEF and promote weight gain.

Studies comparing the thermic effect of food in lean and obese individuals have been difficult to analyze due to the fact that there is no standardization of the test.[44] Considerations in the experimental design for these types of studies include (1) whether a mixed or single-component test meal should be performed; (2) whether the quantity of the meal should be equal for all subjects or based on a proportion of daily energy expenditure; and (3) what time period after the meal is ingested should be used. Despite the problems raised by these questions, many researchers have reported their findings comparing lean and obese individuals.[44] Although there is no consensus, many studies suggest that obese individuals may have a lower rise in metabolic rate in response to a test meal compared to those of normal weight.

The possible explanation for a lower TEF in obese subjects is the fact that obese individuals are insulin resistant and have a lower rate of glucose uptake by skeletal muscle in the postprandial state. Felber and Golay[45] noted that the thermic effect of glucose is lower in obese and non–insulin-dependent diabetic individuals. In addition to glucose uptake, plasma concentration of the thermogenic hormone norepinephrine (NE) rises in response to oral glucose ingestion.[45] Protocols utilizing the euglycemic-hyperinsulinemic clamp technique reveal a lower rate of thermogenesis in insulin-resistant obese subjects compared to lean individuals. This was apparently due to a reduced plasma norepinephrine response to glucose.[46,47] However, this defect may only be secondary to insulin resistance and not present prior to the development of obesity. Whether individuals who are genetically at risk for the development of obesity have an impaired thermic response to a meal before developing obesity is still unknown.

Thermic Effect of Exercise

The component of daily energy expenditure that is most variable for each individual is the calories expended during the day in spontaneous activity and exercise. Estimates of energy expended in physical activity range from 300 kcal/day for sedentary individuals to greater than 5000 kcal/day for athletes in training.[48] Although obese individuals may have differences in RMR and/or TEF, which could account for 200 kcal/day, the variability in the thermic response to exercise could easily mask those differences.

The calories expended in response to a given workload appear to be similar for both lean and obese individuals. Unlike the resting or basal metabolic rate, which is proportional to only the lean body mass, the calories expended in performing work are based upon the total body weight of an individual. It takes twice as many calories for a 200-lb individual to walk 3 mph as it does a 100-lb person. No data suggest that obese individuals are more efficient during exercise but several studies indicate that both their spontaneous physical activity is decreased and that during physical activity there may be an economy of movement in order to perform a specific task, resulting in a lower energy expenditure than predicted.[49,50]

Is there any relationship between thermic response to exercise and food intake? There does appear to be a small interaction between exercise and food intake. Segal et al[51] reported that the thermic response to exercise was greater after a meal (<10 kcal) but the effect is small and is probably not clinically significant.

Of greater interest is the relationship between exercise and the resting metabolic rate. It is well recognized that in addition to the rise in calorie expenditure during exercise, metabolic rate rises for a period of time after completion of a bout of exercise. This rise persists for up to 12 hours and is proportional to the intensity of the exercise.[52] This rise in RMR is thought to be due to replenishment of muscle glycogen stores but is also secondary to alterations in protein metabolism. A response to a single bout of exercise is an increase in protein catabolism followed by an increase in protein synthesis. Because protein synthesis is costly in terms of energy expenditure, this could easily account for an increase in metabolic rate. The rise in metabolic rate in the acute response to a single bout of exercise is probably not significant for obese individuals because the energy expended is less than 100 kcal.

Another important question is whether individuals who perform daily bouts of aerobic exercise maintain a prolonged increase in metabolic rate. There is evidence for an increase in RMR, yet study results do not agree.[48] The comparisons need to be divided for studies where weight is maintained or weight loss was induced. If individuals are exercising daily and maintaining their body weight, there is usually an increase in food intake compared to sedentary controls. The observed increase in RMR could therefore be due to the increase in food intake and not the exercise per se. Another explanation for an increase in RMR is an exercise-induced increase in lean body mass, which will also raise the resting metabolic rate. In individuals who are chronically exercising, the RMR is probably elevated due to differences in body composition and food intake and probably not directly in response to the exercise itself.

The interaction of calorie restriction and daily aerobic exercise is an important area of research since most experts prescribe a combination of exercise and calorie restriction as a treatment of obesity. When obese research volunteers reduced their maintenance caloric intake by 500 kcal/day, the addition of a daily aerobic exercise program produced a greater loss of body weight and body fat than caloric restriction alone.[53] However, when obese volunteers ingested a severely restricted diet (<800 kcal/day) the addition of a 500 kcal/day aerobic exercise program had no additive effect on weight loss or resting metabolic rate. In fact, one study showed further reductions in the RMR.[54] The most reasonable explanation for these provocative findings is that there may be a reduction in the postexercise metabolic rate to maintain a 24-hour daily energy expenditure as during severe calorie restriction alone. Nevertheless, these data indicate that exercise should not be combined with marked calorie restriction to promote weight loss.

The data presented above indicate that thermic response to exercise is the most variable portion of daily energy expenditure and could easily be increased to maintain energy balance by a daily exercise program. However, researchers do not know what factors regulate spontaneous physical activity and whether there is a regulatory mechanism by which individuals increase their spontaneous movement in response to an increase in food intake.

CONCLUSION

Spontaneously obese individuals show many observed differences in energy metabolism and thermogenesis. However, it is still unclear which factors induce obesity and which help maintain obesity. Present knowledge suggests that there may be genetic differences that predispose certain individuals to excessive weight gain in a society where food is generally high-fat and activity is generally sedentary. The question and the challenge for the future: Can a high-fat-consuming, sedentary society overcome energy metabolism predispositions?

REFERENCES

1. Price RA, Gottesman IL. Body fat in identical twins reared apart: roles for genes & environment. *Behav Genet.* 1991;21:1–7.

2. Stunkard AJ, Sorensen TI, Hanis C, et al. An adoption study of human obesity. *N Engl J Med.* 1986;315:128–129.

3. Rice T, Province M, Perusse L, Bouchard C, Rap DC. Cross trait family resemblance for body fat and blood pressure: familial correlates in the Quebec Family Study. *Am J Hum Genet.* 1994;55:1019–1029.

4. Borecki IB, Rice T, Perusse L, Bouchard C, Rao DC. Major gene influence for the propensity to store fat in trunk versus extremity depots: evidence from the Quebec Family Study. *Obes Res.* 1995;3:1–8.

5. Halaas JL, Gajiwala KS, Maffei M, et al. Weight reducing effects of the plasma protein encoded by the obese gene. *Science.* 1995;269:543–546.

6. Pagliassotti MJ, Cherrington AD. Regulation of net hepatic glucose uptake in vivo. *Ann Rev Physiol.* 1992;54:847–860.

7. Magnusson I, Rothman DL, Gerard DP, Katz LD, Sulman GI. Contribution of hepatic glycogenolysis to glucose production in humans in response to a physiologic increase in plasma glucagon production. *Diabetes.* 1995;44:185–189.

8. Howard BV, Klimes I, Vasquez B, Brady D, Nagulesparan M, Unger RH. The antilipolytic action of insulin in obese subjects with resistance to its glucoregulatory action. *J Clin Endocrinol Metab.* 1984;58:544–548.

9. Felig P, Sherwin R. Carbohydrate homeostasis, liver and diabetes. *Progress in Liver Diseases.* 1976;5:149–171.

10. Freidenberg GR, Reichart D, Olefsky JM, Henry RR. Reversibility of defective adipocyte insulin receptor kinase activity in non–insulin-dependent diabetes mellitus. Effect of weight loss. *J Clin Invest.* 1988;82:1398–1406.

11. Reaven GM. Pathophysiology of insulin resistance in human disease. *Physiol Rev.* 1995;75:473–486.

12. Gibbs EM, Stock JL, McCoid SC, Stukenbrok HA, Pessin JE, Stevenson RW. Glycemic improvement in db/db mice by overexpression of the human insulin regulatable glucose transporter (GLUT4). *J Clin Invest.* 1995;95:1512–1518.

13. Yung RT. Color Atlas of obesity. St. Louis, MO: Mosby Year-Book; 1990:37–47.

14. Lindpainter K. Finding an obesity gene—a tail of mice and men. *N Engl J Med.* 1995;332:679–680.

15. Acheson KJ, Schutz Y, Bessard T, Ravussin E, Jequier E, Flatt JP. Nutritional influences on lipogenesis and thermogenesis after a carbohydrate meal. *Am J Physiol.* 1984;246:E62–E70.

16. Westerterp KR. Food quotient, respiratory quotient, and energy balance. *Am J Clin Nutr.* 1993;57:759S–765S.

17. Fabry P. *Feeding Pattern and Nutritional Adaptations.* Prague: Academia; and London: Butterworths; 1969.

18. Lean MEJ, James WPT. Metabolic effects of isoenergetic nutrient exchange over 24 hours in relation to obesity in women. *Int J Obes.* 1988;12:15–27.

19. Abbott WGH, Howard BV, Ruotolo G, Ravussin E. Energy expenditure in humans: effects of dietary fat and carbohydrate. *Am J Physiol.* 1990;258:E347–E51.

20. Dalloso HM, James WPT. Whole body calorimetry in adult man: the effect of fat overfeeding on 24 h energy expenditure. *Br J Nutr.* 1984;52:49–64.

21. Schutz Y, Flatt JP, Jequier E. Failure of dietary fat to promote fat oxidation: a factor in the development of obesity. *Am J Clin Nutr.* 1989;50:307–314.

22. Katzeff HL, O'Connell M, Horton ES, Danforth E Jr, Young JB, Landsberg L. The impact of over- and underfeeding on energy expenditure in lean and obese man: response to graded infusions of norepinephrine. *Metabolism.* 1986;35:166–175.

23. Neel JV. Diabetes mellitus: a thrifty genotype rendered detrimental by "progress"? *Am J Hum Genet.* 1962;14:353–357.

24. Knowler WC, Bennet PH, Hamman RF, Miller M. Diabetes incidence and prevalence in Pima Indians: a 19-fold greater incidence than in Rochester, Minnesota. *Am J Epidemiol.* 1978;108:497–505.

25. Ravussin E, Valencia ME, Esparza J, Bennett PH, Schulz LO. Effects of a traditional lifestyle on obesity in Pima Indians. *Diabetes Care.* 1994;17:1067–1074.

26. Anon. Indirect calorimetry. *Baillieres Clinical Endocrinology & Metabolism.* 1987;1:911–935.

27. Ravussin E, Lillioja S, Anderson TE, Christin L, Bogardus C. Determinants of 24-h energy expenditure in man: methods and results using a respiratory chamber. *J Clin Invest.* 1986;78:1568–1578.

28. Schoeller, DA, Ravussin E, Shultz E, Acheson KJ, Baertschi P, Jequier E. Energy expenditure by double-labeled water: validation in humans and proposed calculation. *Am J Physiol.* 1986;250:R823–R828.

29. Zurlo F, Ferraro RT, Fontvieille AM, Rising R, Bogardus C, Ravussin E. Spontaneous physical activity and obesity: cross-sectional and longitudinal studies in Pima Indians. *Am J Physiol.* 1992;263:E296–E300.

30. Welle S, Forbes GB, Statt M, Barnard RR, Amatruda JM. Energy expenditure under free-living conditions in normal weight and overweight women. *Am J Clin Nutr.* 1992;55:14–21.

31. Prentice AM, Black AE, Coward WA, et al. High levels of energy expenditure in obese women. *Br Med J.* 1986;292:983–987.

32. Ravussin E, Burnard B, Schultz, Y, Jequier E. Twenty-four hour energy expenditure and resting metabolic rate in obese, moderately obese and control subjects. *Am J Clin Nutr.* 1982;35:366–373.

33. Katzeff HL, Daniels RJ. Sympathetic nervous system activity in man. *Int J Obes.* 1985;9(suppl 2):131–139.

34. Danforth E Jr, Burger AG. The impact of nutrition on thyroid hormone physiology and action. *Annu Rev Nutr.* 1989;9:201–227.

35. Kush RD, Young JB, Katzeff HL, et al. Effect of diet on energy expenditure and plasma norepinephrine in lean and obese Pima Indians. *Metabolism.* 1986; 35:1110–1120.

36. Danforth E Jr. The role of thyroid hormones and insulin in the regulation of energy metabolism. *Am J Clin Nutr.* 1983;38:1006–1017.

37. Landsberg L, Young JB. Caloric intake and sympathetic nervous system activity. Implications for blood pressure regulation and thermogenesis. *J Clin Hypertension.* 1986;2:166–171.

38. Ravussin E, Bogardus C. Relationship of genetics, age and physical fitness to daily energy expenditure and fuel utilization. *Am J Clin Nutr.* 1989;49(suppl 5):968–975.

39. Ravussin E. Energy metabolism in obesity: studies in the Pima Indians. *Diabetes Care.* 1993;16(suppl 1):232–238.

40. Ravussin E, Lillioja S, Knowler WC, Bogardus C. Reduced rate of energy expenditure as a risk factor for body weight gain. *N Engl J Med.* 1988;318:467–472.

41. Sims EA, Danforth E Jr, Horton ES, Bray GA, Glennon JA, Salans LB. Endocrine and metabolic effects of experimental obesity in man. *Rec Prog Horm Res.* 1973;29:457–496.

42. Leibel RL, Rosenbaum M, Hirsch J. Changes in energy expenditure resulting from altered body weight. *N Engl J Med.* 1995;332:621–628.

43. Katzeff HL, Danforth E Jr. Decreased thermic effect of a mixed meal during overnutrition in human obesity. *Am J Clin Nutr.* 1989;50:915–921.

44. DíAlessio DA, Kavle EC, Mozzoli MA, et al. Thermic effect of food in lean and obese men. *J Clin Invest.* 1988;81:1781–1789.

45. Felber JP, Golay A. Regulation of nutrient metabolism and energy expenditure. *Metabolism.* 1995;44(suppl 2):4–9.

46. Rowe JW, Young JB, Minaker KL, Stevens AL, Palotta J, Landsberg L. Effect of insulin and glucose infusions on sympathetic nervous system activity in normal man. *Diabetes.* 1981;30:219–225.

47. Ravussin E, Bogardus C, Schwartz RS, et al. Glucose-induced thermogenesis and insulin resistance in man. *Int J Obes.* 1985;9(suppl 2):103–109.

48. Calles-Escandon J, Horton ES. The thermogenic role of exercise in the treatment of morbid obesity: a critical evaluation. *Am J Clin Nutr.* 1992;55:533S–537S.

49. Widdowson EM, Edholm EG, McCance RA. The food intake and energy expenditure of cadets in training. *Br J Nutr.* 1954;8:147–155.

50. Rising R, Harper IT, Fontvielle AM, Ferraro RT, Spraul M, Ravussin E. Determinants of energy expenditure: variability in physical activity. *Am J Clin Nutr.* 1994;59:800–804.

51. Segal KR, Gutin B, Nyman AM, Pi-Sunyer FX. Thermic effect of food at rest, during exercise and after exercise in lean and obese men of similar body weight. *J Clin Invest.* 1985;76:1107–1112.

52. Sedlock DA, Fissinger JA, Melby CL. Effect of exercise intensity and duration on post-exercise energy expenditure. *Med Sci Sports Exerc.* 1989; 21:626–636.

53. Hill JO, Sparling PB, Shields TW, Heller PA. Exercise and food restriction: effects on body composition and metabolic rate in obese women. *Am J Clin Nutr.* 1987;46:622–630.

54. Phinney SD, LaGrange BM, O'Connell M. Effects of aerobic exercise on energy expenditure and nitrogen balance during very low calorie dieting. *Metabolism.* 1988;37:758–765.

CHAPTER 9

Body Fat Content and the Balance Between Fat and Alcohol Oxidation and Consumption

Jean-Pierre Flatt

INTRODUCTION

Body weight maintenance ultimately boils downs to the question: How fat must one be in order to burn as much fat as one eats? Or, what conditions must be met for one to burn as much fat as one eats? The outcome depends on many factors, but this question emphasizes the fact that fat consumption is one of the most important factors in weight maintenance. In contrast to the inherited traits that predispose one toward obesity, fat consumption is amenable to change. The idea that high-fat diets promote obesity is widely accepted[1] and it is therefore important to understand why food energy in the form of fat may have a different influence on body weight than food energy in the form of carbohydrates and protein.

This chapter explains this hypothesis and reviews other factors important in determining the answer to this question. Basic facts about the nature and metabolic roles of protein, carbohydrate, and fat are presented in order to promote a more realistic perception of their role as nutrients and in metabolism.

To maintain a constant weight, the body must: (1) burn a mixture of fuels whose average composition is exactly the same as the mixture of proteins, carbohydrates, and fats in the diet, and (2) take in foods in amounts that supply the same average number of calories as the calories spent. If this adjustment is not perfect, the error is translated almost entirely into gains or losses of body fat. When one considers that most adults experience many years in their lives during which their weight maintains itself within ±1 to 2 kg, and that such a gain or loss reflects a difference of only 1% to 2% between energy intake and energy expenditure, the adjustment of fuel oxidation to nutrient intake is indeed remarkably good, in sedentary as well as in active, in lean as well as in obese people. This is all the more intriguing because extensive variations in daily food consumption and physical activity occur as a matter of course. The main difference between individuals is the degree of adiposity that prevails when they reach approximate weight maintenance, i.e., how fat must they become in order to burn as much fat as they eat.

CHARACTERISTICS OF MACRONUTRIENTS

Proteins

The organic molecules essential for life are made mainly of carbon, hydrogen, and oxygen atoms. Among the three macronutrients—carbohydrates, fats, and proteins—only proteins contain, in addition, a substantial amount of nitrogen (average 16% by weight). There are about 12 kg of protein in the body of an adult. About half is extracellular, much of it in the form of collagen, which constitutes the core protein for the body's structural elements, bone, cartilage, and skin. The other half of the body's proteins are mostly within cells, where they carry out the body's functions, as enzymes, muscle fibers, blood proteins, etc. Proteins are assembled by linking hundreds of amino acids to each other in the special sequence that endows them with their particular properties. The supply of these "building blocks" must be maintained by eating protein-containing foods. These are degraded to amino acids during digestion, absorbed from the gut and transferred to the blood circulation, to be distributed to the body's various tissues and cells. For children, the recommended protein intake is 1.5 g per kg body weight per day, an amount that declines gradually with age. The Recommended Daily Allowance (RDA) for adults is 0.8 g protein/kg body weight/day.[2] These allowances are deliberately set somewhat higher than the minimum amount needed. Western diets generally provide more protein than an individual needs.

Carbohydrates

Glucose is the main form in which carbohydrate is absorbed, exchanged between tissues, and channeled into metabolic pathways. One molecule of glucose contains 6 atoms of carbon, 6 atoms of oxygen, and 12 atoms of hydrogen. (Its chemical formula is thus $C_6H_{12}O_6$.) Glucose must be present in the blood at a sufficient concentration to permit it to diffuse into the cells to support their metabolism. The brain in particular depends on an adequate supply of glucose at all times. If blood glucose levels decline to less than 0.6 g of glucose per liter of plasma the central nervous system does not get enough fuel, a situation known as hypoglycemia, which can become critical.

The most abundant form of edible foodstuff is starch found in grains, potatoes, and other sources. Starches are polymers in which hundreds of glucose molecules are linked together. Starches have provided the bulk of human energy needs during most of our evolution. In affluent societies, a marked increase in fat consumption during this century has reduced the preponderance of carbohydrates in the diet. Furthermore, sucrose and syrups containing glucose plus fructose (produced from starch) that are also used as bulk sweeteners, now provide almost as many calories as does starch in Western diets. Meals commonly supply 50 to 150 g of carbohydrates, which must be hydrolyzed to simple sugars to be absorbed from the intestine. This is a fairly rapid process and the amount of glucose absorbed from the intestine during the one to two hours after a meal is often much greater than the 15 to 20 g of glucose oxidized during that period, or the 15 to 25 g of free glucose present in the whole body (of which about 5 g are present in the blood itself). To avoid excessively high blood glucose levels, or hyperglycemia, and spillage of glucose into the urine, or glucosuria, much of the glucose taken up from the intestine must be rapidly removed from circulation. This is accomplished by conversion of the glucose taken up by cells into glycogen, primarily in liver and muscle. Glycogen molecules are very large glucose polymers (like starches), and they are therefore effectively trapped in the cells that made them. Like starch, glycogen contains 4 kcal per gram. In cells, each gram of glycogen is associated with about 3 g of water, which makes it a rather bulky form of energy reserve (i.e., about 1 kcal per gram similar to a fresh potato). Glycogen accumulation must be limited to prevent excessive swelling of tissues. Glycogen reserves amount to some 200 to 400 g in adults after the overnight fast, about one third of which is in the liver and most of the remainder in muscle. These reserves are not much larger than the amounts of carbohydrate (CHO) consumed in one day (Figure 9–1).[3] It is obviously important that they not be used up too rapidly if carbohydrate intake is unusually low during a few days.

Fats

Oils and fats in plants and animals are lipids known as triglycerides, as they contain three fatty acid molecules linked, or "esterified," to one molecule of glycerol. The most common fatty acids contain 16 to 18 carbon atoms and 32 to 36 hydrogen atoms but only 2 atoms of oxygen; thus they have no affinity for water and do not dissolve. Glycerol resembles a half molecule of glucose and accounts for about 10% of the weight of triglycerides, or 5% of their energy. It is readily converted into glucose. More complex types of lipids also exist, including cholesterol; they are functionally important because they make up cell membranes, but the amounts present are too small to be visible. Because lipids are insoluble in water, oils and fats do not markedly influence the composition of the body's aqueous compartments, regardless of whether the fat in recently consumed meals, or for that matter, the body's total fat reserves, are small or large. To be transported in

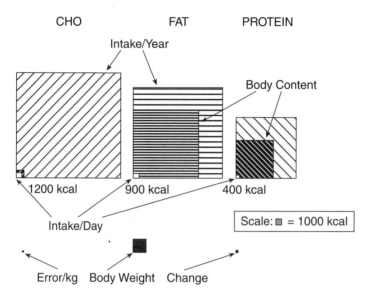

Figure 9–1 Energy reserves and daily and yearly nutrient turnover. *Source:* Reprinted with permission from J.P. Flatt, McCollum Award Lecture, 1995: Diet, Lifestyle and Weight Maintenance, *American Journal of Clinical Nutrition,* Vol. 62, pp. 820–836, © 1995, American Society of Clinical Nutrition.

the blood, fats must be in the form of tiny droplets surrounded by a thin protein coating, allowing them to remain in suspension as an emulsion. Such microscopic fat droplets, called chylomicrons, appear in the blood plasma after fatty meals, making the plasma "lactescent," i.e., like milk, whose white appearance is also due to the presence of emulsified fat droplets. Fat is stored in special cells, which become grossly enlarged by a central fat droplet, becoming much bigger than most of the body's other cells. Fat cells can expand or shrink considerably, but once formed, only their size, not their number can be reduced by fasting. There is a thin layer of metabolically active cytoplasm around the central fat droplet in these adipocytes, and a delicate network of capillary blood vessels between them. In mammals, triglycerides are stored in fat depots known as adipose tissue, where they make up about 90% of the weight of this "lard." Fats and oils provide approximately 9 kcal of energy per gram (or 120 kcal per tablespoon). Energy can thus be stored at about 8 kcal per gram of adipose tissue. This more compact form of energy compared to glycogen (about 1 kcal per gram of hydrated glycogen, as noted above) makes it possible for individuals to carry a substantial energy reserve. In lean adults, fat reserves typically amount to some 10 kg, an energy reserve of 90,000 kcal, enough to survive about two months of near-total food deprivation. This great facility in storing energy as fat has its drawbacks. Because of the size of these fat stores, differences between the amount of fat consumed and the amount oxidized in one day are much too small to be perceived (Figure 9–1). Thus, there was no way, and no reason for evolution to develop accurate mechanisms for regulation of the fat balance, and one can see that the fact that fat is kept out of the aqueous compartment explains why obesity can occur so readily.

Conversion of Carbohydrate into Fat

Conversion of carbohydrate into fat allows animals to build up fat reserves even when their feed contains very little fat. It has therefore long been believed that excess carbohydrate can readily be converted into stored body fat. However, it is now well-established that the occasional consumption of unusually large amounts of carbohydrate (e.g., 500 g in one meal) can be handled by a temporary expansion of glycogen stores.[4] To induce rates of fat synthesis exceeding concomitant rates of fat oxidation, the body's total glycogen stores must first be raised considerably (i.e., from the usual 4 to 6 g/kg body weight to more than 8 g of glycogen per kg body weight).[5] This requires deliberate and sustained overconsumption of large amounts of carbohydrates. Since fat synthesis is essentially negligible under conditions of unrestricted access to food,[6] one can conclude that there are signals that spontaneously restrain food intake to prevent glycogen levels from rising beyond a certain range. The still-common belief that glucose is readily turned into fat can therefore be dismissed. The frequently made argument that the high metabolic cost for synthesizing fat from glucose (about 25% of the glucose calories channeled into lipogenesis) is a cause for greater energy dissipation on high-carbohydrate diets is thus quite unreasonable. It must be appreciated, however, that carbohydrate ingestion reduces the need to use fat as a fuel, and that carbohydrate intake is an important factor in determining how much fat will be burned, and how much retained.

MAIN FEATURES OF METABOLISM AND METABOLIC REGULATION

Energy Expenditure

Overall substrate oxidation rates are dictated by the need to regenerate the adenosine triphosphate (ATP) used in performing the body's metabolic functions, in maintaining temperature, and in moving. ATP is a key intermediary in metabolism that liberates the energy needed to drive chemical reactions and to contract muscle fibers; ATP regeneration is tightly coupled to carbohydrate, protein, and fat oxidation. ATP utilization depends primarily on an individual's size and physical activity. For several decades much emphasis was given to the possibility that obesity may be caused by unusually low rates of metabolism. This impression was created by expressing rates of energy expenditure per kg body weight, instead of considering total energy expenditure. The idea was reinforced by the tendency of overweight individuals to underreport food consumption to a greater degree than lean individuals. A method for the measurement of energy expenditure in free-living individuals has now become available in which the rates of elimination of the heavy (non-radioactive) isotopes of hydrogen and oxygen are measured over several days after ingestion of a dose of doubly labeled water (DLW). Studies using DLW have demonstrated unambiguously that energy turnover is higher in sedentary obese than in sedentary normal-weight individuals.[7] To maintain their body weight, overweight individuals need to eat more than lean subjects carrying out similar physical tasks: from 12 to 20 additional kcal per day for each kg additional weight, depending on the level of physical activity.

Energy Requirements

Energy requirements are often said to equal the amount of food energy needed to maintain energy balance. This is based on the implicit assumption that maintaining energy balance is the key goal. This is not the case, however. The reasons are made obvious by considering the definition of energy requirements used in the Report of a Joint FAO/WHO/UNU Expert Consultation on energy and protein requirements,[8] in which "energy requirement" is defined as "the level of energy intake from food that will balance energy expenditure when the individual has a body size and composition, and level of physical activity, consistent with long-term good health; and that will allow for the maintenance of economically necessary and socially desirable physical activity. In children and pregnant or lactating women the energy requirements includes the energy needs associated with the deposition of tissues or the secretion of milk at rates consistent with good health."

Metabolic Efficiency

When compared to daily energy turnover, the amount of energy retained during growth and during the development of obesity is rather small, amounting to a difference of only a few percent between intake and expenditure. Because a positive energy balance can, in principle, be attributed to excessive intake or to reduced expenditure, there has been considerable interest in the possible significance of even small differences in metabolic efficiency for the development or the prevention of obesity.

Metabolic efficiency can be defined in many ways, which can result in totally different assessments. For example, the energy deposited in the carcass can be compared to the total amount of food energy consumed, which is an important practical consideration in judging feed efficiency in the production of meat. This "gross nutrient efficiency" depends primarily on the amount of excess energy consumed relative to maintenance energy expenditure. In situations characterized by rather small changes in body size over time, as is the case in humans, gross nutrient efficiency is close to zero, or even negative on days on which food intake is less than energy expenditure. It is clearly useless to attempt characterization of potential metabolic differences between lean and obese persons. A more meaningful approach is to assess energy retention relative to the amount consumed in excess of maintenance requirements. The accuracy of such an approach is limited, particularly in humans, because the maintenance energy requirement accounts for a large fraction of the energy consumed, and because this requirement keeps changing as body weight and physical activities vary during the weeks needed to produce measurable changes in body composition. Even small errors in estimating maintenance requirements have a considerable impact on the net efficiency value that one strives to determine. The reliability of such evaluations is questionable.

Whatever differences in ATP dissipation and synthesis there may be, they are all reflected in measured resting metabolic rates. As mentioned earlier, these are closely correlated with the size of the fat-free mass and the fat mass, though a certain degree of variability among individuals remains. The importance often attributed to such differences is founded on the presumption that changes in energy expenditure will not be offset by changes in energy intake. Under conditions where energy intake could be "clamped" to some particular level, a 5% difference in resting energy expenditure would be offset by a difference in body weight of 5 to 8 kg in a sedentary individual, or less in a physically active individual. However, when access to food is not restricted, energy balance is determined overwhelmingly by factors influencing food intake, and by the adjustments in food intake that serve to compensate for recent substrate imbalances, regardless of the overall rate of energy turnover.[9] Pregnancy, for instance, leads to the deposition of a few kg of additional fat in spite of an increase in resting energy expenditure.[2]

In dealing with commonly exaggerated claims about the importance of differences in metabolic efficiency on body weights it is helpful to consider the analogy offered by comparing small, fuel efficient cars and inefficient large vehicles. Regardless of their differing fuel efficiencies, both types of cars will reach their destination as long as gasoline can be bought without restriction. Given that access to foods is essentially unrestricted in affluent societies, differences in energy expenditure are similarly of limited importance, whereas the phenomena that adjust intake to utilization are decisive. Differences in resting metabolic rates are minor among healthy individuals. Arguments about their possible role in promoting or preventing obesity and in playing a role in body weight maintenance are therefore hollow, if they are not linked to a rational consideration of factors controlling energy intake. They often are not linked, however, and end up creating a conceptual trap that unfortunately continues to affect the way people think about the causes of obesity.

Protein Metabolism and Nitrogen Balance

In adults, some 250 to 300 g of protein are lost every day through wear and tear. In addition, some 70 g are secreted into the gut, or lost as sloughed off cells from the intestinal lining. About two thirds of the amino acids liberated by protein breakdown are reutilized for protein resynthesis, and the rest are degraded to intermediates that flow into the metabolic pathways by which carbohydrate and fat are oxidized to carbon dioxide and provide energy for the regeneration of ATP. The nitrogen (N) in the amino groups that is liberated in the process is disposed of by conversion to urea, which is excreted in the urine. Consumption of a certain amount of protein is therefore necessary to replenish the amino acid pools sustaining protein synthesis, so that synthesis can keep pace in replacing the lost and degraded proteins.

By measuring the difference between the amounts of nitrogen in the foods consumed and the amounts excreted, it is possible to monitor changes in the body's nitrogen and hence in its protein content. One gram of nitrogen corresponds to $100/16 = 6.25$ g of protein. Measurements of nitrogen balance have shown that it tends to oscillate around zero, as the body strives to maintain a stable protein content, except during growth and pregnancy, or during recovery from malnutrition and disease, when the body's protein content increases. This, of course, depends on the diet providing enough protein and energy. Amino acids consumed in excess of those needed to sustain protein synthesis are not stored, but degraded. The contribution made by amino acids to ATP regeneration during periods of weight maintenance is thus equal on average to the amount of dietary energy consumed in the form of proteins. This typically amounts to 12% to 18% of total dietary energy, being rarely less than 10% or more than 20% when typical mixed foods are consumed. Given that the body spontaneously tends to maintain a nearly constant protein content, changes in body weight as well as weight maintenance are primarily determined by the intake and utilization of carbohydrates and fats.

Carbohydrate and Fat Metabolism

The brain depends almost exclusively on glucose to obtain its energy, requiring about 5 g of glucose per hour, or 120 g per day in an adult.[10] Humans have evolved regulatory mechanisms that allow the body to maintain stable blood glucose levels, as well as glycogen reserves adequate to sustain them. This is accomplished with the help of hormones.

Insulin, which is released from the pancreas when blood glucose levels rise after food consumption, promotes glucose transport into cells and the storage not only of glucose taken up from the intestine, but of amino acids and fat as well. Insulin activates glycogen formation and protein synthesis in the liver and in muscles, as well as fat deposition in adipose tissue. There are some metabolic costs involved in this storage, which amount to about 10% of the energy content of the foods consumed. This is known as the thermic effect of food (TEF) and explains why energy expenditure increases somewhat after meals. The action of insulin in reducing blood substrate levels is facilitated by the fact that it also inhibits their release from the body's fuel reserves.

The storage induced by insulin during nutrient absorption from the gut is counterbalanced between meals by hormones that activate the release of fuel from the body's glycogen and fat stores. Thus glucagon and epinephrine activate the breakdown of glycogen and the rate of glucose release by the liver, so that concentrations of about 1 g per liter of plasma (or 100 mg per 100 ml) are maintained between meals. (In a solution containing that amount of glucose, a faint sweetness can just be detected.) Maintenance of this glucose level is contingent on the presence of sufficient glycogen reserves in the liver and on the transport from peripheral tissues to the liver of sufficient precursors from which it can make glucose, through the process of "gluconeogenesis." The glucogenic precursors present in amino acid mixtures allow the liver to make about 0.5 g of glucose per gram of amino acids oxidized, whereas only 0.1 g of glucose can be made per gram of fat oxidized to carbon dioxide, because only the glycerol part of triglycerides is a precursor for gluconeogenesis.

Because the body's glycogen reserves are not much greater than the amount of glucose usually consumed and oxidized in one day, the body's regulatory mechanisms must be able to promptly adjust glucose oxidation to changes in glucose availability. The effectiveness of these mechanisms is demonstrated by the ease with which people tolerate substantial decreases or increases in daily carbohydrate intake.[11] This ability to adapt to changes in the relative proportions of carbohydrate and fat in the diet is possible because most of the body's tissues (the brain being the most notable exception) can interchangeably use glucose or fatty acids as substrate for energy production and because adipose tissue can readily provide fatty acids when needed, or accept fatty acids for storage if they are present in excess of demand. Indeed, a few days of fat deposition or mobilization hardly affects the size of the fat stores, which are greater than 10 kg (9000 kcal) in most adults, not uncommonly reaching 20 kg and more in overweight and obese subjects, an energy reserve 100 to 200 times greater than all of the body's glycogen stores. When access to food is unrestricted, the metabolic regulation that serves to maintain adequate glycogen stores is complemented by the fact that substantial losses or accumulation of glycogen influence food intake. Thus inadequately low blood glucose levels or the imminent threat of hypoglycemia induce an extremely powerful urge to find foods and to eat. On the other hand, spontaneous food intake in free-living individuals is inhibited long before the glycogen storage capacity is maximally filled, and glycogen stores are in effect kept several hundred grams below the level at which rapid conversion of carbohydrate to fat would be induced. Freely eating subjects get used to avoiding such extreme situations, however,[12] and the issue is whether, and to what extent, common fluctuations in glycogen levels may influence food intake, thereby contributing to the adjustment of carbohydrate intake to carbohydrate demands and of food intake to energy expenditure. In mice with unrestricted access to food, gains or losses of glycogen on one day tend to cause decreases or increases in food intake on the following day.[3,13] This component of food intake regulation was recently detected in humans as well,[14] but as in mice, it explains only a small part of the variations in daily food consumption.

When the ingestion of carbohydrate-containing foods increases the availability of carbohydrates, the body promptly abandons its parsimonious use of glucose. Carbohydrate oxidation thus increases rapidly after meals. This can be recognized by measuring and comparing the relative amounts of carbon dioxide produced and of oxygen consumed by an individual. This is easily and commonly done by placing a Plexiglas hood over a subject's head and analyzing the air drawn through the system. When fats are oxidized, 0.7 liters of carbon dioxide are produced per liter of oxygen consumed, whereas when glucose is oxidized one liter of carbon dioxide is produced for every liter of oxygen consumed. The increase in the carbon dioxide/oxygen ratio (respiratory quotient, or RQ) observed after meals reveals a prompt shift toward the predominant use of glucose (Figure 9–2).[15] This rise is related to the amount of carbohydrate consumed. It is noteworthy that the presence of fat in the meal has little if any effect on postprandial substrate oxidation. This is imputable in part to the relatively slow rate of fat absorption from the gut, but primarily it is due to the fact that dietary fats appear in the circulation in the form of chylomicrons, which are targeted for deposition in adipose tissue, rather than as free fatty acids (FFAs), the form in which fat is released from adipose tissue and made available to cells for energy generation. As shown by Figure 9–2, fat oxidation is inhibited after meals, and this is the case even when fat is the major macronutrient in the foods consumed.[16] It is clear that carbohydrate intake promotes carbohydrate oxidation, but fat intake does not (or does only slightly) promote fat oxidation.

Fat Balance

Considering that total energy expenditure is determined primarily by body size and physical activity and that the body's metabolic regulation strives to maintain nitrogen balance and stable glycogen reserves, fat oxidation is determined to a large extent by the gap between total energy expenditure and the amounts of energy ingested in the form of carbohydrates and proteins.[13] Fat intake, on the other hand, depends on the proportion of energy present as fat in the foods selected and on how much food one is induced to eat by eating habits and by the availability of appetizing foods, or driven to eat to maintain stable glycogen levels. Fat oxidation and fat intake are therefore determined independently.

Some adjustment of fat oxidation to fat intake results from the fact that postprandial inhibition of fat oxidation is attenuated because fat ingestion tends to delay intes-

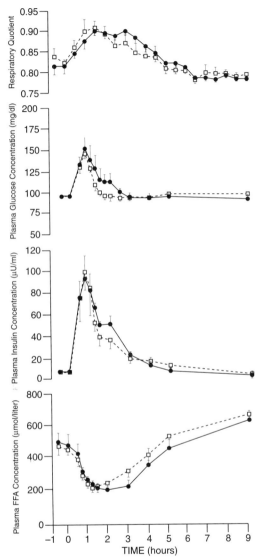

Figure 9–2 Changes in the non-protein respiratory quotient, in blood glucose, and in plasma insulin and free fatty acid (FFA) levels observed in 7 young men in response to a low-fat breakfast providing white bread, jam, and dried meat (73 g carbohydrate, 6 g fat, and 30 g protein ●——●), and after consuming the same breakfast on another day with a supplement of 50 g of margarine (41 g of additional fat □----□). Means ± S.E. *Source:* Reproduced from *The Journal of Clinical Investigation,* 1985, Vol. 76, pp. 1019–1024 by copyright permission of The American Society for Clinical Investigation.

tinal absorption. Furthermore, to the extent that the presence of fat in the foods consumed results in a lesser intake of carbohydrates, glycogen levels will be lower, causing a greater demand for fatty acid release from adipose tissue and higher rates of fat oxidation. However, these indirect effects will not necessarily produce an exact compensation. Furthermore, short-term errors in the fat balance are too small to affect the size of the body's fat stores, FFA levels, fat oxidation, or food intake. The weakness of mechanisms serving to adjust fat oxidation to fat intake, and vice versa, explains why large errors in maintenance of the fat balance occur. Errors in the fat balance, of course, imply errors in the overall energy balance, and if the fat balance is not accurately regulated, neither is the energy balance. How is it, then, that fat oxidation can nevertheless become adjusted to fat intake over the long run, as demonstrated by the fact that people tend to maintain stable body weights even though they eat food mixtures with widely differing fat contents?

The explanation derives from the fact that cumulative fat gains (or losses) over extended periods of time will cause changes in the size of the adipose tissue fat mass, and that such changes have the effect of increasing (or decreasing) fatty acid release from adipose tissue. This in turn affects FFA levels in the circulation, which enhances (or reduces) fat oxidation.[17,18] In time this tends to bring about the oxidation of a fuel mix whose average fat content matches the fat content of the diet. This is why most individuals ultimately reach a state where not only carbohydrate and protein oxidation, but fat oxidation rates as well are commensurate with the amounts of macronutrients usually consumed.

THE BODY'S CARBOHYDRATE AND FAT ECONOMIES AND WEIGHT MAINTENANCE

Since carbohydrate disposal by lipogenesis is insignificant under habitual dietary conditions, and since glucose cannot be made from fatty acids, glucose and fat belong to two separate substrate pools. The fact that the body's energy reserves are kept in two distinct forms, in amounts that differ by two orders of magnitude, has a number of consequences, whose nature and implications are made evident in Figure 9–3.[3] The small reservoir represents the body's limited capacity for storing glycogen; the large reservoir stands for the body's ability to store large amounts of fat. A small turbine represents the exclusive use of glucose by the brain, which accounts for approximately 20% of total flux under resting conditions. The relative proportions of glucose and of fatty acids used by the rest of the body (the large turbine) are assumed to be influenced by the availability of glucose and free fatty acids, which may be thought of as proportional to the levels to which the two reservoirs are filled at a given time.

Replenishment of the body's glycogen and fat stores occurs from time to time through consumption of meals (illustrated by the contents of the small containers

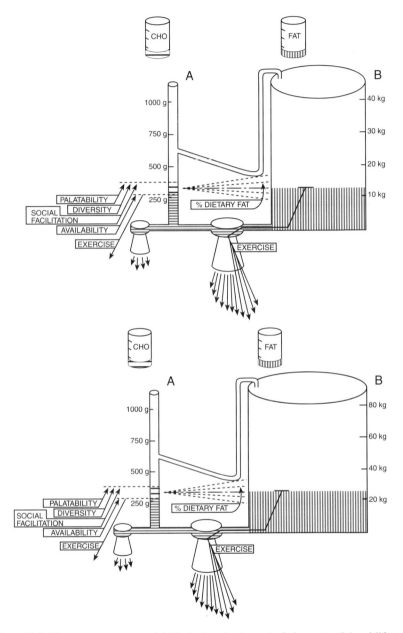

Figure 9–3 Two-compartment model illustrating the impact of circumstantial and lifestyle factors on adiposity. Further explanations are given in the text. (A) Glycogen storage capacity, and (B) fat storage capacity. *Source:* Reprinted with permission from J.P. Flatt, McCollum Award Lecture, 1995: Diet, Lifestyle and Weight Maintenance, *American Journal of Clinical Nutrition,* Vol. 62, pp. 820–836, © 1995, American Society of Clinical Nutrition.

shown above the reservoirs), of which the fraction corresponding to the diet's fat content is delivered into the large reservoir. Food consumption is determined by the habitual pattern of meals, complemented when necessary by physiological regulatory mechanisms, which ensure that glycogen reserves are sufficient to avoid hypoglycemia, while also preventing them from building up to levels at which de novo lipogenesis would be induced, i.e., through the conduit from the small to the large reservoir. Additions to the large reservoir cause only insignificant changes in the body's fat content, whereas they lead to marked changes in the body's glycogen reserves. Raising the level in the small reservoir causes its outflow to increase after meals, as seen in Figure 9–2 by the rise in the RQ, which reflects the postprandial increase in glucose oxidation. As the glycogen reserves become depleted, glucose oxidation declines progressively, allowing a concomitant increase in fat oxidation. These meal-induced cycles cause glycogen levels to oscillate up and down within a particular operating range, with glucose utilization being essentially equal to glucose intake over a few of these cycles. When outflow from the large reservoir (= fat oxidation) is not commensurate with inflow (= fat intake), its content (= adipose tissue mass) will change slowly over time. Ultimately, the content of the large reservoir will reach the level that causes the contribution of the large reservoir to the flow through the big turbine to be equal on average to the amounts habitually delivered into it. A steady state is then reached.

These interactions explain how the body's glycogen content and the size of its fat mass influence the composition of the fuel mix oxidized, and why this is bound to lead in time to the situation in which glucose and free fatty acids are oxidized in the same relative proportions as the diet's carbohydrate and fat content. One can also see that both the fat content of the diet and the range within which glycogen levels are maintained are important in determining the body fat content at which the weight-maintenance plateau tends to become established (i.e., the steady-state level in the large reservoir). When the proportion of carbohydrate and fat in the diet is altered, changes in body composition must occur, until a new body composition is attained for which the relative amounts of glucose and fat in the fuel mix oxidized are again commensurate with the relative proportions of carbohydrate and fat in the diet. If an expansion of the adipose tissue mass is to be avoided when the fat content of the diet is raised, the range within which glycogen levels operate must be appropriately lowered. This is what happens if energy intake is "clamped" at a constant level: glycogen levels will change until glucose oxidation is equal to that provided by the new diet.[11] When access to food is unrestricted, however, the reduction in the glycogen levels may not necessarily occur to the extent needed to allow the appropriate increase in fat oxidation and the appropriate decrease in glucose oxidation. In most cases, more food is needed to maintain stable glycogen levels on a diet that provides more fat, but less carbohydrate. With a higher energy intake, fat will be accumulated, until the fat mass has become large enough to raise FFA levels and fat oxidation sufficiently to match the new dietary fat intake. The insight provided by the model thus leads one to expect that gradual increments in the diet's fat content will quite naturally lead to progressively higher degrees of adiposity, which indeed is the case.[1]

When animals are provided high-fat diets, their body fat content generally increases.[3] This is illustrated in Figure 9–4 for mice fed ad libitum. As the fat content of the diet that they receive becomes higher, there is a progressive rise in the average fat content at which their weight becomes stable. The large variation between animals must be noted. Also noteworthy is the fact that the body fat content of mice kept in groups of four per cage is much higher than when they are kept alone. This "housing effect" causes a very substantial shift in the average dose-response

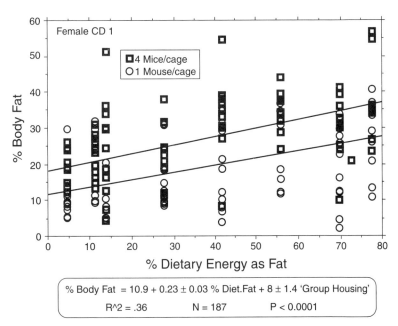

Figure 9–4 Effect of housing conditions on the relationship between dietary fat content and body fat content in female CD1 mice, kept either in groups of 4 mice per cage (upper line) or alone (lower line), and provided ad libitum with diets containing 18% of metabolizable energy as protein, the percentage of energy as fat shown on the abscissa, and the balance as starch plus sucrose (1:1). The equations for the correlations are: % Body Fat (groups) = 18.1 + 0.25 ± 0.04 % Dietary Fat ($R^2 = 0.3$; $P < 0.001$; N = 90), and % Body Fat (alone) = 11.6 + 0.21 ± 0.04 % Dietary Fat ($R^2 = 0.25$; $P < 0.0001$; N = 97), respectively. The equation describing a multiple regression analysis of the data shows that group housing raises body fat content by about 8%. *Source:* Reprinted with permission from J.P. Flatt, McCollum Award Lecture, 1995: Diet, Lifestyle and Weight Maintenance, *American Journal of Clinical Nutrition,* Vol. 62, pp. 820–836, © 1995, American Society of Clinical Nutrition.

relationship, but the influence of the diet's fat content in raising adiposity remains. The leverage of dietary fat in humans is an important indication to keep in mind, even as this effect is sometimes difficult to recognize among all the other factors that contribute to obesity in people.

The two-compartment model of Figure 9–3 also helps to show the impact of various other circumstantial factors on weight maintenance. The availability of appetizing foods and their diversity,[19] as well as good company,[20] are known to increase meal size. Consumption of larger meals has the effect (illustrated by arrows in the figure) of raising the upper limit to which glycogen levels are raised. Another arrow shows that constant food availability, by promoting food consumption between meals, has the effect of attenuating the decline in the glycogen reserves between meals (illustrated by another arrow). The combined effect of these environmental factors is to raise the range within which glycogen levels are habitually maintained, inhibiting fat oxidation. To overcome this inhibition, the content of the large reservoir has to rise to a higher level to bring about a rate of fat oxidation that matches fat intake.

Regular physical activity is effective in preventing or limiting excessive buildup of body fat.[21] This is brought about by two effects: (1) It increases substrate oxidation in skeletal muscle, which uses both glucose and free fatty acids, attenuating the impact of tissues preferentially using glucose and resulting in a decrease in the overall RQ; and (2) exercise lengthens the meal-to-meal interval, considering calories expended rather than number of hours elapsed, thereby causing greater glycogen depletion between meals and longer periods during which the RQ can be relatively low. In addition, physical training enhances the ability of muscle to switch to the predominant use of fat rather than glucose during prolonged efforts.[22]

The effect of inheritance on body composition and on the susceptibility to develop obesity can be extremely powerful.[23,24] Such a permanent difference in the system can be mimicked in the model by expanding or shrinking the diameter of the large reservoir. This is akin to altering the impact of the adipose tissue mass on fat oxidation, since different amounts of fat must be present to reach the level that brings about a given rate of fat oxidation. This can lead to considerable differences in the fat accumulation needed to achieve weight maintenance (e.g., twice as much in the case illustrated in the lower half of Figure 9–3). However, this permanent change in the model prevents neither the usual regulatory interactions, nor the influence of the circumstantial variables described by the various arrows. In fact, their leverage needs to be taken into account to a greater extent among individuals genetically predisposed to obesity, as suggested by the fact that weight gain was greatest among women presumed to be predisposed to obesity (because at least one of their parents was overweight) if they were used to consuming a high-fat diet.[25]

THE STEADY STATE OF WEIGHT MAINTENANCE

Weight maintenance occurs when not only protein and glucose oxidation but fat oxidation as well is equal on average to protein, carbohydrate, and fat intake, i.e., when the amount and composition of the fuel mix oxidized match the macronutrient content of the foods consumed.

The RQ/FQ Concept

Information on the composition of the fuel mix oxidized can be obtained by measuring the respiratory quotient (Figure 9–5). Because proteins are oxidized with an RQ of 0.835 and contribute a fairly constant, but minor proportion of the substrate mix oxidized, the RQ is not greatly affected by variations in the protein content of the fuel mix oxidized. The RQ thus describes the relative proportions of carbohydrate and fat.

Since the regulation of fuel metabolism works to prevent excessive glycogen accumulation, the 24-hour RQ will be higher than usual on days during which more food is consumed than needed for energy balance. On the other hand, RQs will be relatively low on days with low food intake, because endogenous fat must

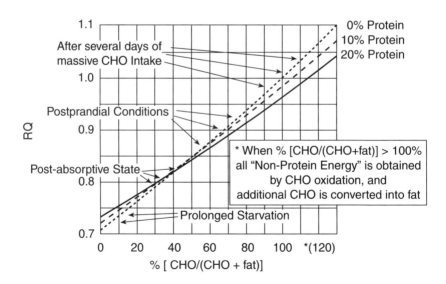

Figure 9–5 Relationship between the overall RQ and the relative contributions made by carbohydrate and fat to the fuel mix oxidized, when protein contributes 0%, 10%, or 20% of total energy.

then make a contribution to the fuel mix oxidized.[26] Long-term weight stability can only occur when the average RQ corresponds to the carbohydrate-to-fat ratio of the diet (Figure 9–6).[13] The left panel illustrates that the RQ for which energy balance is achieved depends on the diet's carbohydrate-to-fat ratio. To facilitate the interpretation of data on the adjustment of fuel composition to nutrient intake, it is convenient to compare respiratory quotient values to the food quotient (FQ), which describes the ratio of carbon dioxide produced to oxygen consumed during the biological oxidation of a representative sample of the diet.[27] The relationship between the RQ and the energy balance can be made independent of diet composition and of differences in rates of energy turnover, by relating the ratio of energy intake over energy expenditure to the RQ/FQ ratio (right panel of Figure 9–6).

Nutrient Imbalances and Corrective Responses

A variety of mechanisms are known that limit excessive variations in food intake. However, in spite of all the known phenomena that contribute to the regulation of food intake (and in spite of those yet to be discovered), daily protein, carbohydrate, fat, and energy balances routinely deviate substantially from zero.[28,29] Body weight stability therefore implies that gains or losses of protein, glycogen, and fat tend to elicit corrective responses that compensate for these deviations, thereby helping to sustain a "steady state" of weight maintenance.[13] Three types of corrective responses are possible: (1) changes in energy dissipation, (2) changes in food intake, and (3) shifts in the composition of the fuel mix oxidized. The latter are readily and quickly brought about, thanks to powerful endocrine and enzymatic regulatory mechanisms,

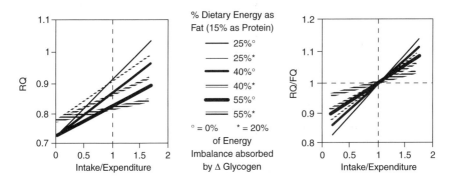

Figure 9–6 Relationships between the RQ, the RQ/FQ ratio, and the energy balance, assuming that carbohydrate balances are equilibrated, or that 20% of the energy imbalances are absorbed by gains or losses of glycogen (dotted lines). *Source:* Reprinted with permission from J.P. Flatt, The RQ/SQ Concept and Weight Maintenance, in *Progress in Obesity Research,* A. Angel, ed., pp. 49–66, © 1996, John Libbey & Company Ltd.

such as those that elicit increased carbohydrate oxidation after eating, as reflected by the prompt postprandial rise in the RQ shown in Figure 9–2. These regulatory responses are dedicated primarily to the goal of maintaining adequate glycogen stores. They have the effect of minimizing deviations from the carbohydrate balance, and cause errors in the overall energy balance to be accommodated primarily by gains or losses of fat.[29] RQ adjustments do not bring about corrections for deviations from energy balance, however. Such corrections must be accomplished by altering the rates of energy dissipation and/or by eliciting increases or decreases in food intake. Energy expenditure is primarily a function of body size and physical activity and changes only modestly in response to energy imbalances, primarily because the metabolic costs incurred in the handling and storage of nutrients are proportional to the amounts consumed. This TEF amounts to about 10% of the food energy consumed. Since changes in energy expenditure attenuate the effect of excessive or insufficient food intake on the energy balance only slightly, maintenance of energy balance during consecutive days depends on appropriate up and down regulation of food intake around the average intake needed for weight maintenance.[3,13]

Regulation of Food Intake and Energy Balance

When the fuel mix oxidized has the same average composition as the nutrient distribution in the diet, adjustments in food intake serving to maintain either protein, carbohydrate, or fat balance are sufficient, in principle, to achieve overall energy balance as well. (In fact, "energy" and "energy balance" are abstract notions, and one should not expect that the energy balance could itself be the target of biological regulation.) In view of the importance of maintaining stable glycogen reserves, deviations from the carbohydrate balance appear much more likely to be influential in eliciting changes in food intake from one day to the next than deviations from the protein and/or fat balances.[12,13,30] Regulation of food intake serving primarily the purpose of maintaining stable glycogen reserves allows maintenance of energy balance, but only when the size of the body's glycogen and fat reserves has reached the particular configuration that complements the body's metabolic fuel regulation in a way that brings about the oxidation of a metabolic fuel mix whose composition matches the nutrient distribution in the diet.

When presented with foods of different macronutrient contents, experimental animals select favorable proportions of nutrients from the choices provided, indicating that the regulation of food intake goes beyond merely influencing the total amount of energy consumed. In humans, who eat a variety of foods that provide mixtures of macronutrients, there seems to be little selection of particular items of the diet for physiologic or metabolic reasons,[31] and the items consumed are influenced by availability, preferences, cost, and conscious selection and/or avoidance.

The regulation of food intake in humans is difficult to elucidate, because numerous circumstantial factors and individual preferences influence food intake. These can readily override physiological signals because substantial short-term deviations from the energy balance are easily tolerated. The average standard deviation for food intake in individuals is about ±22%.[32] Frequent consumption of meals in portions that are not adjusted to individual needs, and the conscious efforts to control food intake, further contribute to the difficulty in gaining a realistic perception of the role of physiological factors controlling food intake in humans. Lack of understanding about the regulation of food intake in humans does not alter the fact that this regulation creates powerful, though often undetected, underlying drives. These drives elicit adjustments in food intake necessary to correct for deviations from energy balance and to limit rates of weight gain even in the face of unrestricted food availability and poor dietary habits. In fact, the large variations in food intake reflected by the individual standard deviation averaging ±22%[32] imply that the amounts of food that one finds enjoyable to eat are far greater than needed to maintain energy balance. This suggests that influences inhibiting food consumption must restrict eating on frequent occasions, and that they are able to do so even when the diet's energy density is high. The power of food intake regulation is illustrated in children who do not yet seek to consciously control their food intake, and whose body weights nevertheless remain generally in a desirable range, in spite of considerable variations in energy expenditure. The strong tendency to regain weight lost by dieting further illustrates this power, as does the spontaneous reduction in food intake that brings about weight loss after periods of deliberate overeating.[33,34] It is the very strength of these drives that makes weight maintenance difficult when body composition differs markedly from that for which the steady state tends to become established spontaneously.

STRATEGIES FOR WEIGHT CONTROL

In metabolic terms, the goal of weight control is to achieve an average RQ equal to the diet's FQ without the need for an undesirable expansion of the adipose tissue mass to satisfy this condition.[9] This goal is more readily achieved by living on a diet high in carbohydrates but low in fat, as it is obviously easier to achieve an average RQ lower than the diet's FQ when the FQ is relatively high. Regular physical exercise provides additional leverage to keep the average RQ as low as the FQ, because exercise promotes fat oxidation more than glucose oxidation.

Restricting Fat Consumption

Since the body will spontaneously and effectively maintain protein and carbohydrate balances, but cannot regulate the fat balance as accurately, it makes sense to direct voluntary efforts at this relatively soft target. Putting emphasis on the fat balance provides a more specific goal than one based on monitoring overall caloric exchanges. Because it is obviously easier to ensure that fat oxidation will be at least equal to fat intake when fat intake is kept small, the key measure is to avoid fatty foods and to satisfy one's hunger by eating foods providing most of their energy in the form of carbohydrates. Several studies have shown that this leads to some loss of body fat (typically 2 to 4 kg), even when food consumption is not restricted and when the low-fat food items offered are designed to be comparable in palatability than the fattier food items that they replace.[35,36]

Awareness of the fact that fatty foods have a particularly high caloric density, and that low-fat diets provide more bulk, has long led dietitians to recommend low-fat diets for weight control. During the last decade, recommendations to reduce fat intake have been increasingly promulgated in dietary guidelines published by government agencies and medical or health-related associations. Limiting fat intake (particularly consumption of the saturated fats present in meats and dairy products) is indeed a key measure in lowering blood cholesterol levels and in minimizing the development of atherosclerosis. These arguments for restricting fat intake are complemented by the realization that the steady state of weight maintenance can be expected, for metabolic reasons, to be achieved with less adipose tissue on board when the diet's fat content is low (as shown in Figure 9–3). Selecting low-fat foods does not entail the discomfort of hunger, as much as it requires avoidance of a whole range of desirable foods.

Alcohol Consumption and Fat Balance

Slightly more than 5% of the food energy consumed in America is provided by alcohol and among individuals regularly consuming alcoholic beverages, alcohol can easily make up more than 10% of daily energy intake.[37] Another fact illustrating that alcohol provides a significant influx of energy for many individuals is the fact that in order to raise blood alcohol levels to the legal limit of .08%, a dose of alcohol has to be consumed that is roughly equivalent to 20% of daily resting energy expenditure. People are well aware of the "beer belly syndrome," but its implications about the effect of alcohol on the energy balance are complicated by seeing the frequent emaciation among chronic alcoholics. Among chronic alcoholics, alcohol may account for nearly half of total energy intake, and its pharmacological effects then inhibit food intake, leading in time to emaciation and malnutrition.

The consumption of alcohol leads to a slight increase in energy expenditure (Figure 9–7). This is due to the fact that oxidation of ethanol does not yield as much ATP per molecule of oxygen consumed than the oxidation of carbohydrate or fat. The effect is more pronounced in habitual alcohol consumers, because regular consumption of alcohol induces oxidative enzymes in the liver that are not

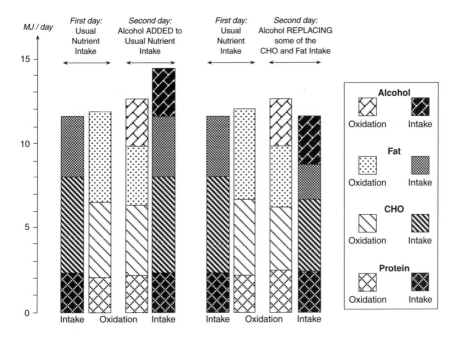

Figure 9–7 Effect of alcohol consumption on 24-hour substrate oxidation in young men. The subjects were studied twice during two consecutive days spent in a respiratory chamber, which allowed determination of daily substrate oxidation and substrate balances, since nutrient intake was precisely controlled. During the second day the volunteers received measured portions of alcohol with their meals, either as a supplement to the usual nutrient intake provided on the first day, or with a corresponding decrease in the amounts of carbohydrate (CHO) and fat provided. The major effect of alcohol consumption was to reduce fat oxidation, whereas protein and carbohydrate oxidation remained essentially unchanged. *Source:* Adapted from P.M. Suter et al., *New England Journal of Medicine,* 1992, Vol. 326, and pp. 983–987. Copyright 1992. Massachusetts Medical Society. All rights reserved.

---

linked to ATP production. These reactions can dissipate at most 25% of the energy provided by ethanol.[38] Studies by Suter et al[39] show that consumption of alcohol and its metabolism do not alter carbohydrate and protein oxidation, but markedly reduce fat oxidation. (Compare the columns showing substrate oxidation on the first and second day of observation in Figure 9–7.) It is therefore not surprising that alcohol consumption does not elicit a compensatory reduction in food intake.[40] The availability of alcoholic beverages tends to increase total energy intake, particularly when diets with high-fat contents are consumed.[37] Finally, one should note that since alcohol has primarily a fat-sparing effect, energy consumed in the form of alcohol should be counted along with fat, rather than with carbohydrate, in calculating the relative proportions of carbohydrate and fat of the diet.

Exercise

Physical activity causes great changes in the body's metabolism, during the exertion itself and thereafter. The overall effect of exercise on fuel utilization and food intake can be judged by considering that the steady state of weight maintenance is reached with a lesser expansion of the adipose tissue mass in physically active individuals.[21] This simple fact integrates all the separate effects of exercise and demonstrates that its overall effect is to promote fat oxidation more than carbohydrate oxidation. Exercise is thus a substitute for greater adiposity, and greater adiposity a substitute for lack of exercise in achieving an average RQ as low as the FQ, and an overall rate of fat oxidation commensurate with fat intake.[41]

STRATEGIES FOR WEIGHT REDUCTION

New and old methods and regimens for weight reduction are constantly promoted, some based on sound principles, others on unsupported or misleading claims. Some of the major metabolically based rationales are summarized below.

The reduction in energy expenditure caused by weight-reducing diets is often greatly overstated. Daily energy expenditure includes a component elicited by food intake itself, i.e., the thermal effect of food, which dissipates about 10% of the food energy consumed. The TEF will, of course, be smaller, for instance by 100 kcal for a 1000 kcal reduction in food intake. The reduction still creates a 900-kcal difference. It is quite obvious that the greater the reduction in energy intake, the greater the energy deficit, and claims questioning this point are rather unreasonable. In addition, energy expenditure is correlated with body size.[7] Once weight has been lost, weight-maintenance energy will, of course, be reduced, by 12 to 15 kcal per day per kg of weight lost.

Avoidance of Dietary Fat

A low-fat diet generally allows the steady state of body weight maintenance to become established at a lower degree of adiposity (Figure 9–4).[1] A sharp reduction in fat intake can therefore be expected to lead to a reduction of the adipose tissue mass in individuals previously consuming substantial amounts of fat. It is important to have reasonable expectations about the possible rates of weight change. For an individual accustomed to a diet providing 40% of total calories as fat, a reduction in fat intake to 30% of total calories will cause a reduction in energy intake of 10%, if protein and carbohydrate consumption remain constant. It would create an energy deficit of some 150 to 300 kcal per day, depending on body size and usual energy turnover, and cause a fat loss of 15 to 30 g per day. Unfortunately, a weekly reduction of the adipose tissue mass by one fourth to one half pound is not likely to create much enthusiasm in individuals who need to shed a lot of weight. These numbers also illustrate that the admonition to eat carbohydrate freely while cutting fat intake, though perhaps reasonable for individuals aiming to maintain weight, is counterproductive for overweight subjects, as it attenuates the impact of a reduction in fat intake on the energy balance. To be effective as a measure for weight correction, a reduction in fat intake must be substantial and complemented by efforts to limit (or at least not increase) carbohydrate intake.

Avoidance of foods with a substantial fat content has the advantage of restricting food choices, which can to some extent attenuate the obesity-promoting influence of the wide food variety provided by mixed diets. This advantage is currently being eroded by the rapid increase in the variety of marketed low-fat substitutes. Consumption of such substitutes, instead of the fattier "real things" that they replace may allow individuals to curb fat intake, but does not reeducate food preferences, thus opening the way for the resumption of the previous dietary habits and weight gain.[42]

Balanced Weight Reduction

Many weight reduction diets prescribe intakes of 1000 to 1500 kcal/day without stressing major shifts in the relative proportions of carbohydrates, fats, and proteins. In order to ensure an adequate protein intake, selection of foods with a relatively high protein content is important, even in such "balanced" weight reduction diets. Given that weight loss is less rapid, the likelihood of staying on course long enough to achieve marked weight reduction is generally less than with the more severely restricted PSMF and VLCD regimens discussed below, on which discomfort due to hunger is often rated to be less.[43] However, balanced weight reduction diets have the considerable advantage of emphasizing reasonable food selection and control of portion size, and of developing knowledge about foods and control of eating behavior, which are essential for long-term success in weight control.

Acute Weight Reduction

The only way to reduce the body's fat content is to use it as a fuel, unless one opts for surgery such as liposuction. Since fat oxidation is limited to the gap between total energy expenditure and carbohydrate plus protein intake, extensive restriction of carbohydrate intake is essential to induce rapid fat oxidation. Near-total avoidance of carbohydrate forces the body to meet most of its energy needs by burning fat. Depending on body size and activity, this may induce the oxidation of 150 to 250 g of fat per day. Thus many weight-reducing diets emphasize avoidance of carbohydrates. But this will be beneficial only to the extent that enhanced fat oxidation is not compensated by high fat intakes. Total starvation creates the greatest energy deficit and a spectacularly rapid initial weight loss, due to a decrease in the extracellular volume during the first days of carbohydrate deprivation. Prolonged starvation can be tolerated for many weeks, as the liver will produce ketone bodies to replace glucose as a fuel for the brain.[10] Quite remarkably, hunger is substantially attenuated after a few days. The great disadvantage of total starvation is that it causes major losses of body protein (some 100 g per day initially, declining to about half that amount after three weeks). Such losses can be effectively minimized by consuming protein. Protein-sparing modified fasts (PSMFs)[44] and very-low-calorie diets (VLCDs)[45] have been developed, which take advantage of the relative suppression of hunger associated with total starvation, while seeking to prevent significant losses of lean body mass. To maintain or approach nitrogen balance during periods of severely negative energy balance, rather high protein intakes are necessary. This fact has sometimes been obscured by comparing the average dose of protein needed to achieve nitrogen balance on a VLCD with the adult RDA for protein, which is set at two standard deviations above the average protein intake needed for nitrogen balance when energy needs are met. In PSMF regimens, 1.2 to 1.5 g protein kg/IBW/day are usually prescribed in the form of lean meat and fish,[44] whereas somewhat lower doses of 70 g protein/day are considered to be sufficient with the VLCD formulas, because they also provide 50 to 70 g of carbohydrates per day. In less obese subjects, in obese adolescents, and in adults engaging in substantial physical activity, slightly more carbohydrate or glucogenic precursors are necessary for maintenance of nitrogen balance.

When proteins of high biological value are provided, complemented with adequate supplements of minerals, vitamins, potassium, and salt, the PSMF and VLCD regimens provide efficient programs for rapid weight loss, though they often lead to gallstone formation.[45] These regimens are most appropriate for markedly obese subjects, who appear to be best able to reduce their need for glucogenic precursors, and for whom there is a special incentive to lose weight as rapidly as possible. Losing fat at a rate of one third to one half pound per day still requires several months to achieve the substantial reduction in adipose tissue that obese individuals may wish to achieve, but at least it offers some hope and motivation. It stands to reason that long periods of severe nutritional restriction can present some dangers to health and that these regimens should be undertaken under medical supervision to ensure adequate intakes of all the nutrients needed (i.e., protein, minerals, electrolytes [notably potassium, which is a prescription item], and vitamins), as well as safe management of drug dosages (which often need to be readjusted) and sound advice about how to cope with individual problems.[44,45] See Chapter 15 on dietary management of weight reduction using these methods.

Weight Regain

While weight reduction depends on defeating the natural tendency to regulate food intake, in weight maintenance one should be able to rely to some extent on spontaneous control of food intake (or at least minimize the struggle against increased intake). It is therefore important to recognize that the logic for nutrient selection during weight maintenance and weight reduction is not the same. This is not commonly appreciated, in part no doubt because such notions are not germane to considerations based merely on the overall energy balance. Failure to appreciate the differences pertaining to weight maintenance and to weight reduction can be conducive to rapid regain of weight lost. Avoidance of carbohydrate in trying to achieve acute weight reduction (e.g., PSMF or VLCD) drastically reduces food choices and compels the organism to operate with low glycogen reserves, which enhances fat oxidation. This allows adaptation to the starvation state where hunger is less intense after a few days, but only as long as carbohydrate intake is kept extremely low (≤ 50 g per day). After such a bout of weight reduction, when carbohydrate intake is no longer as severely curtailed and weight tends to be regained, the dieter may remember that rapid weight loss was achieved by avoiding carbohydrates while eating meat and fish. This reinforces the common belief that carbohydrates are major culprits in causing weight gain. The dieter may be enticed to more liberally consume foods known for their low carbohydrate, but high protein content (i.e., meats, fish, cheese, and nuts). However, now that carbohydrate intake is not severely restricted, this bias is counterproductive, because most of these food items are high in fat, thwarting the central strategy for weight maintenance, which is to prevent a positive fat balance by limiting fat intake.

CONCLUSION

Avoidance of errors in the fat balance has received much lower priority in biological evolution than the need to maintain appropriate glycogen stores and a suitable lean body mass. Protein and carbohydrate balances are thus automatically maintained in all individuals, whether thin or fat, sedentary or athletic. To avoid weight gain, it is therefore necessary and sufficient to burn as much fat as one eats. This is made difficult when consumption of diets with substantial amounts of fat is combined with a sedentary lifestyle. If one fails to limit fat intake, or to maintain glycogen levels low enough to facilitate fat oxidation, or to exercise enough to increase fat oxidation in muscle, the adipose tissue mass will expand, until this has the effect of raising fat oxidation to the rate required to match fat intake.

How fat one must be to burn as much fat as one eats is determined by the particular set of inherited traits, circumstantial conditions, lifestyle, and eating pattern of each individual. As long as circumstantial factors remain unchanged, this "body configuration" tends to be restored if it is temporarily disturbed. It thus appears as if the organism prefers to operate at a particular body weight, which has led to the concept of defense of body weight at a predetermined "setpoint." However, these concepts do not take into account the influence of circumstantial factors without invoking a mysterious "resetting of the setpoint." When one understands that weight maintenance becomes established whenever the particular body composition has been achieved that allows the RQ to be equal to the FQ,[3,9] such ad hoc assumptions are not needed to explain body weight stability. Obesity thus appears to be not so much caused by a defect in the ability to regulate the energy balance, than by a tendency to maintain energy balance, but only in the presence of an unacceptably high amount of adipose tissue.

There is insufficient information on what level the percentage of total energy intake consumed in the form of fat must be reduced to prevent obesity, and this limit is likely to vary for different individuals. The 30% target proposed by current guidelines will not by itself be sufficient to prevent excess weight among individuals prone to develop obesity. However, even if limiting fat intake to 30% does not guarantee or restore ideal body weights, this measure can be expected to have some impact, particularly because a cap on fat intake could substantially alter the dietary habits of obese subjects, who often have a predilection for fatty foods. It is certainly also feasible to reduce fat intake to 25%, or even to 20% of total caloric intake, but this requires a sustained commitment to an increasingly exclusive selection of food items, differing substantially from the assortment of foods preferred in Western societies. In addition to the metabolic leverage thereby achieved, and the reduction in caloric density of the allowed foods, this can have the very significant advantage of facilitating weight control by reducing the diversity of the food offerings provided by mixed diets, if this advantage is not lost to the ever increasing availability of low-fat substitutes. In attempting to control body weight by markedly reducing fat in the diet, it is important to remember that energy consumed in the form of alcohol should be included with that provided by fat, since alcohol intake selectively reduces fat, but not carbohydrate oxidation.[39]

Finally, it is important to understand why the incidence of obesity in the United States has increased from 25% to 33% during the last decade,[46] even though dietary fat content was essentially stable during this period. As illustrated in Figure 9–3, the size that the adipose tissue mass has to reach for fat oxidation rates to be commensurate with fat intake is determined not only by inherited regulatory traits, exercise habits, and dietary fat content, but also by the range within which glycogen levels are habitually maintained. The impact of differences in this range can be surmised to be considerable, though this is generally ignored, because data on glycogen levels are not available. The range within which glycogen levels are habitually maintained is markedly influenced by food palatability, diversity, and availability, as well as by social interactions and exercise habits. Thus the effects of eating habits and lifestyle factors on the incidence of obesity is likely to be mediated in part through their influence on glycogen levels, and thereby on fat oxidation. It seems reasonable to consider that an upward shift in the range within which glycogen levels are habitually maintained, brought about by changes in the food supply and by a further decline in physical activity, could explain the recent increase in the incidence of obesity in the United States and Europe.[3]

ACKNOWLEDGMENTS

The collaboration of K.S. Sargent and D. Demers is gratefully acknowledged. This publication was made possible in part by grant number DK 33214 from the National Institutes of Health. Its contents are solely the responsibility of the author and do not necessarily represent the official views of the National Institutes of Health.

REFERENCES

1. Lissner L, Heitmann BL. Dietary fat and obesity: evidence from epidemiology. *Eur J Clin Nutr.* 1995;49:79–90.
2. *Recommended Dietary Allowances*, 10th ed. Washington, DC: National Academy Press; 1989.
3. Flatt JP. McCollum Award Lecture, 1995: diet, lifestyle and weight maintenance. *Am J Clin Nutr.* 1995;62:820–836.
4. Acheson KJ, Schutz V, Bessard T. Nutritional influences on lipogenesis and thermogenesis after a carbohydrate meal. *Am J Physiol.* 1984;246:E62–E70.
5. Acheson KJ, Schutz V, Bessard T, Anantharank K, Flatt JP, Jequier F. Glycogen storage capacity and de novo lipogenesis during massive carbohydrate overfeeding in man. *Am J Clin Nutr.* 1988;48:240–247.
6. Hellerstein MK, Christiansen M, Kaempfer S. Measurement of de novo hepatic lipogenesis in humans using stable isotopes. *J Clin Invest.* 1991;87:1841–1852.
7. Prentice AM, Black AE, Coward WA, Cole TJ. Energy expenditure in overweight and obese adults in affluent societies: an analysis of 319 doubly-labelled water measurements. *Eur J Clin Nutr.* 1996;50:93–97.
8. FAO/WHO/UNU. *Energy and Protein Requirements.* Geneva: World Health Organization; 1985.
9. Flatt JP. Importance of nutrient balance in body weight regulation. *Diabetes Metab Rev.* 1988;4:571–581.
10. Cahill GFJ. Starvation in man. *Clin Endocrinol Metab.* 1976;5:397–415.
11. Shetty PS, Prentice AM, Goldberg ER. Alterations in fuel selection and voluntary food intake in response to isoenergetic manipulation of glycogen stores in humans. *Am J Clin Nutr.* 1994;60:534–543.
12. Russek M. Current status of the hepatostatic theory of food intake control. *Appetite.* 1981;2:137–143.
13. Flatt JP. Dietary fat, carbohydrate balance, and weight maintenance: effects of exercise. *Am J Clin Nutr.* 1987;45:296–306.
14. Stubbs RJ, Harbron CG, Murgatroyd PR, Prentice AM. Covert manipulation of dietary fat and energy density: effect on substrate flux and food intake in men eating ad libitum. *Am J Clin Nutr.* 1995;62:316–329.
15. Flatt JP, Ravussin E, Acheson KJ, Jéquier E. Effects of dietary fat on postprandial substrate oxidation and on carbohydrate and fat balances. *J Clin Invest.* 1985;76:1019–1024.
16. Griffiths AJ, Humphreys SM, Clark ML, Fielding BA, Frayn KN. Immediate metabolic availability of dietary fat in combination with carbohydrate. *Am J Clin Nutr.* 1994;59:53–59.
17. Björntorp P, Bergman H, Varnauskas E, Lindholm B. Lipid mobilization in relation to body composition in man. *Metabolism.* 1969;18:840–851.

18. Randle PJ, Hales CN, Garland PB, Newsholme EA. The glucose fatty-acid cycle: its role in insulin sensitivity and the metabolic disturbances of diabetes mellitus. *Lancet*. 1963;i:785–789.

19. Rolls BJ, Rowe EA, Rolls ET, Kingston B, Megson A, Gunary R. Variety in a meal enhances food intake in man. *Physiol Behav*. 1981;26:215–221.

20. de Castro JM, Brewer EM. The amount eaten in meals by humans is a power function of the number of people present. *Physiol Behav*. 1992;51:121–125.

21. Ballor DL, Keesey RE. A meta-analysis of the factors affecting exercise-induced changes in body mass, fat mass, and fat-free mass in males and females. *Int J Obes*. 1991;15:717–726.

22. Gollnick PD. Metabolism of substrates: energy substrate metabolism during exercise and as modified by training. *Fed Proc*. 1985;44:353–357.

23. Sorensen TIA, Holst C, Stunkard AJ. Childhood body mass index: genetic and familial enviromental influences assessed in a longitudinal adoption study. *In J Obes*. 1992;16:705–714.

24. Bouchard C, Després J-P, Mauriège P. Genetic and nongenetic determinants of regional fat distribution. *Endocr Rev*. 1993;14:72–93.

25. Heitman BL, Lissner L, Sørensen TIA, Bengtsson C. Dietary fat intake and weight gain in women genetically predisposed for obesity. *Am J Clin Nutr*. 1995;61:1213–1217.

26. Flatt JP. The RQ/FQ concept and weight maintenance. In: Flatt JP, ed. *Recent Advances in Obesity Research*. In press.

27. Flatt JP. The biochemistry of energy expenditure. *Rec Adv Obes Res*. 1978;2:211–228.

28. Edholm OG, Adam JM, Healy MJ, Wolff HS, Goldsmith R, Best TW. Food intake and energy expenditure of army recruits. *Br J Nutr*. 1970;24:1091–1107.

29. Abbott WGH, Howard BU, Christin L. Short-term energy balance: relationship with protein, carbohydrate, and fat balances. *Am J Physiol*. 1988;255:E332–E337.

30. Mayer J, Thomas DW. Regulation of food intake and obesity. *Science*. 1967;156:328–337.

31. Foltin RW, Rolls BJ, Moran TH, Kelly TH, McNelis AL, Fischman MW. Caloric, but not macronutrient, compensation by humans for required eating occasions with meals and snack varying in fat and carbohydrate. *Am J Clin Nutr*. 1992;55:331–342.

32. Bingham SA, Gill C, Welch A. Comparison of dietary assessment methods in nutritional epidemiology: weighed records v. 24h recalls, food-frequency questionnaires and estimated-diet records. *Br J Nutr*. 1994;72:619–643.

33. Roberts SB, Young VR, Fuss P. Energy expenditure and subsequent nutrient intakes in overfed young men. *Am J Physiol*. 1990;259:R461–R469.

34. Tremblay A, Després JP, Thériault G, Fournier G, Bouchard C. Overfeeding and energy expenditure in humans. *Am J Clin Nutr*. 1992;56:857–862.

35. Lissner L, Levitsky DA, Strupp BJ, Kalkwarf HJ, Roe DA. Dietary fat and the regulation of energy intake in human subjects. *Am J Clin Nutr*. 1987;46:886–892.

36. Kendall A, Levitsky DA, Strupp BJ, Lissner L. Weight loss on a low fat diet: consequence of the imprecision of the control of food intake in humans. *Am J Clin Nutr*. 1991;53:1124–1129.

37. Tremblay A, St-Pierre S. The hyperphagic effect of high-fat and alcohol persists after control for energy density. *Am J Clin Nutr*. 1996;63:479–482.

38. Prentice AM. Alcohol and obesity. *Int J Obes*. 1995;19:S44–S50.

39. Suter PM, Schutz Y, Jéquier E. The effect of ethanol on fat storage in healthy subjects. *N Engl J Med*. 1992;326:983–987.

40. de Castro JM, Orozco S. Moderate alcohol intake and spontaneous eating patterns of humans: evidence of unregulated supplementation. *Am J Clin Nutr.* 1990;52:246–253.

41. Flatt JP. Integration of the overall effects of exercise. *Int J Obes.* 1995;19:S31–S40.

42. Mattes RD. Fat preference and adherence to a reduced-fat diet. *Am J Clin Nutr.* 1993;57:373–381.

43. Wadden TA, Stunkard AJ, Day SC, Gould RA, Rubin CJ. Less food, less hunger: reports of appetite and symptoms in a controlled study of a protein-sparing modified fast. *Int J Obes.* 1987;11:239–249.

44. Bistrian BR. Clinical use of a protein-sparing modified fast. *JAMA.* 1978;240:2299–2302.

45. Wadden TA, Stunkard AJ, Brownell KD. Very low calorie diets: their efficacy, safety, and future. *Ann Intern Med.* 1983;99:675–684.

46. Kuczmarski RJ, Flegal KM, Campbell SM, Johnson CL. Increasing prevalence of overweight among US adults. *JAMA.* 1994;272:205–211.

CHAPTER 10

Diet Composition and the Regulation of Food Intake and Body Weight

Victoria Hammer Castellanos
Barbara J. Rolls

INTRODUCTION

Physicians and scientists have worked for decades to uncover the causes of obesity and to develop effective treatments. Different types of dietary treatments for obesity have been tried, some with more success than others. Over the years, various macronutrients in food (carbohydrate/sugar or fat) have been targeted as either the cause of obesity or the solution to successful weight loss in obese individuals. For example, low-carbohydrate diets (including low-sugar diets), high-fiber diets, and low-fat diets have all been in vogue at different times over the last 45 years. These diet plans have been especially popular among dieters when they are so-called "free" diets, such that dieters are allowed to eat as much as they like of certain groups of foods and calorie intake per se is not limited. Currently, low-fat diets are thought to be the solution to weight loss because they seem to require little, if any, conscious energy restriction.

This chapter briefly examines the evolution of theories about the effect of diet composition on the regulation of food intake and body weight, and then reviews the evidence regarding the usefulness of low-fat diets for weight loss and weight maintenance. Finally, particular attention is given to research evidence that supports a view that diets of low-energy density (not just low-fat diets per se) can be helpful in weight reduction and maintenance, and that the success of these diets should be attributed in large part to a spontaneous reduction in dietary energy intake.

BACKGROUND SUMMARY

In the 1950s and 1960s, several weight loss diets emerged advocating free intake of foods high in protein and fat but restricting consumption of foods high in carbohydrate. One of the first was Marriot's diet in 1949,[1] to be followed by The Prudent Diet,[2] Gordon's diet plan,[3] Donaldson's antiobesity routine,[4] Yudkin's Low-Carbohydrate Diet,[5] and others.[6] These diets were based on the premise that carbohydrates, sugar in particular, have low satiety value and that sugar creates some sort of "artificial appetite."[6] It was believed that consumption of non-carbohydrate foods would remain about the same as in the typical eating regimen, such that the reduction in dietary carbohydrate would result in a significant energy deficit,[5,7] and there was some evidence that people did eat less when their diet choices were limited only to high-fat and high-protein foods.[5,8] Some advocates of these diets also speculated that fat may have metabolic advantages over carbohydrate and protein.[5,9] To date, no metabolic advantage has been demonstrated for the use of low-carbohydrate diets for weight reduction, and any enhanced weight loss demonstrated on these diets was likely due to electrolyte loss and large shifts in water balance.[10,11] Although a low-calorie, low-carbohydrate diet could be used for weight loss, a diet with such severe restrictions is not likely to be followed for long periods of time, and a diet high in fat would not be advisable in light of the strong link between dietary fat and risk of chronic diseases.[12]

Interest in the use of fiber supplements and high-fiber foods to satisfy appetite emerged in the 1970s and 1980s. Several reasons led researchers to believe that a fiber-rich diet might reduce overall food intake and help control body weight without the necessity of counting calories. Fiber has been shown to affect gastric emptying, small intestine motility, and rates and completeness of fat, carbohydrate, and protein absorption in the gut.[13] High-fiber foods also require more chewing, taking longer to eat.[14] Although numerous clinical trials have been conducted, methodological problems in many of these studies limit their usefulness in determining whether or not dietary fiber does affect food intake and body weight.[15,16] In general, the use of fiber supplements and the manipulation of fiber in single foods has not been shown to have more than a small effect on energy intake and body weight. It appears that a greater effect may be achieved when high-fiber foods are used as part of an overall diet that is low in energy density. The role of dietary fiber and low-energy diets in weight management will be discussed later.

It is a widely held belief that dietary fat has a greater satiety value than dietary carbohydrate due to differences in the rate of gastric emptying.[17] However, the notion that fat, on an energy basis, leaves the stomach more slowly than carbohydrate has been challenged by work in non-human primates,[18] although comparable experiments have not been performed in humans. The presumed high satiety value of fat was thought to contribute to the success of low-carbohydrate (high-fat) diets by decreasing ad libitum energy intake.[5,8] Some advocates of low-carbohydrate diets also believed that these diets were more palatable than diets with other types of food restrictions, promoting long-term dietary compliance. It is ironic that current thinking suggests that high-fat diets are a cause of obesity.

At present, the most popular method of dieting is to restrict dietary fat.[19] Many nutritionists and other health care professionals are advocating the permanent adoption of a low-fat diet to achieve weight loss and successful maintenance at a lower body weight. It has been suggested that a low-fat diet alone, independent of any conscious energy restriction, will result in significant and permanent weight loss.[20,21] As a result, a new type of "free" diet has emerged, this one allowing free consumption of fat-free or low-fat foods. But, some data from the National Health and Nutrition Examination Survey III (NHANES III) suggests that simply reducing the percent of calories from fat may not lead to successful weight loss. Over the last decade, Americans cut their fat intake from 36% to 34% of calories, but energy intake increased 100 to 300 kcal/day[22] and prevalence of overweight increased 8% over that same period of time.[23] The NHANES III data indicates that although people are eating a lower percentage of their calorie intake as fat, they may not be consuming fewer grams of fat and their energy intake continues to exceed energy expenditure.

The idea that dietary fat contributes to obesity is partly attributable to survey studies that demonstrated a correlation between dietary fat content and degree of overweight in a given population.[24–29] In some of these studies, the amount of fat consumed appears to be a more important determinant of body weight than total energy intake.[24–28] This has led to speculation about how high dietary fat intake might contribute to obesity. It has been hypothesized that fat causes people to overeat (i.e., eat more energy than is required to maintain body weight) because it enhances the palatability of food. It has also been suggested that high-fat foods are overeaten because they are energy dense and a small quantity of food contains a large amount of energy, or that palatability and energy density work together to promote obesity on a high-fat diet.[30] Fat may also contribute to obesity apart from its effect on palatability and energy density. Recent research indicates that while certain groups of people are sensitive to the energy content of a food whether the energy is provided by either fat or carbohydrate, other groups of people (obese individuals and those concerned with their food intake and body weight) may be relatively insensitive to the satiety value of fat.[31] Other research has suggested that the body has little ability to increase fat oxidation to compensate for a high-fat intake, leading to storage of excess dietary fat as body fat.[32] The effect of diet composition on metabolism and its relevance to body weight regulation has been discussed in Chapter 8 and will not be addressed here. The following discussion will examine how the macronutrient composition of the diet affects food intake and thereby affects body weight.

CURRENT RESEARCH AND UNDERSTANDING OF MACRONUTRIENT COMPOSITION OF DIETS, FOOD INTAKE, AND BODY WEIGHT

Numerous investigators have studied various aspects of the effects of diet composition on food intake and body weight regulation. Several different research methodologies have been employed, each of which yields somewhat different types of information. In survey or epidemiological studies, the researcher attempts to study people in their natural environment without influencing their behavior. This research approach has been used to identify which diet characteristics are associated with maintenance of a healthy body weight and which are associated with obesity or weight gain. In contrast to survey studies, intervention studies implement change in free-living populations in order to study the effects of that change. In this case, intervention studies have examined how changes in diet composition may affect food intake, body weight, body composition, and other parameters. Laboratory-based studies have been used to examine the effects of very specific dietary manipulations under highly controlled conditions. In some studies, one food or meal was manipulated, whereas in other studies the diet was manipulated over the course of several days or weeks. In some of the laboratory-based studies, fat or sugar substitutes have been used as a means to manipulate diet composition. Taken together, these different types of studies give us some clues as to how diet composition affects food intake and body weight.

Survey Studies

Relationship between Diet Composition and Body Weight

Several survey studies have examined specifically the relationship between diet composition and body weight. Large survey studies, such as NHANES I and the Nurses Health Study, collected extensive diet and health data, using various measures of self-reported food intake, such as the 24-hour recall, food diaries (two to seven days), or food frequency questionnaires, to determine the usual intake of energy and various nutrients in the study population. Based on these self-reports of food intake, many researchers have found a positive association between measures of overweight (i.e., body mass index, percent ideal body weight, percent body fat) and the percentage of fat in the diet.[24–29] Data from some of these studies[24–28] suggest that the relationship between dietary fat and degree of overweight may be independent of the relationship between dietary fat intake and overall energy intake. Several studies[24,26,29] also found a negative correlation between carbohydrate intake and degree of overweight, although one study[25] showed a greater intake of added sugars in obese individuals. Diets low in dietary fiber have also been associated with higher body weights (Table 10–1).[25,26]

The results are mixed from several longitudinal survey studies[29,33,34] that related diet composition and maintenance of a stable body weight over time. In women aged 30 to 55 participating in the Nurses Health Study cohort,[29] fat intake was positively associated with weight gain in the first two years of follow-up but in the subsequent four years fat intake was negatively associated with weight gain. In

Table 10–1 Diet Records Indicated That Obese Individuals Ate Diets That Were High in Fat and Added Sugar and Low in Total Carbohydrate and Dietary Fiber (N = 78).

	Males		Females	
Variables	Lean	Obese	Lean	Obese
Body fat (%)	11.1	29.2*	16.7	42.7*
Energy intake (kcal)	2,523	2,575	1,775	1,980
Nutrients (% of energy)				
Fat	29.1	33.1*	29.6	36.3*
Carbohydrate	55.1	50.9*	51.9	46.3*
Added sugar (% of sugar energy)	25.2	38.0*	31.4	47.9*
Fiber (g)	26.9	20.9*	22.7	15.7*

*Significantly different from the lean, $p < 0.05$.

Source: W.C. Miller et al., Dietary Fat, Sugar, and Fiber Predict Body Fat Content, Copyright The American Dietetic Association. Adapted by permission from *Journal of the American Dietetic Association,* Vol. 94, No. 6, pp. 612–615, © 1994.

these nurses, dietary carbohydrate was negatively correlated with weight gain over all six years of the study, but sucrose was positively associated with weight gain in the first two years and negatively associated over the last four years of the study. The follow-up study for NHANES I[34] showed an inverse relationship between the percentage of fat in the diet and weight gain in women under 50, but a positive association between fat intake and weight gain in all men free of morbidity. On the other hand, Klesges and coworkers[33] reported a positive association between the proportion of energy as fat and weight change over a three-year period in both men and women. Neither of the two latter studies[33,34] considered the relationship of weight change and other food components, such as carbohydrate, sugar, or fiber. The evidence suggests that a high-fat diet is associated with weight gain, but because the results of these studies were mixed and other nutrients were not consistently studied, the relationship between diet composition and weight maintenance is inconclusive.

In general, the results from survey studies have led to the suggestion that there is a causal relationship between dietary fat and obesity, but by their nature, they do not demonstrate causality. In several studies the data suggest a relationship between dietary fat and obesity independent of energy intake, but interpretation of self-reported food intake data should be made with caution due to the possibility of large sources of error and systematic bias.[35–40] It has been shown that food intake, in general, is underreported[38] and that self-reports of food intake become less accurate as dietary intake increases.[37] Some research[38–40] has also indicated that obese individuals are especially prone to underreporting their food intake. In addition to the problems inherent in self-reported food intake, some of these studies fail to control for likely confounding variables such as activity level and smoking status. Studies that do account for activity level do so through self-report, which may interject another type of bias into the data, i.e., obese individuals may tend to overestimate their activity level.[40] Thus, it is possible that limitations in methodology for determining energy intake and expenditure might have led researchers in some of these studies to erroneously conclude that dietary fat is associated with obesity independent of energy intake.

Taken together, the results of the survey studies support a hypothesis that there are certain nutrients, and perhaps certain diets, associated with overeating.[41] More specifically, they suggest that a high-fat (low-carbohydrate), and perhaps low-fiber and/or high added sugar, diet is associated with excessive energy intake. As dietary fat provides over twice as much energy per gram as dietary carbohydrate and dietary fiber provides little or no metabolizable energy, a high-fat, high-sucrose, low-fiber diet could also be described as energy dense. At least one study[42] has shown (via diet records) that obese individuals show a clear preference for foods of high-energy density and exclude nearly all foods of low-energy density from their diet. In addition, a large clinical sample of obese men and women found that fat was the major nutrient source in their 10 favorite foods.[43]

Laboratory-based research offers support for an enhanced preference for high-fat foods in obese individuals. In sensory tests, obese individuals have shown a preference for higher levels of fat in certain foods than lean individuals.[44] Drewnowski and colleagues[45] found that obese and formerly obese individuals preferred higher levels of fat in mixtures of dairy products and sugar than did lean individuals. However, in subsequent research, Drewnowski et al[46] found that only a subset of obese persons, those with a history of large weight fluctuations, showed an enhanced fat preference. A positive relationship between sensory preferences for fat in a variety of foods and percentage of body fat has also been demonstrated in people within a normal weight range.[47] Taken together, these studies indicate that enhanced preference for fat could be important in the development and maintenance of obesity. Additional research is needed to understand how individual preferences for dietary fat and other macronutrients influence diet selection, and in turn, how composition of the diet that is selected affects the volume of food and amount of energy that is eaten.

Dietary Intervention Studies

Changes in Body Weight Associated with a Reduction in Dietary Fat

Dietary intervention trials to study heart disease and cancer give us the opportunity to study the effects of reducing the fat content of the diet in a free-living non-obese population (obese individuals were mainly excluded from participation) and usually not consciously trying to restrict energy intake. These studies typically have similar designs: (1) baseline dietary intake is determined for free-living individuals through one or more measures of self-reported food intake, i.e., food diaries and food frequency questionnaires; (2) after determination of initial diet characteristics and body weight, the intervention group(s) receives instruction on how to reduce dietary fat intake; and (3) to evaluate compliance and the efficacy of the diet, diet composition is reevaluated and changes in body weight and other physiological parameters are assessed at various time points throughout the study, which typically lasts from several months to two years.

One of the longest and most thoroughly documented intervention trials has been the Women's Health Trial.[48-51] In the vanguard group, 303 women, between the ages of 45 and 69, participated.[48] At the start, the average percentage ideal body weight (IBW) was 111.2, with 48% of the group having body weights 101% to 120% of IBW and with women exceeding 150% of IBW excluded. The treatment consisted of a comprehensive dietary and behavioral program to lower fat intake from a mean baseline of 39% to 20% of energy intake. According to food records, this goal was achieved, with a 59% reduction in total fat intake (to approximately 22% of calories from dietary fat) and a 25% reduction in energy intake during the first 12 months. Although weight loss per se was neither encouraged nor discouraged, the authors noted that many women used the program as an opportunity to lose weight. After six months of intervention, the average weight loss was approximately 3.1 kg, with 2.4 kg of that loss occurring during the first three months. Despite continued reports of low energy and fat intake, only 1.9 kg of that weight loss was maintained at the end of two years (Figure 10–1). Data analysis suggested that changes in percent of energy from fat were more strongly predictive of weight change than were changes in total energy intake, although the average energy intake reported is so low (1300 to 1350 kcal/day at 6, 12, and 24 months), one might question the accuracy of this data.

There are many additional examples of intervention studies aimed at reducing dietary fat in non-obese individuals (<120% to 130% IBW, depending on the study) in order to reduce health risks for certain diseases. We will review a sampling of these studies,[52-62] to determine how the macronutrient composition of the diet affected energy intake and body weight. Because the majority of these studies had findings similar to the Women's Health Trial, they will not be discussed individually, but will be described as a group. In these studies, baseline fat intake ranged from 35% to 41% of energy from fat. Following the intervention, fat intake was reduced to anywhere from 13%[59] to 32%[57] of calories from fat. When dietary fat intake was reduced, the food records reflected a spontaneous reduction in energy intake.[52-55,58-62] As one might expect, a reduction in body weight was also consistently seen in association with a reduction in dietary fat and calories. In

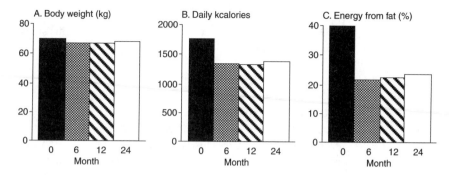

Figure 10–1 Average weight loss was 3.1 kg (A) during the first six months of the Women's Health Trial. Subjects maintained only 1.9 kg of that loss at 24 months post-intervention despite reports of continued low-energy (B) and low-fat (C) intake. *Source:* Adapted with permission from L. Sheppard, A.R. Kristal, and L.H. Kushi, Weight Loss in Women Participating in a Randomized Trial of Low-Fat Diets, *American Journal of Clinical Nutrition,* Vol. 54, pp. 821–828, © 1991, The American Society for Clinical Nutrition.

short studies, lasting less than three months, average weight loss ranged from 1.4 to 2.8 kg.[60,61] In longer studies,[52–59,62] where subjects on a reduced-fat diet were followed from six months to two years, average weight loss ranged from 1 to 6 kg. Where data are available at intermediate time points,[52–54,58] as in the Women's Health Trial[48] (Figure 10–1), the weight loss appeared to occur within the first several (three to six) months and then remained fairly stable for the remainder of the study.

Two additional studies worth discussing in more detail are the Lifestyle Heart Trial by Dean Ornish and colleagues[63] and the Waianae Diet Program.[64] These studies employed the most severe dietary restrictions and reported the most dramatic effect on body weight of any of the studies discussed here. Both studies included obese individuals.

The diet used in the Lifestyle Heart Trial is the same diet that has been advocated in Ornish's recent book *Eat More, Weigh Less.*[21] It is essentially a vegan diet that allows one cup of nonfat milk or yogurt and one egg white per day. Male and female subjects with a wide range of body weights participated in the study. After 12 months of intervention, three-day diet records indicated that fat was reduced from 31.5% to 6.8% of the diet. The diet records indicated approximately a 150 kcal/day reduction in energy intake from baseline, and subjects had an average weight loss of 10 kg after one year. The authors give us no indication whether initial body weight was related to the amount of weight lost.

The Waianae Diet Program used a similarly low-fat diet. This study of Native Hawaiians related consumption of the traditional Hawaiian diet (<7% of calories from fat) to obesity and other risk factors of cardiovascular disease. Twenty obese men and women (body mass index 27.7 to 48.7) participated in a 21-day trial in which Native Hawaiian food was prepared and served at a test site. In this study, average energy intake decreased by 1000 kcal/day and the average weight loss over 21 days was 7.8 kg.

Although these studies suggest that reducing dietary fat to approximately 7% of calories will result in significant weight loss, especially for obese people, achieving this degree of dietary fat reduction requires extreme diet and lifestyle changes. Maintaining diet palatability at this level of dietary fat also requires substantial effort in meal planning and preparation. This was not an issue in the Hawaiian study because it was very short and all of the food was prepared for the subjects at a test site. Thus, this study offers no indication of the practicality of this type of dietary change under non-study conditions. It is likely that only the most highly motivated individuals would be able to maintain this type of diet regimen for any length of time.

It is important to keep in mind that the intervention studies discussed above relied heavily on self-reports as a source of data on macronutrient and total energy intake. Given the limitations of these methods for measuring food intake,[35-40] these studies should be interpreted cautiously. It is also important to remember that, except for the Lifestyle Heart Trial[63] and Waianae Diet Program,[64] most of the subjects in these studies were not significantly overweight at the beginning of the intervention period. It would seem logical that individual weight loss on a reduced-fat diet is related to initial degree of overweight, but because the purpose of these studies was not weight reduction, this type of data analysis was not done. Nevertheless, data from these intervention studies do suggest that a reduction in dietary fat may help adults who are within 30% of their ideal body weight to achieve and maintain a somewhat lower body weight without conscious restriction of dietary energy. The effect of the fat reduction is likely to be proportional to its magnitude, such that dietary fat may need to be reduced to a level below 30% of calories in order to produce a noticeable benefit for weight maintenance or weight loss.

REDUCING DIETARY FAT FOR THE PURPOSE OF WEIGHT LOSS

Several intervention studies have been done to look specifically at the use of low-fat diets for weight loss in obese individuals, both as a way to lose weight without consciously restricting calories and as part of a low-calorie diet. In one study,[65] researchers compared weight loss of two groups with an equal dietary fat restriction (25 g per day), but with one group also restricted to a specific energy level (1200 or 1500 kcal for females or males, respectively). At the end of the 16- to 20-week program, researchers found that both groups lost weight but the energy restricted group lost significantly more weight (4.6 kg on low-fat only vs 8.8 kg on low-fat with energy restriction). Both groups lost similar amounts of lean body mass, with a greater loss of body fat in the low-calorie group (Figure 10–2). Follow-up data collected 9 to 12 months later showed that both groups had gained weight such that there was no longer a difference between the groups.

Researchers at the University of Minnesota[66,67] had somewhat different findings in their 18-month weight loss study. When moderately obese women in one group were instructed to restrict fat intake to a specific gram amount (20 g) while the women in the other group were instructed to limit their intake to 30% fat on a 1000 or 1200 kcal per day diet, both groups reduced their energy intake by the same amount and both lost the same amount of weight (4.4 kg on low-fat vs 3.8 kg on energy restriction) in the first six months. Average weight returned to baseline levels in both groups over the succeeding 12 months despite continued intervention.[67] Although the use of a low-fat diet resulted in modest weight loss in the initial four to six months of both of these studies,[65,67] in neither study was the weight loss continued or even totally maintained. Thus, neither of these studies provide evidence that an obese individual could achieve a large weight loss or continue to lose weight over a long period of time by restricting only dietary fat.

The results from these studies[65–67] indicate that for obese people, adoption of a low-fat diet in the absence of a conscious caloric restriction may result in modest weight loss over a period of a few months. On the other hand, there is some indica-

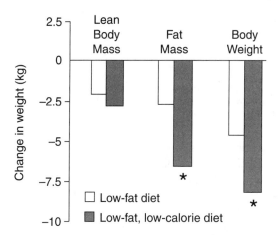

Figure 10–2 Changes in body weight and body composition after 16 to 20 weeks on either a low-fat or a low-calorie diet. Both groups lost similar amounts of lean body mass, with a greater loss of body fat in the low-calorie group. *Source:* Adapted with permission from D.G. Schlundt et al., Randomized Evaluation of a Low Fat Ad Libitum Carbohydrate Diet for Weight Reduction, *International Journal of Obesity,* Vol. 17, p. 626, © 1993, Macmillan Press Ltd.

tion that instructing overweight people to restrict fat *and* calories may be a more effective strategy for weight loss than instructing them to restrict only fat, especially in light of the availability of many new low-fat, high-calorie foods. Whether the enhanced weight loss achieved with caloric restriction will be maintained over the long run is not clear. Certainly it has been demonstrated that most people regain weight that is lost on calorie-restricted diets.[68]

EFFECT OF MACRONUTRIENT COMPOSITION ON EFFICIENCY OF WEIGHT GAIN AND WEIGHT LOSS

It has been put forward by some in the popular press[21] and the scientific community[32] that in weight regulation, the type of calories an individual eats is more important than the total amount of calories eaten, i.e., that the energy content of fat and carbohydrate may not be metabolically equivalent. It appears that excess energy from dietary fat is more efficiently stored as body fat than excess energy from carbohydrate, but the metabolic efficiency of various macronutrients during weight loss or weight maintenance is less clear.

The effects of diet composition on weight gain are clearer than the effects on weight loss. In the Vermont studies of the effects of long-term overeating,[69] it was observed that naturally lean subjects had great difficulty gaining weight when overfed a mixed diet of carbohydrate and fat compared to a similar group fed the extra calories as fat only. At least part of the increased efficiency of weight gain on a high-fat diet can be explained by the fact that it simply costs less energy to store energy from fat compared to extra calories from carbohydrate. The cost of deposition of dietary fat into adipose tissue is only 3%, whereas when dietary carbohydrate is converted to fat the obligatory cost is 23% of original calories from carbohydrate.[70] Additional aspects of fat and carbohydrate metabolism, which may explain differences in efficiency for weight gain during positive energy balance, have been discussed in Chapter 8 and will not be reiterated here.

Very few controlled studies have been done to examine how the macronutrient content of nutritionally adequate diets (excluding very-low-calorie diets) may affect weight loss or weight maintenance when energy intake is matched. In a study where a 1200-kcal weight loss diet contained 10%, 35%, or 45% of calories from fat, with variations in both protein and carbohydrate, there was no significant difference in total weight loss or in loss of lean body mass over a 10-week period.[71] Nor did a similar study show a significant difference in weight loss or body composition between high protein 26% or 45% fat diets (30% protein protein, 1200 kcals/day for 12 weeks).[72] Another study[73] examined the effect of macronutrient content of the diet on body composition and energy expenditure after 12 weeks of weight reduction and 6 weeks of maintenance. In this study, a low-fat diet (15%

fat, 60% carbohydrate) was compared to a low-carbohydrate diet (50% fat, 25% carbohydrate). These reducing diets were designed to promote a weight loss of 1 kg/wk, with energy levels individually prescribed to approximately 75% of each subject's resting metabolic rate. Results showed that composition of the diet did not significantly influence body composition or energy expenditure during weight loss or maintenance following weight loss. Even though body composition and energy expenditure were not different, greater weight loss was observed with the low-carbohydrate than with the low-fat diet (−10.6 vs −8.1 kg, respectively). However, the authors do suggest that compliance may have been different between diets. More studies of this type need to be conducted in order to fully understand how diet composition affects weight loss and body composition. This is especially important because these results differ from the results of similar studies performed in rats, where low dietary fat during weight loss was associated with a greater loss of adipose tissue.[74] Nevertheless, to date, research conducted in humans suggests that the fat-to-carbohydrate ratio does not affect body composition or metabolic efficiency in a diet designed to promote slow weight loss.

There is some question as to whether macronutrients have differential effects on energy expenditure and metabolic efficiency at weight maintenance. Several short-term studies[75–80] examined the effects of high- vs low-carbohydrate diets on various aspects of energy expenditure, i.e., 24-hour expenditure or resting metabolic rate. None of these studies showed a difference in energy requirements from diets differing in fat and carbohydrate content. In addition to calorimetry studies, which are fairly short in duration, Leibel and coworkers[81] reviewed data from long-term feeding studies to determine the metabolic efficiency of diets that varied widely in fat and carbohydrate content. They determined the energy requirements of 16 people (13 adults, 3 children) fed liquid diets of precisely known composition. The subjects were fed each diet for 15 to 56 days while living in a metabolic ward—where activity level was controlled and where it was possible to collect precise data on energy intake and daily body weight. These researchers found that even with extreme changes in the fat-to-carbohydrate ratio (fat varied from 0% to 70% of total energy intake), there was no significant variation in energy need as a function of percentage of fat intake. These findings are in contrast to those of Prewitt and coworkers,[82] who conducted a study to determine the energy requirements of free-living women on a high- or low-fat diet. Subjects were initially fed a baseline diet of 37% fat for 4 weeks, and subsequently fed a 20% fat diet for 20 weeks. In this study, subjects apparently had to consume increasing amounts of low-fat food over the course of the study in order to maintain their body weight, leading the authors to suggest that the low-fat diet increased their energy requirements. Another interpretation is possible. Problems with the experimental design, e.g., inaccurate assessment of the diet composition coupled with decreased dietary adherence and/or increased physical activity over time (the study ran from January to June in a northern climate), could account for the appearance of metabolic inefficiency on the high-carbohydrate diet.

Although there is little evidence that diet composition affects metabolic efficiency when energy intake does not exceed energy expenditure, perfect energy balance is not likely to be achieved on a day-by-day basis. Weight maintenance is likely to occur when periods of positive energy balance are compensated for by periods of negative energy balance. It is reasonable to suggest that the abundant availability of high-fat, energy-dense foods will increase the probability of occurrence of periods of positive energy balance. During these periods of excess energy intake, dietary fat can be very efficiently stored as body fat. Reductions in the percent of energy from dietary fat could decrease or perhaps prevent episodes of positive energy balance and weight gain.

Results of the intervention studies suggest that weight loss associated with reductions in dietary fat is most likely the result of a concurrent decrease in energy intake. It is apparent that many individuals spontaneously decrease energy intake when the fat content of the diet is reduced, and possible explanations for this will be discussed below. Metabolic studies offer little or no evidence that weight loss might be attributed to differences in metabolic efficiency between high-fat and high-carbohydrate diets. If weight loss is desirable, it is likely that body weight can be lost while following a variety of nutritious diets. Thus, selection of a weight reduction diet can be designed around the preferred food patterns and nutritional needs of individuals. After weight loss is achieved, a low-fat diet may be useful to minimize periods of positive energy balance and fat deposition.

Laboratory-Based Studies

Macronutrient Composition of a Specific Food or Meal

Laboratory-based studies provide us with yet another type of information on how diet composition may affect food intake and body weight. Numerous studies have compared the effects of single foods or meals that vary in macronutrient content on subsequent food intake. Other studies have examined how variations in the macronutrient composition of the diet as a whole can affect food intake and body weight. Because the dietary manipulations in these studies are highly controlled and food intake can be accurately measured, laboratory-based research allows us to investigate what aspects of dietary composition may affect food intake.

When low-carbohydrate diets were commonly being used for weight loss, it had been suggested by some advocates of those diets that carbohydrate, sugar in particular, has low satiety value.[6] More recently, it has been suggested that fat may be readily overeaten because it is not very satiating compared to other nutrients, particularly carbohydrate.[83,84] An accepted technique for studying satiety is to administer a fixed amount of a given food or nutrient (a preload) and, after a predetermined delay, measure the effects on subsequent food intake and subjective ratings of hunger.

A thorough review of preload studies comparing the satiety value of carbohydrate and fat has been published recently elsewhere.[85] In general, little evidence exists that carbohydrate has a greater satiety value than fat. Most of the studies[86-89] that have been conducted revealed no differences in the effects of fat and carbohydrate in foods on food intake, although some studies[90] were not designed to be sensitive to subtle differences in macronutrient content. Three experiments[31,83,91] have shown differences between the effects of fat and carbohydrate in foods on satiety. Two studies[83,91] suggested that under certain conditions a high-carbohydrate breakfast suppressed subsequent food intake more than a high-fat breakfast, but under slightly different conditions there was no difference. Another study[31] examined the satiating efficiency of yogurts varying in fat and carbohydrate by using a dose-response paradigm, which is the most sensitive test of differences in satiety. This study showed that certain groups of people (lean men) appear to be very good at compensating for calories from either carbohydrate or fat, while other groups of people (obese individuals and those who consciously restrict their food intake) showed less precise energy compensation in general and a relative insensitivity to the satiety value of fat. Although the results from this study did indicate that fat in yogurt had a significantly lower satiating efficiency than carbohydrate in some individuals, the effect was small and does not suggest that the energy from fat goes undetected by satiety mechanisms. It remains to be determined whether this relative insensitivity to fat in foods is associated with the overconsumption of fat and energy and whether it could be important in the etiology of obesity.

The studies that have just been discussed are preloading studies, where a fixed amount of a food is eaten and the effect of that food on subsequent intake is studied. Such a study design is used to examine the effects of macronutrients on satiety. The term "satiety" refers to the effects of a food or a meal after eating has ended. A different type of study is used to look at how different macronutrients affect "satiation," or the processes involved in the termination of a meal. This study design requires that ad libitum food intake be measured when individuals are presented with foods high in one macronutrient vs another. These types of studies considered food consumed at a single meal as well as total food consumed over periods of many weeks.

One research group[92,93] has looked at the effects of high-fat vs high-carbohydrate foods on spontaneous food intake during an afternoon snack or a supper meal. In one study,[92] lean men consumed a low- or high-energy lunch followed two hours later by the opportunity to eat freely from a selection of high-fat/low-sucrose snacks or high-sucrose/low-fat snacks. The energy density of the high-fat foods averaged twice that of the high-carbohydrate foods. Researchers found that regardless of the lunch size, people ate significantly more calories when offered the high-fat snacks than when they were offered the high-sucrose snacks. There appeared to be some compensation for the differences in energy density, as the subjects consumed a somewhat greater volume of high-sucrose foods than they did of high-fat foods. Similar results were found in an almost identical study in which obese women were offered either a high-fat or high-carbohydrate supper in place of the snack.[93] In both studies, researchers concluded that high-fat foods have a weak effect on satiation and suggest that high-fat foods may lead to over-consumption, probably due to their higher energy density.

Macronutrient Composition of the Diet as a Whole

Tremblay and coworkers[94] looked at the effect of a high-fat diet vs a high-carbohydrate diet on spontaneous food intake over the course of a two-day experiment. Menus were matched, but the proportion of ingredients was altered in order to adjust the fat and carbohydrate composition. The energy density of the high-fat diet was higher than the energy density of the high-carbohydrate diet. In two separate experiments, subjects ate more calories on the high-fat diet (450 to 500 more kcal/day). Although in one experiment subjects ate a slightly greater volume on the high-carbohydrate diet, essentially they consumed similar amounts of each diet and showed very little tendency to compensate for the differences in energy density.[94] Thomas and coworkers[80] found similar results in a seven-day experiment such that people ate significantly more energy on a high-fat diet when diet composition was fixed (160 kcal/day more on the high-fat diet).

Two longer-term feeding studies (2 and 11 weeks) out of Cornell University[20,95] are cited most frequently as indicating that ad libitum consumption of low-fat foods can reduce fat intake and produce weight loss. In both of these studies, female subjects were offered diets in which every food item had a fixed proportion of fat and carbohydrate. The low-fat diets in these studies included commercially available reduced-fat foods, primarily margarines, salad dressings, and mayonnaise, as well as traditionally low-fat foods. As the proportion of dietary fat increased in the diets, so did the energy density.

In the first of these studies,[95] all food was provided over the course of 14 days to women divided into two groups, those <101% IBW and those >101% IBW. The subjects were fed three diets: 15% to 20%, 30% to 35%, or 45% to 50% of calories from fat. Subjects could eat as much or as little as they liked, and spontaneous food intake was measured in order to assess the effect of dietary fat on daily energy intake. The results showed that daily energy intake increased as the proportion of fat increased in the diet, with energy intake being 2087, 2352, and 2614 kcal/day on the low-, medium-, and high-fat diets, respectively,[95] but, by calculation, the weight of the food eaten did not significantly differ between the diets. Over the two-week periods the diets did not produce any significant weight changes. Overweight subjects demonstrated more variation in caloric intake across the three diets, especially with a greater energy intake on the high-fat diet.

In a second study,[20] the design was similar but the intervention period was extended to 11 weeks. In this study, individuals <101% IBW were excluded and only two levels of dietary fat were studied, 20% to 25% and 35% to 40% of calories from fat. With free access to food on both diets, the women consumed an average of 286 kcal/day less on the low-fat diet. Weight loss was significantly greater on the low-fat diet, although subjects lost weight on both diets (low-fat: −2.54 kg, high-fat: −1.26 kg). Over the course of the 11-week study, there appeared to be a trend for subjects on the low-fat diet to compensate for the energy dilution by increasing the volume of food consumed. This trend toward compensation was not significant and the study ended before it could be determined whether the volume of low-fat foods consumed would increase to the point that daily energy intake would be sufficient to prevent further weight loss. As with the shorter study from this research group,[95] when the total weight of food consumed in the study was calculated,[20] there were no significant differences between the two diets.

The results of these feeding studies, comparing the effect of carbohydrate vs fat on satiation, suggest that the energy density of the diet appears to be critical. Unless controlled for, energy density increases with the level of dietary fat, so that if there is a tendency to maintain the volume or weight of food consumed at a constant level, high-fat diets will be associated with elevated energy intakes. It is likely that through their experiences with foods, individuals learn appropriate portion sizes for the satisfaction of hunger. In the studies in which the fat content of the entire meal or diet was manipulated covertly,[20,94,95] the subjects appeared to adopt a strategy of eating similar portion sizes across conditions. Thus, the weight of the food was maintained at a more constant level than energy intake. The results from two recent studies[96,97] are consistent with this observation. When subjects were fed diets with increasing levels of fat and energy density (20%, 40%, and 60% fat diets having 115, 133, and 168 kcal/100 g, respectively) for 7 or 14 days, they ate a virtually identical amount of food on each diet. Because they ate the same amount of food on each diet, there was a stepwise increase in energy intake as dietary fat increased. It could be argued that the major determinant of energy intake in these longer-term feeding studies is the energy density, not the fat content of the available foods.

In order to separate the effects of energy density on food intake from the effects of macronutrients, high-carbohydrate and high-fat diets should be compared that are of equal energy density. To date, no studies have been published in which solid foods have been used in this type of experimental design, but one study[98] has compared high-carbohydrate and high-fat liquid diets of equal energy density. Trappist nuns were given a liquid diet in which the carbohydrate-to-fat ratio (24% vs 47% fat) of the diet was altered and the energy density was matched. The liquid diet provided 75% of the nuns' intake. In this study it was found that the mean daily energy intake remained constant between conditions, and the fat content of the diet did not influence energy intake.

Only one study has been published in which solid foods have been used in this type of experimental design.[99] When subjects were allowed to eat freely on low-, medium-, or high-fat diets with the same energy density, energy intake was very similar despite the large difference in the composition of the diets. There was no evidence of a tendency for energy intake to increase in parallel to the fat content of the diet, which has occurred in studies where the dietary energy density was not matched.[20,94–97] Thus, fat and carbohydrate appeared to be equally satiating when the energy density of the diet was matched.

COULD ENERGY DENSITY BE THE KEY?

In light of the evidence that energy density may be the major determinant of energy intake when diets vary in macronutrient content, several studies[100–103] have specifically looked at the effect of energy density on food intake. When researchers used liquid diets to manipulate energy density, they found that some people appeared to have the ability to adjust the volume consumed to compensate for a dilution in energy density, while others did not.[100–102] In one study,[100] obese people were found to compensate very poorly for changes in energy density, while there was no difference between obese and lean individuals in another study.[101] In 1983, Duncan and colleagues[103] used solid foods to look at the effect of energy density on satiation. They fed lean and obese subjects a diet of low-energy density comprised of traditionally low-fat food (fruits, vegetables, and grains) and a diet of high-energy density (high in fat and simple sugars) for five days (0.7 vs 1.5 kcal/g). The diet of low-energy density had a fiber content of 7 g/1000 kcal compared to 1 g/1000 kcal on the more energy-dense diet. The diets had equal acceptance ratings by the subjects, and they could eat the foods ad libitum. The results showed that both obese and non-obese groups significantly reduced their energy consumption on the low-energy diet. Nearly twice as many calories were consumed on the diet of high-energy density compared to the diet of low-energy density (3000 vs 1570 kcal/day). No data were supplied regarding weight change during the test periods.

In this study,[103] the energy density of the entire diet was altered in part by using high-fiber foods such as fruits, vegetables, and grains. In fact, it is difficult to significantly reduce the energy density or the fat content of a diet without increasing dietary fiber intake. This raises the question of how fiber in foods might interact with the overall energy density of the diet to affect food intake. For example, in *Eat More, Weigh Less,*[21] Dean Ornish suggests that 33% more food must be consumed for maintenance of energy intake after a reduction in dietary fat from 40% to 10% of calories. That is true if one considers a straight gram for gram substitution of carbohydrate for fat, but many carbohydrate foods are also high in fiber and/or water. In order to maintain caloric intake with such a 30% reduction in dietary fat, it would likely require an increase in food volume that greatly exceeds

Table 10–2 Two Dinner Menus of Equal Caloric Content but Differ Dramatically in Fat Content and Energy Density (Menu A: 58% of Calories from Fat and 2.40 kcal/g; Menu B: 12% of Calories from Fat and 0.85 kcal/g)

Menu A. High-Energy Density		*kcal*
Fettuccine Alfredo	8 oz	464
Garlic bread	2 slices	162
w/margarine	2 tsp	90
Fresh vegetable salad	2/3 cup	20
w/ranch-style dressing	1 T	96
Cheesecake	3 oz	254
TOTAL	452 g	1086 kcal

Menu B. Low-Energy Density		*kcal*
Spaghetti w/low-fat marinara	15 oz	483
French bread	3 slices	243
Fresh vegetable salad	2 cups	60
w/fat-free dressing	3 T	58
Italian-style vegetables	1 cup	74
Fresh strawberries	2 cups	90
w/sweetened light cream	2 T	78
TOTAL	1279 g	1086 kcal

the 33% estimate. Thus, it is not surprising that a severe reduction in dietary fat consistently results in an initial decrease in energy intake and body weight. To illustrate the point that a low-fat diet can be of high volume (low in energy density), Table 10–2 compares a high-fat and low-fat dinner menu. In this example, over twice as much food must be consumed in the low-fat meal in order to take in the amount of calories in the high-fat meal. Further studies must be done to understand the relationships between fiber, energy density, and food intake. It is safe to say that frequent consumption of foods that are naturally high in fiber and low in calories is likely to be helpful for weight maintenance and perhaps for weight loss.

These studies in which dilutions in dietary energy were specifically examined,[100–103] and a study that controlled energy density while manipulating macronutrient content of the diet,[98] provide support for the hypothesis that energy density of foods is a major determinant of food intake. Although more naturalistic studies need to be conducted using solid foods, and the role of dietary fiber must be determined, the evidence indicates that energy density has a much greater effect on food intake than does macronutrient composition.

Intense Sweeteners and Fat Substitutes

Modern food technology has provided many different techniques for sugar and fat replacement in foods. Undoubtedly, a variety of these techniques were used to help achieve desired macronutrient and caloric manipulations in the studies previously discussed. The replacement of fat or the use of intense sweeteners usually results in the dilution of energy density in food. Thus, to some extent, by examining the effects of low-fat diets and/or energy dilution, we have some idea how the replacement of fat or sugar may affect food intake. Up to this point, we have not discussed studies that have looked specifically at how intense sweeteners and fat substitutes affect food intake. Although a thorough review of these studies is beyond the scope of this discussion, an overview is useful. Extensive reviews on intense sweeteners and fat substitutes have been published elsewhere.[104–106]

Intense sweeteners have been available for decades. Saccharin was the first widely available sweetener. It has largely been replaced by aspartame, which is used to reduce sugar in a wide range of foods and drinks. Acesulfame K, another intense sweetener, has also been approved for use. Other sweeteners, ranging from 400 to 10,000 times sweeter than sucrose, are awaiting approval. Recently there has been considerable debate about the effectiveness of intense sweeteners as an adjunct to weight control. This debate began with reports that sweet taste can increase appetite and food intake.[107,108]

Although there have been reports of increased hunger ratings associated with intense sweeteners, a number of investigators have found the most widely used sweetener, aspartame, is generally associated with decreased or unchanged ratings of hunger. Even when aspartame increased ratings of hunger, there was no evidence of an effect on regulation of food intake and body weight. Aspartame has not been found to increase food intake; indeed, several studies have shown that consumption of aspartame-sweetened food or drinks was associated with either no change or a reduction in energy intake.[105,106]

Data from long-term studies of the use of sugar substitutes are limited. Laboratory studies in which aspartame replaced sugar indicate that if the calorie reduction is substantial—that is, if a number of sugar-free foods are consumed during the day, compensation for this reduction will be incomplete and daily energy intake will be reduced.[109–111] Other studies suggest that the substitution of only a few sugar-reduced foods may not reduce daily energy intake.[105,106] Thus, by itself, the casual use of foods with sugar substitutes is unlikely to be of benefit in weight control. On the other hand,[112] in one study, foods that incorporated sugar substitutes formed a valuable part of a balanced weight control program that included behavioral interventions and exercise in addition to dietary modification. The use of aspartame-sweetened products increased satisfaction with the diet by providing a range of palatable foods with reduced energy, and aspartame use was associated with better long-term control of body weight.

In contrast to intense sweeteners, fat substitutes are relatively new to the food supply. Although the percentage of fat in the American diet has decreased over the last 10 years, fat continues to comprise approximately 34% of the calories in the average diet in the United States,[22] which is above the maximum level recommended (30%) in the dietary guidelines for Americans. Because taste is the primary determinant of food choices, and since eating habits are difficult to change, a key to fat reduction may be to provide reduced-fat foods that mimic the full-fat versions. In one assessment[51] of dietary changes associated with several years of successful compliance with a low-fat diet, it was found that trimming fat from foods and substituting low-fat foods for the higher-fat versions were the most effective strategies for long-term fat reduction.

A wide range of fat substitutes, including gums, emulsifiers, starches, and proteins is used to produce palatable low-fat or fat-free products. Approved for consumption by the Food and Drug Administration in 1996 are zero-calorie (nonabsorbable) fat substitutes having the same physical and sensory properties as traditional fats. These fat substitutes are suitable for a wide range of applications, including frying and baking. Thus, the potential for a change in the nutrient composition of the food supply is enormous.

Since fat substitutes represent a new technology, there is little information on their effects on food intake and food selection. Several recent studies in which olestra (a zero-calorie fat substitute) was covertly incorporated into a meal or several meals showed that both children[113] and lean young men[114] compensated for the calorie reduction later in the test day so that there was no reduction in daily energy intake. Olestra consumption was associated with a dose-dependent reduction in fat intake and a reciprocal increase in carbohydrate intake. In other words, subjects did not eat more fat to make up for the fat replaced by olestra. It seems likely that the most important health benefit associated with the use of fat substitutes will be a reduction in the percentage of calories from fat in the diet.

The role of fat substitutes in weight reduction has not yet been examined. In one study,[115] it was suggested that the incorporation of olestra into food reduces the feelings of "deprivation" associated with low-fat diets and also reduces the number of foods that are considered "tempting." Studies are needed to determine whether fat substitutes have long-term value for dietary modification or weight control.

Whether sugar and/or fat substitutes will reduce energy intake may be dependent on the way the consumer uses them. These products can aid with compliance to and satisfaction with low-energy diets by increasing the range of palatable foods available for consumption. However, there may be no beneficial changes in energy intake if a consumer uses the consumption of such reduced-energy foods as a license to eat other high-fat foods or if low-fat but high-calorie foods are overeaten. The consumer should also be aware that although some fat-reduced and sugar-reduced foods are low in calories, others may not have significantly less

ORIGINAL
Strawberry Yogurt
Nutrition Facts

Serving Size 1 container (170g)

Amount per Serving	
Calories 180	Calories from Fat 15

	% Daily Value*
Total Fat 1.5 g	3%
Cholesterol 10 mg	3%
Sodium 105 mg	4%
Total Carbohydrate 33 g	11%
Sugars 27 g	
Protein 8 g	16%

FAT-FREE
Strawberry Yogurt
Nutrition Facts

Serving Size 1 container (170g)

Amount per Serving	
Calories 160	Calories from Fat 0

	% Daily Value*
Total Fat 0 g	0%
Cholesterol <5 mg	1%
Sodium 105 mg	4%
Total Carbohydrate 33 g	11%
Sugars 26 g	
Protein 7 g	14%

FAT-FREE & SUGAR-REDUCED
Strawberry Yogurt
Nutrition Facts

Serving Size 1 container (170g)

Amount per Serving	
Calories 90	Calories from Fat 0

	% Daily Value*
Total Fat 0 g	0%
Cholesterol <5 mg	1%
Sodium 85 mg	4%
Total Carbohydrate 16 g	5%
Sugars 8 g	
Protein 5 g	10%

Figure 10–3 A national brand of fat-free strawberry yogurt has 20 fewer calories per serving than the original formulation, but the fat-free, sugar-reduced version has only half as many calories as the original. Thus, some fat- and sugar-modified foods are significantly reduced in calories while others are not.

calories than the original products (Figure 10–3). Further studies of the psychological and physiological effects of sugar and fat substitutes are critical for developing appropriate nutritional counseling strategies to promote acceptance of and adherence to dietary modifications.

Alcohol

It is beyond the scope of the present review to examine the complex relationships between alcohol intake and the regulation of body composition. However, it is important to note that alcohol is also an energy-dense nutrient (7.1 kcal/g), and alcohol consumption should be considered when advising clients. Between 55% and 72% of males and females between the ages of 18 and 60 consume at least three drinks per week.[116] For Americans, the estimated alcohol contribution of calories from alcohol is about 4% of total energy,[117] but in some adult drinkers, alcohol may account for between 10% to 15% of their total caloric intake.[118] One could easily imagine a situation where alcohol could account for an even greater percentage of total energy intake, i.e., three drinks per day provides approximately 600 kcal or 30% of a 2000-kcal diet. Whether calories provided by alcohol are utilized efficiently is a question of current controversy. A number of epidemiological studies[119,120] have reported an inverse relationship between the amount of alcohol consumed and body mass index. At the same time, there are suggestions[121] that alcohol intake may actually promote fat deposition and adiposity. Until consensus is reached, it is reasonable to advise clients to account for energy provided by alcohol in their diets aimed at weight loss or maintenance. Also, because people tend to lose their inhibitions when they consume alcohol, individuals should be aware of its potential role in compromising compliance to a low-energy diet.

CONCLUSION

It seems clear that obesity is often associated with consumption of a high-fat diet. Currently, the most popular method for weight reduction in the United States is to reduce consumption of dietary fat. Research suggests that reducing the fat content of the diet in the absence of a conscious energy restriction will likely result in a small degree of weight loss. This weight loss appears to be due, in large part, to a spontaneous reduction in energy intake. Studies done in individuals within 20% or 30% of IBW showed an average weight loss of 1 to 6 kg over the course of several months to two years with a reduction in dietary fat.[48,52–62] In studies where data are available at intermediate time points,[48,52–54,58] body weight decreased for several months after the dietary change and then stabilized at a somewhat lower weight. This research indicates that reducing dietary fat alone may result in a modest weight reduction in people who are moderately overweight.

It is difficult to know the effect of dietary fat reduction on weight loss in obese individuals. In the two studies looking at fat restriction *only* as a means of weight loss,[65,67] a 4- to 5-kg weight loss was achieved over the course of five to six months. In one of the studies,[65] greater weight loss was achieved when both dietary fat *and* calories were restricted. These studies offer no evidence that weight loss will be sustained for periods longer than six months or that more than a modest weight loss can ultimately be achieved. It may be necessary for individuals to make a conscious effort to restrict calories if they are seeking a large weight loss or a sustained weight loss over a long period of time—although without relevant clinical research, nothing definitive can be said.

There is little indication that the macronutrient composition of a nutritionally adequate weight reduction diet is important. Research indicates that weight loss is not dependent on the composition of the diet as long as total energy is reduced.[71,73] If weight loss is desirable, it is likely that body weight can be lost while following a variety of nutritious diets. Thus, selection of a weight reduction diet can be designed around the preferred food patterns and nutritional needs of individuals. Limiting fat intake may make it easier to reduce calories because the dieter will be able to consume a greater, and perhaps more satisfying, volume of food.

It has been suggested that the most beneficial aspect of altering the composition of the diet in terms of weight control may be in the maintenance phase.[122] Although no dietary principle is applicable to all individuals, it is reasonable to suggest that the abundant availability of an energy-dense diet will increase the probability of occurrence of periods of positive energy balance.[122] Reductions in the percentage of energy from dietary fat could decrease or, perhaps, prevent episodes of positive energy balance and weight gain.

Laboratory-based research suggests that weight loss on a low-fat diet is due, at least in part, to the inability of humans to compensate completely for changes in the energy density of the diet.[30,96,97,103] A spontaneous reduction in energy intake consistently occurs when the energy density of the diet, as a whole, is reduced. A diet of low-energy density is usually characterized as low in fat and high in complex carbohydrates and fiber. Many fat- and sugar-reduced foods, which are also reduced in calories, are currently available. These products may be helpful for weight loss and/or weight maintenance in that they increase the range of foods available that are of low-energy density. It is important to note that the substitution of only a few low-energy foods may not reduce daily energy intake and is unlikely to be of benefit in weight control.

Guidelines for Practice

In the interest of developing more effective methods for helping people achieve and/or maintain a healthy body weight, several guidelines can be formulated from the diverse literature regarding the effect of diet composition on food intake and body weight.

- For weight loss, the critical aspect of a diet is the reduction in energy intake, not macronutrient composition. Thus, a weight reduction diet can be designed around the preferred food patterns and nutritional needs of individuals. A diet of low-energy density (described below) may be a good choice because it requires the development of eating habits conducive to weight maintenance.

- Maintenance of a desirable body weight is most likely to be achieved on a low-fat diet of low-energy density. Episodes of positive energy balance are minimized on such a diet, and, when they do occur, dietary fat is not readily available for efficient deposition into adipose cells.
- Adoption of a diet of low-energy density will likely lead to a spontaneous reduction in energy intake that will be helpful to achieve weight loss or weight maintenance. The energy density of the diet may best be reduced by a combination of the following:
  - reduction in dietary fat
  - increase in intake of high-fiber, low-energy foods, namely fruits and vegetables
  - reduction in intake of energy-dense foods, regardless of their composition (it may be helpful to substitute low-energy foods made with sugar or fat substitutes for the high-energy version)
  - reduction in alcohol consumption

REFERENCES

1. Marriott HL. A simple weight reducing diet. *Br Med J.* 1949;2:18.
2. Joliffe N. *The Prudent Diet*, 3rd ed. New York: Simon & Schuster; 1963.
3. Gordon ES, Goldberg M, Chosy GJ. A new concept in the treatment of obesity. *JAMA.* 1963;186:50–60.
4. Donaldson BF. *Strong Medicine*. London: Cassell; 1963.
5. Yudkin J. The treatment of obesity by the "high-fat" diet. The inevitability of calories. *Lancet.* 1960;2:939–941.
6. Craddock D. *Obesity and Its Management*. London: Churchill; 1973.
7. Yudkin J. The low-carbohydrate diet in the treatment of obesity. *Postgrad Med.* 1972:151–154.
8. Stock AL, Yudkin J. Nutrient intake of subjects on low carbohydrate diet used in treatment of obesity. *Am J Clin Nutr.* 1970;23:948–952.
9. Kekwick A, Pawan GLS. Calorie intake in relation to body-weight changes in the obese. *Lancet.* 1956;2:155–161.
10. Dwyer JT, Lu D. Popular diets for weight loss: from nutritionally hazardous to healthful. In: Stunkard AJ, Wadden TA, eds. *Obesity: Theory and Therapy*, 2nd ed. New York: Raven Press; 1993:231–252.
11. Rabast U, Vornberger KH, Ehl E. Loss of weight, sodium and water in obese persons consuming a high- or low-carbohydrate diet. *Ann Nutr Metab.* 1981;25:341–349.
12. National Research Council. *Diet and Health: Implications for Reducing Chronic Disease Risk*. Washington, DC: National Academy of Sciences; 1989.
13. Leeds AR. Dietary fibre: mechanisms of action. *Int J Obes.* 1987;11:3–7.

14. Haber GB, Heaton KW, Murphy B, Burroughs L. Depletion and disruption of dietary fibre. Effects on satiety, plasma-glucose and serum-insulin. *Lancet.* 1977;2:679.

15. Stevens J. Does dietary fiber affect food intake and body weight? *J Am Diet Assoc.* 1988;88:939–945.

16. Levine AS, Billington CJ. Dietary fiber: does it affect food intake and body weight? In: Fernstrom JD, Miller GD, eds. *Appetite and Body Weight Regulation: Sugar, Fat, and Macronutrient Substitutes.* Boca Raton, FL: CRC Press; 1994:191–200.

17. Guthrie HA. *Introductory Nutrition.* 7th ed. St. Louis: Times Mirror/Mosby College Publishing; 1989.

18. McHugh PR, Moran TH. Calories and gastric emptying: a regulatory capacity with implications for feeding. *Am J Physiol.* 1979;236:R254–R260.

19. Calorie Control Council. *Calorie Control Commentary.* Vol 15. Atlanta, GA: Calorie Control Council; 1993.

20. Kendall A, Levitsky DA, Strupp BJ, Lissner L. Weight loss on a low-fat diet: consequence of the imprecision of the control of food intake in humans. *Am J Clin Nutr.* 1991;53:1124–1129.

21. Ornish D. *Eat More, Weigh Less.* New York: HarperCollins Publishers; 1993.

22. Centers for Disease Control and Prevention. Daily dietary fat and total food-energy intakes—NHANES III, Phase 1, 1988–91. *JAMA.* 1994;271:1309.

23. Kuczmarski RJ, Flegal KM, Campbell SM, Johnson CL. Increasing prevalence of overweight among US adults. *JAMA.* 1994;272:205–211.

24. Miller WC, Lindeman AK, Wallace J, Niederpruem M. Diet composition, energy intake, and exercise in relation to body fat in men and women. *Am J Clin Nutr.* 1990;52:426–430.

25. Miller WC, Niederpruem MG, Wallace JP, Lindeman AK. Dietary fat, sugar, and fiber predict body fat content. *J Am Diet Assoc.* 1994;94:612–615.

26. Dreon DM, Frey-Hewitt B, Ellsworth N, Williams PT, Terry RB, Wood PD. Dietary fat:carbohydrate ratio and obesity in middle-aged men. *Am J Clin Nutr.* 1988;47:995–1000.

27. Romieu I, Willett WC, Stampfer MJ, et al. Energy intake and other determinants of relative weight. *Am J Clin Nutr.* 1988;47:406–412.

28. Tucker LA, Kano MJ. Dietary fat and body fat: a multivariate study of 205 adult females. *Am J Clin Nutr.* 1992;56:616–622.

29. Colditz GA, Willet WC, Stampfer MJ, London SJ, Segal MR, Speizer FE. Patterns of weight change and their relation to diet in a cohort of healthy women. *Am J Clin Nutr.* 1990;51:1100–1105.

30. Rolls BJ, Shide DJ. Dietary fat and the control of food intake. In: Fernstrom JD, Miller GD, eds. *Appetite and Body Weight Regulation: Sugar, Fat, and Macronutrient Substitutes.* Boca Raton, FL: CRC Press; 1994:167–177.

31. Rolls BJ, Kim-Harris S, Fischman MW, Foltin RW, Moran TH, Stoner SA. Satiety after preloads with different levels of fat and carbohydrate: implications for obesity. *Am J Clin Nutr.* 1994;60:476–487.

32. Flatt JP. The difference in the storage capacities for carbohydrate and for fat, and its implications in the regulation of body weight. *Ann NY Acad Sci.* 1987;499:104–123.

33. Klesges RC, Klesges LM, Haddock CK, Eck LH. A longitudinal analysis of the impact of dietary intake and physical activity on weight change in adults. *Am J Clin Nutr.* 1992;55:818–822.

34. Kant AK, Graubard BI, Schatzkin A, Ballard-Barbash R. Proportion of energy intake from fat and subsequent weight change in the NHANES I epidemiologic follow-up study. *Am J Clin Nutr.* 1995;61:11–17.

35. Block G. A review of validations of dietary assessment methods. *Am J Epidemiol.* 1982;115:492–505.

36. Wolper C, Heshka S, Heymsfield SB. Measuring food intake, an overview. In Allison DB, ed. *Handbook of Assessment Methods for Eating Behaviors and Weight-Related Problems.* Thousand Oaks, CA: Sage Publications; 1995:215–240.

37. Gibson RS. *Principles of Nutritional Assessment.* New York: Oxford University Press; 1990.

38. Schoeller DA. How accurate is self-reported dietary energy intake? *Nutr Rev.* 1990;48:373–379.

39. Bray GA, Zachary B, Dahms WT, Atkinson RL, Oddie TH. Eating patterns of massively obese individuals. *J Am Diet Assoc.* 1978;72:24–27.

40. Lichtman SW, Pisarska K, Berman ER, et al. Discrepancy between self-reported and actual caloric intake and exercise in obese subjects. *N Engl J Med.* 1992;327:1893–1898.

41. Mela DJ. Exploring the many causes of obesity. *J Am Diet Assoc.* 1994;94:1366–1367.

42. Strain GW, Hershcopf RJ, Zumoff B. Food intake of very obese persons: quantitative and qualitative aspects. *J Am Diet Assoc.* 1992;92:199–203.

43. Drewnowski A, Kurth C, Holden-Wiltse J, Saari J. Food preferences in human obesity: carbohydrates versus fats. *Appetite.* 1992;18:207–221.

44. Drewnowski A. Fats and food acceptance: sensory, hedonic and attitudinal aspects. In: Solms J, Booth DA, Pangborn RM, eds. *Food Acceptance and Nutrition.* Vol 1. New York: Academic Press; 1987:189–204.

45. Drewnowski A, Brunzell JD, Sande K, Iverius PH, Greenwood MRC. Sweet tooth reconsidered: taste responsiveness in human obesity. *Physiol Behav.* 1985;35:617–622.

46. Drewnowski A, Kurth CL, Rahaim JE. Taste preferences in human obesity: environmental and familial factors. *Am J Clin Nutr.* 1991;54:635–641.

47. Mela DJ, Sacchetti DA. Sensory preferences for fats: relationships with diet and body composition. *Am J Clin Nutr.* 1991;53:908–915.

48. Sheppard L, Kristal AR, Kushi LH. Weight loss in women participating in a randomized trial of low-fat diets. *Am J Clin Nutr.* 1991;54:821–828.

49. Insull W Jr, Henderson MW, Prentice RL, et al. Results of a randomized feasibility study of a low-fat diet. *Arch Intern Med.* 1990;150:421–427.

50. Gorbach SL, Morrill-LaBrode A, Woods MN, et al. Changes in food patterns during a low-fat dietary intervention in women. *J Am Diet Assoc.* 1990;90:802–809.

51. Kristal AR, White E, Shattuck AL, et al. Long-term maintenance of a low-fat diet: durability of fat-related dietary habits in the Women's Health Trial. *J Am Diet Assoc.* 1992;92,5:553–559.

52. Kasim SE, Martino S, Kim P, et al. Dietary and anthropometric determinants of plasma lipoproteins during a long-term low-fat diet in healthy women. *Am J Clin Nutr.* 1993;57:146–153.

53. Retzlaff BM, Dowdy AA, Walden CE, et al. Changes in vitamin and mineral intakes and serum concentrations among free-living men on cholesterol-lowering diets: the Dietary Alternatives Study. *Am J Clin Nutr.* 1991;53:890–898.

54. Boyd NF, Cousins M, Beaton M, Kriukov V, Lockwood G, Tritchler D. Quantitative changes in dietary fat intake and serum cholesterol in women: results from a randomized, controlled trial. *Am J Clin Nutr.* 1990;52:470–476.

55. Baer JT. Improved plasma cholesterol levels in men after a nutrition education program at the worksite. *J Am Diet Assoc.* 1993;93:658–663.

56. Henkin Y, Garber DW, Osterlund LC, Darnell BE. Saturated fats, cholesterol, and dietary compliance. *Arch Intern Med.* 1992;152:1167–1174.

57. Bloemberg BPM, Kromhout D, Goddijin E, Jansen A, Obermann-de Boer GL. The impact of the guidelines for a healthy diet of the Netherlands Nutrition Council on total and high density lipoprotein cholesterol in hypercholesterolemic free-living men. *Am J Epidemiol.* 1991;134:39–48.

58. Hyewon LH, Cousins M, Beaton M, et al. Compliance in a randomized clinical trial of dietary fat reduction in patients with breast dysplasia. *Am J Clin Nutr.* 1988;48:575–586.

59. Brown GD, Whyte L, Gee MI, et al. Effects of two "lipid-lowering" diets on plasma lipid levels of patients with peripheral vascular disease. *J Am Diet Assoc.* 1984;84:546–550.

60. Buzzard IM, Asp EH, Chlebowski RT, et al. Diet intervention methods to reduce fat intake: nutrient and food group composition of self-selected low-fat diets. *J Am Diet Assoc.* 1990;90:42–50, 53.

61. Hunninghake DB, Stein EA, Dujovne CA, et al. The efficacy of intensive dietary therapy alone or combined with lovastatin in outpatients with hypercholesterolemia. *N Engl J Med.* 1993;328:1213–1219.

62. Boyar AP, Rose DP, Loughridge JR, et al. Response to a diet low in total fat in women with postmenopausal breast cancer: a pilot study. *Nutrition and Cancer.* 1988;11:93–99.

63. Ornish D, Brown SE, Scherwitz LW, et al. Can lifestyle changes reverse coronary heart disease? *Lancet.* 1990;336:129–133.

64. Shintani TT, Hughes CK, Beckham S, O'Connor HK. Obesity and cardiovascular risk intervention through the ad libitum feeding of traditional Hawaiian diet. *Am J Clin Nutr.* 1991;53:1647S–1651S.

65. Schlundt DG, Hill JO, Pope-Cordle J, Arnold D, Virts KL, Katahn M. Randomized evaluation of a low fat ad libitum carbohydrate diet for weight reduction. *Int J Obes.* 1993;17:623–629.

66. Shah M, McGovern P, French S, Baxter J. Comparison of a low-fat, ad libitum complex-carbohydrate diet with a low-energy diet in moderately obese women. *Am J Clin Nutr.* 1994;59:980–984.

67. Jeffery RW, Hellerstedt WL, French SA, Baxter JE. A randomized trial of counseling for fat restriction versus calorie restriction in the treatment of obesity. *Int J Obes.* 1995;19:132–137.

68. Brownell KD, Rodin J. The dieting maelstrom: is it possible and advisable to lose weight? *Am Psychol.* 1994;49:781–791.

69. Sims EAH, Danforth E Jr, Horton ES, Bray GA, Glennon JA, Salans LB. Endocrine and metabolic effects of experimental obesity in man. *Recent Prog Horm Res.* 1973;29:457–496.

70. Flatt JP, Ravussin E, Acheson XJ, Jequier E. Effects of dietary fat on post-prandial substrate oxidation and on carbohydrate and fat balances. *J Clin Invest.* 1985;76:1019–1024.

71. Alford BB, Blankenship AC, Hagen RD. The effects of variations in carbohydrate, protein, and fat content of the diet upon weight loss, blood values, and nutrient intake of adult obese women. *J Am Diet Assoc.* 1990;90:534–540.

72. Golay A, Eigenheer C, Morel Y, Kujawski P, Lehmann T, de Tonnac N. Weight loss with low or high carbohydrate diet? *Int J Obes.* 1996;20:1067–1072.

73. Racette SB, Schoeller DA, Kushner RF, Neil KM, Herling-Iaffaldano K. Effects of aerobic exercise and dietary carbohydrate on energy expenditure and body composition during weight reduction in obese women. *Am J Clin Nutr.* 1995;61:486–494.

74. Boozer C, Brasseur A, Atkinson RL. Dietary fat affects weight loss and adiposity during energy restriction in rats. *Am J Clin Nutr.* 1993;58:846–852.

75. Lean MEJ, James WPT. Metabolic effects of isoenergetic nutrient exchange over 24 hours in relation to obesity in women. *Int J Obes.* 1988;12:15–27.

76. Hurni M, Burnand B, Pittet P, Jequier E. Metabolic effects of a mixed and a high-carbohydrate diet in man, measured over 24 hours in a respiration chamber. *Br J Nutr.* 1982;47:33–43.

77. McNeill G, Bruce AC, Ralph A, James WPT. Inter-individual differences in fasting nutrient oxidation and the influence of diet composition. *Int J Obes.* 1988;12:455–463.

78. Abbott WGH, Howard BV, Ruotolo G, Ravussin E. Energy expenditure in humans: effects of dietary fat and carbohydrate. *Am J Physiol.* 1990;258:E347–E351.

79. Hill JO, Peters JC, Reed GW, Schlundt DG, Sharp T, Green HL. Nutrient balance in humans: effects of diet composition. *Am J Clin Nutr.* 1991;54:10–17.

80. Thomas CD, Peters JC, Reed GW, Abumrad NN, Sun M, Hill JO. Nutrient balance and energy expenditure during ad libitum feeding of high-fat and high-carbohydrate diets in humans. *Am J Clin Nutr.* 1992;55:934–942.

81. Leibel RL, Hirsch J, Appel BE, Checani GC. Energy intake required to maintain body weight is not affected by wide variation in diet composition. *Am J Clin Nutr.* 1992;55:350–355.

82. Prewitt TE, Schmeisser D, Bowen PE, et al. Changes in body weight, body composition, and energy intake in women fed high- and low-fat diets. *Am J Clin Nutr.* 1991;54:304–310.

83. Blundell JE, Burley VJ, Cotton JR, Lawton CL. Dietary fat and the control of energy intake: evaluating the effects of fat on meal size and postmeal satiety. *Am J Clin Nutr.* 1993;57:772S–778S.

84. Schutz Y, Flatt JP, Jequier E. Failure of dietary fat intake to promote fat oxidation: a factor favoring the development of obesity. *Am J Clin Nutr.* 1989;50:307–314.

85. Rolls BJ, Hammer VA. Fat, carbohydrate and the regulation of energy intake. *Am J Clin Nutr.* 1995;62(55 suppl):1086S–1095S.

86. de Graaf C, Hulshof T, Westrate JA, Jas P. Short-term effects of different amounts of protein, fats, and carbohydrates on satiety. *Am J Clin Nutr.* 1992;55:33–38.

87. Warwick ZS, Hall WG, Pappas TN, Schiffman SS. Taste and smell sensations enhance the satiating effect of both a high-carbohydrate and a high-fat meal in humans. *Physiol Behav.* 1993;53:553–563.

88. Rolls BJ, Kim-Harris S, McNelis AL, Fischman MW, Foltin RW, Moran TH. Time course of effects of preloads high in fat or carbohydrate on food intake and hunger ratings in humans. *Am J Physiol.* 1991;260:R756–R763.

89. Foltin RW, Fischman MW, Moran TH, Rolls BJ, Kelly TH. Caloric compensation for lunches varying in fat and carbohydrate content by humans in a residential laboratory. *Am J Clin Nutr.* 1990;52:969–980.

90. Caputo FA, Mattes RD. Human dietary responses to covert manipulations of energy, fat and carbohydrate in a midday meal. *Am J Clin Nutr.* 1992;56:36–43.

91. Cotton JR, Burley VJ, Westrate JA, Blundell JE. Dietary fat and appetite: similarities and differences in the satiating effect of meals supplemented with either fat or carbohydrate. *J Human Nutr Diet.* 1994;7:11–24.

92. Green SM, Burley VJ, Blundell JE. Effect of fat- and sucrose-containing foods on the size of eating episodes and energy intake in lean males: potential for causing overconsumption. *Eur J Clin Nutr.* 1994;48:547–555.

93. Lawton CL, Burley VJ, Wales JK, Blundell JE. Dietary fat and appetite control in obese subjects: weak effects on satiation and satiety. *Int J Obes.* 1993;17:409–416.

94. Tremblay A, Lavallee N, Almeras N, Allard L, Despres Jean-P, Bouchard C. Nutritional determinants of the increase in energy intake associated with a high-fat diet. *Am J Clin Nutr.* 1991;53:1134–1137.

95. Lissner L, Levitsky DA, Strupp BJ, Kalkward HJ, Roe DA. Dietary fat and the regulation of energy intake in human subjecs. *Am J Clin Nutr.* 1987;46:886–892.

96. Stubbs RJ, Ritz P, Coward WA, Prentice AM. Covert manipulation of the ratio of dietary fat to carbohydrate ratio and energy density: effect on food intake and energy balance in free-living men, eating ad libitum. *Am J Clin Nutr*. 1995;62:330–337.

97. Stubbs RJ, Murgatroyd PR, Prentice AM. Covert manipulation of dietary fat and energy density: effect on substrate flux and food intake in men eating ad libitum. *Am J Clin Nutr*. 1995;62:316–329.

98. van Stratum P, Lussenburg RN, van Wezel LA, Vergroesen AJ, Cremer HD. The effect of dietary carbohydrate: fat ratio on energy intake by adult women. *Am J Clin Nutr*. 1978;31:206–212.

99. Stubbs RJ, Harbron CG, Prentice AM. Covert manipulation of the dietary fat to carbohydrate ratio of isoenergetically dense diets: effect of food intake in feeding men ad libitum. *Int J Obes*. 1996;20:651–660.

100. Campbell RG, Hashim SA, Van Itallie TB. Repsonses to variations in nutritive density in lean and obese subjects. *N Engl J Med*. 1971;285:1402–1407.

101. Wooley OW. Long-term food regulation in the obese and nonobese. *Psychosom Med*. 1971;33:436–444.

102. Spiegel TA. Caloric regulation of food intake in man. *J Comp Physiol Psychol*. 1973;81:24–37.

103. Duncan KH, Bacon JA, Weinsier RL. The effects of high and low energy density diets on satiety, energy intake, and eating time of obese and nonobese subjects. *Am J Clin Nutr*. 1983;37:763–767.

104. Rolls BJ. Role of fat substitutes in obesity prevention and treatment. Progress in obesity research. In *7th International Congress on Obesity*. Eds. Angel A, Anderson H, Bouchard C, Lau D, Leiter L, Medelson R. London: John Libby; 1995.

105. Rolls BJ. Effects of intense sweeteners on hunger, food intake and body weight: a review. *Am J Clin Nutr*. 1991;53:872–878.

106. Drewnowski A. Intense sweeteners and the control of appetite. *Nutr Rev*. 1995;53:1–7.

107. Blundell J, Hill AJ. Paradoxical effects of an intense sweetener (aspartame) on appetite. *Lancet*. 1986;1:1092–1093.

108. Rogers PJ. Appetite control and the use of intense sweeteners. *Nutr & Food Sci*. 1993;6:13–15.

109. Porikos KP, Booth G, Van Itallie TB. Effect of covert nutritive dilution on the spontaneous intake of obese individuals: a pilot study. *Am J Clin Nutr*. 1977;30:1638–1644.

110. Porikos KP, Hesser MF, Van Itallie TB. Caloric regulation in normal weight men maintained on a palatable diet of conventional foods. *Physiol Behav*. 1982;29:293–300.

111. Porikos KP, Pi-Sunyer FX. Regulation of food intake in human obesity: studies with caloric dilution and exercise. *Clin Endocrinol Metab*. 1984;13:547–561.

112. Kanders BS, Lavin PT, Kowalchuk MB, Greenberg I, Blackburn GL. An evaluation of the effect of aspartame on weight loss. *Appetite*. 1988;11:73–84.

113. Birch LL, Johnson SJ, Jones MB, Peters JC. Effects of a nonenergy fat substitute on children's energy and macronutrient intake. *Am J Clin Nutr*. 1993;58:326–333.

114. Rolls BJ, Pirraglia PA, Jones MB, Peters JC. Effects of olestra, a non-caloric fat substitute, on daily energy and fat intake in lean men. *Am J Clin Nutr*. 1992;56:84–92.

115. Foreyt JP, Goodrick GK. Potential impact of sugar and fat substitutes in American diet. *J Nat Cancer Inst Mono*. 1992;12:99–103.

116. Brooks S, Williams G, Stinson F, Dufour MC. Diet and alcohol consumption in the general population: preliminary findings. *Alcohol Health and Research World*. 1989;13:272–276.

117. Hoffman CJ. Dietary intake of calcium, iron, folacin, alcohol, and fat for college students in central Michigan. *J Am Diet Assoc*. 1989;89:836–838.

118. Williamson DF, Forman MR, Binkin NJ, Gentry EM, Remington PL, Trowbridge FL. Alcohol and body weight in United States adults. *Am J Public Health*. 1987;77:1324–1330.

119. Colditz GA, Giovannucci E, Rimm EB, et al. Alcohol intake in relation to diet and obesity in women and men. *Am J Clin Nutr*. 1991;52:49–55.

120. Hellerstedt WL, Jeffrey RW, Murray DM. The association between alcohol intake and adiposity in the general population. *Am J Epidemiol*. 1990;132:594–611.

121. Suter PM, Schutz Y, Jequier E. The effect of ethanol on fat storage in healthy subjects. *N Engl J Med*. 1992;326:983–987.

122. Hill JO, Drougas H, Peters JC. Obesity treatment: can diet composition play a role? *Ann Intern Med*. 1993;119:694–697.

CHAPTER 11

Reproduction and Body Weight: Menarche, Pregnancy, Lactation, and Menopause

Barbara J. Moore
Ruth Kava

INTRODUCTION

Differences in body weight between male and female infants have been detected at birth.[1] Differences in body fat content emerge soon thereafter and are accentuated at various developmental periods throughout life. The changes in body composition, particularly in the body fat compartment, that occur throughout life in the human female in developed countries are the focus of this chapter. Because of adaptations to seasonal, periodic, or chronic food shortage, it should be expected that maturation, development, and changes in body composition associated with reproduction in women in less-developed countries will differ markedly from what is described here.

This chapter discusses the changes in body fat that accompany menarche and adolescence. This is followed by a review of changes in the body fat compartment that normally occur during pregnancy, taking into account the current recommendations for weight gain during pregnancy. The role of pregnancy-induced changes in body fat in the support of lactation and the impact of the high energy demand of lactation on body fat are discussed. The chapter ends with a consideration of the changes in body fat associated with menopause.

The term "body fat compartment," in the context of this discussion, refers to the body weight minus the weight of all lean tissue (primarily muscle, bones, blood, and the internal organs). In some cases, especially if animal studies are referenced, it is possible to quantify the amount of fat stored in specific adipose tissue depots under certain reproductive conditions or in certain developmental stages. Wherever possible, the sites in which fat is typically deposited during normal development and aging in the female will be discussed because there is some evidence that site-specific fat depostion is related to risk for certain chronic diseases. Finally, despite the limitations of doing so, body weight change will sometimes be used as a proxy for body fat change, especially in connection with pregnancy and lactation in which more direct measures of body fat are often lacking.

Wherever possible, this chapter includes what is known about the relevant developmental changes in females from minority populations in the United States, particularly if those changes differ from those seen in their white counterparts in the corresponding reproductive or developmental condition. It should be noted that there is a paucity of such information available. Throughout the chapter, the most compelling areas in which further research is needed will be identified, especially where opportunities exist to promote health, prevent disease, or reduce risk for disease.

INFLUENCE OF MENARCHE ON BODY WEIGHT, BODY COMPOSITION, AND THE RISK OF ADULT OBESITY

Adolescence, Puberty, and Menarche

Adolescence spans the period between childhood and adulthood and incorporates both physiological and psychological maturation. Although commonly associated with the teenage years, the physical changes that herald the attainment of full reproductive capability in women may actually begin well before age 13. Early biological changes that precede menarche (the onset of the menstrual cycle) include the initiation of breast development, pubic hair growth, and a rapid increase in height that may begin as early as 9.5 years, but typically occurs by 10.5 years.[2] The attainment of the most rapid longitudinal growth rate (peak height velocity) typically precedes the onset of menses by about 6 to 12 months.[3] Menarche actually occurs well into puberty, and thus does not indicate the onset of puberty as is sometimes mistakenly assumed. In the United States, the mean age of menarche is 12.5 years, with the normal range extending from 10 to 16.5 years.[2] By menarche, the young woman has reached about 95% of her adult height. Forbes[4] found that in a group of 113 healthy white girls, maximum stature was achieved by one year after menarche. However, the subjects were followed only up to 80 months post-menarche, so any later changes in stature would not have been documented. Hediger et al[5] found that girls in late adolescence (from about 1.5 years after menarche to 18 years of age) continued longitudinal growth, although at a slower rate than before menarche.

Pubertal girls do not reach peak rate of weight gain until approximately six months after peak height velocity has been attained, and this maximal rate may coincide with menarche.[3] During the period of peak weight velocity, girls gain around 5.5 to 10.6 kg/year. After this period, rate of gain decreases. Depending on the duration of weight accretion, in all, a gain of 5 to 10 kg may be expected between menarche and attainment of full adult weight.[3]

Changes in Body Fat: Quantity and Distribution

Augmented body weight and height are two very obvious changes occurring around the time of menarche, but more pertinent to a discussion of obesity are the concurrent changes in body composition. In the years preceding menarche, absolute increases in lean weight are greater than those in body fat.[4] However, as longitudinal growth slows, incremental gain in body fat continues, so that while preadolescent girls typically have a body composition of about 15% to 18% fat, this increases to about 28% by 18 years of age.[3,6]

Frisch and Revelle[7] and Frisch[8] proposed that the increased percent of body fat underlies the initiation of menarche. These investigators argue that there is a critical percent body fat that must be attained before menarche occurs. In part, this theory is based on observations of women who become amenorrheic after the severe weight loss of anorexia nervosa, or because of extraordinary physical exertion, as is typical of ballet dancers and elite athletes. Other investigators have disputed this hypothesis on the grounds that the original estimations of body fat were calculated, not measured, and highly variable[4,9]; and also that when such women are refed, menses resume before body composition is normalized.[10] Chronic undernutrition decreases circulating levels of gonadotrophins; even short-term periods of fasting suppress the secretion of these hormones.[10] Again, refeeding restores hormone levels before body composition is normalized, suggesting that energy intake may be more important than body weight or fat for resumption or menstrual cycling. However, recent support for the Frisch hypothesis was provided by a report that leptin, an adipocyte-derived cytokine that regulates adiposity, accelerates the rate of maturation when injected into female mice.[11] This may be a mechanism by which adipose tissue mass can trigger maturational events.

Several investigators[12,13] have noted that not only is there an accretion of body fat in girls during adolescence, but that the distribution of this fat may differ, depending on when during adolescence the adipose compartment is expanded. Such changes may have important health effects, as it is well known that obese women who have a centrally distributed or truncal adiposity are at a greater risk of developing diabetes and heart disease than are those whose fat is distributed on hips and thighs.

De Ridder et al[9] studied 68 healthy Dutch schoolgirls for three years, both before and after menarche. They found that early in puberty, changes in body fat distribution were largely determined by changes in fat at the waist level. In addition, body fat mass was inversely related to the rate of pubertal development toward menarche. In other words, the greater the fat mass, the shorter the interval between the development of secondary sexual characteristics and menarche.

Van Lenthe et al[14,15] also studied the relationship between age at menarche and fatness. In their longitudinal study of 98 healthy white schoolgirls, they examined changes in fat distribution as indicated by skinfold anthropometry. Girls with an early menarche had a more centrally distributed fat mass than did the girls who matured later, even when the data were adjusted to take into account differences in fatness per se. Van Lenthe notes, "Rapid maturation seems to have long-term consequences for obesity and should therefore be considered a risk indicator for the development of obesity."[15(p18)]

One study providing evidence to the contrary is that of Troisi et al[16] who conducted a large (n = 44,487) cross-sectional study of pre- and postmenopausal women 40 to 65 years of age who were free of cancer, cardiovascular disease, and diabetes. These workers found only a weak positive association between age at menarche and waist-to-hip ratio (WHR). In other words, early menarche was not associated with increased WHR. Although this study was large, it relied on self-reported values for WHR and for this reason, its findings are suspect.

Health Consequences of Adolescent Obesity

A recent report by McGill et al[17] provides chilling evidence of the link between obesity and increased risk for cardiovascular disease and diabetes. They performed autopsy analyses of 1532 young persons aged 15 to 34 years. They quantified atherosclerosis of the aorta and right coronary artery; postmortem blood cells were analyzed for glycohemoglobin and postmortem serum for lipoprotein cholesterol and thiocyanate (as an indicator for smoking). Adiposity was assessed by measurement of the thickness of the panniculus adiposus and by body mass index (BMI). Glycohemoglobin levels exceeding 8% were associated with "substantially more extensive" fatty streaks and raised lesions in the right coronary artery in persons more than 25 years of age. Both thickness of the panniculus adiposus and BMI were associated with more extensive fatty streaks and raised lesions in the right coronary artery. These findings could not be explained by either a less-favorable lipoprotein profile or smoking. To our knowledge, these results appear unique and demonstrate for the first time that increased adiposity accelerates the progression of atherosclerosis and possibly is related to diabetes predisposition in youth.[17]

Dietz[18] has characterized adolescence as a critical period for the development of obesity, particularly for women, because obesity that begins during this period is more likely to persist into adulthood. He cites data indicating that about 30% of obese adult women were obese in early adolescence, while only 10% of obese adult males were also obese in their teens.

In perhaps the longest follow-up to date (>50 years), Must et al[19] examined the relationship between adolescent overweight and adult morbidity and mortality. The Harvard Growth Study began in 1922, when the subjects were between 13 and 18 years old. In this study, 52% of the subjects who had been obese as adolescents

(BMI >75th percentile) were still overweight when they were examined again in 1988. Although there was no increased risk of mortality among the women who had been obese adolescents, they did have an increased risk of arthritis, and reported greater difficulty with activities of daily living. It must be mentioned, however, that the definition of obesity as BMI >75th percentile in this study may have skewed the results. If, as in other work, obesity had been defined as BMI greater than the 90th or 95th percentile, there may well have been a significant effect of adolescent obesity on cardiovascular disease and mortality—but this possibility is speculative only. Further, in another analysis of the same study, Casey et al[20] reported significant correlations between women's BMI at 18 years of age and at 30, 40, and 50 years. Another caveat is that the analyses of both Must et al and Casey et al were based on relatively small numbers of survivors. The original Harvard Growth Study included 1857 schoolchildren who were studied annually for at least eight years. By 1988, Must et al found only 53 women who had been obese adolescents,[19] and Casey et al reported data for only 35 to 59 women.[20]

Not only can obesity have long-term negative health consequences for the adolescent, it may also have negative social and economic sequelae. Gortmaker et al[20] followed young people age 16 to 24 for seven years. They found that young women who started out with a BMI >95th percentile wound up with less education, were less likely to be married, had lower household income, and had higher rates of household poverty than women who had not been overweight at the start of the study.

One need not wait for adulthood to see negative consequences of adolescent obesity on health. Rocchini[22] found that obese adolescents were more likely than non-obese peers to exhibit hypertension and abnormal lipoprotein profiles, thus increasing their risk of cardiovascular disease. Both of these risk factors are decreased when obese adolescents lose weight.

A more recent study by Caprio et al[23] examined the distribution of body fat and its association with a number of risk factors for cardiovascular disease in 14 obese (BMI = 30 ± 1.3) and 10 lean (BMI = 21 ± 0.5) adolescent girls. The subjects were matched for both age and stage of development. Magnetic resonance imaging (MRI) was used to determine the size of fat depots. Obese girls had two- to three-fold greater intraabdominal and subcutaneous fat depots than did lean girls. In the obese subjects, the size of the intraabdominal fat depot was significantly positively correlated with basal insulin and plasma triglyceride levels, but inversely correlated with high-density lipoprotein (HDL) cholesterol level. The size of the femoral (thigh) adipose depot was inversely significantly related to triglyceride and low-density lipoprotein (LDL) cholesterol in the obese girls. Thus, even during adolescence, these authors found that a central distribution of adipose tissue in obese girls led to a significant elevation of those factors linked to increased cardiovascular disease in adults. The concern here, of course, is the early age of onset of such factors that may lead to the earlier development of cardiovascular disease. In light of the data of McGill et al[17] described above, it is likely these individuals face a future of reduced productivity in their prime adult years and an increased disease burden.

Counseling Pitfalls to Avoid: Eating Disorders

When dealing with the adolescent girl, the counselor is faced with the necessity of treading a fine line between encouraging weight control when it is appropriate to do so, and scrupulously avoiding the development of eating disorders. In the current social milieu, when physical thinness may be seen by the adolescent as the only positive goal, the nutrition counselor will be faced with the sometimes difficult task of emphasizing health concerns over concerns about physical appearance. Adolescents are notoriously indifferent to the long-term consequences of behavioral choices. The psychological and social development of young girls includes increasing independence from the nuclear family and increasing attention to and dependence upon peer influence. Intense interest in and concerns about physical appearance and body weight increase the adolescent's vulnerability to ill-advised methods of weight control. An attempt should be made to introduce an appreciation for long-term health and avoidance of negative sequelae to obesity. Thus, an emphasis on healthy lifestyle, one that includes not only a balanced diet and the basics of portion control, but also appropriate physical activity, should be introduced and reinforced. Since the maintenance of weight loss may be improved by concurrent physical activity, there is good reason to emphasize the combination when counseling young girls and women.[24] Recent recognition of the possible negative psychological effects of dwelling only on weight as an index of success, and of utilizing dietary restriction as the main means to that end make it imperative to structure counseling to achieve a more realistic and inclusive view of body weight and total lifestyle.[25]

In addition to developmental factors relating solely to the girl being counseled, the family milieu may also need to be taken into account for the adolescent. Children of obese parents are more likely to be obese, and thus are at a greater risk of obesity-related problems. Also, as Dietz[26] points out, a child's obesity may play an adaptive role within the family, and may thus be very difficult to treat independently.

The health care professional should note that physical activity drops markedly in both males and females during adolescence, but the decrease is greater in females. As shown in Figure 11–1, the Surgeon General's Report on Physical Activity[27] describes female adolescents as "much less" physically active than their male counterparts.

The accretion of excess body fat is fundamentally a matter of energy balance— where energy consumed in food consistently exceeds energy expended. Among

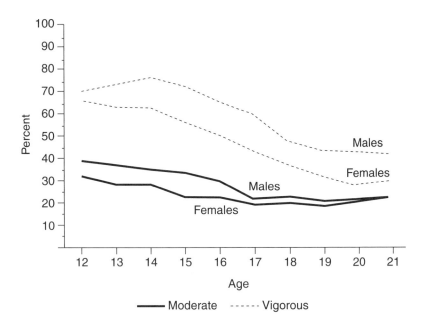

Figure 11–1 Physical activity levels of adolescents and young adults, by age and sex. The solid bar indicates moderate activity and the stippled bar indicates vigorous activity. *Source:* Reprinted from the 1996 Surgeon General's Report on Physical Activity and Health, Centers for Disease Control and Prevention.

U.S. teenagers, the reduced energy expenditure for physical activity contributes to the increasing prevalence of overweight and obesity in this age group.[28] Regrettably, it is not uncommon for teenage girls to use diet pills, laxatives, and cigarette smoking to control their weight and to forego increased physical activity. This is particularly disturbing because the strategies they adopt for the purpose of weight control are harmful, and because the American Heart Association has identified physical inactivity, per se, as a risk factor for cardiovascular disease. As C. Everett Koop noted in a recent (1996) communication to the authors, "It is particularly disturbing to see physical activity levels diminish in our young people since this certainly sets them up to become a part of the epidemic of obesity that is taking hold in America."

PREGNANCY AND LACTATION

It is widely accepted that fat deposition normally occurs during pregnancy in women and that these fat stores are intended to serve as a reservoir of energy needed for milk production after delivery of the infant. There are numerous anecdotal reports throughout the literature that pregnancy in many women triggers the onset of overweight and obesity. For example, in a retrospective analysis of 128 women in a Swedish Obesity Unit, Swedish researchers Rossner and Ohlin found that 73% of their "severely obese" patients had retained more than 10 kg (22 lb) in connection with a pregnancy.[29]

A careful examination of the data pertinent to the issue of how parity impacts body weight indicates that cross-sectional data yield different information from longitudinal data, and studies that rely on recalled height and weight tend to distort the information. In prospective longitudinal studies in which height and weight are measured, most studies demonstrate only a modest increment in body weight associated with pregnancy when compared to properly age-matched nonpregnant controls or when compared to parity-matched nonpregnant controls.[30-32] However, a small subpopulation of women do appear to be at increased risk for significant weight gain during pregnancy.[33] The challenge to the health professional is to identify those women at risk and counsel them properly during pregnancy and the postpartum period. Because it is so difficult to treat obesity successfully once it has been established, it would be extremely helpful to understand the cause of weight gain in these high-risk women and to identify strategies that would prevent it from occurring.

Brown et al[34] conducted a survey of 41,184 postmenopausal women participating in a population-based study, the Iowa Women's Health Study. The women were asked to report lifetime parity, weight at 18, 30, 40, and 50 years and current height. Although this study is large, its retrospective design and reliance on recalled data, which are notoriously unreliable,[30] must be treated with caution. The results indicated that on average, the women gained over 11 kg between the ages of 18 and 50 years.[34] It is important to keep in mind this fairly large increase in weight that occurs with aging as we attempt to tease out what portion, if any, of that weight gain is attributable to pregnancy. Parity was associated with an increase in body weight but results differed depending on the number of live births. Women with lifetime parity of one or two live births had lower mean body weight and BMI, and a lower proportion of overweight (defined as BMI >27) than either nulliparous women or women with three or more lifetime births. These workers concluded that there was strong association between aging and body weight but that the association between parity and both weight gain and overweight was weak.

Ohlin and Rossner have succinctly summed up the dilemma that faces the health professional concerning changes in body composition that may accompany reproduction in women: "Whereas the obstetrician is anxious that the weight development of the mother does not in any way compromise the safety of the fetus and the newborn, the specialist in nutrition and medicine is concerned if an excessive weight retention in connection with a pregnancy results in future overweight, obesity and ensuing medical complications."[35(p271)] The growth and development of the fetus must be safeguarded as measures are taken to counsel women to avoid significant weight gain as a consequence of pregnancy. It is well known that inadequate maternal weight gain is associated with low birth weight in the infant and increased risk of perterm delivery.[36] The corollary of this is that maternal weight is a significant predictor of infant birth weight,[37] so increased maternal weight has a desirable effect on birth weight. Yet clinics that focus on obesity treatment observe that many of the severely obese women who seek treatment state that their weight problems originate in past pregnancies.[29] Despite these widespread anecdotal reports, whether pregnancy predisposes women to obesity remains unclear.

Recommended Weight Gain During Pregnancy

Weight gain recommendations were formulated by the Institute of Medicine (IOM) in 1990.[38] These new guidelines, shown in Table 11–1, are based on observed (rather than calculated) weight gains of women and take into account the prepregnancy body weight, or more specifically, the prepregnancy body mass index (BMI) of the mother. (Note: BMI is calculated as body weight [expressed in kilograms] divided by [height (in meters) squared].)

Note that even obese women are advised to gain weight during pregnancy; indeed, weight loss for overweight and obese women is ill-advised because of its impact on the developing fetus. Dewey et al[38] has proposed that after lactation is well-established, a moderate weight loss regimen that includes increased physical activity may safely be pursued provided the energy deficit results in weight loss that does not exceed 2 kg (4.4 lb) per month.[39] The IOM recommendations for lactation caution that this rate of loss is unlikely to adversely affect milk volume, but that such women should be alert for any indications that the infant's appetite is not being satisfied.[40]

Table 11–1 Prepregnancy BMI and Recommended* Weight Gain During Pregnancy

Prepregnancy BMI (kg/[m²])	Recommended Weight Gain (lb)
<19.8 (underweight)	28 to 40
19.8 to 26.0	25 to 35
26.1 to 29.0 (overweight)	15 to 25
>29.0	minimum 15, but not much more

Note: for twin pregnancy, weight gain should be 35 to 45 lb.
*Institute of Medicine 1990 recommendations.[38]
Source: Data from Nutrition During Pregnancy, Part I: Weight Gain, © 1990, Institute of Medicine, National Academy of Sciences, National Academy Press.

Young adolescents and black women are encouraged to strive for gains at the upper end of the range that corresponds to their prepregnancy BMI, and short women (ht <157 cm) should strive for gains at the lower end of the range.[38] Although these recommendations have been criticized by some who fear they may be too lenient and may promote obesity,[41] others have welcomed them as a realistic alternative to the inappropriately restrictive guidelines in the past that caused unnecessary stress and guilt in women whose weight gain commonly exceeded those limits.[33,42,43]

A recent study of 6690 women found that those women who gained weight within the IOM guidelines had better pregnancy outcomes.[43] Those who gained less than the IOM recommendations experienced an increased incidence of infants that were small for gestational age. Gains above the recommendations were associated with increased risk of infants who were large for gestational age and Caesarean deliveries. This study should help allay concerns about the appropriateness of the guidelines with respect to birth outcome. However, the impact of the guidelines on the subsequent development of maternal obesity, especially in minority populations is less clear.

Effects of Pregnancy on Maternal Body Weight

Using body weight as a proxy for body fat, many of the earlier studies examining the impact of pregnancy on weight retention have included only a small number of subjects and nearly all suffered from the methodological flaw of relying on recalled (rather than measured) prepregnancy weights. A five-year prospective cohort study of 2788 women by Smith et al[45] is distinctive in that 53% of the study subjects were black. Subjects were recruited through community-based sampling and were 18 to 30 years of age at the time of baseline examination in 1985 and 1986. Subjects were nulliparous at entry and throughout the five-year study; nulliparous at entry but primiparous after five years; or parous at entry and had one more pregnancy during the five-year study period. All parous subjects were at least 12 months postpartum when examined at the end of study.

The average weight gain of the primiparas was significantly greater than that of nulliparas, but in white women the average gain was 4.5 kg whereas in black women it was 8.8 kg (these values were adjusted for baseline weight, age, education, smoking status, physical fitness, baseline physical activity, and change in activity).[45] After taking into account the fact that nulliparas gained weight over the five-year study period, excess gain associated with the first pregnancy was 3.0 kg in black women and 1.8 kg in white women. The latter figure is in reasonable agreement with the 1.5 kg gain in white women attributed to pregnancy by Lederman.[30] The larger average gain in black women is in agreement with the observations of Parker and Abrams[44] and the greater variability of gain in this group as evidenced by a larger standard deviation is also consistent with the observations of others.[42]

Rossner and Ohlin[29] reported results of the Stockholm Pregnancy and Weight Development Study, which examined the effects of pregnancy on future weight development in 1423 women. This study had a retrospective and a prospective component. Data were collected retrospectively from routine pregnancy records and then extended prospectively to 6 and 12 months after delivery. The mean weight retention associated with a pregnancy one year after delivery was estimated to be 0.5 kg, which is lower than other large prospective studies. It is possible that the discrepancy can be explained by the fact that prepregnancy body weight was not measured although it is also possible that this figure is more appropriate for the Swedish population. These workers found that 14% of the women gained more than 5 kg,[29] lending support to the idea that even among a relatively homogeneous Swedish population, there is a subpopulation that is vulnerable to high gain associated with pregnancy.

Keppel and Taffel[42] studied a sample of women who participated in the National Maternal and Infant Health Survey and who had live births in 1988. Although this study relied on recalled weight and did not include a suitable control for weight gain associated with aging, the ethnic differences found in this study merit mention. In this study, 206 subjects were black and 1323 were white. The data were stratified by prepregnancy BMI and weight gain during pregnancy in order to examine the impact of the IOM guidelines for weight gain on subsequent weight retention. Overall, the proportion of white women who retained 9 lbs or more was 25.3% whereas for black women it was 44.7%. The proportion of white women who retained 14 lbs or more was 13.6% but for black women it was 30.7%. It appeared that even when black women achieved weight gains within the range recommended by the IOM based on maternal prepregnancy BMI, 45% of them experienced weight retention of 9 lbs or more. Although the sample size in this study is not large, these results and those of Smith et al[45] and Parker and Abrams[44] signal the need to focus more attention on the "balancing act" that pregnancy may represent to the African American population. On the one hand, lower weight gain is associated with a higher incidence of low birth weight babies in this population, yet on the other, these women seemed to be faced with a greater threat of excessive weight retention even when they gain within the recommended guidelines. The data of Smith et al[44] described above would suggest that the proportion of this large weight retention in black women that can be ascribed to pregnancy per se is rather small—perhaps 3 kg. The implication is that factors other than childbearing may play a significant role. This should be a fertile area for future research. In the meantime, the health care professional should pay close attention to lifestyle factors that may need to be addressed in order to minimize postpartum weight retention.

The First Pregnancy—A Risk Factor for Subsequent Risk for Obesity?

Management of the first pregnancy may be of critical importance for averting subsequent maternal obesity, especially in African American populations. The study by Smith et al[45] described above showed that both black and white primiparous women showed significantly greater increases in waist-to-hip ratio (WHR) than did nulliparas, indicating an adverse redistribution of body fat during pregnancy. Note that these subjects were studied at least one year postpartum, but this finding may be attributable, in part, to a loss of abdominal muscle tone as a consequence of pregnancy.

The increase in WHR was independent of weight change in both black and white primipara. Within parity groups, black women had larger absolute increases in WHR than white women. Indeed, the increases in WHR were at least twice as large among black multiparas as those in white multiparas.[45] It is generally accepted that an increased WHR reflects the central deposition of body fat and is considered a risk factor for the development of cardiovascular disease. The finding that after a first pregnancy, women experience increases in body weight and central body fat distribution that persist and that cannot be accounted for by aging alone merits further investigation because it may predispose these women to an increased risk of heart disease. Whether the increased central adiposity in black women, especially black multipara, predisposes these women to a high risk of cardiovascular disease is an important research question as well.

Pregnancy in Older Women

Williamson et al[46] examined the effect of childbearing on the weight gain of older mothers. Whereas Smith et al[45] looked at women age 18 to 30, Williamson conducted a prospective study of childbearing in 2547 older women, 25 to 45 years of age. These women had been weighed in the First National Health and Nutrition Examination Survey (1971–1975) and were re-weighed an average of 10 years later. The data were adjusted for duration of follow-up, age, body mass index, initial parity, education, smoking, drinking, employment status, marital status, illness, physical activity, and dieting to lose weight. When women who gave birth during the study were compared to women who did not (both parous and nulliparous), the mean excess weight gain attributable to childbearing was 1.4, 1.0, and 1.8 kg for women having one, two, and three live births, respectively. If nulliparous women were removed from the comparison, the estimates increased to 1.7, 1.7, and 2.2 kg, respectively. Unlike Smith et al,[45] they did not find a more pronounced effect of childbearing among primiparas, possibly explained by the greater length of time for recovery of prepregnancy body weight in the longer study by Williamson. Alternatively, the difference in results of these studies may be attributable to the younger age or higher proportion of non-white subjects in the Smith study. Williamson et al[45] found that parous women who had ceased child-bearing before the study was initiated tended to gain less weight on average than either nulliparous women or most groups of women who continued bearing children. They reported that the risk of gaining more than 13 kg was increased by 40% to 60%, and the risk of becoming overweight was increased by 60% to 110% in women who bore children during the 10-year study period.[46]

Taken together, these studies suggest that the average weight gain associated with pregnancy is quite modest. Nonetheless, some women are at risk for excessive weight gain and may even become overweight as a consequence of pregnancy. In younger women, that risk may be greater for women going through a first pregnancy as compared to subsequent pregnancies. The data suggest that excessive weight gain during the pregnancy itself seems to signal such high-risk individuals and the high gain is usually evident in the first trimester. These studies should alert the health professional to look for these critical periods of weight gain, especially in black women, and in older women who are bearing children. The data point to the need for additional studies in members of other ethnic groups who may respond to pregnancy (and parity) differently than white women. There is a need to understand the underlying mechanisms of this increased adiposity and central adipose tissue distribution associated with pregnancy as well as the impact this may have on long-term morbidity and mortality.

Childrearing vs Childbearing

"We are unable to infer directly that childbearing, per se, is the cause of the excess weight gain. . . . Other factors, possibly related to changes in diet and physical activity, that are themselves associated with child rearing, rather than childbearing, may be the true causes of the excess long-term weight gain."[46(p568)] This statement by Williamson et al raises an important issue that has not received adequate attention in the research community. What are the important factors associated with childrearing that may predispose women to an increased risk of excessive weight gain? Rossner and Ohlin,[29] in the Stockholm Pregnancy and Weight Development Study, found that weight increase during pregnancy was the strongest predictor for sustained weight retention one year later, but they looked at other factors as well. Their data ruled out prepregnancy weight as a predictor and found that lactation pattern had only a minor influence. They found that smoking cessation was an important predictor for sustained weight increase as was a change in lifestyle (eating habits, meal patterns, and physical activity). In fact, they concluded that "eventual body weight after pregnancy is more determined by the changes in association with that particular pregnancy than with the lifestyle before."[29(p267S)] The health care professional is therefore well advised to offer concrete and practical information on healthy eating and increased physical activity if there is any indication that significant weight gain is a possibility.

Effect of Body Composition on Pregnancy Outcome

Pregnant and lactating women are believed to be particularly vulnerable to suboptimal folate status due to the increased folate metabolism associated with fetal growth during pregnancy and milk production during lactation.[47] The consequences of inadequate folate intake may be an increased risk of neural tube defects (NTDs) in the developing fetus and this risk has been considered great enough for the Food and Drug Administration to have recently taken steps to fortify foods in the U.S. food supply and thereby ensure adequate intake in most women of childbearing age. Against this background of changing public health policy, two separate studies[48,49] have shown that the risk of NTDs increases with prepregnancy weight, and that this finding is independent of folate intake. The mechanism by which obesity is linked to the development of NTDs is unclear at this time but is of vital importance as the prevalence of obesity among women increases. This is yet another area that merits further investigation. In the meantime, ensuring optimal folate intake in obese women who are pregnant or who are contemplating pregnancy is essential.

LACTATION AND BODY COMPOSITION

In women, the energy requirements of lactation exceed those of pregnancy, and are met through a combination of increased intake and withdrawal from the maternal stores of body fat.[40] During lactation, it is important to encourage the consumption of nutrient-dense foods because, as Abrams and Berman note, "although the RDA [recommended dietary allowance] for energy increases only 17%, RDAs for vitamins and minerals increase between 20% and 100%. Thus, most women do not require a great deal more quantity of food, but they do require better quality."[50(p589)]

After a pregnancy, weight loss is a major concern of many American women. It is important for the health professional to be aware of the need to balance the requirements for adequate milk supply to the breastfeeding infant with maternal desires to restrict energy intake for the purposes of weight reduction. In practice, this balance may not be difficult to maintain; Abrams and Berman[50] point out that the infant's demand for milk is the most important determinant of milk production. Neither moderate postpartum weight loss (up to 2 kg per month)[38] nor regular exercise[39] appear to affect breast milk output. On the other hand, the lactational demands for increased intake of certain nutrients (calcium, magnesium, zinc, folate, and vitamin B_6) will not readily be met if care is not taken to ensure the quality of the maternal diet. Any deficit will most assuredly be met from maternal stores.[50]

The energy demands of milk production have been estimated to be approximately 800 kcal per day, and during lactation it is recommended that energy intake increase by only 500 kcal. Therefore, it can be expected that the deficit is made up from maternal energy stores and/or reductions in energy expenditure for physical activity. Although most breastfeeding mothers will experience gradual weight loss, about 20% of these women will maintain or even gain weight.[40,50]

Dewey et al[51] reported that mothers who breastfed for more than 12 months lost an average of nearly twice as much (4.4 kg) weight as those who breastfed for less than 3 months (2.4 kg). Changes in triceps skinfold thickness suggest that some of this lost weight was fat although body composition was not measured in their study. They noted that the majority of the difference in weight loss and in triceps skinfold took place from three to six months postpartum and concluded that lactation enhances weight loss postpartum if breastfeeding continues for at least six months.[51] These results agree with those of Ohlin and Rossner.[32]

Dewey et al[50] have pointed out that the above results agree with the findings of some investigators but not all. They attribute the failure to find enhanced weight loss among lactating women to methodological differences among the studies. The finding of enhanced weight loss among women who lactate for six months or more is consistent among investigators who use a strict definition of breastfeeding and conduct the study for more than six months. Finally, Dewey et al[51] point out that breastfeeding women are less likely to deliberately restrict calories in an effort to lose weight whereas dieting is common practice among non-lactating postpartum mothers. To ensure an unbiased comparison, dieters must be carefully excluded from both the lactating and the non-lactating control group.[51] From these studies we conclude that breastfeeding is desirable from two important perspectives. It delivers optimal nutrition to the infant and facilitates maternal efforts to return to prepregnancy body weight. Although a small proportion of breastfeeding women gain weight, among those who breastfeed for more than six months, the proportion is small. To optimize weight loss and fat loss, at least as indicated by triceps skinfold thickness, breastfeeding should be prolonged for as long as possible during the first year after delivery.

BODY COMPOSITION AND MENOPAUSE

Changes in body composition during menopause have received little scientific attention yet it is clear to many women that this period is marked by significant weight gain. Whether this change is a consequence of inevitable physiological processes and whether it plays an important role in predisposing postmenopausal women to cardiovascular disease are two important questions that need to be addressed. The role of the increasingly common use of hormone replacements on total fat deposited as well as on fat distribution is another area of concern.

Heymsfield et al[52] reviewed the research examining perimenopausal changes in body composition and energy expenditure. They concluded that in addition to the increase in body weight typically seen with aging, changes in body composition occur with age and the changes are independent of weight gain. They pointed out that the weight gain that is typical of aging and the increases in body fat content are associated with the development of cardiovascular disease, diabetes, certain malignancies, osteoporosis, arthritis, and several other clinical conditions. The resulting decrease in mobility and limitation of independence can seriously erode the quality of life for the postmenopausal woman.[52]

A disruption of energy balance is the cause of obesity at any stage of life, i.e., energy intake from foods consistently exceeds energy expenditure. The excess calories are stored as fat. It is widely assumed by laypersons that a reduction in energy expenditure is a necessary consequence of aging. Hence, many perceive an increase in body fat as an inevitable consequence of aging. Yet there is evidence to the contrary.

To examine this question Heymsfield et al[52] divide energy expenditure into three mains components: (1) resting metabolic rate (RMR), which is the rate of energy expended at rest and in a postabsorptive condition; (2) thermic effect of food, which is the incremental increase in energy expended after a meal is fed; and (3) energy expended for physical activity, which is variable over the course of the day. In the average person, by far the largest component of total energy expenditure is RMR. In premenopausal women, Webb[53] and Solomon et al[54] observe a cyclic variation in RMR. A spike in metabolic rate that may amount to more than 350 kcal/day is associated with the luteal phase of the menstrual cycle. This spike is not observed in postmenopausal women, i.e., the RMR is therefore reduced after menopause. This factor may contribute to the positive energy balance and consequent increased fat deposition that marks menopause.

Several factors change simultaneously in the perimenopausal period, and isolating the factor(s) primarily responsible for the development of positive energy balance is a challenge to the researcher. Physical activity usually decreases during this period of life and decrements in lean body mass are a consequence of decreased activity. This in turn will have a depressing effect on RMR. The interesting question is whether RMR can be maintained at a premenopausal level if sufficient physical activity is sustained to preserve lean body mass.

In a nonrandomized, longitudinal, prospective study of 35 healthy, nonsmoking, premenopausal women, Poehlman et al[55] examined the effects of menopause on RMR, body composition, fat distribution, physical activity, and fasting insulin levels. The subjects were recruited through advertising and screened for eligibility by telephone. Hence these may not be typical of the general population. Metabolic tests were conducted between days 5 and 12 of the follicular phase of their menstrual period at the beginning of the study and these tests were repeated six years later. At this point, 18 women were postmenopausal and 17 had normal menstrual function. Three women were perimenopausal and had to be excluded. None of the women received hormone replacement therapy.

At the end of the study, the average age, weight, and energy intake of the two groups of women did not differ, but there were significant (p <0.01) declines in fat-free mass, RMR, leisure time physical activity, and fasting insulin levels in the postmenopausal group. Both fat mass and waist-to-hip ratio were significantly elevated in this group as well. In this study, the observed decline in the fat-free mass was 3 kg (6.6 lb) yet RMR declined by only 100 kcal/day, suggesting that health professionals should suggest strategies to defend fat-free mass as one ages in order to sustain RMR. One such strategy is to engage in physical activity to defend or even increase fat-free mass (primarily muscle, but also bone) but most workers observe a decline in activity as women go through menopause.[56]

A similar decline in physical activity was reported by Wing et al.[57] In the Healthy Women Study, these workers prospectively studied 485 women who were premenopausal and aged 42 to 50 years, and then studied them again three years later. The women were healthy and were not taking estrogens or any of a wide array of drugs at the start of the study. By the end of three years, 279 women were still premenopausal. The "naturally postmenopausal" group (n = 61) had stopped menstruating for at least 12 months and did not undergo surgical menopause or hormone replacement therapy. The balance of women were perimenopausal, hormone users, or had undergone hysterectomies. In this study, weight gain of the two groups of interest—pre- and postmenopausal women—was somewhat more than 2 kg and the magnitude of gain was similar in each group. Efforts to predict weight gain were "largely unsuccessful."[57]

The health care professional might note that the largest gainers were black women, women who lived alone, and women who decreased their activity levels. Menopausal status was the best predictor of adverse changes in lipid profiles, but weight gain in both groups of women was significantly associated with increases in total cholesterol, triglycerides, blood pressure, and fasting insulin levels.[58] Furthermore, the greater the gain, the greater the magnitude of these adverse changes, which are associated with cardiovascular disease.

Ley et al[58(p953)] state, "compared with premenopausal women, fat distribution in postmenopausal women is changing towards that of a man." In a study of healthy white volunteers, Ley et al[58] reported a 20% greater fat mass in postmenopausal women (n = 70; none receiving sex steriod therapy) when compared to premenopausal women (n = 61). This study did not control for age as did the study by Poehlman et al[55] described above, but it did include measurements of body composition using dual-energy X-ray absorptiometry (DEXA). The results showed a greater proportion of upper body (android) fat and a declining proportion of lower body (gynoid) fat in postmenopausal women as compared to premenopausal (and younger) controls. BMI of the postmenopausal group was also significantly greater.[58] The health care professional is cautioned that these workers view these changes as consistent with the notion that menopause is a risk factor for cardiovascular disease in women.[58]

Owens et al[59] studied the same subjects studied by Wing et al[57] in order to more closely evaluate the effects of physical activity on both weight change and the risk factors for cardiovascular disease during the perimenopausal period. They postulated that high levels of physical activity (evaluated using the Paffenbarger Physical Activity Questionnaire) would have a protective effect. Their hypothesis was confirmed; high levels of activity reported at baseline was associated with less weight gain over the three-year study period. Just as important, women who increased their activity levels during the three-year period had the smallest increases in weight and the smallest decrement in HDL cholesterol (both HDL-C and HDL2-C).[59]

Effects of Body Composition on Dyslipidemia

Using cross-sectional data from the Second National Health and Nutrition Examination Survey, Denke et al[60] evaluated the contribution of body weight (presumably as a proxy for body fat) to undersirable changes in blood lipid levels, especially those associated with increased risk for cardiovascular disease. They concluded that "although age and hormonal status are important affecters of lipoprotein risk factors, body weight also worsens the degree of dyslipidemia in white women."[60(p401)] In younger (premenopausal) women, excess body weight was associated with higher total, non-HDL, and LDL cholesterol levels, higher triglyceride levels, and lower HDL cholesterol levels. The effects of excess body weight in perimenopausal and postmenopausal women were also observed but were less pronounced than in younger women.[60] Because these changes are associated with increased risk for cardiovascular disease, it is important to understand how changes associated with menopause modulate and influence lipoprotein levels in older women.

Interaction of Parity and Menopause

Kritz-Silverstein et al[61] studied 1275 women between the ages of 50 and 89 who lived in Rancho Bernardo, CA. They found that HDL cholesterol levels were not related to pregnancy in women with four or fewer pregnancies. However, in women with five or more pregnancies, HDL levels were significantly lower. These women were more likely to be overweight and have elevated waist-to-hip ratio (WHR), and had gained more weight since age 18. They were also more likely to be diabetic. After adjusting for these factors, the lower HDL levels in women with five or more pregnancies remained statistically significant.[62] These data suggest that as women age, those with a history of multiple pregnancy may be especially well advised to control weight gain and to sustain increased physical activity and other lifestyle factors that will help prevent the adverse changes in lipoprotein levels that signal increased risk for cardiovascular disease.

Can Intervention Be Successful?

Simkin-Silverman et al[62] conducted a five-year randomized clinical trial that tested the hypothesis that adverse changes in lipid profiles and weight gain during menopause can be prevented with an intensive dietary and behavioral intervention. This intervention—called the Women's Healthy Lifestyle Project (WHLP)—focused on healthy women between the ages of 44 and 50 and sought to reduce total fat, saturated fat, and cholesterol intake, prevent weight gain, reduce obesity, and increase physical activity levels. The BMI of the study subjects covered the range from 20 to 34. All women were menstruating at the start of the study and none were taking hormone replacement therapy.[62]

The women who agreed to participate in this study were randomly assigned to the intervention (n = 253) or "assessment only" (n = 267) groups. The intervention consisted of 15 group meetings during the first 20 weeks and both groups received clinic assessments at 6, 18, 30, 42, and 54 months. The intervention group was further subdivided according to BMI at entry so that a weight loss goal could be appropriately assigned. Women with BMI less than or equal to 24.44 were given a 5 lb weight loss goal; a 10 lb goal was assigned to women with a BMI of 24.45 to 26.44; and the remainder were given a 15 lb weight loss goal.[62]

Intervention subjects were given a 1300 or 1500 kcal meal plan for four weeks. They were taught to use pocket diaries to monitor calorie, fat, and saturated fat intake as well as cholesterol. Starting at week three, participants were given education and guidance on how to gradually increase their physical activity level to 1000 kcal/wk. Those already active were encouraged to expend 1500 kcal/week, or if they already exceeded that level, to maintain their activity pattern.[62]

After the 20-week intervention period, the maintenance program consisted of three monthly group meetings, followed by three bimonthly meetings. Support was provided thereafter by group, mail, or telephone contact every two to three months, with attention sometimes being provided individually to subjects with "adherence difficulties" as evidenced by increases in either LDL-C or weight gain.[62]

As compared to the assessment only control group, the results of this intensive intervention showed significant increases in physical activity in the intervention group as well as significant decreases in total energy, total fat, saturated fat, and cholesterol intake. With one exception, the changes in lipid profiles were all favorable (reduced risk for cardiovascular disease) as were the changes in systolic and diastolic blood pressure and fasting glucose. Body weight decreased by an average of 4.8 kg and body fat decreased by 4.9%. Improvements were seen in BMI, waist circumference, and waist-to-hip ratio (WHR). The exception noted above was that HDL-C decreased in the intervention group despite increases in physical activity, but it should be noted that the HDL to total cholesterol ratio improved.[62]

The authors point out that the participants in this trial are predominantly white, married, employed, and highly educated.[62] The latter factor may be important in explaining the high degree of compliance achieved in this study. Nonetheless, this study demonstrates that modest weight loss can be achieved in this age group at a critical period in development. It also demonstrates a number of beneficial effects of that weight loss, with the notable exception of a decrease in HDL-C. One can only speculate that the magnitude of this decrease would have been greater if increases in physical activity had not been achieved. The study is ongoing and the long-term results will eventually be available.

Is Hormone Replacement Therapy Helpful or Harmful?

Kritz-Silverstein and Barrett-Connor[63] reported on 671 women aged 65 to 94 years who were initially enrolled in the Rancho Bernardo study between 1972 and 1974 and who had participated in a 1988 to 1991 follow-up clinic visit. These women fell into three groups: those who had never used hormone replacement therapy (n = 194), those who had used hormones intermittently (n = 331), and those who used hormones continuously (n = 146) for the 15 years between baseline and follow-up. Height and weight were measured at both clinic visits. At follow-up, waist and hip circumference were measured for calculation of waist-to-hip ratio (WHR) and body fat was measured using bioelectric impedance. When the results were adjusted for potentially confounding covariates, no significant differences were found between estrogen users and nonusers in terms of BMI, weight change, BMI change, WHR, or fat mass. These workers concluded that hormone replacement therapy, whether used intermittently or continuously for 15 or more years, is not associated with the weight gain and central adiposity commonly reported in postmenopausal women.[63] Troisi et al[15] also failed to find elevated WHR in women who were current users of hormone replacement therapy, although this study relied on self-reported WHR values.

Using dual photon absorptiometry to measure body composition, Aloia et al[64] conducted a longitudinal prospective randomized study of normal-weight (BMI averaged between 24 and 25) women. The primary purpose of the study was to evaluate and compare the effects of dietary calcium with and without hormone replacement on bone status in women who were at least six months postmenopausal. A secondary purpose was to evaluate body composition in all three groups. This study divided 118 women into three groups: (1) a placebo control group; (2) a vitamin D and calcium supplementation group (1700 mg/day); and (3) an estrogen/progesterone/vitamin D and calcium group. The hormone replacement regimen consisted of conjugated equine estrogens of 0.625 mg daily for 25 days per month plus 10 mg medroxyprogesterone per day from day 16 to 25.[64]

These workers could find no evidence of a protective effect of hormone replacement therapy on any variable other than bone mineral density. Despite a rapid rate of loss of lean body mass, weight gain was observed in all three groups. Although not statistically significant, the greatest weight gain and the greatest increase in percent body fat was seen in the hormone replacement (HRT) group, and more of this added fat was deposited in the central or truncal region of the body[64]—a region that is associated with increased risk for diseases related to obesity, especially cardiovascular disease.

Aloia et al[63] could detect no changes in activity or food intake that could explain the greater fat gain in the HRT group. They were disturbed by the postmenopausal decrements in lean body mass in all groups and surprised by the lack of efficacy of HRT in preventing this loss. They suggested that "weight-loading exercise" be encouraged in order to help protect lean body mass.[64] Because the finding of increased body fat associated with menopause confirms earlier findings of this same group using a different technique to measure body composition, they concluded that modification in diet or exercise should probably be recommended to women entering menopause. Because of the need to understand and prevent the loss of lean body mass, they also assert the influence of androgens should be studied.[65]

Taken together, these studies show that menopause is indeed marked by significant weight gain and undesirable changes in body composition, especially increases in central adiposity and decreases in lean body mass. But on balance, the results to date do not suggest that HRT is a significant contributor to the weight gain associated with menopause or to the undesirable changes in body composition that are associated with increased cardiovascular disease risk. On the contrary, there is evidence that HRT may provide protection against cardiovascular disease, with one study reporting a 50% reduction in risk or a coronary event in women using unopposed oral estrogen.[65] Another report from the Postmenopausal Estrogen/Progestin Interventions (PEPI) Trial[66] found similar results with unopposed estrogen as the optimal regimen to raise HDL cholesterol in women without a uterus, and a combination of estrogen (0.625 mg/day) plus cyclic micronized progesterone (200 mg/day for 12 days per month) as the optimal regimen in women with a uterus.[66]

Effect of Ethnicity on Weight Gain Associated with Menopause

Williamson et al[67] found that black women tended to gain more weight between the ages of 45 and 55 years than did white women. Interestingly, Hamman et al[68] reported no weight gain at the time of menopause in Pima Indian women. We are unaware of other studies of the effects of ethnicity on either menopausal weight gain, fat deposition, or fat distribution. Clearly this question should be examined using studies of longitudinal design and controlling for the use of hormone replacement therapy. Currently, health professionals should be advised that meno-pausal weight gain may be a significant issue for women of non-white racial back-grounds.

Effect of Body Compostion on Bone Mineral Density

With aging, all components of the fat-free body decline: brain, skeletal muscle and skeletal bone mass, and calcium content.[52] But a recent study by Tremollieres et al[69] showed that elevated BMI (but not body weight per se) was associated with a preservation of vertebral bone mineral density as assessed by dual photon absorptiometry. This protective effect of weight on bone is likely related to excess adipose tissue. These workers studied 155 "early postmenopausal" women who were followed for 31 months. They observed higher plasma levels of dehydro-epiandrosterone sulfate levels in the women with elevated ($\geq$25) BMI, which may be a consequence of conversion of estrogen from adrenal precursors and/or in-creased production of adrenal androgens. Hormonal as well as mechanical factors of increased strains on the skeleton may be involved.[69] This information is note-worthy because of the increasingly common occurrence of osteoporosis in women who are postmenopausal. This may represent the sole health benefit of obesity— an association with a preservation of bone mineral density in postmenopausal women. Weight loss, on the other hand, beginning at age 50 increases the risk of hip fracture in older white women.[71,72]

CONCLUSION

The following summarizes points the health care professional should consider when counseling the obese female at various stages of development. Where ap-propriate, developmental stages and factors that may place the individual at in-creased risk for obesity are noted. Points of possible intervention at each develop-mental stage are also indicated.

Adolescence

1. Age at menarche: the earlier the age of onset, the higher the risk of obesity.
2. Current age in relation to menarche: is the client likely to be past the peak of height velocity? If not, care must be taken to avoid restricting energy intake so that the child falls off her own growth curve. Fewer than 1500 kilocalories daily is not advised in growing individuals.
3. Family history and risk factors: is there a family history of cardiovascular disease, hypertension, diabetes (type II)? If so, greater vigilance and perhaps more aggressive intervention is warranted.
4. Patient's lifestyle: emphasize both healthy eating and increased physical ac-tivity. Dietary restriction may be inappropriate or ill-advised in teens who

are seriously preoccupied with body image and fatness and who may be at increased risk for eating disorders. Indeed, a referral for psychological counseling may be warranted.

5. Family dynamics: the presence of parental obesity indicates increased risk for obesity in the adolescent. Is the adolescent obesity a consequence of or adaptation to familial dysfunction? Are the parents or caregivers willing and able to provide support for the necessary behavioral changes? If such support is absent, only strategies that can be implemented by the adolescent can be considered.

6. Watch for signs of laxative abuse and incipient eating disorders. If in doubt, refer for psychiatric evaluation.

Pregnancy

1. Although the average increase in body weight associated with pregnancy is small, a proportion of white women (5% to 10%) are at risk for significant weight gain. For African American women, this proportion may be as high as 15%. Other ethnic groups, such as Hispanic women, may be similarly at increased risk.

2. Weight gain associated with healthy outcome, from the perspective of maternal body weight and body composition, is quite variable.

3. Significantly increased gain, above the normal pattern, is more often manifest during the first trimester, rather than the second or third.

4. Women who enter pregnancy at elevated body weight are advised to gain less weight than average. See Table 11–1.

5. Postpartum, identify women who experience difficulty returning to prepregnancy weight. Pay careful attention to lifestyle, especially physical activity and eating habits, and encourage extending breastfeeding to beyond six months if this method of feeding is chosen.

6. Breastfeeding mobilizes maternal body fat laid down during pregnancy to support the energy costs of milk production.

7. Optimal folate intake in an obese woman who is pregnant or who is contemplating pregnancy is essential because of the increased risk of neural tube defects observed among the obese.

8. For reasons of lifestyle, as well as a consequence of physiological changes, the first pregnancy may be a period of increased risk for both excessive weight gain and for the central deposition of body fat, which may predispose to cardiovascular disease.

Lactation

1. Body weight will significantly decrease immediately postpartum but complete return to prepregnancy body weight may take six to nine months.

2. The pattern of weight loss during lactation is highly variable and changes in body weight do not reliably reflect changes in body fat.
3. In women who breastfeed, some will lose weight, some will gain, and some will not experience a significant change in weight.
4. Extended breastfeeding, beyond six months and up to a year, is reliably associated with reductions in maternal body fat.
5. Once lactation is well established, physical activity may be safely pursued, and in most cases should be encouraged.
6. A caloric deficit producing weight loss of more than 2 kg (4.4 lb) per month is not recommended.
7. Efforts to lose weight should be carefully monitored to ensure that the infant is able to feed to appetite.

Menopause

1. Significant weight gain associated with menopause is common. This weight gain is an indication of increased body fat.
2. The distribution of body fat associated with menopause is in the abdominal region and is associated with undesirable changes in blood lipids, lipoproteins, blood pressure, and other risk factors for cardiovascular disease.
3. Women with a histroy of multiple pregnancies are at particular risk for the above adverse changes, many of which can be improved with increased physical activity.
4. Interventions designed to prevent increases in body weight during menopause must be comprehensive: increased physical activity, dietary counseling on portion control and low-fat food selection, as well as, when appropriate, weight loss. Such interventions must include long-term follow-up and vigilance on the part of the individual client as well as the health care professional if weight gain is be avoided.
5. For women at risk for osteoporosis, several studies have shown that obesity is protective of bone mineral density. Because of the increased risk for major chronic diseases associated with obesity, such women should consider adopting both weight-bearing (e.g., walking) and strength training exercise to preserve and increase lean body mass and promote increased bone mineral density. These forms of exercise have the added benefit of offsetting the increase in body fat content that is commonly observed in women passing through menopause.

REFERENCES

1. Catalano PM, Drago NM, Amini SB. Factors affecting fetal growth and body composition. *Am J Obstet Gyn.* 1995;172:1459–1463.

2. Tanner JM. *Growth at Adolescence*. 3rd ed. Boston, MA: Blackwell Scientific Publications, Inc; 1962.

3. Story M, Alton I. Becoming a woman: nutrition in adolescents. In: Krummel DA, and Kris-Etherton PM, eds. *Nutrition in Women's Health*. Gaithersburg, MD: Aspen Publishers Inc; 1996:1–34.

4. Forbes, GB. Body size and composition of perimenarchal girls. *Am J Dis Child*. 1992;146:63–66.

5. Hediger ML, Scholl TO, Schall JI, Cronk CE. One-year changes in weight and fatness in girls during late adolescence. *Pediatrics*. 1995;96:253–258.

6. St. Jeor ST, Silverstein LJ, Shane SR. Obesity. In: Krummel DA, Kris-Etherton PM, eds. *Nutrition in Women's Health*. Gaithersburg, MD: Aspen Publishers Inc; 1996:353–382.

7. Frisch RE, Revelle R. Height and weight at menarche and a hypothesis of menarche. *Arch Dis Child*. 1971;46:695–701.

8. Frisch RE. The right weight: body fat, menarche and fertility. *Proc Nutr Soc*. 1994;53:113–129.

9. De Ridder CM, Thijssen JHH, Bruning PF, et al. Body fat mass, body fat distribution, and pubertal development: a longitudinal study of physical and hormonal sexual maturation of girls. *J Clin Endocrinol Metab*. 1992;75:442–446.

10. Cameron JL. Nutritional determinants of puberty. *Nutr Rev*. 1996;54:S17–S22.

11. Chehab FF, Mounzih K, Lu R, Lim ME. Early onset of reproductive function in normal mice treated with leptin. *Science* 1997;275:88–90.

12. Beunen GP, Malina RM, Lefevre JA, et al. Adiposity and biological maturity in girls 6–16 years of age. *Int J Obes*. 1994;18:542–546.

13. Garn SM, LaVelle M, Rosenberg KR, Hawthorne VM. Maturational timing as a factor in female obesity. *Am J Clin Nutr*. 1986;43:879–883.

14. Van Lenthe FJ, Kemper HCG, van Mechelen W, et al. Biological maturation and the distribution of subcutaneous fat from adolescence into adulthood: the Amsterdam growth and health study. *Int J Obes*. 1996;20:121–129.

15. Van Lenthe FJ, Kemper HCG, van Mechelen W. Rapid maturation in adolescence results in greater obesity in adulthood: the Amsterdam growth and health study. *Am J Clin Nutr*. 1996;64:18 24.

16. Troisi RJ, Wolf AM, Mason JE, Klingler KM, Corditz GA. Relation of body fat distribution to reproductive factors in pre- and postmenopausal women. *Obes Res*. 1995;3:145–151.

17. McGill HC Jr., McMahan CA, Malcom GR, et al. Relation of glycohemoglobin and adiposity to arteriosclerosis in youth. *Arterioscler Thromb Vasc Biol*. 1995;15:431–440.

18. Dietz WH. Critical periods in childhood for the development of obesity. *Am J Clin Nutr*. 1994;59:955–959.

19. Must A, Jacques PF, Dallal GE, Bajema CJ, Dietz WH. Long-term morbidity and mortality of overweight adolescents. *New Engl J Med*. 1992;327:1350–1355.

20. Casey VA, Dwyer JT, Coleman KA, Valadian I. Body mass index from childhood to middle age: a 50-year follow-up. *Am J Clin Nutr*. 1993;56:14–18.

21. Gortmaker SL, Must A, Perrin JM, Solbol AM, Dietz WH. Social and economic consequences of overweight in adolescence and young adulthood. *New Engl J Med*. 1993;329:1008–1012.

22. Rocchini, AP. Adolescent obesity and cardiovascular risk. *Ped Annals*. 1992;21:235–240.

23. Caprio S, Hyman LD, McCarthy S, et al. Fat distribution and cardiovascular risk factors in obese adolescent girls: importance of the intra-abdominal fat depot. *Am J Clin Nutr*. 1996;64:12–17.

24. Skender ML, Goodrick GK, Del Junco, DJ, et al. Comparison of 2-year weight loss trends in behavioral treatments of obesity: diet, exercise, and combination intervention. *J Am Diet Assoc.* 1996;96:342–346.

25. Polivy J. Psychological consequences of food restriction. *J Am Diet Assoc.* 1996;96:589–592.

26. Dietz, WH. Childhood and adolescent obesity. In: Frankle RT, Yang MU, eds. *Obesity and Weight Control.* Gaithersburg, MD: Aspen Publishers Inc; 1988:345–359.

27. US Department of Health and Human Services. *Physical Activity and Health: A Report of the Surgeon General.* Atlanta, GA: Centers for Disease Control and Prevention; 1996.

28. Troiano RP, Flegal KM, Kuczmarski RJ, Campbell SM, Johnson CL. Overweight prevalence and trends for children and adolescents. The National Health and Nutrition Examination Surveys, 1963 to 1991. *Arch Pediatr Adolesc Med.* 1995;149:1085–1091.

29. Rossner S, Ohlin A. Pregnancy as a risk factor for obesity: lessons from the Stockholm Pregnancy and Weight Development Study. *Obes Res.* 1995;3:267S–275S.

30. Lederman SA. The effect of pregnancy weight gain on later obesity. *Obstet Gyn.* 1993;82:148–155.

31. Prentice AM, Poppitt SD, Goldberg GR, et al. Energy balance in pregnancy and lactation. In: Allen L, King J, Lonnerdal B, eds. *Nutrient Regulation during Pregnancy, Lactation, and Infant Growth.* New York: Plenum; 1994;11–26.

32. Ohlin A, Rossner S. Maternal body weight development after pregnancy. *Int J Obes.* 1990;14:159–173.

33. Abrams B. Prenatal weight gain and postpartum weight retention: a delicate balance. *Am J Public Health.* 1993;83:1182–1183.

34. Brown JE, Kaye SA, Folsom AR. Parity-related weight change in women. *Int J Obes.* 1992;16:627–631.

35. Ohlin A, Rossner A. Factors related to body weight changes during and after pregnancy: the Stockholm Pregnancy and Weight Development Study. *Obes Res.* 1996;4:271–276.

36. Siega-Riz AM, Adair LS, Hobel CJ. Maternal underweight status and inadequate rate of weight gain during the third trimester of pregnancy increases the risk of preterm delivery. *Am J Clin Nutr.* 1995;126:146–153.

37. Brooks AA, Johnson MR, Steer PJ, Pawson ME, Abdalla HI. Birth weight: nature or nurture? *Early Hum Develop.* 1995;42:29–35.

38. Institute of Medicine. *Nutrition During Pregnancy, Part 1: Weight Gain.* Washington, DC: National Academy of Sciences, National Academy Press; 1990.

39. Dewey KG, Lovelady CA, Nommsen-Rivers LA, McCrory MA, Lonnerdal B. A randomized study of the effects of aerobic exercise by lactating women on breast-milk volume and composition. *New Engl J Med.* 1994;330:449–453.

40. Institute of Medicine. *Nutrition During Lactation.* Washington, DC: National Academy of Sciences, National Academy Press; 1991.

41. Manson, JE, Colditz GA, Stampfer M. Parity, ponderosity, and the paradox of a weight-preoccupied society. *JAMA.* 1994;271:1788–1790.

42. Keppel KG, Taffel SM. Pregnancy-related weight gain and retention: implications of the 1990 Institute of Medicine guidelines. *Am J Public Health.* 1993;83:1100–1103.

43. Moore BJ, Greenwood, MRC. Pregnancy and weight gain. In: Brownell, KD, Fairburn CG, eds. *Eating Disorders and Obesity: A Comprehensive Textbook.* New York: Guilford; 1995:51–55.

44. Parker JD, Abrams B. Differences in postpartum weight retention between black and white mothers. *Obstet Gyn.* 1993;81:768–774.

45. Smith DE, Lewis CE, Caveny JL, et al. Longitudinal changes in adiposity associated with pregnancy. *JAMA*. 1994;271:1747–1751.

46. Williamson DF, Madans J, Pamuk E, et al. A prospective study of childbearing and 10-year weight gain in US white women 25 to 45 years of age. *Int J Obes*. 1994;18:561–569.

47. O'Connor DL. Folate status during pregnancy and lactation. In: Allen L, King J, Lonnerdal B, eds. *Nutrient Regulation during Pregnancy, Lactation, and Infant Growth*. New York: Plenum; 1994:157–172.

48. Shaw GM, Velie EM, Schaffer D. Risk of neural tube defect—affected pregnancies among obese women. *JAMA*. 1996;275:1093–1096.

49. Werler MM, Quik C, Shapiro S, Mitchell AA. Prepregnant weight in relation to risk of neural tube defects. *JAMA*. 1996;275:1089–1092.

50. Abrams BF, Berman CA. Nutrition during pregnancy and lactation. *Obstetrics*. 1993;20:585–597.

51. Dewey KG, Heinig MJ, Nommsen L. Maternal weight-loss patterns during prolonged lactation. *Am J Clin Nutr*. 1993;58:162–166.

52. Heymsfield SB, Gallagher D, Poehlman E, et al. Menopausal changes in body composition and energy expenditure. *Exp Geront*. 1994;29:377–389.

53. Webb P. 24-hour energy expenditure and the menstrual cycle. *Am J Clin Nutr*. 1986;44:616–619.

54. Solomon SJ, Kurzer MS, Calloway DH. Menstrual cycle and basal metabolic rate in women. *Am J Clin Nutr*. 1982;36:611–616.

55. Poehlman ET, Toth MJ, Gardner AW. Changes in energy balance and body composition at menopause: a controlled longitudinal study. *Ann Intern Med*. 1995;123:673–675.

56. Poehlman ET, Toth MJ, Bunyard LB, et al. Physiological predictors of increasing total and central adiposity in aging men and women. *Arch Intern Med*. 1995;155:2443–2448.

57. Wing RR, Matthews KA, Kuller LH, Meilahn EN, Plantinga P. Weight gain at the time of menopause. *Arch Intern Med*. 1991;151:97–102.

58. Ley CL, Lees B, Stevenson JC. Sex- and menopausal-associated changes in body-fat distribution. *Am J Clin Nutr*. 1992;55:950–954.

59. Owens JF, Matthews KA, Wing RR, Kuller LH. Can physical activity mitigate the effects of aging in middle-aged women? *Circulation*. 1992;85:1265–1270.

60. Denke MA, Sempos CT, Grundy SM. Excess body weight: an under-recognized contributor to dyslipidemia in white American women. *Arch Intern Med*. 1994;154:401–410.

61. Kritz-Silverstein D, Barrett-Connor E, Wingard DL. The relationship between multiparity and lipoprotein levels in older women. *J Clin Epidemiol*. 1992;45:761–767.

62. Simkin-Silverman L, Wing RR, Hansen DH, et al. Prevention of cardiovascular risk factor elevations in healthy premenopausal women. *Prev Med*. 1995;24:509–517.

63. Kritz-Silverstein D, Barrett-Connor E. Long-term postmenopausal hormone use, obesity, and fat distribution in older women. *JAMA*. 1996;275:46–49.

64. Aloia JF, Vaswani A, Russo L, Sheehan M, Flaster E. The influence of menopause and hormonal replacement therapy on body cell mass and body fat mass. *Am J Obstet Gyn*. 1995;172:896–900.

65. Barrett-Connor E, Bush TL. Estrogen and coronary heart disease in women. *JAMA*. 1991;266:1861–1867.

66. The Writing Group for the PEPI Trial. Effects of estrogen or estrogen/progestin regimens on heart disease risk factors in postmenopausal women. The Postmenopausal Estrogen/Progestin Interventions (PEPI) Trial. *JAMA*. 1995;273:199–208.

67. Williamson DF, Kahn HS, Remington PL, Anda RF. The 10-year incidence of overweight and major weight gain in US adults. *Arch Intern Med.* 1990;150:665–672.

68. Hamman RF, Bennett PH, Miller M. The effect of menopause on serum cholesterol in American (Pima) Indian Women. *Am J Epidemiol.* 1975;102:164–169.

69. Tremollieres FA, Pouilles JM, Ribot C. Vertebral postmenopausal bone loss is reduced in overweight women: a longitudinal study in 155 early postmenopausal women. *J Clin Endocrinol Metab.* 1993;77:683–686.

70. Langlois JA, Harris T, Looker AC, Madans J. Weight change between age 50 years and old age is associated with risk of hip facture in white women aged 67 years and older. *Arch Intern Med.* 1996;156:989–994.

71. Jensen LB, Quaade F, Sorensen OH. Bone loss accompanying voluntary weight loss in obese humans. *J Bone Miner Res.* 1994;9:459–463.

CHAPTER 12

Social Aspects of Obesity: Influences, Consequences, Assessments, and Interventions

Jeffery Sobal
Carol M. Devine

INTRODUCTION

Weight is both a physical and a social characteristic. This chapter uses concepts and theories drawn from the social sciences (psychology, sociology, anthropology, and others) to examine body weight and obesity from four perspectives (Figure 12–1). Social influences on weight will be discussed first, followed by an examination of the social effects of obesity, social assessments of obesity, and social theories underlying weight loss interventions. Considering social causes and effects is important in understanding the role of social patterns and processes in obesity. Considering social assessments and social theories in interventions will enhance the ability of health professionals to deal with weight issues.

SOCIAL INFLUENCES ON WEIGHT

Social influences contribute to the prevalence, patterns, and changes in body weight, with people in different cultures and in different positions within society systematically varying in weight. Stunkard observed that "social factors must be considered as among the most important, if not the most important, influence on the prevalence of obesity today."[1(p4)] That suggests that "just as you are what you eat, you also are what you weigh."[2] Social factors include large-scale social contexts that influence weight by providing a socio-cultural environment within which people eat and engage in activity, as well as specific social characteristics of individuals that operate to determine their personal weight patterns.

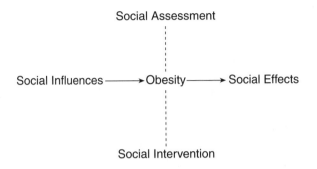

Figure 12–1 A model for conceptualizing social perspectives on obesity.

Social contexts are often the ultimate influences on weight, with culture and historical era providing social environments within which body weight exists. These larger environments provide the setting for individual variations and changes in weight as well as overall values and attitudes affecting weight levels within society.

Cultural systems are the primary influence on weight because culture permeates all aspects of life as a determinant of fundamental ways of living.[3] Culture is the system of categories, rules, and plans that governs the structure, processes, and ideals of a society. Culture sets the context for eating and activity levels, and also provides meaning and interpretation of body weight. Thinness is culturally valued as an ideal in contemporary postindustrial societies, and fatness is rejected and stigmatized. Change of a culture from traditional to modern and acculturation of individuals from traditional cultures into modern societies are typically associated with increases in body weight and obesity.[3] (Culture is discussed further in Chapter 3.)

Historical trends clearly exist in body weight in the United States.[4] During the last several decades body weight ideals for women have increasingly emphasized thinness.[5,6] These increases in pressures to be slim have been suggested as contributors to chronic dieting and eating disorders. The prevalence of overweight has recently increased in the United States, with 25% of adults overweight in 1980 while 33% were overweight in 1990.[7,8] The discrepancy between ideal and actual weight has contributed to the rising prevalence of eating disorders, the development an antidiet movement in the United States, and the emergence of the size acceptance movement that rejects societal emphasis on thinness.[9]

Social characteristics of individuals are key predictors of their weight status. Social scientists often use a constellation of characteristics of individuals to consider the social epidemiology of a condition, including age/lifestage, sex/gender, race/ethnicity, socioeconomic status (income, education, occupation), employment, household composition, marriage, parenthood, and geographic location (urban-rural residence and region). Social science theories provide perspectives about how these characteristics influence weight that offer insights beyond those theories using only a biomedical model.[10,11] Patterns in the social epidemiology of weight are presented in Exhibit 12–1. Overall patterns are discussed, but it is important to note that these characteristics all interact with each other.

Age and lifestage are related to the incidence of major weight gain, with the highest major gain occurring in both men and women between 25 and 34 years of age. Weight increases more slowly thereafter and then declines in the years past age 55.[12] While this pattern is partly biological, it is also socially structured into a normative weight trajectory that people follow as they progress through their life course. People engage in what they consider to be age-appropriate behaviors and have expectations that they will gain weight as they get older and then lose weight when they become elderly. Concern about body weight changes as people move through lifestages, with a peaking of concern about weight and appearance developing in adolescence and young adulthood. With maturity, concerns about weight and appearance decline and are supplanted by concerns about weight and health. Finally, there is a reversal and people become concerned about weight loss among

---

Exhibit 12–1 The Social Epidemiology of Obesity

Social Contexts

Culture: People in developed societies are fatter than developing societies
History: Fatness is increasing in the United States, but idealized weights are
   decreasing

Social Characteristics

Age/lifestage: Fatness increases during adulthood, declines in the elderly
Sex/gender: Women are fatter
Race/ethnicity: African American women are fatter
SES/socioeconomic status
   Income: Lower-income women are fatter
   Education: Less-educated women are fatter
   Occupational prestige: Women in less prestigious jobs are fatter
Employment: Women who are not employed are fatter
Household composition: Older people who live with others are fatter
Marriage: Married men are fatter
Parenthood: More parous women are fatter
Residence: Rural women are fatter
Region: People residing in the South are fatter

the aged. A life course perspective[13] provides insights into weight transitions and trajectories as individuals undergo life changes in the process of aging.

Gender is a social role that has both biological and social influences on weight. While males and females have physiologically determined sex differences in their fat stores and gender roles of men and women include expectations and interpretations that determine behaviors leading to weight gain or loss. In the United States, women are more concerned about appearance than men are, and weight is a major issue in managing appearance.[14] Women, especially younger women, almost universally seek to look thin, while men, primarily younger men, often desire to gain weight to appear big and powerful. Women pay more attention to weight, have more stringent weight standards applied to them and internalized by them, and engage in more efforts to avoid being overweight and to become and remain slim.[15,16]

Ethnicity is the subcultural identity held by individuals within a larger society. Ethnicity may include some biological race differences that influence weight, but more importantly it involves subcultural values and behaviors associated with fatness and thinness. The prevalence of obesity differs among different racial and ethnic groups in the United States.[17] Black and Latino women are more likely to be classified as overweight than white women.[18,19] To the extent that ethnic groups acculturate into a larger society, they tend to lose their prior ethnic behaviors and values about weight and become more similar to their new society. For example, ethnic differences existed in the body weights of European immigrants to the United States, but these differences decreased as they acculturated into the larger U.S. society.[20] Values about ideal weight differ among major ethnic groups in contemporary U.S. society, with African Americans, Hispanic Americans, Native Americans, and Pacific Islanders usually valuing thinness less than white Americans.[3,18]

Socioeconomic status is the position that a person occupies in the stratification system of a society. In the United States, women of lower socioeconomic status are significantly more likely to be obese.[21] Socioeconomic status has several components that influence weight, including income (which provides resources that can be used in weight management), education (which provides knowledge useful in weight management), and occupational prestige (which provides lifestyle related to weight management). Weight also influences socioeconomic status, with the stigma of obesity retarding social mobility of obese individuals.[22] Women and members of some ethnic and racial minority groups are found disproportionately in lower socioeconomic strata. Socioeconomic status accounts for some but not all of the differences in weight status between some racial groups.[18] The trend toward an increased prevalence of overweight over time is more marked among members of lower socioeconomic groups.[23]

Employment is a major social role for most adults, with almost all men and the majority of women currently participating in the labor force. Work influences health through exposure to health risks, opportunities for health care, and health

attitudes and beliefs.[24] Work involves time demands that influence eating and activity behaviors, carries expectations about appropriate body weights for specific
positions, offers social pressure and social support from coworkers, and provides
resources that can influence health care, physical activity patterns, and food
choices. Entering the work force, changing jobs, losing a job, and retiring are employment role transitions that may be important in body weight changes. Relatively little analysis has focused on employment and weight, but some studies
reveal employed women are thinner than those not in the labor force.[25]

Household composition provides a context for social interactions that a person
experiences at home. Living alone does not provide social facilitation for eating or
social support for health behaviors, and many studies of older people show that
those who live alone are at risk of poor diets and high levels of thinness.[26,27] Little
analysis of the relationship between obesity and living situation has been done,[28]
and research on body weight and household size and composition is needed.

Marriage is important in the lives of most people, and marital status and marital
role changes are important influences on weight.[29] Obese people, especially women,
have a difficult time finding a marital partner, and thus it is more difficult for them to
enter the marital role.[30,31] People entering the marital role tend to gain weight, married
men are more likely to be obese than those who are not married, marital partners gain
and lose weight in synchrony, and people leaving marriage tend to lose weight.[25,32]
Family responsibilities create expectations and demands that influence eating behaviors and activity level and are involved in weight changes, as seen in eating and exercise changes that occur with entry into the marital role.[33]

Being a parent is another family role associated with body weight. Among
women, weight changes associated with parenthood begin in pregnancy. Pregnancy-related weight retention has been estimated to average 1 kg per birth,[34] and
postpartum weight retention is higher among black women than among white
women.[35,36] While there are biological influences on weight through childbearing,
the social role of childrearing is also an important influence on parents' weight
through changes in the family food system and activity levels associated with parenthood.[37] The food and nutrition roles associated with motherhood are perceived
by women to influence their access to food and meal patterns, as well as their
motives and opportunities for self-care.[38] The social expectations and demands of
the parental role are important influences upon weight, and body image ideals
associated with the parental role differ from those of non-parents. For example,
the traditional maternal role of nurturing is often associated with a larger body
size. Transitions in social roles over the life course often occur concurrently with
biological transitions, especially changes such as menarche and pregnancy among
women. Social norms related to weight may have a greater salience at times when
people are experiencing role transitions.[39]

Geographic residence is weakly associated with weight. Rural women are
slightly heavier than women living in metropolitan areas, although the effect is

weak and largely accounted for by demographic differences between rural and metropolitan residents.[40] Variations in body weight also occur between residents of various geographic regions, although those patterns have not been extensively investigated. Residents of the South are most likely to be overweight.[41,42]

In summary, social influences provide underlying causes for weight changes in society through the social environments in which people live and the roles that they play. The effects of social contexts and social characteristics are important to consider for understanding levels of body weight and changes in weight.

PSYCHOLOGICAL AND SOCIAL EFFECTS OF OBESITY

Considerable attention has been given to the physiological effects of obesity, with much research on how obesity operates as a risk factor for mortality and morbidity such as hyperlipidemia, hypertension, and hyperinsulinemia.[43] A growing consensus in the literature on the psychological and social effects of obesity is also emerging, finding that obesity has some psychological effects and has many social consequences.[44] Many of the social problems associated with obesity occur in routine daily relationships, as well as in professional relationships, including those with health professionals.

Psychological Effects

Psychological consequences of obesity, weight loss, and weight loss attempts can be examined along several dimensions, including psychopathology, affect/ depression, and self-esteem. Psychological dysfunction does not exhibit a higher incidence among obese individuals than the general population.[45] Similarly, obese individuals have not been shown to have differing personality traits.[46] This suggests that obesity and weight loss are not associated with problems in major cognitive and personality attributes.

Weight change is an important symptom of clinical depression. In cross-sectional population studies depressive symptoms are only weakly associated with body weight.[47] Longitudinal analysis reveals depression is related to weight gain among young adults and weight loss among older people, especially individuals of lower socioeconomic status.[48] Being obese appears to have no direct effect on depression (except for people of high socioeconomic status), although obese individuals are more likely to engage in dieting and have worse physical health, which both contribute to depression.[49]

Dieting to achieve weight loss has been suggested to lead to "dieting depression,"[50] characterized by irritability and nervousness. Later investigations suggest that positive changes in affect may occur with weight loss,[51] although a return to baseline levels of depression and dissatisfaction with appearance have been associated with weight regain in follow-up.[52] This suggests that attempts to lose weight may have some positive and some negative effects on mood that may vary among different individuals, different methods of weight loss, and even in different social contexts of dieting.[53] One review of the consequences of dieting found no existing evidence of severe psychological reactions to dieting, but the authors identified several unresolved methodological problems with the measurement and timing of dieting.[54] The persistence of these effects and the influence of dieting on long- vs short-term changes in affect need further investigation and clarification.

Self-esteem is the personal evaluation that individuals have of themselves, and has been shown in some studies to be diminished among obese individuals while other investigations show no problems associated with self-esteem.[55] One aspect of self-esteem is negative body image, where obese individuals misperceive and disparage their bodies because of their weight. Several studies demonstrate that obese people devalue their bodies[56] as they internalize societal values that emphasize slimness, compare themselves to slim ideals portrayed in the mass media, and are subject to negative evaluations in social interactions. Other studies have suggested that reduced self-esteem is associated with dieting attempts.[57]

Self-efficacy is an assessment of one's ability to accomplish a certain goal.[58] Self-efficacy in weight control has been identified as a predictor of weight loss.[59] The weight gain-and-loss pattern of repeated "yo-yo" dieting and weight cycling that has been the experience of many obese people can lead to a cumulative loss of self-efficacy about one's ability to lose weight or to maintain weight loss. This may contribute to the negative association that has been observed between prior weight control attempts and subsequent weight loss success.[59,60]

Social Effects

Social consequences of obesity occur in relationships where obese individuals are stigmatized by others, and in role access where obese people are denied entry into desirable social positions. The prejudicial values against obesity in contemporary society are enacted in stigmatization and discrimination.

Stigmatization of obese individuals occurs as relationships with others who are prejudiced against obese people lead to derogation, devaluation, and derision of individuals because of their weight. Obesity is stigmatized aesthetically as ugliness, religiously as sinfulness, criminally as badness, and medically as sickness.[61] When the stigma of obesity is compared with other stigmatized conditions in contemporary society, it is apparent that few other characteristics are more severely or openly stigmatized as obesity.[62] The pain of social attitudes toward obesity occurs as people are hassled, harangued, harassed, and hurt in stigmatizing acts by others who consider weight fair game for stigmatization. The effects of stigmatization are internalized, especially by women.[63] The social costs of obesity tend to be greater for women because weight and appearance are more closely related to self-esteem among women, and women have traditionally lacked means of achieving social status besides physical appearance.

Stigmatization of obese individuals may influence the size, quality, and composition of their social networks. Obese children have been reported to be less liked and more often rejected by friends.[64] Obese adults limit and are limited in their social participation and involvement in social networks.[65] However, some investigations report that obese people do not have fewer or less positive social contacts and relationships.[66] Because of the importance of social networks and social support in quality of life and health, additional work needs to be done to more fully examine the social relationships of obese individuals.

Stigmatization can be dealt with by assisting obese individuals to cope with stigmatizing acts, and a four-component model can be used to help people cope with stigmatization.[67] People who may be stigmatized can: (1) recognize stigmatization by increasing awareness and understanding; (2) ready themselves by anticipating and preparing for stigmatizing situations; (3) react to stigmatization in ways that minimize its problems; and (4) repair any problems that are caused by stigmatization.

Health professionals tend to have negative attitudes toward obese people, similar to those of the general public. Stigmatization and discrimination against obese individuals occurs in a broad spectrum of health professionals, including psychologists, counselors, nurses, and others, but because of their prestige and power in the medical system, physicians' attitudes toward obesity are especially significant. Physicians frequently stigmatize obese people as medical students,[68] medical residents,[69] and in medical practice.[70] The stigmatization of obese individuals influences the diagnostic activities of physicians[71] and other health professionals[72] who exhibit bias against obese individuals in their diagnoses of medical problems (including those unrelated to weight) and their application of medical therapy. On a positive note, some programs for medical students have successfully decreased stigmatization of obese patients[73] using education that increases knowledge, sensitivity, and empathy.

Discrimination occurs as obese people are prevented or hindered from entering roles or positions in society because of their weight and not for reasons related to their ability to perform those roles. Discrimination limits access to roles in many social arenas, including education, employment, marriage, housing, and health care.[30,67,74] Such discrimination is particularly harmful because it obstructs obese people from entering important and desirable roles in society, such as student, employee, and spouse. Such discrimination can have major impacts on people for their entire lives.

Legal considerations exist in discrimination against obese individuals. A number of discrimination cases have been litigated with varying results, especially in connection with employment discrimination. Obesity has often been ruled as not constituting grounds for denial or termination of employment, although not all cases have reached that conclusion.[75] A major legal issue is whether obesity is a disability and existing disability laws are applicable to obese individuals,[76] and it has not currently been resolved whether the 1990 Americans with Disabilities Act (ADA) act is applicable to obese people.[30]

Alterations in body weight have been suggested to lead to disruptions in family relationships, especially among women who have lost large amounts of weight through surgery,[77] because the high weight levels of some family members play a role in the dynamics of family functioning.[78] Weight and weight change are not strongly associated with marital quality in the general population,[79] however, suggesting that marital effects of obesity may occur in a relatively few dysfunctional family relationships.

In summary, obesity has some psychological effects that tend to be a result of internalized negative societal values about weight and unpleasant social relationships that obese individuals have in everyday interactions. Stigmatization of obesity is prevalent and severe in contemporary society, and social prejudices are often enacted in discrimination against obese individuals. Health professionals often engage in stigmatization and discrimination against obese people, but educational programs may be useful in helping to overcome bias among health professionals. Discrimination has led to legal actions, which have not yielded consistent results and have not been fully resolved.

SOCIAL ASSESSMENT AND MEASUREMENT OF WEIGHT AND OBESITY

Physiological assessments used in practice and measurements used in research on obesity focus on body fat levels, assessing parameters such as body weight, skinfolds and other measures of fatness, waist-to-hip ratios to assess body fat distribution, weight history and fluctuations, and co-morbidity. By contrast, social assessments and measurements of obesity focus on the meaning, beliefs, knowledge, and attitudes about weight and obesity. Exhibit 12–2 presents a summary of selected questions and scales that may be used in the social assessment of weight. Questions about reported weight rather than measured weight measure people's awareness of their weight and congruence with actual weight. Assessments of perceived weight, desired weight, self-rated weight, or weight satisfaction capture their evaluation of their current weight. Ratings of silhouettes or photographs are also used in social assessments.[80,81] Social assessments of weight may go further in probing clients' weight satisfaction to include weight at important life transitions, and the ability to wear a particular size of clothing or a particular garment.[82]

Assessment of the social context of weight is crucial in evaluating a person's comfort level with their current weight and interest in participation in a weight management program.[83] The Institute of Medicine of the National Academy of

Exhibit 12–2 Social Assessments of Weight and Obesity

Questions about Social Aspects of Weight

Self-reported weight: How much do you weigh without shoes? How tall are you?

Weight history: How long have you been at this weight? How has your weight changed?

Usual weight: How much do you usually weigh?

Desired weight: How much would you like to weigh?

Reasonable weight: What weight do you think you could reasonably maintain for a year?

Desired change: Would you like to gain weight, lose weight, or stay the same?

Perceived weight: Do you think your weight is too high, too low, or about right?

Self-defined weight: How would you describe your weight?

Weight satisfaction: How satisfied are you with your weight?

Body satisfaction: How satisfied are you with your shape/body?

Clothing size: What size clothing do you wear now?

　What size clothing would you like to be able to wear?

　What sizes of clothing do you own that you want to wear again some day?

Questions about the Social Context of Weight

Demographics: Gender, age, generation, socioeconomic status (education, occupation, income), employment, ethnicity, marital status, household composition, parenthood, residence, region

What are your major social roles and responsibilities in life?

　How do you think your roles and responsibilities affect your weight?

What is going on in your life right now?

Is your weight a particular concern at this time?

　What are some of the reasons for your concern at this time?

Who are the people who are closest to you? How do they feel about your weight?

　How much would the people who are close to you like you to weigh/look?

What happened the last time you tried to lose/gain weight?

　What things that made it difficult? What things that made it work?

What are your hopes for how your life might change if you lost/gained weight?

　What would you expect would really happen if you lost/gained weight?

What kinds of personal resources do you have that would help you lose/gain weight?

Instruments to Assess Social Aspects of Weight

Obesity Knowledge Quiz (OKQ)	Price et al, 1985[109]
Knowledge about Obesity (KAO)	Harris 1983[110]
Attitudes Toward Obese Persons Scale (ATOP)	Allison et al, 1991[111]
Attitude Toward Weight Gain During Pregnancy (ATWGDP)	Palmer et al, 1985[112]
Beliefs about Obese Persons Scale (BAOP)	Allison et al, 1991[111]

continues

Exhibit 12–2 continued

Weight Locus of Control Scale (WLOC)	Saltzer, 1982[83]
Dieting Readiness Test (DRT)	Brownell, 1990[113]
Dietary Restraint Scale (DRS)	Herman & Polivy, 1984[114]
Obesity-Related Problems Scale (OP)	Sullivan et al, 1993[115]
Fat Phobia Scale (FPS)	Robinson et al, 1993[116]
Dating Obese Persons Scale (DOPS)	Sobal et al, 1995[31]
Anti-Fat Attitudes Scale (AFAS)	Crandall & Biernat, 1990[117]

Sciences has proposed criteria for assessing the fit between weight management programs and consumers of such programs,[84] including assessments of personal, situational, and cultural factors. Similar assessments of environmental, psychosocial, behavioral, temporal, and biomedical issues are proposed in other models for evaluating people for participation in weight management programs.[85]

Other important social assessments of weight include measurement of knowledge, attitudes, and beliefs about weight and weight change. Instruments that assess concepts from social science theories related to weight are available, such as assessments of Weight Locus of Control.[83] As shown in Exhibit 12–2 scales to measure dieting and dietary patterns associated with weight have also been developed. Finally, it is important to assess the problems associated with being obese, including stigmatization and discrimination, and instruments have been developed for doing so such as the Dating Obese Persons Scale and Anti-Fat Attitudes Scale (Exhibit 12–2).

As the importance of considering social aspects of weight becomes increasingly recognized, additional social assessments will undoubtedly be developed to add to the current inventory of measures and assessments. This chapter focuses on scales, questions, and other assessments specific to obesity. A range of other assessments and measures that deal with eating disorders and disordered eating[86] may also be relevant.

SOCIAL INTERVENTIONS AND OBESITY

Interventions for obesity have been classified in many ways. Some are almost purely biomedical, such as the administration of drugs and the performance of surgery. Most, however, involve changing eating and activity behaviors. Such behavior changes are explicitly or implicitly grounded in one or more social science theories. It is important to consider theories underlying interventions because the theory drives the implementation of interventions. This section presents several major approaches to weight management interventions and the social science theories that underlie them.

Behaviorist theory approaches weight change and maintenance through behavioral learning based on the work of psychologists such as B.F. Skinner. Since the landmark work of Stuart,[87] behavior modification in either its pure form or some adaptation has been a key ingredient of many weight loss interventions.[88] Behaviorism assumes that specific eating and activity behaviors are learned through operant (or less often classical) conditioning that involves shaping behavior using rewards and punishments. Changing eating or activity behaviors occurs as further conditioning reshapes behavior patterns.

Cognitive theories have been applied in weight loss interventions. Psychodynamic theory has not been successful in dealing with obesity. More recent cognitive approaches have assumed that the way people conceptualize and think about eating and activity is important in maintaining and changing those behaviors. Cognitive restructuring is often incorporated into behavioral programs to assist people in reframing the way they deal with food and eating. Cognitive work seeks to overcome self-defeating thoughts and cope with maladaptive beliefs.[89]

A wide variety of social psychological theories focus on how a person's knowledge, attitudes, beliefs, and perceptions operate to shape eating, activity, and weight patterns.[55] The Health Belief Model focuses on perceived susceptibility and severity of health threats from obesity that are involved in weight management.[90] The Theory of Reasoned Action (which has been expanded into the Theory of Planned Behavior) considers how people rationally evaluate their attitudes and subjective perceptions of social norms to influence their intent to engage in weight-related behaviors.[91] Social Learning Theory considers how concept of self leads one to make weight-related decisions based on an internal locus of control oriented toward self-control or external locus of control oriented toward chance or the influence of powerful others.[83,92] Social Cognitive Theory proposes that behavior, cognition, and the environment interact as people develop outcome expectations and efficacy expectations that lead them to engage in behaviors related to body weight.[93,94] The Transtheoretical model suggests that people can be classified according to their stage of readiness to engage in weight-related behaviors.[95]

Social support theories approach weight as an aspect of social relationships. This assumes that individuals' behaviors are shaped by their interactions with others, and that those relationships are involved in body weight levels. The psychological concept of social facilitation as well as sociological theory about social networks have been incorporated into eating and activity interventions that enlist significant others to assist in weight management. Weight loss programs for couples have been used in weight management,[96] and other aspects of social support have been incorporated into weight management programs.[97,98]

Family systems theory suggests that individual behaviors are integrated parts of larger family systems. The body weight of individuals is seen as playing a role in the person's family dynamics, and failure to consider the function of an obese person in the family context is seen as a crucial omission in conceptualizing weight management.[78] This perspective may be more useful in predicting consequences of weight changes than behavior changes involved in weight loss itself.[79]

Ecological theories suggest that eating, activity, and obesity are situated in larger community, societal, and cultural contexts, and that the dynamics of those contexts must be recognized and dealt with in weight management interventions. One way ecological theories have been used has been in worksite and community weight management programs, where the intervention attempted to change the food environment, activity levels, and values about weight of entire worksites and communities.[99] This approach suggests that obese individuals and behaviors that support obesity are embedded within larger social units, and that by changing the context, the weight of the individuals also would change.

Theories about social structure and social processes underlie public policy approaches to weight management. Providing communities with institutional and organizational structures changes their capacity to deal with weight issues and provides opportunities for individuals in the community. Examples of changes in public policy that support weight management include insurance coverage for nutrition education and counseling and membership in fitness clubs, community standards for food service and physical activity in schools, and community funding of safe walking trails and bicycle paths.

The focus on social aspects of weight such as the quality of life and stigmatization has led to efforts that entirely reject weight loss and encourage size acceptance in conjunction with a healthy lifestyle.[9,100] Avoidance of restrained eating (through dieting) because it may itself lead to binging and weight gain[101] has led to non-dieting approaches as an alternative to standard strategies of dieting and behavior modification.[102]

Many other theoretical approaches from the social sciences are applicable to body weight. The number of theories is large, their applications are varied, and there is insufficient space to review them all here. However, it is essential to examine the theoretical assumptions that are made about weight by a particular program or strategy. The way the problem is conceptualized will determine what is assessed, which (if any) interventions are chosen, and how the interventions are implemented. Clear assessment of specific situations and clear specification of assumptions and theoretical approaches should lead to better choices regarding weight management in the future.

Historically, efforts to design weight management interventions have focused on biomedical assessments of degree of obesity and degree of medical risk. Future activities in this area will benefit from assessing personal desire to lose weight, the biological, social, and psychological risks and benefits of intervention, and individual, social, and environmental resources that will increase choices for a positive experience and outcome.

CONCLUSION

This chapter reviews social science aspects of obesity, considering how social factors operate as causes and consequences, and how those who deal with weight issues can consider social factors in assessments and interventions. Physiological factors such as genetics, endocrinology, and metabolism are essential to consider as determinants of obesity, and the energy-balance behaviors of eating and activity levels must be examined in explanations of how people become obese and maintain their weight. However, examination of the social causes of obesity, the social prevalence and patterns of obesity, the meaning of obesity, and the experiences of obese individuals requires the use of social science perspectives.

Comprehensive analysis of weight must consider social influences and social effects, and professionals who deal with weight management can benefit from conducting social assessments and being clear about the social theories underlying their interventions (Figure 12–1). The social sciences offer powerful conceptual and methodological tools for extending current work on obesity that offer insights that are not available when only biomedical perspectives are used. As biological science advances and more is understood about the physiology of obesity, new psychological, social, cultural, and ethical questions related to obesity will emerge. Social concepts and analyses will be needed to address these emerging issues.

The population of the world is getting fatter, with the average weight of most populations increasing and the number of obese people rising in both developed and developing countries.[103] Simultaneously, ideals about body weight are increasingly emphasizing slimness while rejecting obese individuals and subjecting them to stigmatization and discrimination.[9] Medical and commercial weight loss interventions are increasing as the multibillion dollar weight loss industry grows and spreads worldwide. However, success of weight loss interventions is low and weight loss is rarely maintained.[104–108] Strategies for dealing with weight have focused on biomedical approaches and may benefit from the inclusion of social science perspectives.

REFERENCES

1. Stunkard AJ. The social environment and the control of obesity. In: Stunkard AJ, ed. *Obesity.* Philadelphia: WB Saunders; 1980:438–462.
2. Sobal J. Social influences on body weight. In: Brownell KD, Fairburn CG, eds. *Comprehensive Handbook of Eating Disorders and Obesity.* New York: Guilford Press; 1995:73–77.
3. Brown PJ. Cultural perspectives on the etiology and treatment of obesity. In: Stunkard AJ, Wadden TA, eds. *Obesity: Theory and Therapy.* New York: Raven Press; 1993:163–178.
4. Seid RP. *Never Too Thin.* New York: Prentice Hall; 1989.
5. Garner DM, Garfinkel PE, Schwartz D, Thompson M. Cultural expectations of thinness in women. *Psychol Rep.* 1980;47:483–491.

6. Wiseman C, Gray JJ, Mosimann JE, Ahrens AH. Cultural expectations of thinness in women: an update. *Int J Eating Dis.* 1992;11:85–89.

7. Kuczmarski RJ. Prevalence of overweight and weight gain in the United States. *Am J Clin Nutr.* 1992;55:495S–502S.

8. Kuczmarski RJ, Flegal KM, Campbell SM, Johnson CL. Increasing prevalence of overweight among US adults: The National Health and Nutrition Examination Surveys 1960 to 1991. *JAMA.* 1994;272:205–211.

9. Sobal J. The medicalization and demedicalization of obesity. In: Maurer D, Sobal J, eds. *Eating Agendas: Food and Nutrition as Social Problems.* London: Aldine de Gruyter; 1995:67–90.

10. Engel GL. The need for a new medical model: a challenge for biomedicine. *Science.* 1977;196:129–136.

11. Engel GL. The clinical application of the biopsychosocial model. *Am J Psychiatry.* 1980;137:535–544.

12. Williamson DF, Kahn HS, Remington PL, Anda RF. The 10-year incidence of overweight and major weight gain in US adults. *Arch Intern Med.* 1990;150:665–672.

13. Devine C, Olson C. Women's dietary prevention motives: life stage influences. *J Nutr Ed.* 1991;23:269–274.

14. Hayes D, Ross CE. Concern with appearance, health beliefs, and eating habits. *J Health Soc Behav.* 1987;28:120–130.

15. Rodin JL, Silberstein L, Streigel-Moore R. Women and weight: a normative discontent. In: *Nebraska Symposium on Motivation.* Lincoln: University of Nebraska Press; 1984:267–307.

16. Pliner P, Chaiken S, Flett GL. Gender differences in concern with body weight and physical appearance over the life span. *Personality Soc Psychol Bull.* 1990;16:262–273.

17. Kumanyika S. Special issues regarding obesity in minority populations. *Ann Intern Med.* 1993;119:650–654.

18. Kumanyika S. Obesity in black women. *Epidemiol Rev.* 1987;9:31–50.

19. Pawson IG, Martorell R, Mendoza FE. Prevalence of overweight and obesity in US Hispanic populations. *Am J Clin Nutr.* 1991;53:1522S–1528S.

20. Stunkard AJ. Environment and obesity: recent advances in our understanding of the regulation of food intake in man. *Fed Proc.* 1968;27:1367–1373.

21. Sobal J, Stunkard AJ. Socioeconomic status and obesity: a review of the literature. *Psychol Bull.* 1989;105:260–275.

22. Sobal J. Obesity and socioeconomic status: a framework for examining relationships between physical and social variables. *Med Anthropol.* 1991;13:231–247.

23. Flegal KM, Harlan WR, Landis JR. Secular trends in body mass index and skinfold thickness with socioeconomic factors in young adult women. *Am J Clin Nutr.* 1988;48:535–543.

24. Verbrugge LM. Women's sex roles and health. In: Berman PW, Ramsey ER, eds. *Women: A Developmental Perspective.* Washington, DC: Government Printing Office; 1982:49–78. NIH Pub. No. 82-2298.

25. Sobal J, Rauschenbach B, Frongillo E. Marital status, fatness, and obesity. *Soc Sci Med.* 1992;35:915–923.

26. Davis MA, Murphy SP, Neuhaus JM, Lien D. Living arrangements and dietary quality of older US adults. *J Am Diet Assoc.* 1990;90:1667–1672.

27. McIntosh WA, Shifflett PA, Picou JS. Social support, stressful events, strain, dietary intake and the elderly. *Med Care.* 1989;27:140–153.

28. Gerrior SA, Guthrie JF, Fox JJ, Lutz SM, Keane TP, Bastiotis PP. Differences in dietary quality of adults living in single versus multiperson households. *J Nutr Ed.* 1995;27:113–119.

29. Sobal J. Marriage, obesity and dieting. *Marriage Fam Rev.* 1984;7:115–139.

30. Gortmaker SL, Must A, Perrin JM, Sobol AM, Dietz WH. Social and economic consequences of overweight in adolescence and young adulthood. *N Engl J Med.* 1993;329:1008–1012.

31. Sobal J, Nicolopoulos V, Lee J. Attitudes about weight and dating among secondary school students. *Int J Obes.* 1995;19:376–381.

32. Kallen DK, Sussman MB, eds. *Obesity and the Family.* New York: Haworth Press; 1984.

33. Craig PL, Truswell AS. Dynamics of food habits of newly married couples: weight and exercise patterns. *Aust J Nutr Diet.* 1990;47:42–46.

34. Institute of Medicine, National Academy of Sciences. *Nutrition During Pregnancy.* Washington, DC: National Academy Press; 1990:9.

35. Smith DE, Lewis CE, Caveny JL, Perkins LL, Burke GL, Bild GL. Longitudinal changes in adiposity associated with pregnancy. *JAMA.* 1994;271:1747–1751.

36. Keppel KG, Taffel SM. Pregnancy-related weight gain and retention: implications of the 1990 Institute of Medicine guidelines. *Am J Public Health.* 1993;83:1100–1103.

37. Williamson DF, Madans J, Pamuk E, Flegal KM, Kendrick JS, Serdula MK. A prospective study of childbearing and 10-year weight gain in US white women 25 to 45 years of age. *Int J Obes.* 1994;18:561–569.

38. Devine CM, Olson CM. Women's perceptions about the way social roles promote or constrain personal nutrition care. *Women Health.* 1992;19:79–95.

39. Nichter M, Nichter M. Hype and weight. *Med Anthropol.* 1991;13:249–284.

40. Sobal J, Troiano R, Frongillo E. Rural-urban differences in obesity. *Rural Sociology* 1996;61:289–305.

41. Piani AL, Schoenborn CA. Health promotion and disease prevention: United States, 1990. *Vital Health Stat.* 1993;10:1–88.

42. Prevalence of overweight—Behavioral Risk Factor Surveillance System, 1987. *Mortal Morbid Weekly Rep.* 1987;38:421–423.

43. Pi-Sunyer FX. Medical hazards of obesity. *Ann Intern Med.* 1993;119:655–660.

44. Stunkard AJ, Sobal J. Psychosocial consequences of obesity. In: Brownell KD, Fairburn CG, eds. *Comprehensive Handbook of Eating Disorders and Obesity.* New York: Guilford Press; 1995:417–421.

45. Wadden TA, Stunkard AJ. Social and psychological consequences of obesity. *Ann Intern Med.* 1985;103:1062–1067.

46. Leon GR, Roth L. Obesity: psychological causes, correlations, and speculations. *Psychol Bull.* 1977;84:117–139.

47. Istvan J, Zavela K, Weidner G. Body weight and psychological distress in HNANES I. *Int J Obes.* 1992;16:999–1003.

48. DiPietro L, Anda RF, Williamson DF, Stunkard AJ. Depressive symptoms and weight change in a national cohort of adults. *Int J Obes.* 1992;16:745–753.

49. Ross CE. Overweight and depression. *J Health Soc Behav.* 1994;35:63–78.

50. Stunkard AJ, Rush J. Dieting and depression reexamined: a critical review of untoward responses during weight reduction for obesity. *Ann Intern Med.* 1974;81:526–533.

51. Wadden TA, Stunkard AJ, Smoller JW. Dieting and depression: a methodological study. *J Consult Clin Psychol.* 1986;54:869–871.

52. Wadden TA, Stunkard AJ, Liebschutz J. Three-year follow-up of the treatment of obesity by very low calorie diet, behavior therapy and their combination. *J Consult Clin Psychol.* 1988;56:925–928.

53. Smoller JW, Wadden TA, Stunkard AJ. Dieting and depression: a critical review. *J Psychosom Res.* 1987;31:429–440.

54. French SA, Jeffery RW. Consequences of dieting to lose weight: effects on physical and mental health. *Health Psychol.* 1994;13:195–212.

55. Parham ES. Nutrition education research in weight management among adults. *J Nutr Ed.* 1993;25:258–268.

56. Wadden TA, Stunkard AJ. Psychosocial consequences of obesity and dieting: research and clinical findings. In: Wadden TA, Stunkard AJ, eds. *Obesity: Theory and Therapy.* 2nd ed. New York: Raven Press; 1993:163–177.

57. Polivy J, Heatherton TF, Herman CP. Self-esteem, restraint and eating behavior. *J Abnorm Psychol.* 1988;97:354–356.

58. Bandura A. *Social Foundations of Thought and Action: A Social Cognitive Theory.* Englewood Cliffs, NJ: Prentice-Hall; 1986:391.

59. Jeffery RW, Bjornson-Benson W, Rosenthal BS, Lindquist RA, Kurth CL, Johnson SL. Correlates of weight loss and its maintenance over two years of follow-up among middle-aged men. *Prev Med.* 1984;13:155–168.

60. Adams SO, Grady KE, Wolk CH, Mukaida C. Weight loss: a comparison of group and individual interventions. *J Am Diet Assoc.* 1986;86:485–490.

61. Allon N. The stigma of overweight in everyday life. In: Bray GA, ed. *Obesity in Perspective.* Vol 2, Part 2. Washington, DC: US Government Printing Office; 1973:83–102.

62. Weiner B, Perry RP, Magnusson J. An attributional analysis of reactions to stigmas. *J Pers Soc Psychol.* 1988;55:738–748.

63. Crocker J, Cornwall B, Major B. The stigma of overweight: affective consequences of attributional ambiguity. *J Pers Soc Psychol.* 1993;64:60–70.

64. Strauss CC, Smith K, Frame C, Forehand R. Personal and interpersonal characteristics associated with childhood obesity. *J Pediatr Psychol.* 1985;10:337–343.

65. Kuskowska-Wolk A, Rossner S. Decreased social activity in obese adults. In: Baba S, Zimmet P, eds. *World Data Book of Obesity.* New York: Elsevier Science; 1990:265–269.

66. Miller CT, Rothblum ED, Brand PA, Felicio DM. Do obese women have poorer social relationships than nonobese women? Reports by self, friends, and coworkers. *J Pers.* 1995;63:65–85.

67. Sobal J. Obesity and nutritional sociology: a model for coping with the stigma of obesity. *Clin Sociology Rev.* 1991;9:125–141.

68. Blumberg P, Mellis LP. Medical students' attitudes toward the obese and the morbidly obese. *Int J Eating Dis.* 1985;4:169–175.

69. Brotman AW, Stern TA, Herzog DB. Emotional reactions of house officers to patients with anorexia nervosa, diabetes, and obesity. *Int J Eating Dis.* 1984;3:71–77.

70. Maiman LA, Wang VL, Becker MH, Findlay J, Simonson M. Attitudes toward obesity and the obese among professionals. *J Am Diet Assoc.* 1979;74:331–336.

71. Adams CH, Smith NJ, Wilbur DC, Grady KE. The relationship of obesity to the frequency of pelvic examinations: do physician and patient attitudes make a difference? *Women Health.* 1993;20:45–57.

72. Young LM, Powell B. The effects of obesity on the clinical judgments of mental health professionals. *J Health Soc Behav.* 1985;26:233–246.

73. Wiese HJC, Wilson JF, Jones RA, Meises M. Obesity stigma reduction in medical students. *Int J Obes.* 1992;16:859–868.

74. Rothblum ED, Miller CT, Garbutt B. Stereotypes of obese female job applicants. *Int J Eating Dis.* 1988;7:277–283.

75. McEvoy SA. Fat chance: employment discrimination against the overweight. *Labor Law J.* 1992;43:3–14.

76. Baker JO. The Rehabilitation Act of 1973: protection for victims of weight discrimination? *UCLA Law Rev.* 1982;29:947–971.

77. Hafer RJ. Morbid obesity: effects on the marital system of weight loss after gastric restriction. *Psychother Psychosom.* 1991;56:162–166.

78. Ganley RM. Epistemology, family patterns and psychosomatics: the case of obesity. *Fam Process.* 1986;25:347–351.

79. Sobal J, Rauschenbach B, Frongillo E. Obesity and marital quality: analysis of weight, marital unhappiness, and marital problems in a US national sample. *J Fam Issues.* 1995;16:746–764.

80. Massara EB, Stunkard AJ. A method of quantifying cultural ideals of beauty and the obese. *Int J Obes.* 1979;3:149–152.

81. Stunkard AJ, Sorenson TI, Schulsinger F. Use of the Danish adoption register for the study of obesity and thinness. In: Kety S, Rowland L, Sidman R, Mathysse S, eds. *Genetics of Neurological and Psychiatric Disorders.* New York: Raven Press; 1983:115–120.

82. Foster GD. Reasonable weights: determinants, definitions, and directions. In Pi Sunyer FX, Allison DB, eds. *Obesity Treatment: Establishing Goals, Improving Outcomes, and Reviewing the Research Agenda.* New York: Plenum Press; 1995:35–44.

83. Saltzer EB. The weight locus of control (WLOC) scale: a specific measure of obesity research. *J Pers Assess.* 1982;46:620–28.

84. Institute of Medicine, National Academy of Sciences. *Weighing the Options, Criteria for Evaluating Weight-Management Programs.* Washington, DC: National Academy Press; 1995:6.

85. Wadden TA, Foster GD. Behavioral assessment and treatment of markedly obese patients. In: Wadden TA, VanItallie TB, eds. *Treatment of the Severely Obese Patient.* New York: Guilford; 1992:290–307.

86. Allison DB, ed. *Handbook of Assessment Methods for Eating Behaviors and Weight Related Problems.* Thousand Oaks, CA: Sage; 1995.

87. Stuart RB. Behavioral control of overeating. *Behav Res Ther.* 1967;9:177–186.

88. Brownell KD, Wadden TA. Behavior therapy for obesity: modern approaches and better results. In: Brownell KD, Foreyt JP, eds. *Handbook of Eating Disorders: Physiology, Psychology, and Treatment of Obesity, Anorexia, and Bulimia.* New York: Basic Books; 1986;180–197.

89. Collins RL, Rothblum ED, Wilson GT. The comparative efficacy of cognitive and behavioral approaches to the treatment of obesity. *Cognit Ther Res.* 1986;10:299–317.

90. O'Connell JK, Price JH, Roberts SM, Jurs SG, McKinley R. Utilizing the health belief model to predict dieting and exercising behavior of obese and nonobese adolescents. *Health Ed Q.* 1985;12:343–351.

91. Sejwacz D, Ajzen I, Fishbein M. Predicting and understanding weight loss: intentions, behaviors, and outcomes. In: Ajzen I, Fishbein M, eds. *Understanding Attitudes and Predicting Social Behavior.* Englewood Cliffs, NJ: Prentice-Hall, Inc; 1985:101–112.

92. Muhlenkamp AF, Nelson AM. Health locus of control, values, and weight reduction behavior. *J Psychosoc Nurs Ment Health Serv.* 1981;19:21–24.

93. Bernier N, Avard J. Self-efficacy, outcome and attrition in a weight reduction program. *Cognit Ther Res.* 1986;10:319–338.

94. Desmond SM, Price JH. Self-efficacy and weight control. *Health Educ.* 1988;19:12–18.

95. Prochaska JO, DiClemente CC. Common processes of self-change in smoking, weight control, and psychological distress. In: Shiffman S, Wills T, eds. *Coping and Substance Use.* Orlando, FL: Academic Press; 1985:345–363.

96. Black DR, Gleser LJ, Kooyers KJ. A meta-analytic evaluation of couples weight loss programs. *Health Psychol.* 1990;9:330–347.

97. Hoerr S, Kallen D, Kwantes M. Peer acceptance of obese youth: a way to improve weight control efforts? *Ecol Food Nutr.* 1995;33:203–213.

98. Parham ES. Enhancing social support in weight loss management groups. *J Am Diet Assoc.* 1993;93:1152–1156.

99. Taylor CB, Stunkard AJ. Public health approaches to weight control. In: Stunkard AJ, Wadden TA, eds. *Obesity: Theory and Therapy.* 2nd ed. New York: Raven Press; 1993:335–353.

100. Barron N, Lear BH. Ample opportunity for fat women. In: Brown LS, Rothblum ED, eds. *Overcoming Fear of Fat.* New York: Harrington Park Press; 1989:79–92.

101. Polivy J, Herman CP. Dieting and binging: a causal analysis. *Am Psychol.* 1985;40:193–201.

102. Polivy J, Herman CP. Undieting: a program to help people stop dieting. *Int J Eating Dis.* 1992;11:261–268.

103. Gurney MG, Gorstein J. The global prevalence of obesity: an initial review of the available data. *World Health Stat Q.* 1988;41:251–54.

104. Stunkard AJ, McLaren-Hume M. The result of treatment for obesity. *Arch Intern Med.* 1959;103:79–85.

105. Cogan JC, and Rothblum ED. Outcomes of weight loss programs. *Genet Soc Gen Psychol Monogr.* 1992;118:387–415.

106. Garner DM, Wooley SC. Confronting the failure of behavioral and dietary treatments for obesity. *Clin Psychol Rev.* 1991;11:729–780.

107. Wing RR, Jeffery RW. Outpatient treatments of obesity: a comparison of methodology and clinical results. *Int J Obes.* 1979;3:261–279.

108. Stuart RB, Mitchell C, Jensen J. Therapeutic options in the management of obesity. In: Prokop CK, Bradley LA, eds. *Medical Psychology: Contributions to Behavioral Medicine.* New York: Academic Press; 1981:321–353.

109. Price JR, O'Connell JR, Kukulka G. Development of a short obesity knowledge scale using four different response formats. *J Sch Health.* 1985;55:382–384.

110. Harris MB. Eating habits, restraint, knowledge, and attitudes toward obesity. *Int J Obes.* 1983;7:271–286.

111. Allison DB, Basile VC, Yuker HE. The measurement of attitudes and beliefs about obese persons. *Int J Eating Dis.* 1991;10:599–607.

112. Palmer JL, Jennings GE, Massey L. Development of an assessment form: attitude toward weight gain during pregnancy. *J Am Diet Assoc.* 1985;85:946–949.

113. Brownell KD. Dieting readiness. *Weight Control Digest.* 1990;1:5–10.

114. Herman CP, Polivy J. A boundary model for the regulation of eating. In Stunkard AJ, Stellar E, eds. *Eating and Its Disorders.* New York: Raven Press; 1984:141–156.

115. Sullivan M, Karlsson J, Sjostrom L, et al. Swedish obese subjects (SOS)—an intervention study of obesity. Baseline evaluation of health and psychosocial functioning in the first 1743 subjects examined. *Int J Obes.* 1993;17:503–512.

116. Robinson BE, Bacon JG, O'Reilly JO. Fat phobia: measuring, understanding, and changing anti-fat attitudes. *Int J Eating Dis.* 1993;14:467–480.

117. Crandall C, Biernat M. The ideology of anti-fat attitudes. *J Appl Psychol.* 1990;20:227–243.

CHAPTER 13

Weight Management: Framework for Changing Behavior

Janet K. Grommet

INTRODUCTION

Weight management, including both the prevention of overweight and the treatment of obesity, is perhaps the most talked-about public health issue today. The pursuit of efficacious interventions continues to be encumbered in part by the complex etiology of obesity, but despite this challenge, effective interventions have not yet been exhausted.

In this chapter, weight management interventions are predicated on behavioral changes that constitute a healthy lifestyle and potentially influence weight status. Behavioral change relevant to weight management is approached as a client-centered intervention. Behavioral change is framed as a dynamic variable by delineating the sequence of stages in implementing behavioral or lifestyle changes. Intervention strategies are keyed to specific stages of behavioral change to emphasize the idea that change involves both cognitive and affective strategies as well as more familiar action-oriented strategies. Thus, this chapter focuses on maximizing interventions relevant to prevention and treatment.

SETTING THE STAGE FOR INTERVENTION

Considering the Etiology of Obesity

Weight management, and particularly the treatment of obesity, is wrought with many dilemmas. Which came first: hyperinsulinemia or obesity? Or which came first: lack of physical activity or obesity? Or which came first: emotional depression or obesity? These "chicken or egg" scenarios represent the difficulties of causality and imply that if the causes of obesity are understood, then effective treatment modalities can be pursued. For example, if a lack of physical activity is indeed a cause of obesity, then a rational conclusion is that increased physical activity is an efficacious treatment strategy. This question is complicated by the multifactorial etiology of obesity. If hyperinsulinemia, lack of physical activity, and depression all potentially contribute to obesity, then this diversity of causal agents necessitates comprehensive, individualized treatment. For example, the diversity of metabolic components such as hyperinsulinemia, physiological components such as physical activity, and psychological components such as depression suggest a need for multidisciplinary assessment and treatment.

In addition to the difficulty of determining cause and effect and the problem of multifactorial etiology, a third question involves the interaction of causal agents. The hypothesized causal agents may be interdependent. For example, depression may exacerbate the lack of physical activity; or, the lack of physical activity may exacerbate depression. This interplay of complex, diverse, yet interrelated causal agents has made it difficult to effectively treat obesity.

However, many conditions are effectively managed if not cured, even without a knowledge of the intricacies of etiology. For example, the etiology of diabetes mellitus is not fully understood, but the condition can be effectively managed. Someday when the pathophysiology is further elucidated, improved management and even cure may be an option. Similarly, although obesity can be treated without a complete understanding of its etiology, further clarification will undoubtedly enhance treatment.

Redirecting the Focus of Weight Management

Although obesity can be treated without a detailed understanding of its etiology, the efficacy of obesity treatment has been less than stellar.[1] This treatment record, however, is due not only to the unclear etiology but perhaps also to an inappropriate treatment emphasis. Often weight management, including the treatment of obesity, has focused on body weight rather than factors that might influence body weight. That is, the treatment has focused on the outcome rather than the means to the outcome. In diabetes treatment, this would be analogous to focusing exclusively on glucose control and not on the triad of dietary, physical activity, and pharmacological interventions that are a means of managing serum glucose.

In an attempt to refocus the treatment of obesity, some have proposed a "non-dieting" approach that minimizes the emphasis on body weight as well as the emphasis on caloric restriction.[2] Although this implies a liberation from restrictive dieting, the null descriptor of "non-dieting" fails to define the method of treatment. A new paradigm by Robinson et al[3] that focuses on healthy living provides a more apt description. Rather than defining treatment and success in terms of weight loss, this new paradigm focuses on health-related behaviors such as reducing fat intake and increasing physical activity. This reinforces the NIH Technology Assessment Conference Panel's proposal that treatment for obesity should "focus on approaches that can produce health benefits independently of weight loss."[4(p947)]

Another strength of this paradigm is that it recognizes that body weight is not totally under voluntary control. Weight is influenced by a variety of factors, some of which are modifiable and some of which are not. Modifiable factors include the quantity and quality of food; frequency, duration, and intensity of physical activity; and emotional state. These factors reflect a personal environment that an individual creates. Factors that are not modifiable include genetic factors that regulate hormonal and endocrine functions and thus influence appetite regulation, metabolic rate, and fat storage efficiency. The healthy lifestyle paradigm focuses on the modifiable factors. These factors may alter weight and improve health status.

Historically familial studies have suggested a genetic basis for obesity.[5] Recent research, however, has elucidated specific obesity genes and has contributed to a clearer understanding of the pathophysiology of obesity. This work in molecular biology has been a major breakthrough and pharmacological applications are now being pursued. Bouchard[6] estimates that of the multiplicity of factors affecting body weight, genetics accounts for 25% to 40% and environmental factors account for the remainder of the influence on body weight. (See Chapter 6.) Evidence of a genetic basis for obesity may relieve some of the stigma of obesity as the public begins to understand that excess body weight is not solely a result of "lack of willpower." Thus, the pursuit of genetic-based interventions could markedly enhance treatment outcome.

The majority of the influences on body weight derive, at least theoretically, from modifiable factors. The genetic factors probably provide a propensity but are not definitive. Krall and Dawson-Hughes[7] report, for instance, that lean body mass status is inherited. The accretion of body fat is non-genetic, although the distribution of this fat is thought to be influenced by heredity.[6] Thus, weight status results from the interaction of modifiable and non-modifiable factors. Focusing on modifiable factors, namely behavioral changes that constitute a healthy lifestyle, is appropriate to weight management in general, including both prevention and treatment.

CONCEPTS THAT GUIDE WEIGHT MANAGEMENT

Fostering Client-Centered Intervention

Based on the premise that weight management can proceed without a complete understanding of the etiology of obesity and that intervention has been appropriately redirected from body weight per se to a healthy lifestyle, current treatment presumably emphasizes lifestyle management drawing upon concepts from behavioral medicine. Historically, however, the professional treatment of obesity was reduced to physicians' diet orders and/or clinical nutritionists' calorie-controlled diets. These may be thermodynamically correct, numerical solutions, but tend to be authority-centered, meaning that these interventions originated predominantly with the authority or so-called expert.

Recent work in the realm of chronic disease management underscores the value of patient- or client-centered intervention in contrast to authority-centered intervention.[8] The objective is to empower the individual to be responsible for daily management. Since obesity is a condition that cannot be eradicated with one course of therapy, it is appropriately viewed as a chronic condition and the tenets of client-centered intervention are applicable.

Client-centered care is based on a collaborative relationship in which clients participate in exploring and clarifying their individual needs and in proposing solutions to the identified problems. Client-centered intervention thus encourages the individual to be an active participant in treatment rather than a passive recipient and thereby improves the prognosis for effective treatment. Reviewing a 1200 kcal diet with a client exemplifies an authority-centered intervention in that this promotes a passive role for the client. Encouraging the client to identify problem situations facilitates the individual's active participation: "So you seem to be saying that business luncheons are problematic for you. What options might there be for lower-fat luncheons?"

To date, much intervention work has been conducted under the rubric of behavior modification. Behaviorism contends that behavior is a learned response to specific antecedents and that positive consequences reinforce the behavior. As applied to weight management,[9] antecedents or stimuli to eating are identified to reduce the number of cues and to minimize the effect of cues on eating. Behavior modification emphasizes modifying or changing behaviors that presumably mediate weight status. This provides a more informed approach to treatment than the aforementioned numerical solution of a 1200 kcal diet. Behavior modification, however, offers a treatment plan but does not necessarily address how the plan will be implemented. Thus, in some settings, behavior modification has been a client-centered intervention whereas in other situations behavior modification has been authority-centered.

An individual, for example, may complete behaviorally oriented food records that elicit antecedent information such as time of eating, location of eating and with whom, physical position while eating, activity while eating, emotional state, and degree of hunger prior to eating as well as food type and quantity. This data could then be used to help the individual identify cues to eating, to explore ways to reduce the number of cues, and to explore non-food responses to the cues. The active involvement of the individual in identifying and exploring eating cues and in proposing other responses is indicative of client-centered intervention.

Alternatively, when the food record is presented as an assignment to be submitted to the professional for review, the behavior modification strategies become authority-centered. Furthermore, when the professional responds to the food records with a behavioral solution such as, "You will need to keep all your food in the kitchen behind cabinets to eliminate 'visual cues,' " the individual may or may not find this advice relevant. This is a behaviorally sound concept but unless it is based on the needs of the individual, the advice is a presumptive solution to an assumed problem. Behavior modification is the basis for a treatment plan, and the plan can encourage personal growth of the individual when the interaction is client-centered, or it can be delivered as a "bag of tricks" when the interaction is authority-centered.

A client-centered approach is relevant to working with an individual patient, a small group of clients, or in a community-wide intervention. Successfully identifying relevant needs improves the prognosis for change but other factors must also be addressed. A middle-aged executive, for example, may note that overeating at dinner is a problem and may recognize that this is a food response to the stress of the workday. A large, immediately satisfying dinner has served over the years to help this individual "unwind" from work. Having identified work-related stress as the stimuli, the individual determines that a non-food response would be more appropriate and plans to walk for 20 minutes after work to "unwind" and then to eat dinner in a more relaxed state when controlled portion sizes will be more achievable. Although this is a seemingly logical, personalized remedy, this solution still may not be implemented. Factors other than the context of client-centered interventions must be considered, namely when and how behavioral changes are made.

Clarifying the Process of Behavioral Change

Effective treatment of obesity presumes that the individual will need to change. Something, or some things, will need to change for the individual to attain a healthy lifestyle and lose weight; but behavioral changes relevant to managing weight are perhaps more complex than stimulus-response. Thus, the concept of behavioral "chains" attempts to address the complexity of behavior by acknowledging that behavior may result from a cascade of antecedents. And, in fact, intervening early in the cascade of events offers the individual more control than attempting to modify a behavior that results from a culmination of events.

Sequential Stages

Expanding this concept of behavior modification, however, may be useful to both prevention and treatment of obesity. For instance, rather than envisioning behavior as a reaction or even the result of a chain reaction, behavior may be viewed as the result of an intention.[10] Thus, in an attempt to understand how an individual initiates and sustains intentional behavioral changes, Prochaska and Norcross[11] elucidated a sequence of five steps or stages manifest in making a behavioral change. These stages include precontemplation, contemplation, preparation, action, and maintenance and are defined as follows[12]:

- **Precontemplation** is the stage in which an individual has no intention to change behavior in the foreseeable future. An individual in this stage is unaware or under-aware of a personal problem. Some individuals in this stage may deny the existence of a problem whereas others may be resistant to change.
- **Contemplation** is the stage in which an individual is aware that a problem exists and is seriously thinking about working on it, but the individual has not yet made a commitment to take action. An individual may remain in this stage for an extended period of time until ready to act.
- **Preparation** is a stage in which an individual commits to taking action and forms a behavioral goal. An individual in this stage intends to take action immediately and perhaps is already making small behavioral changes as a prelude to the next stage.
- **Action** is the stage in which an individual actively modifies behavior, experiences, or environment to resolve a problem. Action involves the most overt behavioral changes and requires considerable commitment of time and energy.
- **Maintenance** is the stage in which an individual works to prevent relapse and to consolidate the gains attained during the action stage, thus stabilizing the behavioral change.

This delineation of stages of change underscores the idea that that behavioral change is not an event but a process. Thus, many individuals in society may be contemplating or thinking about making a dietary change such as reducing fat intake; some individuals will move from contemplating this change to preparing, taking action, and maintaining the changed behavior. The stages of change are consistent with the old adage that "saying it" and "doing it" are two different things. "Saying it" corresponds to the contemplation and preparation stages. "Doing it" corresponds to the action and maintenance stages. Prochaska et al[13] report that these steps or stages are common to a host of health-related problems including weight control, high-fat diets, and exercise; and they provide evidence that the stages reflect the process of self-mediated as well as professionally assisted change. That is, individuals who lose weight on their own maneuver through the same sequence of stages as do individuals in organized treatment programs.

Sporny and Contento[14] reported that classification of individuals to specific stages of change also corresponded with fat intake. For instance, in examining individuals' interest in low-fat eating, individuals classified as being in the contemplation stage consumed significantly more fat than individuals classified as being in the action stage, i.e., 39% and 34% of calories, respectively. Individuals in the maintenance stage consumed the least amount of fat at 32% of calories.

Although Sporny and Contento's sample did not purposefully include overweight individuals, their work would seem relevant to weight management. They provide empirical evidence that the stage the individual is in within the behavioral change process affects nutrient intake.

Laforge et al[15] assessed individuals according to the stages of change model as a preliminary step in planning community-based interventions to promote increased fruit and vegetable consumption for the National Cancer Institute's Five-A-Day Campaign. The stages of change corresponded with fruit/vegetable consumption, with individuals in the initial stages consuming the least amount and those in the action and maintenance stages representing greater fruit/vegetable consumption. In a random sample of more than 400 individuals, the distribution of individuals across stages was as follows: precontemplation (38%), contemplation (29%), preparation (18%), action (2%), and maintenance (13%). Thus, prior to the intervention, two thirds of the population either had no intention of consuming five fruit/vegetable servings per day (i.e., precontemplation stage) or only expressed an intention to adopt the practice of eating five fruit/vegetable servings per day (i.e., contemplation stage). Far fewer individuals were in the latter stages of action or maintenance.

Greene et al[16] assigned individuals to stages of change based on the individual's interest in avoiding high-fat foods. In a random sample of more than 600 individuals, the distribution across stages was as follows: precontemplation (18%), contemplation (14%), preparation (8%), action (12%), and maintenance (48%). In this study, approximately one third of the individuals were classified in the early stages of precontemplation and contemplation compared with two thirds as reported by Laforge et al.[15] The difference in stage distribution in these cross-sectional studies by Laforge et al[15] and by Greene et al[16] may be attributed to differences in dietary habits related to fruit/vegetable consumption and fat intake. On the other hand, the absolute number is not as critical as is the point that in both studies a sizeable portion of the population was not ready to make behavioral changes. In fact, in both of these studies only a minority of the individuals were in the action stage. Consequently, assessing the needs of an individual, including their stage of change, may enhance treatment.

For example, enrollment in a weight management program does not verify that an individual is ready to take action. Indeed an individual may enroll in a program at the insistence of a significant other but personally be resistant to making changes (i.e., precontemplation stage). Or an individual may enroll in a program and be seriously thinking about making changes but not yet committed to making those changes (i.e., contemplation stage). Intervention programs such as behavior modification programs, however, tend to be action oriented; and thus individuals in the precontemplation and contemplation stages may derive limited benefit from treatment. The individual in the precontemplation stage may terminate treatment early by dropping out of treatment. The individual in the contemplation stage may experience modest weight loss. This seemingly modest progress, however, may mask the significant work that has ensued as this individual progressed from contemplation to preparation to action. Thus, focusing treatment primarily on the action stage not only underestimates the requisite work needed for changing behavior but may be appropriate only for a minority of individuals. As Laforge et al[15] note, action-oriented interventions may "underserve" or "misserve" a significant number of individuals.

Viewing behavioral change as a sequence of stages reinforces the idea that maintenance is a specific stage of change. Individuals who succumb to "going on a diet" and then "going off the diet" have difficulty sustaining weight loss since they generally view dieting as a short-term, remedial intervention. In contrast, when an individual is ready to act, the individual devotes time and energy to implementing behavioral changes. This constellation of changes related to food intake and physical activity constitutes a lifestyle, a long-term venture. Maintenance involves the consolidation of these changes so they become habit, not happenstance. Consequently, maintenance is an active stage and is not the absence of change.[17]

Spiral of Sequential Stages

A corollary to Prochaska and DiClemente's[17] work indicates that behavioral change is sequential but not necessarily linear as indicated by the concepts of precontemplation, contemplation, preparation, action, and maintenance.[11] Change is more appropriately depicted as a spiral pattern as shown in Figure 13–1 rather

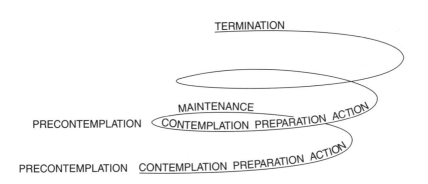

Figure 13–1 Spiral pattern of change. *Source*: From *Systems of Psychotherapy: A Transtheoretical Analysis*, by J.O. Prochaska and J.C. Norcross. Copyright © 1994, 1984, 1979, Brooks/Cole Publishing Company, Pacific Grove, CA 93959, a division of International Thomson Publishing Inc. By permission of the publisher.

than as a straight line, since change is not perfectly maintained. An individual, for example, may temporarily relapse and thus repeat some sequence of the stages.

Although relapse is often regarded as a negative event, depicting behavioral change as a spiral helps cast relapse in a positive light. The spiral pattern conveys that perfection is unrealistic and that relapse is to be expected. When relapse is expected as part of the change process, plans can be made to minimize the relapse. Furthermore, by examining the circumstances that precipitate relapse in the targeted behaviors, the individual can learn from relapse.[18] In essence, the spiral pattern of behavior change indicates that relapse can be a lapse in the change process but need not be a collapse of the process.

The now-classical study on recidivism and weight management by Schachter[19] initially met with surprise since the weight loss of individuals who lost weight on their own exceeded reports of individuals in organized treatment programs. In this study a remarkable 62.5% of the individuals with a history of obesity achieved weight loss, defined as weight loss ≥10% and current weight ≤10% overweight. Men, on the average, lost 39.1 lbs in 13.4 years and women lost 29.0 lbs in 8.3 years.

Inferences regarding the spiral of stages of change can be drawn from this work, since the weight loss was reportedly the result of one or many attempts to lose weight. Over time these individuals apparently managed to implement behavioral changes relevant to weight management (i.e., active stage) and eventually maintained the behaviors required to sustain the weight loss (i.e., maintenance stage). In the process, however, individuals quite probably relapsed to less favorable behaviors, perhaps re-entered the spiral of change at the contemplation stage, recommitted themselves to certain behavioral changes, and then progressed through the subsequent stages of action and maintenance.

This is in contrast to outcome evaluations in the literature that typically describe results of single, time-limited attempts to manage weight. Prochaska et al,[20] for instance, in specifically applying the stages of change model to individuals in a 10-week treatment program, noted that fewer individuals were in the contemplation stage at week five than at week one of the program. Conversely, more individuals were in the action stage at week five than at week one, suggesting that individuals were progressing through the process of change. However, according to Prochaska et al[20] a 10-week program was too brief an intervention for individuals to successfully negotiate the action stage and confidently enter maintenance. Thus, both the work of Schachter[19] and the work of Prochaska et al[20] suggest that effective weight management is consistent with a lifestyle rather than a time-limited action.

Coordinating Strategies and Stages

Envisioning behavioral change as a sequence of stages in a spiral pattern provides insight into the process of changing behavior. Yet a further challenge is to facilitate progress through the stages. Prochaska and Norcross[11] delineated the therapeutic strategies most effective in helping individuals move from one stage to another. In essence, those who successfully move through the stages of change invoke cognitive (thinking-related) and affective (feeling-related) strategies in the early stages and behavioral (action-oriented) strategies in the latter stages. Recognizing that strategies shift across the stages may contribute to improved treatment outcomes.

Precontemplation

Precontemplation would appear to be a difficult stage to influence since by definition individuals in this stage are unaware or under-aware of a problem and thus have no intention to change behavior. As precontemplators, these individuals are processing little information about the problem since they do not perceive the existence of a problem. Frequently practitioners presume that giving sufficient information to individuals will motivate them to act. For individuals in the precontemplation stage, however, the physician's articulate monologue regarding the health risks of obesity or the clinical nutritionist's soliloquy regarding fat content of animal products will have limited impact. Rather than inundating these individuals with facts, more useful strategies relate to "consciousness raising." Both cognitive and affective issues must be brought to the awareness of the individual in the precontemplation stage.

Prochaska et al[13] suggest that initial interventions be targeted toward emphasize acknowledging the benefits of changing. That is, acknowledging the benefits or pros of a healthy lifestyle may be more effective than describing pathophysiology. To make this personally relevant, the benefits may be directly tied to observations about the individual rather than generic benefits. Noting the benefits of a healthy lifestyle illustrates "consciousness raising" in that this is an attempt to bring thoughts regarding the problem to the individual's awareness.

"Consciousness raising" may also deal with affective issues. In fact, ignoring the individual's resistance to change or denial of a problem may serve to conspire with the individual's precontemplation. Such "game playing" is an ineffective intervention. Rather than colluding with the individual in precontemplation, the practitioner might gently acknowledge the individual's resistance or denial. This is a particularly critical strategy; and it is perhaps underused by many practitioners, such as physicians and clinical nutritionists, who are traditionally schooled in content-laden curricula and are perhaps more accustomed to examining the content of an issue than the affect.[21] Acknowledging the individual's resistance or denial may be effectively done by focusing on the "here and now." That is, the practitioner might focus on identifying the individual's present feeling to assist in bringing this affect to the individual's awareness. For example, "I appreciate your interest in losing 20 lbs, but you seem hesitant to identify some food changes that we might consider." This is an attempt to help the individual explore the resistance and thus facilitate movement from precontemplation to contemplation.

Verbal and non-verbal skills that enhance the practitioner's ability to facilitate behavioral or lifestyle changes are discussed in Chapter 14. Skills that enhance the practitioner's ability to understand problems from the client's perspective illustrate client-centered care. These skills include both content and affective responses that are germane to the "consciousness raising" strategies. The content and affective responses discussed in Chapter 14 assist the individual in "owning" the problem and thus moving from precontemplation to contemplation.

Contemplation

Individuals in the contemplation stage also benefit from both cognitive and affective "consciousness raising" since by definition they are aware of the problem but not yet committed to resolving it. Thus, the verbal skills of content and affective responses discussed in Chapter 14 are also relevant at this stage. These skills encourage the individual to continue working through the contemplation stage by encouraging the individual to explore further and thus clarify the problem behavior.

The cognitive focus in contemplation, however, differs from the focus in precontemplation. Prochaska et al[13] reported that once progress has occurred, effective intervention then targets decreasing barriers or obstacles to changing, whereas cognitive issues for precontemplators appropriately focused on increasing awareness via emphasis on the benefits of changing, this stage now addresses the barriers to making changes. Sporny and Contento[14] reported linear trends across the stages of change relative to several psychosocial variables. In their work, individuals' perception of the barriers to change tended to decrease as they moved through the stages. Thus, working collaboratively with the individual to identify and then minimize barriers to behavior change is a useful approach.

Focusing on affective issues continues to be paramount in this stage. As individuals become more aware of the problem from a cognitive or educational perspective as well as from an affective or emotional perspective, they are able to reevaluate the problem and themselves. The individual, in essence, calculates a personal cost/benefit analysis by comparing the costs and benefits of changing a targeted behavior. Prochaska and Norcross[11(p468)] note, "Movement from precontemplation to contemplation, and movement through the contemplation stage, involves increased use of cognitive, affective, and evaluative processes of change. To better prepare individuals for action, changes are required in how they think and feel about their problem behaviors and how they value their problematic lifestyles."

Preparation

Preparation is a transition stage and represents a shift from predominantly cognitive and affective strategies to behavioral strategies. D'Augelli et al[22] reported a similar sequence when noting that effective counseling addresses *understanding* and *action*. The initial emphasis on *understanding* helps the practitioner understand the problem from the individual's perspective and helps the individual explore and clarify the problem behavior. Work can then progress to focusing on *action*. This concept regarding effective intervention or counseling strategies can be succinctly presented as follows: counseling = understanding + action. The preparation stage serves as a juncture and the individual begins making small behavioral changes in this stage.

Action

Although the action stage is often approached prematurely by practitioners, this stage is perhaps the most familiar stage in the process of behavioral change. In this stage the individual is ready to modify behaviors. Thus, the cardinal strategies of behavioral intervention are now appropriate. To increase the prognosis for effective change, the individual must develop incremental goals that will guide the action. Danish and D'Augelli[23] recommend converting problem behaviors into positively stated goals to increase the prognosis for change. See Chapter 14 and Appendix 14–A on the goal setting process.

Kalodner and DeLucia[24] review behavioral strategies appropriate to the action stage of weight management including stimulus control, counterconditioning, and contingency management strategies. Stimulus control strategies are aimed at changing the antecedents to specific problem behaviors related to food and exercise. Counterconditioning strategies are designed to directly modify the problem behaviors by changing the response to stimuli, preferably by substituting healthy alternatives. Contingency management strategies attend to the consequences of the behavior and are designed to provide positive consequences to increase or reinforce the new behaviors. Self-monitoring of behavior is often a component of contingency management.

By definition the action stage involves the most overt changes. Prochaska and Norcross[11(p469)] note, "action is a particularly stressful stage of change. . . . Knowing that there is at least one person who cares and is committed to helping serves to ease some of the distress and dread of taking life-changing risks." Thus, social support in addition to active behavioral strategies is appropriate for this stage. Social support seems to have beneficial influence on the change process. Prochaska et al,[20] for instance, report that social support was the strongest pretreatment variable for predicting weight loss.

Social support, however, is often invoked inappropriately by practitioners, just as behavioral strategies are often invoked prematurely. Less-experienced practitioners may inappropriately invoke this strategy by suggesting that an individual bring a significant other to treatment sessions. For example, "Because your wife does most of the cooking for you, she should come to your next session." For an individual in precontemplation, the presence of the significant other may feel like coercion rather than support. Until the individual "owns" the problem, including others in the process because of their presumed support may be risky. Family members and friends may act as saboteurs rather than supporters. Thus, social support strategies are not as simplistic as "bring someone with you."

Parham[25] explores the association of social support and weight management to identify effective means of enhancing support. Social support in weight management generally refers to emotional or esteem support, as opposed to other forms of social support such as tangible aid (e.g., money) or information. Two basic strategies are available for enhancing social support in weight management: helping the individual to more effectively elicit support from others and improving the sources of support that significant others provide. Thus, both "give" and "take" aspects influence the quality of social support.

Maintenance

Maintenance builds on the positive changes of the action stage. As previously noted, maintenance is not the absence of change but the consolidation of the gains attained during the action stage. Prochaska and Norcross[11(p469)] note, "Perhaps most important is the sense that one is becoming more of the kind of person one wants to be." Thus, in the maintenance stage individuals continue to use active behavioral strategies and integrate these changes into daily living to reflect a healthy lifestyle. When these changes are valued by the individual and significant others, the changes are more likely to be sustained.

To determine behavioral differences, Kayman et al[26] interviewed overweight women who had regained after having lost weight (relapsers), normal-weight women who were formerly overweight (maintainers), and normal-weight women who had always achieved average weight (controls). Although the maintainers used numerous strategies to lose weight, each maintainer applied these strategies specifically to her own lifestyle thus reflecting the tenets of client-centered intervention. For example, few of the women successfully maintained weight loss via a package of strategies from a class or with the help of a physician or nutritionist, although these resources were available. Rather, the maintainers made decisions to lose weight, reminiscent of the commitment that characterizes the preparation stage, and then they devised personal weight loss plans to fit their lives.

These plans, reminiscent of the action stage, usually included regular activity or exercise and a new eating style of reduced fat, reduced sugar, and increased fruit and vegetable consumption resulting in fewer calories than previously consumed. The maintainers reported that they did not completely restrict favorite foods and made efforts to avoid feelings of deprivation while changing food patterns. Maintainers reported setting attainable goals so they could manage their personally devised weight loss plans. Some used ideas from earlier weight loss experiences, suggesting that they learned from relapse and re-entered the spiral of behavioral change. The maintainers persisted until new eating patterns were established, suggesting that they valued the attained behaviors; they were eventually able to de-emphasize food in their lives, suggesting that the strategies became integral components of their lifestyle.

In contrast, few of the relapsers reported exercising but reported having lost weight by taking appetite suppressants, fasting, or following restrictive diets, suggesting little commitment to making behavioral changes. While restricting food intake, they did not permit themselves the food they enjoyed; they focused on selecting special diet foods that were different from the foods the family consumed. Thus, the relapsers felt deprived on the restrictive diet and resorted to old behavior patterns. Many of the relapsers reported regaining weight in response to a negative life event that made preparing special food difficult. In essence, the relapsers focused on changing body weight rather than changing behaviors in accordance with a healthy lifestyle.

In comparing the maintainers and the relapsers, the behaviors of the maintainers depicted progression from preparation to action and ultimately to maintenance. The stages of change model, however, would suggest that the maintainers entered the spiral of change as a heterogeneous group with some initially in the precontemplation stage and others in the contemplation stage. Thus, in addition to the overt behavioral changes reported by Kayman et al,[26] many of the maintainers presumably prefaced these changes by engaging in cognitive and affective work that facilitated their commitment to change.

The experiences of the relapsers are instructive. In spite of the attempts to lose weight, individuals in this group will presumably re-cycle to the precontemplation stage because they appear unaware or under-aware of behavioral problems and thus have no intention of changing behaviorally. Although the tendency is to immediately focus such individuals on behavioral changes (actions), the stage of change model would suggest that intervention focus on "consciousness raising" strategies to address the resistance and/or denial of problems. These individuals need to move sequentially through the stages of change to make behavioral changes relevant to weight management. Therefore, initially exploring an individual's resistance to exercise may be therapeutically more useful, for example, than prescribing an exercise routine as this would support the individual in initiating the process of behavioral change.

CONCLUSION

The complex etiology involving both modifiable and non-modifiable factors undoubtedly encumbers prevention and treatment of obesity. Intervention as addressed in this chapter focuses on modifiable factors, namely behavioral changes that are consistent with a healthy lifestyle and potentially influence weight status.

To facilitate behavioral change, client-centered interventions are encouraged that empower the individual to be an active participant in the management of weight rather than a passive recipient of treatment. Behavioral change is postulated as a process, not an event, as commonly regarded. Stages of change in accordance with Prochaska and Norcross's[11] model provide a framework for the dynamics of behavioral change: precontemplation, contemplation, preparation, action, and maintenance. Studies suggest that a sizeable number of individuals present as precontemplator or contemplators, thus common action-oriented interventions such as behavior modification may underserve or misserve these individuals. Intervention strategies specifically keyed to the stages of change facilitate an individual's movement through the stages. Strategies relevant to the early stages emphasize cognitive and affective interventions (understanding) whereas later strategies focus on behavioral interventions (action).

Redirecting the focus of weight management from body weight to embracing a healthy lifestyle is both biologically and therapeutically sound. This refocusing may be followed by other refinements in intervention. For example, a change from authority-centered to client-centered intervention acknowledges that the client has expertise regarding the behavior to be changed since this is the context of the individual's life. Additionally, the traditional emphasis on action-oriented intervention needs to be reconsidered. The enhancement of interventions for weight management is perhaps not so dependent on developing further action strategies but rather on strategies related to the prelude to action (i.e., precontemplation and contemplation) and the postlude (i.e., maintenance). Thus, interventions related to weight management, although challenging, have not yet been exhausted.

ACKNOWLEDGMENT

This chapter was supported by a Faculty Research Grant from the Research Committee of the CW Post Campus of Long Island University, Brookville, NY.

REFERENCES

1. Garner D, Wooley S. Confronting the failure of behavioral and dietary treatments for obesity. *Clin Psychol Rev.* 1991;11:729–780.
2. Chiliska D. *Beyond Dieting—Psychoeducational Interventions for Chronically Obese Women: A Non-Dieting Approach.* New York: Brunner/Mazel, Inc; 1994.
3. Robinson JI, Hoerr SL, Petersmarck KA, Anderson JV. Redefining success in obesity intervention: the new paradigm. *J Am Diet Assoc.* 1995;95:422–423.
4. NIH Technology Assessment Conference Panel. Methods for voluntary weight loss and control. *Ann Intern Med.* 1992;116:942–949.
5. Stunkard AJ, Harris JR, Pedersen NL, McClearn GE. The body mass index of twins who have been reared apart. *JAMA.* 1990;322:1483–1487.

6. Bouchard C. Current understanding of the etiology of obesity: genetic and nongenetic factors. In: Bouchard C, ed. *The Genetics of Obesity*. Boca Raton, FL: CRC Press; 1994:223–233.

7. Krall E, Dawson-Hughes B. Soft tissue body composition: familial resemblance and independent influences on bone mineral density. *J Bone Miner Res*. 1995;10:1944–1950.

8. Silberman CE. Providing patient-centered care. *Health Manage Q*. 1992;14:12–16.

9. Ferguson JF. *Learning to Eat: Behavior Modification for Weight Control*. Palo Alto, CA: Bull Publishing; 1975.

10. Ajzen I. From intentions to actions: a theory of planned behavior. In: Kuhl J, Beckman J, eds. *Action Control: From Cognition to Behavior*. New York: Springer-Verlag; 1985:11–39.

11. Prochaska JO, Norcross JC. *Systems of Psychotherapy: A Transtheoretical Analysis*. 3rd ed. Pacific Grove, CA: Brooks/Cole Publishing Co; 1994:453–492.

12. Prochaska JO, DiClemente CC, Norcross JC. In search of how people change. *Am Psychol*. 1992; 47:1102–1114.

13. Prochaska JO, Velicer WF, Rossi JS, et al. Stages of change and decisional balance for 12 problem behaviors. *Health Psychol*. 1994; 13:39–46.

14. Sporny LA, Contento IR. Stages of change in dietary fat reduction: social psychological correlates. *J Nutr Ed*. 1995;27:191–199.

15. Laforge RG, Greene GW, Prochaska JO. Psychosocial factors influencing low fruit and vegetable consumption. *J Behav Med*. 1994;17:361–374.

16. Greene GW, Rossi SR, Reed GR, Willey C, Prochaska JO. Stages of change for reducing dietary fat to 30% of energy or less. *J Am Diet Assoc*. 1994;94:1105–1110.

17. Prochaska JO, DiClemente CC. Transtheoretical therapy: toward a more integrative model of change. *Psychother Theor Res Pract*. 1982;9:276–288.

18. Marlatt GA, Gordon JR, eds. *Relapse Prevention: Maintenance Strategies in the Treatment of Addictive Behaviors*. New York: Guilford Press; 1985:32–33.

19. Schachter S. Recidivism and self-cure of smoking and obesity. *Am Psychol*. 1982;37:436–444.

20. Prochaska JO, Norcross JC, Fowler JL, Follick MJ, Abram DB. Attendance and outcome in a work site weight control program: processes and stages of change as process and predictor variables. *Addict Behav*. 1992;17:35–45.

21. Grommet JK, Jemmott JM. Impact of low-calorie foods on nutrition education. In: Altschul AM, ed. *Low-Calorie Foods Handbook*. New York: Marcel Dekker, Inc; 1993:397–398.

22. D'Augelli AR, D'Augelli JF, Danish SJ. *Helping Others*. Monterey, CA: Brooks/Cole Publishing Co; 1981:9–10.

23. Danish SJ, D'Augelli AR. *Helping Skills II: Life Development Intervention*. New York: Human Sciences Press, Inc; 1983:9–35.

24. Kalodner CR, DeLucia JL. Components of effective weight loss program: theory, research, and practice. *J Counsel Dev*. 1990;68:427–433.

25. Parham ES. Enhancing social support in weight loss management groups. *J Am Diet Assoc*. 1993; 93:1152–1156.

26. Kayman S, Bruvold W, Stern JS. Maintenance and relapse after weight loss in women: behavioral aspects. *Am J Clin Nutr*. 1990;52:800–807.

CHAPTER 14

Practitioner Counseling Skills in Weight Management

Idamarie Laquatra
Steven J. Danish

INTRODUCTION

Helping clients develop strategies to deal with their eating patterns and physical activity is a major challenge for dietitians. As more information emerges about the change process, it has become clear that dietitians must possess knowledge and skills that stretch beyond a comprehensive understanding of nutrition.

Dietitians and all health professionals involved in weight management must be equipped with counseling skills.[1] Often drawn to the profession because of their desire to help others, health practitioners have a zeal for learning facts. The dietetics curriculum includes courses in nutrition, biochemistry, physiology, and diet therapy, but rarely do dietitians receive courses or training in counseling skills. Health professionals usually acquire their counseling skills on the job, by observing other professionals who may or may not have mastered the appropriate listening and behavior change approaches. Most courses in health care are presented in a lecture-type format, resulting in little experiential learning. While dietitians and other professionals may assume they can counsel, what they normally do is provide information.[2]

Seasoned dietitians react with surprise when they discover that the words they use are tools, just as dietary recall and food frequency lists are tools. They express relief when they learn a process that returns the responsibility for change to the client. They exhibit renewed enthusiasm for their jobs when they learn skills that help to individualize their approach to dietary problems. New entrants to the health professions usually have less "unlearning" to do, but they may face obstacles in the workplace if there is little support for incorporating counseling in weight management.

WHY WEIGHT MANAGEMENT PROFESSIONALS SHOULD LEARN COUNSELING SKILLS

Accepting the rationale for learning counseling skills requires acquiring knowledge about the change process and recognizing the growing movement to individualize nutrition therapy. The dietitian is the representative professional mentioned throughout this chapter, but the counseling skills and examples discussed are valuable for all health practitioners involved with weight management.

The Change Process

The stages of change model is useful in weight management. The model details five stages of behavior change: precontemplation, contemplation, preparation, action, and maintenance.[3] During the precontemplation stage, the client has no intention of changing and may even be unaware of the problem. Examples might include a client who is gaining weight but has not developed elevated blood lipids or blood pressure, or a woman whose bones are thinning but has not experienced a fracture or had a bone density test. The contemplation stage is marked by client awareness of the problem but no commitment to change. Perhaps the client knows he has high blood cholesterol, but has not decided to do anything about it. Clients in the preparation stage have made a commitment to change. Symptoms of disease can push clients into this stage. For example, shortness of breath and pain are frightening and can result in a commitment for change. In the action stage, clients undertake efforts to change and observe the results of some of their efforts. Reducing saturated fat or adjusting insulin to food intake represent change efforts in this stage. The maintenance stage involves stabilization of behaviors and developing skills to avoid or deal with relapses. Clients who lose weight face formidable obstacles during the maintenance phase; however, clients making any type of change will encounter challenges that can either strengthen or weaken maintenance efforts.

The strategies clients use in each stage of change differ.[4] During the precontemplation and contemplation stages, the client's awareness begins to increase. During the preparation stage, self-evaluation takes place in the process of building commitment. The action stage is filled with skills for behavior change, including setting goals, making decisions, weighing the risks vs the benefits of changing behaviors, and building support systems. Maintenance involves permanent incorporation of the change into the value and belief systems, and the development of strategies to prevent regression.

Clients may not be ready to take action during the initial session, yet the majority of strategies dietitians use (giving information, offering advice, developing a diet) are geared to clients ready to act.[4] When dietitians use these strategies with clients who are not ready to act, they often feel discouraged. They spend an enormous amount of time and energy instructing the client on what to eat and what not to eat, yet the client still does not change.

How can dietitians assess where clients are in the change process? Only by using effective listening skills that create a trusting atmosphere can dietitians evaluate the client's awareness and view of the problem. Research supports the idea that the quality of the interaction between the expert and client plays an important role in the change process. Good interactions increase satisfaction with counseling. Carl Rogers[5] described the core conditions of helping as empathy, genuineness, and unconditional positive regard. Empathy is the ability to perceive accurately the meaning and feelings of another person, and to communicate this understanding. Genuineness refers to the degree to which the counselor honestly communicates feelings toward the client. Unconditional positive regard, or warmth, is defined as the acceptance of the client without placing conditions on that acceptance. When the core conditions exist, the interaction that results between the expert and the client is of high quality.

Change vs Adherence

The adherence literature is filled with studies showing the lack of relationship between adherence and the characteristics of the client (age, gender, race, religion, education, marital status, family, ethnic background, socioeconomic status) and characteristics of the illness (acute vs chronic).[6–9]

Adherence has traditionally been defined as following advice, recommendations, or a prescribed regimen. Perhaps this view of adherence explains why levels of adherence to medical regimens and dietary regimens are so low. Clients usually use only those procedures that suit their lifestyle,[10] yet in the medical and nutrition professions, there is a long history of first determining what the best treatment is for a particular disease and then matching the client to that treatment.[11] Clients play a passive role until the time comes for implementing the behavior changes. Clients are expected to follow the recommendations (which they had no or little input in designing) to achieve results. In essence, dietitians have been taught to tell clients what to eat and what not to eat and clients must make the necessary changes to incorporate the information. Dean Ornish stated, "You can't feel free if someone is telling you to do something, even if it is supposedly for your own good. That goes back to Adam and Eve, when God said, 'Don't eat the apple.' We saw how effective that was— and that was God talking."[12] Research shows that successful weight loss maintainers are involved in developing their own strategies.[13,14]

The traditional definition of adherence also seems very narrow. Rather than focusing on adherence to a particular regimen, it is more positive and accurate to think in terms of the change process itself. Clients may only be able to make one small change at a time. While initially this may not have clinical impact, over time it can result in beneficial effects. Would a client making only the initial small steps be classified as nonadherent? According to the traditional definition of adherence, probably so.

Finally, adherence represents a lower motivational process. According to Kelman,[15] there are three levels of motivation: compliance (adherence), identification, and internalization. Compliance occurs when an individual participates in the program to gain rewards or avoid punishment (lose weight, reduce cholesterol, avoid a heart attack, etc.). The client performs the required behaviors to avoid a negative occurrence such as being admitted to the hospital. When the emergency passes so do the behaviors. Compliance rarely results in maintenance.

A higher-level process is identification. Clients adopt behaviors to obtain the approval of the dietitian or because they like or respect the dietition. Problems occur with maintenance when the dietitian no longer exerts an influence; that is, when clients finish the program and end contact with the dietitian.

The highest level of motivational process is internalization. This occurs when clients develop and adopt strategies for change because the rationale agrees with their value system. Because the change is intrinsically rewarding, clients are more likely to maintain use of the change strategies in diverse environments. The Modification of Diet in Renal Disease (MDRD) Study found that participants who maintained change were those who *liked* their eating patterns.[16] Interviews with individuals who lost at least 20 lbs and maintained the loss for a minimum of three years revealed their success was intimately tied to the decision to lose weight for themselves.[14]

The Individualization of Nutrition Therapy

A welcome change is under way in the nutrition community. In the treatment of diabetes and obesity, specific "one size fits all" diets are being abandoned in favor of individualized nutrition therapy. The approach to renal disease fosters the self-management approach. Furthermore, most clients, no matter what their diagnosis, prefer to be involved in planning their dietary strategies.[17]

In diabetes treatment, for example, there is no one diabetic or American Diabetes Association diet anymore. The Diabetes Control and Complications Trial demonstrated the benefits of blood glucose control and the effectiveness of individualized nutrition therapy in achieving glycemic goals.[18] The dietitian's role in diabetes treatment entails helping the client develop strategies for change in nutrition and exercise habits to improve metabolic control.[19,20]

The National Institutes of Health issued a conference statement evaluating methods for voluntary weight loss and control.[21] The panel found that for most weight loss methods, persons lose weight while participating in such programs, but after completing the program, they tend to regain weight over time. Additionally, the panel noted considerable diversity of response within each of the broad categories of weight loss strategies. Our interpretation of these findings is that giving a specific diet program to everyone does not work, and that there is no one "right" approach. Studies on maintenance of weight loss and detailed interviews with successful maintainers support this interpretation.[13,14]

The individualization of nutrition therapy requires more from the dietitian. The dietitian must know the effects of nutrition on the course of disease and use this knowledge as a framework during nutrition counseling. He or she must also integrate information from the client: What is the client's perception of the problem? What does the client want to do? Does the client feel it is important to change? Will changing behaviors be a priority? What obstacles hinder change?

THE COUNSELING PROCESS

Traditionally, dietitians learned specific dietary interventions for different disorders. Counseling in this context meant teaching the diet to the client. Dietitians have expressed a desire for more information and training in counseling.[22]

Danish[23] described counseling as a two-part process: (1) the development of rapport, empathy, and a trusting relationship; and (2) the implementation of behavior-change strategies. The goals of each part differ. The goal of establishing an effective helping relationship is to learn about the nature of the problems from the client's viewpoint and to promote self-exploration by the client. In the second part of counseling, the goal is to help clients design specific, realistic behavior-change strategies that are within their perceived capabilities and that are directed at their problems.

Obviously, the first part of counseling is the foundation for the second. A counselor cannot initiate treatment and expect clients to change their behaviors until an effective relationship is developed and the counselor has a clear understanding of the problem. Attending to the second part of the counseling process without the strong foundation afforded by the first part results in dealing with the problem as being separate from the client, or worse yet, providing solutions to the wrong problems. Behavior-change strategies designed under these circumstances are not likely to succeed.

The skills involved with the first part of counseling, developing a helping relationship, are packaged in a training program developed by Danish et al.[24] The program has been tested extensively and results in positive effects on clients, counselors, and the helping interaction. Dietitians and dietetic students have been successfully trained to use the skills in the program. In addition to increasing their repertoire of skills brought into the nutrition counseling session, the program encourages dietitians to develop a realistic philosophy about helping people change.

BUILDING THE FOUNDATION FOR BEHAVIOR CHANGE

Continuing Responses

The skills basic to the development of a high-quality interaction between the expert and the client are called "continuing responses." Continuing responses are the behaviors embodied in Rogers' construct of empathy.[5] Continuing responses are statements that summarize or reflect the content or feeling presented by the client. The purpose of continuing responses is to communicate a willingness to help, to encourage the client to continue talking, and to clarify the problem. These responses help dietitians understand exactly what the problem is from the client's perspective. Listed below are three examples, showing how dietitians can summarize, in their own words, the *content* of what the client has said.

Client: I can easily eat low-cholesterol, low-saturated-fat foods at home, but when I visit my relatives, it's hard. They constantly push rich foods on me. I hate to always say no because I don't want to hurt their feelings, especially when they've prepared something special for me. I usually end up eating foods I don't really want at all.

Continuing Response: You just don't have as much control over your behavior when you're visiting relatives as you do when you're at home because saying "no" is hard to do.

Client: It's impossible to follow my low-fat diet now that my kids are living with me. I used to do so well. Now, when I shop and buy them chips, I say to myself, "I won't eat this, it's for the kids." Once it's in the house, I end up eating it too.

Continuing Response: Sounds like your determination at the store melts once you bring the snacks home.

Client: I've lost 60 lbs since January, mostly by eating just one meal a day. Last week, I passed out in the lab and my boss sent me to the doctor. The doctor told me to eat small meals high in carbohydrates. I started to do that, but if I gain weight I'll just die. This is the first time I've ever been successful losing weight on my own.

Continuing Response: You're so determined to succeed that you're almost willing to jeopardize your health. It almost sounds like a fight between your health and your self-esteem.

When the client's statements are summarized, two things happen. First, clients better understand their beliefs. Second, the dietitian develops a better understanding of the problem and the situation surrounding the problem. When the dietitian focuses on the client's feelings, a better understanding of the client as a person occurs. To help clients design effective behavior-change strategies, an understanding of both the person and the problem is necessary. In fact, the key to building a foundation for behavior change is to understand how the client experiences the problem. The dietitian, then, must connect the person and the problem. To understand the client's feelings, the dietitian labels the feeling evident in the client's voice or in the client's words. There are two steps involved. First, the dietitian pinpoints the feeling or *affect* expressed by the client. Second, the feeling is put into a complete sentence. Examples of such responses follow:

Client: I can easily eat low-cholesterol, low-saturated-fat foods at home, but when I visit my relatives, it's hard. They constantly push rich foods on me. I hate to always say no because I don't want to hurt their feelings, especially when they've prepared something special for me. I usually end up eating foods I don't really want at all.

Continuing Response:

- Step 1: Client is feeling torn.
- Step 2: You feel torn because you want to control your eating, but you also don't want to disappoint your relatives.

Client: It's impossible to follow my low-fat diet now that my kids are living with me. I used to do so well. Now, when I shop and buy them chips, I say to myself, "I won't eat this, it's for the kids." Once it's in the house, I end up eating it too.

Continuing Response:

- Step 1: Client feels guilty.
- Step 2: Sounds as though you feel guilty about eating foods you know are high in fat.

Client: I've lost 60 lbs since January, mostly by eating just one meal a day. Last week, I passed out in the lab and my boss sent me to the doctor. The doctor told me to eat small meals high in carbohydrates. I started to do that, but if I gain weight I'll just die. This is the first time I've ever been successful losing weight on my own.

Continuing Response:

- Step 1: Client is afraid of regaining weight.
- Step 2: You're afraid that eating the small meals will make you regain the weight you've worked so hard to lose as well as lose the self-esteem you've worked so hard to gain.

Continuing responses may feel uncomfortable to use at first for a number of reasons. First, previous training in dietetics has conditioned dietitians to use what the clients say to vault into a discussion of the diet. The approach described here forces the health practitioner to listen and respond to the client's statements rather than interjecting information and advice. This approach results in greater client satisfaction with the nutrition counseling session, and improved understanding of the dietary problem and how it is being experienced by the client.

Second, another reason for the discomfort dietitians may feel when using continuing responses results from the decreased amount of talking they do when using these skills. During workshops we have conducted to teach this method, dietitians frequently say they feel most comfortable when they are in control and doing most of the talking during a dietary counseling session.[25] Of interest are the results of a study that showed that counselors who talked most of the time during a counseling session were seen as unhelpful, inattentive, and nonunderstanding.[26]

Third, some dietitians are afraid that using continuing responses puts them in the role of a psychologist. In fact, most of the help individuals receive with their problems comes from family, friends, and neighbors, not professionals. Dietitians are merely assuming the role of a health professional who is concerned about the welfare of their clients, not simply their stomachs or eating behaviors.

Finally, sometimes dietitians hesitate to use the skills because they fear they will say the wrong thing. There are no right or wrong continuing responses. If the response made is off target, the client will clarify. Recall that clarification is one of the purposes of using continuing responses. As with the development of any skill, practice smooths the rough edges and makes the skills come more naturally.

Think about the following questions:

- What is a continuing response?
- When do you think a continuing response would be appropriate?
- What type of continuing response would you make to the following clients?

Client: I really want to lose weight, but I just can't seem to do it on a permanent basis. I've tried a million diets, and I do lose weight, but I always go back to my old habits and regain what I lost plus more. I'm so tired of being fat.

Client: I dread the thought of having to eat out now that I have diabetes. How will I ever be able to choose what to eat? Restaurants don't prepare special food for people with diabetes.

Client: The doctor says I have high blood pressure and that I need to watch my sodium intake and my weight. I don't feel sick at all, so why should I bother changing what I do?

Taking More Control: Leading Responses

Leading responses shift the responsibility for the direction of the counseling session to the dietitian, who begins the process of trying to resolve the dietary problem. Note that the dietitian is responsible for the counseling session; the client is responsible for learning self-management. Dietitians most frequently use two leading responses: (1) questions and (2) advice. *Questions* are responses used to gather new information. There are three types of questions: (1) open, (2) closed, and (3) "why" questions. Open questions begin with the words "what" or "how," and usually cannot be answered with "yes," "no," or one or two words. Statements such as "tell me more about it" are considered open because they allow the client to explore freely. Closed questions can be answered with "yes," "no," or one or two words. They often begin with the following words: is, are, was, were, have, had, do, does, and did. Open questions are preferred to closed questions; however, it is recognized that there are times when closed questions are necessary. Unfortunately, dietitians, despite knowing better, tend to overuse closed questions and rely on them heavily during counseling sessions.[2,27] Note the difference between the open and closed questions below:

- Closed question: Were you able to stick to your diet this week?
  Open question: How did your eating plans go this week?
- Closed question: Do you understand?
  Open question: What questions do you have?

Recall that questions are used to gather *new* information. A common error is asking a question when the answer is already known, either because you do not know what else to say or because you are afraid to say the "wrong" thing. Before asking a question, practitioners should consider whether they already first know the answer. If so, the question should be rephrased into a continuing response. If this is done, the interaction will be both more effective and efficient.

The last type of question is a "why" question. "Why" questions should be avoided because they tend to put clients on the defensive. When dietitians ask "Why?," clients may feel they need to come up with an excuse. Worse still, the "why" question will not result in any additional information when the answer is "I don't know."

Think about the following questions:

- What is the purpose of asking questions?
- Think of your last counseling session. How often did you ask a question when you already knew the answer?
- What open questions can you use for the following client statements? How could you change the questions to a continuing response?

Client: This is the fourth time I've been admitted this year with my blood sugar out of control. You don't have to explain the exchange system to me. I know the diabetic diet inside and out. But knowing it and following it are two different things. Have you ever tried to follow a specific eating pattern each day? It's not easy, I can tell you that.

Client: Things seem so easy when we plan them in your office. Unfortunately, when I'm alone and I start thinking about food, I lose my determination, and the long-term benefit of managing weight or eating better seems to disappear. All I can think about is how fat I will feel if I eat.

Client: Watching the amount of saturated fat I eat is going to be difficult. I travel quite a bit and eat out most of the time. When I'm home, the easiest thing to do is to buy prepared food rather than making it myself.

In addition to questions, dietitians are also familiar with advice, another leading response. *Advice* is a response that provides a possible solution to a problem. Good advice may be about thoughts or acts not yet tried by the client. Good advice is also specific and realistic. Advice should not be given until the dietitian has a very clear idea about what the problem is, what solutions have already been tried, and what solutions should be tried. If advice is given too quickly, without exploration into alternatives previously tried and without an understanding of the problem, the client will counter the advice with "Yes, but . . . " When this happens the dietitian must return to better understanding the client through the use of continuing responses.

Client: I know I need to decrease the amount of soda I drink during the day, but I get so thirsty.

Advice: You might want to try to incorporate more water to quench your thirst.

Client: Yes, but I like the carbonation in the soda.

Advice: What about trying seltzer water?

Client: Yes, but I like something sweet.

Advice: Maybe you could switch to diet soda.

Client: Yes, I guess I could, but the diet sodas don't taste as good to me.

Obviously, the dietitian needs to stop giving advice until there is an understanding of both the problem and the person with the problem.

The Personal Side of Counseling: Self-Referent Responses

Dietitians can make the counseling session more personal by using "self-referent responses." Dietitians use self-referent responses when they express their own feelings to the client or talk about themselves. There are two types of self-referent responses: self-involving and self-disclosing responses.

Self-involving responses provide specific feedback to the client about the dietitian's feelings. The responses are a reaction to what the client said or did.

Client: I've been using these new herbs I saw advertised for weight loss.

Self-Involving Response: I'm concerned that you're using these products without first knowing about their safety and efficacy.

Client: I finally did it! I figured out that every time I feel overly stressed, I start to eat.

Self-Involving Response: It's great that you've been able to pinpoint that.

Client: How would you know what it's like to be overweight? I bet you never had a weight problem in your life. You're so thin.

Self-Involving Response: I'm upset that you've judged my abilities based on what I look like.

Self-disclosing responses give the client information or facts about the dietitian's background and/or previous experiences.

Client: I really seem to have a problem with eating after I get home from work. Even when I'm not terribly hungry, I end up just eating mindlessly.

Self-Disclosing Response: That used to happen to me, too. I found that I used food as a way to relax.

Client: I can't eat just one cookie. When there's a box of cookies, I start out eating one, then two, then the whole box. No other food does this to me!

Self-Disclosing Response: I have the same problem with chocolate-covered peanuts.

Client: I used to live in the Pittsburgh area, and I knew everyone in my neighborhood. Now, I feel so alone. My main entertainment is eating.

Self-Disclosing Response: I used to live in Pittsburgh, too. It's a tough adjustment when you move.

There are benefits and dangers to using both types of self-referent responses. Benefits of self-involving responses include: they can be used to gently confront clients about their behavior because they give specific feedback, and they provide a model for talking about feelings. Self-disclosing responses show the client that the dietitian is human, too, with a past or with likes and dislikes. They can move the counseling from an impersonal to a more personal level. On the negative side, both types of responses can shift the focus from the client to the dietitian. They may intimidate the client, make clients feel as though their problems are not unique, and they can waste time, especially when the client starts asking questions about the dietitian, turning the counseling session into a chat session.

Three questions can be asked to assess whether or not it is appropriate to use a self-referent response:

- What personal needs am I fulfilling by saying this?
- Do I know how the client will respond?
- How will my self-referent response affect the helping relationship?[24]

The responses we have described are not inclusive. Altogether, seven responses have been identified in the Helping Skills I Program as representing the domain of possible responses in a helping interaction.[24] These responses serve as the tools and foundation for building a helping relationship. Listed in Appendix 14–A is a Counselor Evaluation System. Dietitians can evaluate what they say and their understanding of the client by completing Part I and Part II. However, for one to help another, a problem-solving, behavior-change orientation must be established and implemented. The issue becomes, then, how to use these responses to facilitate behavior change.

A FRAMEWORK FOR BEHAVIORAL CHANGE

All too often, clients focus on the problems they are experiencing rather than on the positive outcomes they seek. Counselors, in turn, tend to dwell on these problems and inadequacies. Instead, the focus should be on encouraging personal development and individual strengths. The message communicated is that clients must take an active role in changing their lives and that counselors should teach clients to "take the reins" in their lives.

While the idea of taking an active role in one's life can be easily understood and accepted, it is not so easily accomplished. Many roadblocks stand in the way. For example, focus groups of clients who were trying to change food intake identified pressure from family members, social eating, eating out, and time constraints as obstacles that made changes difficult.[28] These roadblocks are not insurmountable, although they often seem so. Change occurs when people realize that the elimination of roadblocks is under their control, at least in many instances. Often new skills must be learned, new information acquired, or new risks taken. When clients learn how to set goals, they learn that they can approach their lives in an active way. This produces a sense of self-confidence and control. They also learn that the choices they make and the plans they carry out make a difference. Future problems can be handled in a more carefully planned, goal-oriented way. Indeed, such a self-directed person plans ahead to prevent future problems. Self-development then becomes a constant, active process instead of merely a reaction to a problem.

This framework is embodied in the second training program, Helping Skills II: Life Development Intervention.[29] Six skills are taught: (1) goal assessment, (2) knowledge acquisition, (3) decision making, (4) risk assessment, (5) creating social support, and (6) skill development. The program may be applied to the training of all helping professionals. It has been used in the training of dietitians on numerous occasions.[25] It is predicated on the assumption that dietitians work with *people* who have dietary problems, not just with dietary problems.

Goal Setting: An Essential First Step

Once health professionals have gained a clear indication of what the client's problem is through the use of continuing responses, they can help clients identify a goal by encouraging them to verbalize what they would like to do about the problem. Goal setting is a central strategy for encouraging clients to become more self-directed. Through goal assessment, counselors help clients identify, set, and attain goals by breaking down complex behavior changes into a series of small, successive steps. No other counseling approach specifically focuses on teaching clients how to set and reach goals. The positive goal orientation focuses on the strengths of the client. Because the client has the freedom to decide what the goals are and is active in the process of setting them, commitment to change is fostered. There are four parts to goal assessment: (1) goal identification, (2) goal importance assessment, (3) goal roadblock analysis, and (4) goal attainment. Part III of Appendix 14–A is a guide for the goal assessment process, which is explained below.

Goal Identification

The first step in goal assessment is goal identification. By goals, we are referring to actions undertaken to reach some desired end, not the end itself. Goals are different from results. Goals are actions over which the client has control. Clients often have only partial control or no control over results they want. For example, suppose a client has failed in previous attempts to lose weight. He may tell you he wants to lose 30 lbs and maintain the loss for a year. This is not a goal, but a result. Asking "What actions can you take?" helps clients focus on goals rather than results. The overweight client might set a goal to learn how to talk positively to himself and learn how to rebound from temporary setbacks. For a hypertensive client, a goal might be to design lower-sodium menus, whereas the result may be to lower blood pressure. Similarly, clients must set goals related to their own behavior and not the behavior of others. If a client states "I want my partner to stop buying cookies," recognize that the goal is for someone else, not the client. The likelihood of achieving such a goal is slim.

In addition to having control over their goals, clients must state their goals in positive terms and define their goals behaviorally. When goals are not positively stated, the focus is on the negative, and considerable energy is wasted trying not to do something. A positive goal is: "I will eat five servings of fruit and vegetables five days per week." A negative goal is: "I will not eat any ice cream." Negative goals may be converted into positive goals. For example, "I will eat one serving of ice cream one day per week." Setting a negative goal almost always produces a negative result. Negative goals bring to mind the "allowed" and "avoid" lists so prominent when using prescribed diets. When clients see how many items they must avoid, they feel defeated before starting, even if they rarely eat the foods on the "avoid" list. They soon become focused on what *not* to eat rather than on what *to* eat. Goal statements that include words like "not," "avoid," and "limit," should be changed into positive statements so that the image of the goal is something to be achieved and worked toward. Imagine two clients wanting to lose weight; one has the goal to plan meals using the Food Pyramid as a guide and the other has a goal to limit fats and sugars by not eating desserts. Both have the same general goal, but one is stated positively and the other negatively. The client with the positive goal has a positive image and a greater likelihood of success.

The goal should also be behaviorally stated or defined clearly. "I would like to control my night eating by eating less" does not include specific behaviors that indicate exactly what the client will do to achieve the goal. It is unclear what "control my night eating" means or what constitutes "less." Vague statements do not allow the client the satisfaction of truly knowing whether or not the goal has been attained. This lack of clear feedback usually results in frustration and often leads to "quitting." The more behaviorally oriented the goal, and the more clearly the goal is defined, the more likely it is that the goal will be achieved. It is the dietitian's task to help the client delineate exactly what will be done to achieve the goal. A rule of thumb when developing behaviorally stated goals is to answer the questions: What is the action to be taken? How many times will the action occur? When will the action occur? Under what conditions will the action take place? For example, "I will label a container of food for night eating only, four times per week at 9:00 PM when hungry."

Suppose that through the use of continuing responses, it established that a client who snacks heavily at night is truly hungry two hours after dinner, but the problem is a lack of planning what the snack will be. The client decides that controlling night eating means eating a planned snack. Eating the planned snack, then, becomes the action to be taken. The client believes that the snack can be eaten four evenings during the following week (how many times), at 9 PM (when), when he or she experiences hunger (under what conditions). The client's goal has therefore been transformed to something tangible: "Four evenings during the next week, I will eat a planned snack at 9 PM." The goal of "control" is thus converted to the goal of planning.

Goal Importance Assessment

The second element of the goal assessment process is goal importance assessment. Dietitians need to ask, "To whom is the goal most important?" If the goal is more important to the physician or dietitian than it is to the client, it is unlikely it will be achieved. Having clients set their own goals is critical because making dietary changes involves commitment and energy.

Unimportant goals are rarely, if ever, reached. Dietary goals often contain the words "should" or "ought to": "I should watch my weight"; "I really ought to start exercising." "Should" or "ought to" goals generally result in a lesser level of commitment than goals clients *want* to achieve. When clients set goals, dietitians can help them ascertain if the goal is a "should" or a "want." Dietitians can then either help clients change "should" goals to "want" goals or help clients identify "want" goals. When dietitians align themselves with the client's "wants," success is more likely.

Assessing the importance of the goal sets the responsibility for achieving the goal squarely on the shoulders of clients. Dietitians often express frustration and guilt when clients do not change. It is too often forgotten that the client has the ultimate responsibility for changing.

Goal Roadblock Analysis

Being able to set a goal is one thing; being able to reach or attain the goal is another. The third part of goal assessment is analysis of the obstacles or road-blocks that hamper goal achievement. Sometimes, no obstacle stands in the way of goal achievement, and dietitians can immediately help clients develop steps for reaching their goals as soon as a goal is identified. More often, roadblocks hinder goal attainment. A common reason for not reaching goals is "I just wasn't moti-vated." When clients identify a specific goal (goal identification) and determine that the goal is important to them (goal importance assessment), lack of motiva-tion is not the roadblock. There are four major roadblocks: a lack of knowledge, a lack of skill, the inability or fear of appropriate risk-taking, and lack of adequate social support.

A lack of knowledge means that clients are missing some information necessary to achieve the goal. Suppose the client who wanted to eat a planned snack did not know what foods to put together to make a nutritious, satisfying snack. The ob-stacle would therefore be a lack of knowledge.

When clients make dietary changes, the obstacle is frequently more than just a lack of knowledge. However, few practitioners use strategies other than information-giv-ing. The information-giving strategy is based on two tenuous assumptions: (1) if enough facts are communicated, clients will know what to do and behavior change will occur; and (2) if clients recognize that certain practices endanger their health, their behaviors will change.[30] Most of the time, these assumptions are simply not true. It is important to recognize that giving information is important, but only when there is a lack of knowledge that interferes with clients achieving their goals. Usually, how-ever, lack of information is only one of the obstacles preventing behavior change. Also, even when the obstacle is a lack of knowledge, the amount of information given must be carefully considered. Patient education studies have shown that within five minutes, patients forget half the information presented to them. Also, the more infor-mation given, the more is forgotten.[31]

Another roadblock is a lack of skill. Lack of skill can refer to either physical or mental skills. One can identify the roadblock as a skill deficiency when the client does not know "how to." For instance, the client may not know how to budget time to make the snack in advance, and would need help in learning some time manage-ment skills before achieving the goal. Other skills clients might need to be taught include becoming more assertive, making better decisions, learning to talk to themselves positively, and gaining self-control.

If the obstacle is an inability or fear of appropriate risk-taking, the client is *afraid* of something: afraid to fail because of past attempts at controlling intake, afraid to hurt another's feelings by turning down an invitation for food from a friend, or afraid the strategies will have negative consequences for family mem-bers. Helping clients assess the real risks involved gives them more power over the situation. If, after assessing the risk and finding that the costs outweigh the benefits of achieving the goal, clients may decide to abandon the goal. The health practitioner can help clients assess the risks and then help them to increase the benefits of an action and reduce the costs.

When clients lack social support, they must determine what support they need, who can provide them the support (and who cannot), and how to ask for the support. For example, not all spouses are supportive. Some may fear that their relationship will change for the worse if behaviors change. There are two types of support: *tangible* support such as doing the shopping or dishes for a partner, or *emotional* support such as listening to a partner's worries about whether he/she will be able to lose weight. More details on how to help clients attain knowledge, develop skills, assess risks, and find support are given in the Danish and D'Augelli program.[29]

Goal Attainment

If no obstacle stands in the way, dietitians can help clients specify exactly what steps they plan to take to achieve their goal. When clients identify one or more roadblocks, part of the intervention becomes removing the obstacle(s) so that the individual may work toward the goal. Removing the roadblock(s) may become a goal in itself. Much of what the intervention agent does is to teach or coach others, individually or in groups, to set goals, identify and overcome roadblocks, and reach their goals by developing new skills, acquiring new knowledge, learning to take risks, and developing effective support systems.

Attaining the goal involves developing a specific plan, a goal ladder, to reach the goal. A goal ladder breaks the goal down into achievable, small steps. Too often, individuals try to reach the goal all at once. If the goal can be broken down into a number of steps, between eight and ten, the likelihood of achieving it increases tremendously. A sample goal ladder for reaching a goal to eat planned snacks is shown in Appendix 14–B.

Once clients achieve the first goal, other goals can be set. Many times there are a number of small goals that must be achieved to reach an overall goal. For example, a person with a weight problem may set goals for controlling snacking behavior, starting an exercise program, eating at social events, identifying feelings, and dealing with boredom or anxiety.

Putting the Skills into Practice

One of the major reservations health professionals have against using the types of skills discussed in this chapter is a lack of time. Any new skill requires an initial time investment until it "fits"; that is, until using the skill is a natural part of counseling. Also, although time constraints are a very real issue, it is time for health professionals to reassess their roles and realize that they have much more to offer beyond giving information.

Anyone can give information, but not everyone can work with people to effect dietary change. How much time is wasted giving people information they already know or cannot easily digest? Clearly, the view of what constitutes nutrition counseling needs to be broadened. Part IV of the Counselor Evaluation System in Appendix 14–A and the following questions are presented with the hope that they will encourage dietitians and all health professionals to more critically evaluate their counseling sessions:

- During the counseling session, who did most of the talking?
- How did the client react to the continuing responses you used?
- Could you have changed any of the closed questions to open questions?
- Did the client answer with "Yes, but" when you gave advice?
- Did the focus stay on the client during the session?
- Did you give information selectively or not at all if the obstacle to goal achievement was not a lack of knowledge?

CONCLUSION

Changing behavior is not easy, especially dietary behaviors. Behavior change is not a very fast process. Helping clients set and achieve goals can be difficult but rewarding. If skills are used that encourage clients to make and maintain change, dietitians will truly be fulfilling their roles as dietary change agents. Counseling skills are vital to all health professionals in weight management.

REFERENCES

1. Licavoli L. Dietetics goes into therapy. *J Am Diet Assoc.* 1995;95:751–752.
2. Laquatra I. *Helping Skills for WIC Nutrition Education Counselors.* University Park, PA: The Pennsylvania State University; 1983. Dissertation.
3. Prochaska JO, DiClemente CC. Towards a comprehensive model of change In: Miller W, Heather N, eds. *Treating Addictive Behaviors.* New York: Plenum Press; 1986:3–27.
4. Green GW, Rossi SR, Reed GR, Willey C, Prochaska JO. Stages of change for reducing dietary fat to 30% of energy or less. *J Am Diet Assoc.* 1994;94:1105–1110.
5. Rogers CR. A theory of therapy, personality and interpersonal relationships, as developed in the client-centered framework. In: Koch S, ed. *Psychology: A Study of Science.* New York: McGraw-Hill Book Co; 1959; vol 3:184–256.
6. Milas NC, Nowalk MP, Akpele L, et al. Factors associated with adherence to the dietary protein intervention in the Modification of Diet in Renal Disease Study. *J Am Diet Assoc.* 1995;95:1295–1300.
7. Davis MS. Variations in patients' compliance with doctors' advice. An empirical analysis of patterns of communication. *Am J Public Health.* 1968;58:274–288.

8. Francis V, Korsch BM, Morris MJ. Gaps in doctor-patient communication. Patients' response to medical advice. *N Engl J Med.* 1969;280:535–540.

9. Haynes RB. Determinants of compliance. The disease and mechanics of treatment. In: Haynes RB, Taylor DW, Sackett DL, eds. *Compliance in Health Care.* Baltimore: The Johns Hopkins University Press; 1979:49–62.

10. Best JA, Bloch M. Compliance in the control of cigarette smoking. In: Haynes RB, Taylor DW, Sackett DL, eds. *Compliance in Health Care.* Baltimore: The Johns Hopkins University Press; 1979:202–222.

11. Institute of Medicine. *Weighing the Options.* Washington, DC: National Academy Press, 1995:94–95.

12. Ornish D. Changing life habits. In Moyers B. *Healing and the Mind.* New York: Doubleday; 1993:87–113.

13. Kayman S, Bruvold W, Stern JS. Maintenance and relapse after weight loss in women: behavioral aspects. *Am J Clin Nutr.* 1990;52:800–807.

14. Fletcher AM. *Thin for Life.* Shelburne, VT: Chapters Publishing Ltd; 1994.

15. Kelman, HC. Compliance, identification, and internalization: three processes of attitude change. In: Hinto BL, Reitz HJ, eds. *Groups and Organizations. Integrated Readings in the Analysis of Social Behavior.* Belmont, CA: Wadsworth Publishing Company Inc; 1971.

16. Coyne T, Olson M, Bradham K, Garcon M, Gregory P, Scherch L. Dietary satisfaction correlated with adherence in the Modification of Diet in Renal Disease Study. *J Am Diet Assoc.* 1995;95:1301–1306.

17. Trudeau E, Dube L. Moderators and determinants of satisfaction with diet counseling for patients consuming a therapeutic diet. *J Am Diet Assoc.* 1995;95:34–39.

18. American Dietetic Association. Nutrition recommendations and principles for people with diabetes mellitus. *J Am Diet Assoc.* 1994;94:504–506.

19. Monk A, Barry B, McClain K, Weaver T, Cooper N, Franz MJ. Practice guidelines for medical nutrition therapy provided by dietitians for persons with non-insulin-dependent diabetes mellitus. *J Am Diet Assoc.* 1995;95:999–1006.

20. Koehler AN, O'Leary LA, Kramer MK, Caggiula AW, Dorman JS. Dietary intake of patients with insulin-dependent diabetes mellitus compared with nutrition guidelines. *J Am Diet Assoc.* 1995;95:1317–1319.

21. National Institutes of Health Technology Assessment Conference Statement. *Methods for Voluntary Weight Loss and Control.* Bethesda, MD: Office of Medical Applications of Research, National Institutes of Health; March 30–April 1, 1992.

22. Whisenant SL, Smith BA. Eating disorders. Current nutrition therapy and perceived needs in dietetic education and research. *J Am Diet Assoc.* 1995;95:1109–1112.

23. Danish SJ. Developing helping relationships in dietetic counseling. *J Am Diet Assoc.* 1975; 67:107–110.

24. Danish SJ, D'Augelli AR, Hauer AL. *Helping Skills. A Basic Training Program.* 2nd ed. New York: Human Sciences Press; 1980.

25. Danish SJ, Lang D, Smiciklas-Wright H, Laquatra I. Nutrition counseling skills: continuing education for the dietitian. *Top Clin Nutr.* 1986;1:25–32.

26. Kleinke CL, Tully TB. Influence of talking level on perceptions of counselors. *J Couns Psychol.* 1979;26:23–29.

27. Danish SJ, Ginsberg MR, Terrell A, Hammond MI, Adams SO. The anatomy of a dietary counseling interview. *J Am Diet Assoc.* 1979;75:626–630.

28. Iszler J, Crockett S, Lytle L, et al. Formative evaluation for planning a nutrition intervention: results from focus groups. *J Nutr Ed.* 1995;27:127–132.

29. Danish SJ, D'Augelli AR. *Helping Skills II. Life Development Intervention.* New York: Human Sciences Press; 1983.

30. Henderson JB, Hall SM, Lipton HL. Changing self-destructive behaviors. In: Stone GC, Cohen F, Adler NE, et al, eds. *Health Psychology. A Handbook.* San Francisco: Jossey-Bass Publishers; 1979:141–160.

31. Green LW. Educational strategies to improve compliance with therapeutic and preventive regimens: the recent evidence. In: Haynes RB, Taylor DW, Sackett DL, eds. *Compliance in Health Care.* Baltimore: The Johns Hopkins University Press; 1979:157–173.

Appendix 14–A

Counselor Evaluation System*

PART I—EVALUATING WHAT YOU SAY

A. *Counselor's Verbatim Record of Responses:* Write out your responses *verbatim* including mmhmm's, uh-huh's, etc. Number each response and categorize it. Categories include: Mmhmmm; Continuing Response; Open Question; Closed Question; Why Question; Advice-Giving; Information-Giving; Self-Involving Response; Self-Disclosure; Other.

Responses	*Category*	*Rating (+,0,–)*

B. *Counselor's Behavior:*
   1. *Nonverbal Behavior:* Summarize your notable nonverbal behaviors. What impact did your nonverbal behaviors have on the client? *Be specific.*
   2. *Verbal Behavior:*
       a. Total number of responses made: _____
       b. Percentage in each category: *(number in category × 100%)*
          Mmhmmm:_____   Advice-Giving:_____
          Continuing:_____   Information-Giving:_____
          Open Question:_____   Self-Involving:_____
          Closed Question:_____   Self-Disclosing:_____
          Why Question:_____   Other:_____
C. *Self-Assessment of Verbal Responses:*
   1. What responses could have been better phrased? *Exactly* how would you re-state them?
   2. Which responses could or should have been omitted? Why?

PART II—UNDERSTANDING THE CLIENT

A. List the most important specific topics discussed by the client.
B. What feelings does the client have about each topic?

---

*Courtesy of Steven J. Danish, Richmond, Virginia.

C. Describe how these topics are related to each other.

D. Describe how the topics relate to what you know about the client; in other words, connect "the client to the problem."

E. Based on the information above, what is your understanding of the client's concern?

PART III—GOAL ASSESSMENT

A. *Goal Identification:*

1. Using the client's concern/problem identified above, help the client determine whether the goal meets the characteristics of a reachable goal that he/she expressed an interest in attaining.

   a. Is the goal described stated positively? Positively stated goals describe some action the client wants to take. The client can create a mental image of what it is the client wants to have happen rather than something the client doesn't want to have happen. Negatively stated goals often have words like "not," "cannot," "do not," "will not," or other words like "avoid." *Write the client's positively stated goal below.*

   b. Is this goal stated specifically? When a client makes a specifically stated goal, the client knows when it is attained. With a general goal, a client may have trouble knowing when he/she has reached it. Goals that are not specific often have words like "good," "better," "more," or "less" in them. *Write the client's specifically stated goal below.*

   c. Is the goal under the client's control? When a client selects a goal that requires the actions of someone else (friend, family member, employer, teacher, etc.) rather than the client, the client does not have control over whether the goal can be attained. Although a client may ask the other individual to act in a way consistent with the goal, the final determination is up to the individual, not the client. Similarly, setting goals such as "being successful," "winning," or "being happy" are really results, not goals. Goals are the actions a client can take to reach these results. *Write a goal that is under the client's control below.*

2. Describe the dimensions of the goal:

   a. How long has the client wanted to achieve this goal?

   b. What, if anything, has the client done to reach the goal?

   c. Describe the specific situation in which the client came closest to reaching the goal.

   d. Describe the specific situation in which the client felt farthest from the goal.

   e. Why is it important to the client to reach this goal now?

3. Restate the goal. Make sure it meets all the criteria described.

B. *Determining Goal Importance:*
   1. What makes the goal important to the client? Is it more important to the client than to other people in the client's life?
   2. Is the goal something the client *wants* to accomplish or something the client feels *should* or *ought to* be accomplished?
   3. From your perspective, is it worthwhile for the client to achieve the goal? Why?
   4. What does the client gain by reaching the goal?
   5. What does the client gain by *not* reaching the goal?
   6. How likely is it that the client *can* reach the goal?
C. *Roadblocks to Goal Attainment:*
   Why has the client been unable to reach the goal?
   1. Is it a lack of knowledge? If so, what knowledge is needed to reach the goal?
   2. Is it a lack of skills? If so, what does the client need to know how to do to reach the goal?
   3. Is it an inability to take risks? If so, what would assist the client in overcoming the fear of taking the risk?
   4. Is it a lack of social support? If so, what support does the client need and who can provide it?
   5. Is it some combination of a lack of knowledge, lack of skills, inability to take risks, and lack of social support? Describe.
D. *Goal Attainment:*
   1. Identify the steps for achieving the goal using the Goal Ladder. Are the steps small and manageable? If not, divide the most complex step into smaller ones. It is possible to have more than ten steps.

GOAL LADDER

Goal:

Step	*Time Frame (in no. of weeks or by date)*
10	
9	
8	
7	

6

5

4

3

2

1

2. With what step(s), if any, is the client likely to have trouble?
3. What kind of help will assist the client to overcome this trouble?
4. Who can offer this assistance?

PART IV—IF YOU COULD . . .

A. If you could do this session over again, given your understanding of the client's concerns/problems/goals, how would you approach the session differently, if at all (what would you *say* next—be specific) and why?
B. What issues would you like to explore with the client in the next session? How would you pursue this direction?
C. Things I will work on related to my counseling skills:

Appendix 14–B

Goal Attainment

GOAL LADDER

Goal: Four evenings during the next week, I will eat a planned snack at 9 PM.

Step	*Time Frame*
7. I will keep a journal of the snack I ate and the days I am able to do it.	
6. After finishing the snack and cleaning up, I will reward myself by listening to my favorite music for one-half hour.	
5. I will eat my snack at the dining room table.	
4. At 9 PM on the specified nights, I will set aside at least 15 minutes to enjoy my snack.	
3. Right after dinner, I will make my 9 PM snack and put it in the refrigerator.	Monday, Tuesday, Wednesday, and Thursday, April 20–23
2. I will shop for the food to make the snacks.	Monday, April 20
1. I will plan four snacks and choose the four nights to have the snacks.	Sunday, April 19

CHAPTER 15

Multidisciplinary Weight Management

Cathy Nonas

INTRODUCTION

The management of obesity, defined as sufficient excess body fat to incur moderate to high health risks, may seem simple: for a person to lose weight, energy consumption should be less than energy expenditure; for a person to maintain weight, energy intake should equal expenditure. Yet this simplicity is misleading: obesity management is much more difficult in practice than it is in theory. Despite a booming diet business, the prevalence of obesity in the United States continues to climb. There are more than 33 million people in this country who are now obese,[1] an increase of 8% during the 1980s decade.

Even if a diet is successful, weight loss itself is not the panacea. Even more difficult is maintaining a stable weight after successful weight loss. The causes of this recidivism remain elusive. The idea that overweight people should just stop overeating is a simplistic view of an extremely complex disorder that has at least as much to do with biology as it does with environment.

If obesity is so difficult to treat successfully should professionals, as some suggest, stop all treatment? The answer is a resounding "no!" The research literature is clear: obesity is associated with significant health risks. Dieting to lose weight may be merely a cosmetic issue for some people, but for many, dieting is a serious attempt to improve health. Obesity is associated with an increased risk of adult-onset diabetes, elevated serum cholesterol, hypertriglyceridemia, hypertension, gall-bladder disease, stroke, myocardial infarctions, certain cancers, gout, osteoarthritis, and other disorders.[2,3] Obesity is thus defined as sufficient excess body fat to incur moderate to high health risk.

This chapter presents weight management from the viewpoint of a weight management center that offers multidisciplinary long-term services to patients. Because of the center's comprehensive approach, the discussion includes a wide range of issues, examples, and questions related to managing obesity as a chronic disease.

REDEFINING OBESITY

Instead of insisting that diets do not work—they do work during the time they are followed—the overall philosophy of care for the obese patient must be redefined. Obesity should be considered a chronic disorder. In so doing, "diet" or "treatment" or "control" can be changed to "long-term management" of a lifetime disorder. Therefore, intensive therapy or treatment are necessary during times of acute flare-up, or lapse, while at other times, well-controlled weight may be managed by maintaining a healthy lifestyle. How does a management approach redefine the goals of traditional treatment?

Weight Loss

In terms of weight loss, weight management means that the goals are less lofty. Even without the presence of concomitant disease, obesity is associated with risk.[4] Family history, fat distribution, age, and degree of overweight must be taken into account. If improved health is the goal, then weight loss can reduce the current and potential risks associated with obesity. But the amount of weight loss need not be large. Small weight losses can show dramatic health results. A 5% to 15% reduction in body weight can reduce duration of hospitalizations, reduce postoperative complications, decrease blood pressure, and improve blood glucose levels.[5]

Changing Behavior

In terms of modifying behavior, weight management means a periodic review and readjustment of eating and exercise patterns and a creative flow of new ideas between the patient and the health professional on managing potential trouble points. It is important to remember that although some overweight people do not know the basics of nutrition, many have a great deal of nutritional knowledge, and have practiced good nutrition guidelines and have increased activity for periods in the past. Therefore nutritional knowledge may not be needed as much as the need to redesign, or translate, the information into behaviors that result in better food and lifestyle choices. New genetic theories suggest that some people may not respond to satiety signals.[6,7] A person may intellectually understand the concept of fullness, but biologically, the brain does not receive the message. Although some approaches suggest that behavior modification is unlikely to be successful until the biological signals can be corrected,[8] treatment of obesity in association with behavior modification is still more successful than treatment without it.[9] Furthermore, other behavior changes, particularly addictive behaviors such as smoking, usually take many trials before a person can successfully change.[10] Why do people have different expectations for weight management? A weight management program must offer participants the chance and support needed to defend themselves as successfully as possible in an environment that gives short shrift to biological imperfections. Behavior modification should always be part of weight management: a "user-friendly" approach based on socioeconomics, education, culture, gender, and age.

Most important, it is expected that as general lifestyle changes, so will a person's other behaviors. Small behaviors, both positive and negative, may cause large changes over time. For example, a person may have been eating a low-fat diet for three years, but portion size or number of snacks has been steadily increasing. Changing food behavior thus requires not just support but continuous attention and creative revisions.

Treatment

In terms of treatment, weight management means that interventions should vary based on an individual's needs and readiness. Although individualizing treatment makes a program protocol more complex, a tailored intervention improves the success of the program. Maintenance is as much a part of the treatment as weight loss.

Weight Maintenance

In terms of maintenance, continuing contact with a health professional is crucial in weight maintenance.[11] Recycling behavioral and nutritional techniques used for weight loss is not enough. Most patients have had considerable experience with both weight loss and weight gain, but few have learned the skills of weight maintenance. While health professionals monitor patients with other chronic diseases over long periods, weight loss programs have generally not included long-term monitoring of post-obese persons. Although obesity has often been discussed as a chronic disease, treatment programs do little or nothing to manage it as such. The emphasis should be not on achieving perfect weight but on minimizing weight fluctuation and the concomitant risks associated with such fluctuations. Therefore, it is incumbent upon weight management professionals and weight management centers to offer specific solutions and interventions to maintainers through regularly scheduled visits for as long as the patient will attend and through outreach to provide support on an ongoing basis. As with all chronic disease management, lifetime visits may be needed for successful maintenance.

Overall Philosophy

A weight management program should offer action steps for patients to control what is within their reach. A program cannot offer a promise of permanency, or unrealistic expectations, but should offer hope that weight fluctuations can be kept within a more manageable range and that lost weight can be maintained within limits for as long as the patient is willing to work at weight management.

A WEIGHT MANAGEMENT CENTER

The word "management" was carefully chosen for the weight management center. Weight "control" connotes restraint, even domination over something. This is the kind of thinking that can perpetuate typical all-or-nothing responses: "I'm either perfect or I'm bad." On the other hand, management means doing the best job possible under the circumstances. "Managing" weight is a skill that presupposes that an individual, through training and experience, can succeed—albeit with varying degrees of difficulty—to keep weight within a manageable range.

A weight management center, therefore, must set up a relationship between patient and staff similar to that of an athlete and coach: the coach begins by directing the athlete; the athlete begins by adhering to the plan. Eventually it is the athlete who becomes the architect of his or her own training, and the coach continues as the support system. If the athlete does not adhere to the direction agreed upon, the coach and the athlete jointly seek another route to reach the same goal. Similarly, the patient learns the skills of management. If the patient does not respond to one approach, another is tried. When the management goal is near, the patient proceeds independently, becomes the architect, and the staff becomes the background support.

The Management Team

The center must be equipped with health professionals who offer creative programs to enhance the treatment and keep the patient on course. The basic management team consists of a physician, a dietitian, an exercise physiologist, a psychologist, a clinical coordinator, and an office manager. Nurses, medical office assistants, dietitians, or experienced health professionals with master's degrees and certifications in nutrition or exercise physiology (or both) should monitor the patient's progress and continuously assess risks, e.g., sudden diarrhea. Is there a precipitous drop or sudden increase in blood pressure? Dizziness? Headache? Upper right quadrant pain? Depression? Any major or sudden changes that may be diet-related should immediately be cause to refer the patient to the physician. What about adherence to the dietary treatment plan? If the person is not following the individualized plan, should new dietary goals be discussed? Binge eating, body image distortions, social pressures, and life changes all affect feelings of success and failure as well as adherence to, and appropriateness of, the plan. The patient should have intermittent access to individual dietitians and psychologists when necessary and should participate in group proceedings. If a patient requires excessive individual attention, a referral for individual treatment may be necessary.

In order to maintain a flexible structure that can readily be adjusted to meet patient needs, it is helpful for each team member to perform numerous tasks. For example, the dietitian can also monitor blood pressure; the exercise physiologist can perform electrocardiograms (ECGs) or teach T'ai Chi; the physician who has a strong background in both nutrition and research can design evaluation studies; the clinical coordinator may be a nurse with an advanced degree in nutrition or exercise physiology; and the office manager understands CPT codes and billing. In this way, a small permanent staff can become very efficient at meeting patient needs. When more staff is needed, they can be hired on a per diem or part-time basis.

The Program

The center must offer flexible treatments that can be tailored to the individual, not generically prescribed. We have found it best to offer both one-to-one counseling and group counseling. Individual counseling can involve nutrition, exercise, and cognitive therapy. We have found that traditional psychotherapy is important, but may be too complex to offer in a weight management center. Instead, a one-time consultation or continuing group sessions that deal with one topic each session such as "what is blocking me from losing weight" is more practical. Typical therapy tends to be long term and may have no effect on weight. Nutrition, exercise, and some cognitive therapy sessions can be flexible in content, and scheduled times and number of classes should be adjusted for the convenience of both the patient and the center. Class content can also be adjusted. Patient data is valuable for evaluating outcomes. For example, if the class discussion and monitoring support are successful, positive well-being will improve and return visits may lead to successful maintenance. Tangible successes such as reduction in weight, improvement of laboratory tests, and increased fitness can be compared to the type and number of sessions patients attend. For example, do those patients who attend more cognitive therapy sessions lose more weight than those who attend exercise sessions?

The most successful classes are diverse groups that include a combination of nutrition, exercise, and psychoeducation as the base curriculum and specialty classes such as body image, cognitive behavior, cooking, and yoga as extracurricular. Different patients need different forms of support. Not only should patients be encouraged to restructure negative thinking, but they need to be taught self-monitoring tools that help keep them on track or get them back on track if they lapse. Such tools include food records, and food behavior techniques such as breaking the day into manageable pieces, eating only one kind of food during high-stress snack times, and visualization.

The center must be able to manage both the physical weight and weight-related diseases and psychological ramifications of lapses, or "flare-ups." In this way, the center exists to help the patient for life, acknowledging that the disorder does not go away, but does become easier to manage at certain times than at others and that support is especially needed during vulnerable periods.

Patient Flow

After a patient's initial diuresis following reduced calorie intake, weight loss should consist of at least 75% adipose tissue. Current studies indicate that obesity is protective of lean tissue, suggesting that the greater the degree of obesity, the better the dieter is able to conserve body protein during weight loss. A loss of no more than 1% of body weight per week after the initial period of diuresis is the guideline suggested in weight control programs.[12] As the weight changes, the guideline rate of weight loss must be recalculated. Obviously, if weight loss exceeds the guideline, calorie intake should be increased. When lean tissue is compromised, muscle catabolism and hypometabolic states can occur.[13] In a program that individualizes treatment, clinical flow may have a volatile, less structured pattern than in some health care clinics. A patient may report undefined indigestion in the upper portion of the right quadrant of the body: is it gas or a gall-bladder problem? Or a patient may report sudden dizziness. Is it a flu symptom or a consequence of a very-low-calorie diet? Although much of the time the staff serves as gentle cheerleaders, encouraging the patient to keep on track, it is imperative to remain alert to any sudden physical changes that may occur. The entire staff must be skilled at eliciting and interpreting information suggestive of such changes. The hierarchy of clinical care should be carefully maintained, but the staff should function flexibly amidst a medical flow that will vary from day to day.

First Visit

Physicians assess the patient physically and set the medical protocol, taking into account the dietary treatment as well as the patient's medical risks; the protocol might include the number of ECGs within a certain time period, the number of physician visits, specific laboratory tests, etc. An experienced physician will not only assess the appropriateness of the diet based on physical risks, but also on the psychological profile. Has there been a long history of dieting? Of binge eating? Other eating disorders or addictive behaviors? Is the patient taking antidepressants? Is there any history of attempted suicide? The dietitian can be especially useful in assessing the patient's readiness to develop a plan and identifying where nutritional, behavioral, and cognitive problems occur. A nutritional evaluation before the initial physician visit is valuable, as the dietitian can assess what kind of diet is most appropriate given the patient's social conditions as well as the patient's current eating pattern.

Weekly Management

In a center that emphasizes individual care, the medical flow can be difficult to manage. During most patient hours, at least one physician should be available to see patients for follow-up, prescription renewals, initial assessments, and emergencies. Apart from physician visits, every patient sees a clinical assistant weekly for a blood pressure check, weigh-in, and monitoring of symptoms. The clinical assistant must have an adequate knowledge of nutrition, overeating, and disordered eating behaviors. In this way, both physical and psychological symptoms are briefly assessed and referred for further evaluation when necessary.

Who To Treat

Who is overweight? Overweight is defined as a body mass index, or BMI (weight in kilograms divided by height in meters squared), of 27.8 or more in men, 27.3 or more in women, or 20% or more above the midpoint of the middle frame range of the 1983 Metropolitan Life Insurance Company tables of recommended weights for heights.[14] The 20% figure represents the weight at which the risk to health begins when body mass exceeds this threshold value.[15] Obesity is defined as a condition in which adipose tissue storage is excessive.[16] However, overweight and obese are most often used interchangeably because most people who are overweight are also obese.[17] See Chapter 1 for a full discussion of body weight definitions.

Adipose tissue is not uniformly distributed throughout the body. Fat location may determine treatment. The metabolic activity of fat cells at various sites can be quite different. Upper-body obesity, or android obesity, which is estimated by either a waist-to-hip ratio or a waist circumference, is associated with increased health risk. The increased intraabdominal fat, predominately stored in the upper abdomen and chest, drains into the liver. The resulting increased perfusion of free fatty acids to the liver can set the stage for metabolic changes such as non–insulin-dependent diabetes, abnormally high serum lipid levels, cardiovascular disease, hypertension, stroke, and sudden death.[18] Therefore, if a person enters a program weighing 15 lbs above recommended body mass index, but most fat is located in the upper abdominal portion of the body and the family history indicates a high risk of cardiovascular disease, should the practitioner suggest weight loss? Yes. Immediately.

But what about the person with large thighs who is also 15 lbs over recommended weight, has a family history of health, and has no medical complications? Should the practitioner suggest weight loss for this person as well? Maybe, but certainly not with a restrictive diet. Dieting does not necessarily precipitate either binge eating or an eating disorder,[19] but the potential exists to exacerbate a preoccupation with weight and body image. Such a person should have an individual consultation with a registered dietitian to evaluate nutritional balance, to stabilize an eating pattern that might include too many snacks, and to plan increased physical activity. Although a diet has a negative connotation for many people,[20] the word should not be misconstrued as a negative means of managing overweight. Healthful eating is not a harmful objective, nor is achieving a healthy weight an unrealistic goal. Because of the preoccupation with ideal weights in the United States, there are many people who perceive themselves to be overweight who are not. In such cases, dieting for weight loss is inappropriate. Learning how to make healthy food choices should be a major goal for such people. Appropriate treatment may also include some form of psychological help to improve body image. A weight management center's main goal is to encourage optimal health.

Opportunities to learn and apply skills to ensure a well-balanced food intake of appropriate portions and establish a stable exercise pattern are all part of the management program. Many overweight people are preparing to lose weight but are not yet ready.[10] This preparation period is important to long-term success and can be a time to learn decision-making skills such as judging the advantages and disadvantages of choices in food, body movement, social activities, and other areas. If the goal is to encourage optimal health, and weight reduction becomes a long-range goal, then the patient can be successful within the program even without immediate weight loss. See Chapter 13 on changing behavior and Chapter 14 on setting goals in weight management.

MEDICAL MANAGEMENT

To the outside observer, dieting is a simple issue of eating less and losing weight. To the health practitioner, dieting constitutes an additional stress factor that, if not carefully planned and monitored, can worsen rather than improve the condition of the patient. Despite this fact, there is no government or scientific consensus concerning the clinical monitoring of patients in weight loss. Although guidelines have been written, such as the Michigan Task Force to Establish Weight Loss Guidelines[21] and the Institute of Medicine guidelines for evaluating weight loss methods and programs,[22] the weight loss industry remains essentially unregulated. Therefore, the weight management program's three main responsibilities are: (1) ensuring that the health professionals are highly qualified and experienced in weight loss; (2) setting a protocol that is conservative in that it will reduce potential risk factors inherent in dieting while improving the health status of the patient; and (3) offering a realistic and sensible plan so that each patient has a high probability of successfully learning weight management skills.

Although primary care physicians can assess the patient for maintenance of weight, many do not understand the physiology of weight loss. Special medical needs of a patient during weight loss include monitoring liver enzymes, iron status, electrolytes, and other parameters. For example, in an obese person, uric acid levels may be high without symptoms of gout; a physician experienced in weight loss will know that uric acid levels may increase further during the first few weeks of dieting before levels fall.[5] The bariatric physician will decide whether to treat to prevent the possible onset of gout, or to monitor the results of a high-carbohydrate diet planned to avoid ketosis and ameliorate the potential problem.

Adult-onset diabetes is common among obese people, particularly those with a high waist-to-hip ratio.[23] Physicians tend to treat uncontrolled blood sugar with increasing amounts of insulin or oral hypoglycemic agents. The weight loss physician will usually reduce the dose of medication in order to prevent hypoglycemia during dieting even if it means an initial rise in blood sugar, with the understanding that blood sugar will decrease as weight loss occurs. Slightly elevated serum transaminase levels are probably signs of a fatty liver due to obesity, not other underlying ailments. Like uric acid, these enzymes may continue to rise at the beginning of a hypocaloric diet due to the flow of fatty acids to the liver, although they tend to normalize as weight loss continues.[5]

Potassium must also be carefully monitored. Although a serum potassium level of 3.6 may be adequate for weight maintenance, this is not necessarily high enough during weight loss because weight loss can result in loss of electrolytes, not only during the initial diuresis, but over the long term. Noting abnormal electrolyte levels and decreases within normal values is necessary or order to evaluate the need for supplements. A fall in electrolytes can precipitate cardiac arrhythmias, a great risk to the patient.[5]

Finally, not only should arrhythmias be noted on an ECG, but also QT_c prolongation, a sign of lean tissue loss from progressive protein deficit.[24] QT_c prolongation is not associated with abnormal electrolytes, but can be an indication of physical vulnerability in the person who is losing weight too rapidly.[25,26]

Two examples illustrate how this program would apply to patients. Jane F. is a healthy, sedentary, 36-year-old woman who, after having seen the physician for an assessment, was given regular balanced food guidelines for 1000 calories per day. Her initial weight is 174.0 lbs. She is 60 in tall, with a BMI of 33.7. Her body is pear-shaped, with extra weight distributed mostly in her lower body. She presently has no comorbidities. She attends a group class (to be discussed later) and is monitored by the clinical assistant each week for blood pressure, heart rate, weight, and problems that may be associated with the diet. She would like to lose 40 lbs. ECGs and blood tests are prescribed according to the percentage of weight lost such as when the patient has lost 10% of body weight. Because Jane is low risk and her weight loss is slow, her follow-up ECG and blood work tests are scheduled the twelfth week of her diet, when she has lost 18 lbs.

Jerry S. is 45 years old, moderately active, and hypertensive. He has a personal history of atrial fibrillation and a family history of severe coronary artery disease. His initial weight is 310 lbs. His height is 73 in, his waist-to-hip ratio is 1.0, and his BMI is 40.98. He begins a diet that is also 1000 calories per day, but he chooses liquid formula as his weight loss treatment. Compared to previous calorie intake, 1000 calories per day results in a much greater calorie deficit for Jerry S. than it did for Jane F. Jerry is monitored weekly by the physician. His electrolytes and ECG are measured at the first and fourth visits. His guideline rate of weight loss is 3.3 lbs per week, but his diuresis is so great that he drops 30 lbs in the first five weeks (10, 7, 5.5, and 5). His calories are increased to 1300, and he is still consuming all-liquid formula. His weight loss slows to between 2.8 and 3.7 lbs per week. Like Jane F., he attends a weekly class. He is monitored by a clinical assistant each time he comes, and also sees the physician each month. Follow-up electrolytes and ECG are also measured each month, according to standard formula protocol.

DIETARY REQUIREMENTS

Total Calories

Should anyone be prescribed a very-low-calorie diet (VLCD), defined as lower than 800 calories per day?[27] In a study in which patients were randomly assigned to three liquid formula diets providing 420, 660, or 800 calories, the researchers found no significant differences in amount of weight lost during the study period.[28] Furthermore, consuming 800 calories or more may decrease the risks of long-term dieting and require less intensive medical supervision and still result in similar weight loss. Therefore, there seems no reason for a weight management center to prescribe less than 800 calories per day.

The two patients, Jane F. and Jerry S., have different BMIs, and one would not expect them to have the same maintenance calorie requirements. Neither would one give them similar weight loss criteria after an individual assessment.

A 1000 calorie diet, as we saw in the examples, results in very different weight losses for each patient. The 1000 calorie diet can produce a much greater weight loss and put a far greater nutritional stress on a large, active man who has a daily maintenance calorie requirement of 3500 than it can on a 5 ft, sedentary woman with a maintenance calorie requirement of 1800. Therefore, a percent calorie deficit based on BMI rather than a flat calorie prescription is a more appropriate way to calculate the calorie prescription. The maintenance calorie requirement is the first step in evaluating the calorie prescription for the patient. This consists of calculating the resting energy expenditure (REE) multiplied by a physical activity factor.

Resting oxygen consumption measured by indirect calorimetry is expensive and time consuming. The Harris-Benedict equation,[29] which uses age, gender, height, and initial weight, can be used to predict REE. However, the Harris-Benedict equation may underestimate energy requirements of an obese person.

However, as a weight management center should always err on the conservative side, a physical activity factor of 1.5 (moderate activity) is added to this equation to estimate 24-hour expenditure, e.g., REE for women (calories) = 655 + 9.56 × weight (kg) + 1.85 × height (cm) – 4.68 × age × 1.5.

A "moderate" calorie restriction of 500 calories/day[30] would promote a loss of 1 lb per week; a deficit of 1000 calories, 2 lbs per week. However, a guideline weekly weight loss rate of no more than 1% of body weight is suggested.[12] The weight loss exceeds the guideline rate if the calorie deficit is too great. Though this might not be precise on a weekly basis, it will be a good gauge over a two- to three-week time period. If weight is being lost too quickly, increase the calorie prescription.

Protein

Once the calorie prescription for weight loss is set, the composition of the diet must be evaluated. In particular, protein should be prescribed in amounts high enough to sustain nitrogen balance. Therefore, although the recommended daily allowance (RDA) for protein during maintenance is 50 g for women and 63 g for men,[31] scientists suggest 72 to 80 g per day during caloric restriction (or 1.0 to 1.5 g/kg ideal body weight).[32] Research studies have indicated that patients who consume less than 34 g of protein per day exhibit adverse changes in plasma proteins, and are at considerable risk of developing ventricular arrhythmias.[33] Patients who consume a VLCD must be prescribed adequate amounts of complete proteins as deaths related to protein loss reported in the mid-1970s were partially attributed to inadequate amounts of protein of high biological value.[34] Finally, the entire diet should be balanced in such as way as to spare the loss of body proteins.

Carbohydrates

Many researchers have found that when the diet is adequate in carbohydrate, lean tissue is spared more efficiently.[35] This is particularly important to note in light of fad diets that are based on low carbohydrate, high protein, and moderate to high fat percent of calories. Diets should consist of no less than 100 g carbohydrate per day to minimize ketosis, and the carbohydrate sources should consist mostly of high-fiber food choices.

Fat

In 1988, the Surgeon General's office recommended ≤30% of total calories from fat.[36] There are several reasons why 30% is probably too high for an obese population: (1) because fat grams are more dense in calories (9 calories per gram in comparison with 4 calories per gram for protein or carbohydrates), the amount of fat in foods is frequently underestimated; (2) 30% fat diets have not generally been shown to reduce the risk of cancer or heart disease; and (3) too much flexibility might be difficult for the patient to reckon with. Food choices should be preferred by the patient and be palatable. A goal of 20% total fat may be more feasible. As long as a liquid formula or very-low-calorie diet using regular food is prescribed, it is suggested that one meal per day contain at least 10 g of fat to stimulate gall-bladder contraction, thereby reducing the risk of gallstone formation.[37,38]

Micronutrients

Any weight loss program should include at least the RDA for vitamins and minerals. The best way to obtain required vitamins, minerals, and other nutrients is from the food itself. Weinsier et al[39] prescribed a 1000 calorie per day diet, emphasizing a high vegetable and fruit intake. They gave no vitamin supplements. Over 20 weeks, blood levels of vitamins and minerals remained normal and vitamin C levels increased. Many dieters tend to eat "diet" foods that are often low in micronutrients as well as calories, or to follow an unvaried restrictive diet that is lacking in nutrient density. In these cases, taking a multivitamin capsule with minerals is often necessary, particularly to obtain nutrients such as calcium, iron, zinc, linoleic acid, and vitamin E.[40] After surgical procedures such as vertical gastroplasty, chewable vitamins are available to avoid blockage of the stomach opening. Potassium supplements might also be indicated if the serum potassium is on the low side of normal and weight loss is expected to be rapid.

DIETARY TREATMENTS

No matter what a "new" weight loss plan may suggest, there are only a limited number of ways to diet. They all result in a calorie deficit achieved by decreasing food intake or increasing physical activity, or both.[17] Food plans are of four kinds: specific guidelines that can be adhered to, prepackaged/preportioned foods, liquid formula, or part regular food/part liquid formula. Products such as medication can enhance weight loss but should be prescribed in conjunction with new dietary guidelines. Increasing physical activity is important, but by itself does not result in the rate and amount of weight loss most patients need to stay motivated in the early stages of weight management. A healthy diet supports weight loss and prevents the onset of certain diseases. Within this short list of ways to lose weight, however, there are many ways to individualize the regimen to support the patient's needs and preferences.

Although a severely obese person may physically tolerate an 800 calorie diet, it may not be realistic for many reasons. Factors to be taken into account when developing a food plan include:

- the eating patterns of the patient (binge, nibble, eat one big meal, snack from evening to bedtime, etc.)
- past dieting history (how many times on liquid formula, calorie counting, exchanges, high protein/low carbohydrate, high carbohydrate/low protein, medication)
- weight loss goals (health, aesthetics)
- psychosocial and lifestyle factors (depression, work, travel, home, relationships, aging)
- food preference (high fat, high carbohydrate, high volume)

For example, take the person who has tried liquid formula three different times, resulting in successful weight losses each time, but who has subsequently regained the weight very quickly. This person should be steered away from formula a fourth time. Instead, learning how to "normalize" regular food use is important even if it results in uneven weight loss and constant readjustment of the diet. In this case, the first goal may be to find "peace" with food before weight loss can be achieved. This approach reduces the opportunity to fail by self-sabotage, since weight loss is no longer the primary focus and outcome. At times, it is even appropriate to have patients weigh "backwards" (not face the measurement side of the scale), so that feelings of success are not guided by weight.

However, a person who has not had a lot of experience with formula and who feels totally out-of-control with food might be very successful on an initial liquid formula plan. A liquid formula diet may also reduce binge eating as opposed to precipitating it. The time-out from eating regular food often appears to give the binge eater an opportunity to regroup without returning to destructive eating patterns.[16] The percentage of binge eaters in weight control programs ranges from 11% to 50% depending upon the criteria.[41,42]

Conversely, some patients have long histories of rigid dieting where foods are limited to specific amounts of protein, carbohydrate, and fats, as well as calories, while other foods have been eliminated altogether. This type of diet might be more appropriate for a less structured approach, one where dessert or wine is allowed, so that dieting is not an aberration as much as a new way of life. The focus is on food and exercise "policies" that can be integrated into the person's lifestyle forever.

Formula Diets

Formula diets have gone out of fashion in the last few years, but remain a healthy choice for people who need to lose a substantial amount of weight, with or without concomitant disease. An estimated 12 to 15 million people have tried liquid formula,[43] many with excellent results. Most research reports a weight loss of approximately 10 to 20 kg in 12 to 26 weeks, with the preponderance of weight lost in the first 12 weeks. Although there is speculation that VLCDs reduce resting metabolic rate chronically, this is incorrect. Wadden et al studied the long-term effects of dieting and found that a patient following a VLCD will respond with a significant reduction in resting metabolic rate only during the VLCD phase. During the refeeding phase the metabolic rate will increase to a similar state as that of dieters following a 1200 calorie conventional food diet as shown in Figure 15–1.

VLCDs and low-calorie diets (LCDs) can be very helpful to the patient with Type II diabetes. Because the consistency of the nutrients and the specific intervals at which the formula is consumed, glycemic control is improved.[44] A patient

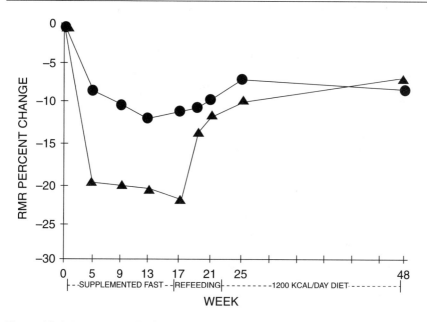

Figure 15–1 Percentage reduction in resting metabolic rate (RMR) in patients randomly assigned to balanced-deficit diet (BDD) (circles) or to a very-low-calorie diet (VLCD) (triangles). A balanced-deficit diet is a nutrient balanced, calorie-deficit diet. The BDD patients consumed approximately 1200 kcal/day throughout treatment, while the VLCD patients consumed 420 kcal/day for 16 of the first 17 weeks, a refeeding diet for weeks 18 through 23, and a balanced-deficit diet providing 1200 to 1500 kcal/day for the remainder of treatment. Mean weight losses of the BDD patients at weeks 17 and 48 were 11.0 kg and 18.2 kg, respectively. Losses for the VLCD patients at weeks 17 and 48 were 23.1 kg and 21.6 kg, respectively. *Source:* Reprinted with permission from T.A. Wadden et al., Long-term Effects of Dieting on Resting Metabolic Rate in Obese Outpatients, *Journal of the American Medical Association,* Vol. 264, pp. 707–711, Copyright 1990, American Medical Association.

may be able to decrease or even discontinue insulin and hypoglycemic agents within a short time of beginning this type of diet.

Liquid formula diets should be used with care depending upon the patient and the program. Percentage of overweight is also important if the formulas cannot be adjusted for additional calories. The literature suggests 30% or more overweight as one criterion.[45] Age is also important because formula may not be appropriate for a person who is young and has not completed growth or who is old enough so that age itself becomes an additional stressor (usually under 18 and over 60 years of age).[46] Obviously, clinical evaluations should be individualized. Most liquid formulas include a set number of calories, usually 800 or below. Rapid weight loss and severe hypocaloric diets should not be prescribed for patients with recent history of myocardial infarctions or unstable cardiac status. People taking potassium-wasting diuretics must be closely monitored since the diuretic effect of a VLCD or LCD will cause increased diuresis and potential electrolyte imbalance. Other contraindications include renal or hepatic disease, acquired immune deficiency syndrome (AIDS), cancer, pregnancy, significant depression, and a history of substance abuse.

Ideally, a formula diet should be adjustable in terms of both calories and macronutrients. Although it is more costly, the authors designed a base formula of protein (76 g), micronutrients (140% of the RDA), fat (12 g), carbohydrate (120 g) and fiber (12 g). Additional fat (8 g each) in the form of corn oil and additional carbohydrates in the form of maltodextrins (38 g each) are mixed with the base as needed (see Figure 15–2).

Therefore, calories can range from 800 to 1500 in all formulas, and percentages of fat and carbohydrate can be manipulated depending upon the medical needs of the patient. That is how Jerry S. was able to increase his calories from 1000 to 1300 and still remain on an all-formula plan.

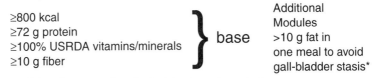

*additional source of maltodextrins for extra calories

Figure 15–2 Suggested guideline for daily liquid formula. This guideline presumes that (1) the formula comes in powder form; (2) that either fat or carbohydrate can be mixed in with the base source as prescribed; and (3) that some fat (at least 3% linoleic acid) and some carbohydrate are also included in the base.

Fluids are particularly important when a liquid diet is being consumed. Sufficient liquid is critical to prevent dehydration, maintain acid-base balance, and prevent formation of kidney stones.[47] The body is two-thirds water, and water loss cannot be replaced through the formula only. Ingestion of at least 2 L of fluid per day is recommended to prevent complications. The monotony of formula diets can be both an advantage and a disadvantage. The consistency and amount of weight loss can be very encouraging. Also, dieters express relief at having all choices removed. In a study of 76 persons who were prescribed a liquid diet for 10 weeks, LaPorte and Stunkard[48] found that 64% had either complete or good adherence to the prescription.

The most common complaints from formula dieters over time are that they need to chew and that they find the restriction on social activities difficult. Weight loss using a formula diet slows in most patients by week 12, probably due to the addition of unplanned regular food as well.[43] This is also the case at our center. However, weight loss rate decreases for all treatments: formula, regular food, and medication. This can be attributed to a reduction in motivation that naturally occurs over time and underscores the need for developing skills to manage and maintain behavior change, emotional coping, and seeking continuing professional and personal support.

In addition, wavering formula dieters may be encouraged to consume moderate amounts of plain raw or steamed vegetables and low-sodium broth or to drink various noncaloric drinks to help them continue on the diet. The advantage of using different diets in one center is that when one diet begins to be less effective, another diet can be attempted.

Part Formula/Part Food

As a Primary Treatment for Weight Loss

If a formula diet is too restrictive for the patient, a combination of food and formula can be a satisfying alternative. It offers an opportunity to participate in social eating while limiting total calories.

Although this plan of liquid formula twice each day and one regular meal might seem the most practical for weight loss, it is often the least successful. The tendency is to substitute formula for meals that could be calorically manageable and to continue eating regular food at the meal that is characteristically when most overeating occurs. For example, our healthy patient, Jane F., has a tendency to overeat in the evening, yet she chooses to use formula for breakfast and lunch and eat a regular food meal for dinner. The problem inherent in this is that she has done little to change the risk of continuing to overeat. In this scenario Jane eats only 600 calories during the day and 1000 or more at night. The result is that she loses weight at an exceptionally slow rate. Considering that she is using formula, albeit only partially, this can be very frustrating. Try as she might to be conscious of calories, that one regular food meal is looked forward to with such zeal that it often becomes too difficult to manage appropriately.

There are three ways to make Jane's food/formula plan more successful:

1. Substitute formula for two meals, but make one of them a substitution for the most caloric meal of the day. For example, Jane might consume formula for breakfast and dinner and eat a regular food lunch.
2. If Jane is intent on one specific food at meal time, preportioned frozen meals can be prescribed. A wide variety of nutritionally sound frozen meals are available that can be supplemented with extra vegetables or skim milk or fruit. In one study of 202 patients, using prepackaged, preportioned food resulted in more weight loss than among another group who were offered financial incentives to lose weight.[49] With preportioned meals, a small serving of extra formula can serve as the dessert—and signal the end to eating regular food.
3. Another alternative is to begin with a formula-only plan for about four weeks and then prescribe the combination of formula and food. The advantage of this route is that patients (1) usually lose a substantial amount of weight in the first few weeks, which encourages further adherence; (2) become used to adhering to the formula; and (3) distance themselves from the regular food meal, making it easier to manage a reduced food intake.

As a Transition from All-Liquid Formula

A partial formula and partial regular food diet is an excellent option for a person who is making the transition from a plan of all-formula to one of food. In this case, the dietitian can introduce foods slowly, using the formula as a buffer if the patient feels out of control with any food choices. Furthermore, the actual transition can take as long or as short a time as the cooperative effort to manage food requires.

For some patients, regular foods such as one or two servings of fruit are added as extra calories when their rate of weight loss is too great on formula alone. This might have been the case for Jerry S. who would have lost weight too quickly if an adjustable-calorie formula were not available. For others, regular food is prescribed in a formula-like manner so that they will become used to regular food without the added burden of having to make choices. Turkey sandwiches or oatmeal with skim milk are two such formula-like regular food items.

The patient's goal in introducing food in this manner is to eat a nutritionally dense, but calorically appropriate diet. To this end, the most common prescription for a transition diet is 600 calories of liquid formula and 400 to 600 calories of regular food. The exact amount and type of formula depends upon the nutrient composition of the regular food. A general recommendation is that the meal choice is low in fat and sodium and equivalent in protein to the formula being replaced.

At the beginning of this transition period, plainly cooked foods are suggested as the patient may be sensitive to spices, or become gaseous from too many raw vegetables. The typical regular food meal might include 4 oz lean meat, poultry, or fish, a baked potato or equivalent starch that is both high in fiber but portion-controlled, and a small amount of steamed vegetables. Over subsequent weeks, more vegetables, fruit, and high-fiber starches are added to replace liquid formula.

Transition from all-formula to all regular food can take from 4 weeks to 12 weeks depending upon the confidence and the adherence of the patient. If food becomes too difficult to control, return to all-formula and start again.

Regular Food

The word diet stems from a Greek word, *dieta,* which means "way of life." Though dieting has a bad connotation these days, the goal for someone who is losing weight by eating regular food would be to integrate a new, healthy, lower-calorie food plan into a normal lifestyle. This is easier said than done.

It is old-fashioned to think that a diet should be so restrictive that the diet becomes an aberration from regular life—something that eventually ends—sending the dieter back to former and weight-gaining lifestyle habits. Although a restrictive diet can be helpful, particularly initially to break the pattern of overeating, ultimately the person has to integrate eating into lifestyle and learn to make "policy" decisions about eating rather than relying on will power.

Jane F., for example, regularly uses "diet behavior" at restaurants when she's trying to be "good." Diet behavior means restraint, but it is not necessarily good management. Jane refuses alcohol, tries hard not to eat any bread and dessert, and eats only half—well, maybe a little more—of her entree. But if she were to make policy decisions and use diet as a way of life, she would start by taking account of what she enjoys most about a restaurant meal. She might say to herself that alcohol, dessert, and the entree are not as enjoyable for her as the bread if it is fresh. Therefore, the way she might manage restaurants is to feel free to eat the bread but order two low-fat appetizers instead of an entree to balance what otherwise could be a high-calorie meal. And she would do this all without feeling deprived.

Most patients entering a weight management program have a great deal of knowledge about nutrition. Many are experts at counting calories. And a number of the patients may have already significantly reduced their fat intake. Some patients have joined weight control programs many times before and can often recite verbatim the classic curricula. Furthermore, most weight control center patients can easily write a 1200 calorie diet. The problem is in the translation, as if when they try to incorporate the diet into their lives, it turns into a different language. The program leader's role is to help the patients take what they know, and show them how to make it work in their own lives.

Weight loss on a regular food diet is usually half that achieved by diets consisting of all-liquid formula.[43] Indeed, the authors' weight management center (Theodore B. VanItallie Center for Nutrition and Weight Management, St. Luke's–Roosevelt Hospital, New York, New York), results are similar. In our center, during the first 10 weeks, average weight loss on regular food is 6 kg but is 13 kg using liquid formula (see Table 15–1). Because a rigid regular food plan is difficult to adhere to for any length of time in a social environment conducive to eating higher-calorie foods in larger portions, significant weight loss on a regular food diet can be challenging. Losing weight using individually designed "policy decisions" instead of adhering to fixed foods can make a diet more "user friendly." Unlike rigid diets that encourage avoidance of food, policy eating forces the patient to create flexible boundaries in different situations so that while there is more choice than on a rigid diet, the direction remains clear. In the Jane F. case, her policy about bread gave her the choice to eat what she enjoyed without deprivation or overeating. She carried her policy even further to give her clear direction: if the bread was not good, she would always order fish or pasta as the entree and glass of wine instead of the bread.

The responsibility of the dietitian is to help the patient create individualized guiding principles that can serve as a backbone of improved eating, no matter what the situation. These principles or policies protect patients from confusion and constant debate. For example, without looking at the menu in an Italian resraurant, what is both supportive of weight goals and satisfying for the patient to order? In a supermarket, what is the primary focus? Calories? Cholesterol? Sodium? Fat? Saturated fat? The dietitian is the one who helps the patient focus on what is most important. Once these guiding principles are internalized, the details can be filled in as the situation dictates. Some of the most common focus points follow.

1. *What about fat?* Assessing whether patients have the correct nutrition information about fat and know how to use that information is important because many

---

Table 15–1 Summary of Weight Loss by Treatment at Week 12 and Week 16

Program	Week 12		Week 16	
	# in Group	Avg Loss (kg)	# in Group	Avg Loss (kg)
Food	126	6.5 ± 4.6	117	7.4 ± 7.9
Formula	87	12.9 ± 7.6	69	13.1 ± 8.8
Medication	43	10.0 ± 5.4	38	11.5 ± 7.6

patients understand only the most obvious information such as that too much red meat and butter is unhealthy. Many of them worry about cholesterol, for example, but not about saturated fat, which can increase serum cholesterol twice as quickly as dietary cholesterol itself.[31] On the other hand, if a patient worries not about total fat but about a recommended daily allowance of no more than 10% saturated fat, then the original intent—weight loss—might be overlooked. Furthermore, it would be easy for a patient to tire of the calculations, and return to high-fat eating. A patient must understand how to identify and measure total fat and be able to manage fat in a food plan. Salmon, for example, may be a fatty fish, but is it bad for you or your diet? Not if measured to meet fat and calorie guidelines.

A further concern about lowering fat content of food is the reliance on no-fat snacks and very large portions of no-fat starchy foods. Many patients, such as Jane F., have already reduced their dietary fat content significantly. Unwittingly, they may have increased their calories from starchy items: a bagel no longer averages two ounces, but five; an ounce of pretzels is 110 calories but pretzels come in different sizes and some are so large that one is equal to an ounce; a small bag of ready-to-eat baby carrots is 200 calories, and popcorn sold at movies ranges from 350 to 900 calories depending upon the size of the bag. Therefore, portion sizes as well as the number of times someone eats are important further considerations. Identifying the size of food portions is an important weight management tool.

2. *Is there concern about volume?* Understanding portion size requires more than a willingness to measure and weigh foods. Weighing and measuring can be tiring and are not always practical. Generally, a patient can learn which categories of foods tend to be high in calories and which categories are low enough to choose ad libitum. Vegetables, for example, do not need to be as carefully portioned as starches. A whole fruit is portion-controlled, yet there is a world of difference among apples and peaches in terms of size and calories, and between apples and peaches in nutritive value. Fish, even fatty fish, is generally low in calories, while most red meats are high in calories. Therefore, the caloric mistake the patient makes in eating eight ounces of salmon instead of four, is much less than the one that is made if the patient eats an equivalent amount of steak.

One of the important principles Jane F. learned was that her calories were not controlled merely because she lowered her fat intake. She tended to grab a plain bagel for breakfast. Lunch would be a sandwich or bean soup and a roll. She ate pretzels in the late afternoon whenever she got hungry. At night she would eat a large bowl of pasta, soaking up the no-fat tomato sauce with a slice of Italian bread (no butter, of course). She would add a small salad on the side for dinner and perhaps a piece of fruit afterward. Because of the large portions, her low-fat eating added up to 2200 calories per day.

Increasing her total intake of vegetables by adding them in large amounts to her spaghetti sauce, reducing her portion of pasta, eating fruit for breakfast, and substituting the bagel for the bread of her sandwich, Jane reduced her daily calories to approximately 1600. The nutritional content was higher than before. And most important, she is now able to continue eating the food she enjoys. Some days she chooses yogurt and fruit instead of a bagel to reduce the calories of her breakfast and increase the vitamin and mineral content.

3. *Is the pattern of eating stable?* An unstable eating pattern is one reason why counting calories is not necessarily helpful. Jane F. usually eats three meals and two snacks per day. But during a time of high stress she starts to eat six snacks per day, compensating for the extra food by eating smaller meals. Before long, her meals are not different from her snacks. Her calories at the end of the day may not be greater than usual, but there is no stable pattern to her eating. This kind of distorted eating is not conducive to long-term weight management because it wears the patient down, making it difficult to care about weight, and eating is not satisfying. With consistent counseling, Jane F. can monitor her eating patterns as well as her food choices, thereby stabilizing them when they become erratic. Another policy decision may be to establish a stable eating pattern rather than to rely on calorie counting in order to maintain or lose weight.

4. *Does overeating occur at a particular time of day?* When is the patient most likely to overeat? Every day at four in the afternoon? After dinner? Only in restaurants? If, for example, a patient eats large quantities of bread and pasta at night, maybe the dinner meal should contain controlled items in the starch category such as small baked potatoes. Or maybe patients get too hungry in the late afternoon, becoming ravenous by the time they return home in early evening. Such patients should eat a more substantial snack in the late afternoon, or have something pre-prepared at home to avoid nibbling indiscriminately on anything that's available when they walk through the door.

5. *What is the tolerance for failure?* Instead of fostering the "all or nothing" behavior that is typical of so many dieters, it is important to teach patients how to make choices, and be able to acknowledge the consequences. For example, it may not be appropriate for the dietitian to suggest that it is all right to buy a whole chocolate cake and expect the patient to eat just one piece when the patient has a history of eating half a cake. On the other hand, if patients enjoy chocolate cake, it would be just as absurd to suggest that they stay away from it altogether. So how does a patient accommodate the desire for chocolate cake and still have weight loss or weight maintenance? The patient makes a policy about it: "If I really want it, get the best, and eat it." That might mean that sometimes the patient will eat cereal and milk and fruit for breakfast, a large salad with tuna for lunch, and chocolate cake and milk for dinner. Or another patient might decide to have a small piece of chocolate cake every night. The policies are individualized, and the dietitian can help the patient experiment until the policy is successful.

6. *Special considerations.* Special considerations include grazing, such as eating snack-type foods all day long; binge eating,[41,42] and night-eating.[50] Binge eating and night-eating are discussed in Chapter 4. Some patients think of their overeating as binge eating when it is not, and are anxious about their night-eating when they only eat a rice cake or a carrot in the middle of the night. Therefore, the dietitian ensures that the patient's characterization of the problem is explained in detail so that the problem—and its management—can be assessed objectively. Formula may be a good alternative if someone is binge eating[8] when weight loss with regular food may be a difficult process. Most weight control centers are not set up to handle the special considerations of binge eating if it does not ebb within the first few weeks of the dietary treatment. Referral to a center specializing in binge eating disorders is then necessary.

Grazing, or snacking all day, can be dangerous for two reasons: remembering everything that was eaten is difficult, and consuming too many calories without any satisfaction is too easy. Consolidating these snacks and creating three meals each day can be very helpful to this type of eater.

MODIFYING BEHAVIOR

Most practitioners are well aware that a patient can hear something over and over again without internalizing it, until one day the patient suddenly sees a way to put the information into use. A typical example of this is one woman who was in a program for four years. She had some success, but was finding it difficult to maintain any weight loss. She attended a six-week workshop for overeaters, hoping that a new voice might help her. Indeed, when she returned she glowingly spoke about how she had had "an epiphany." What was this epiphany? That she should only eat when she was hungry! Obviously, she had been told this many times before, but suddenly, coming from a new voice, she was able to hear it.

There is evidence that modification of food behavior does not work.[8] Indeed, by tracing behavior modification treatment for obesity from its beginnings,[51] although success during treatment has been significant but small,[9] it has had almost no long-term effect.[8,9,51]

Many factors including genetics, fat cell number, metabolic rate, insulin resistance, and lipoprotein lipase activity[52-57] play a significant role in determining whether a person can sustain a substantial weight loss. Medication therapy, such as the use of fenfluramine, dexfenfluramine, and sibutramine also appears to make behavior modification nearly obsolete, since weight loss success is increased by the effect of the medication on body weight regulation.[58-61] However, long-term efficacy (i.e., longer than one or two years) of these medications has not been shown. Our own experience, as well as that of others[62] is that the effects of these medications may be greatest with concomitant changes in food choices and exercise, but that in fact, the effect on weight loss in most cases may be limited to less than 10% of initial weight. Medication may be more useful as a maintenance tool, although this has not been fully studied. Therefore, with or without medication, behavior modification remains one of the most valuable elements in the weight loss and weight-maintenance aspects of weight control.

Environment is one area in which people can exert some, albeit not complete, control. People cannot control the "obesifying" aspects of their environment, such as food availability and food advertising, but they can change their relationship to it. In a practical sense, this means that if patients can learn to manage external cues, they may be able to alter or adjust these effects on body weight. Modifying behavior may not result in weight change; nevertheless, in order to maintain weight, behavior must be modified continually as the environment changes. Behavior modification has often failed in weight loss programs, yet we find it valuable in some stages of weight management. Thinking that modifying some behaviors will result in life-long successful changes in a chronic disorder is naive. Although people do change, they tend to have more difficulty with change in certain areas, and return to old habits.[10] For an obese person, eating behavior is difficult to change for a lifetime, yet the effort to change deserves consistent support. An obese person put in an environment where food cannot be obtained will lose weight. If food is readily available, the person who has a susceptibility to gaining weight must learn how to manage the susceptibility. As with any susceptibility, there are times when one is more vulnerable than at other times; skills in eating management may help during these times.

Until the physiology of obesity is better understood and medication is improved, weight management programs should encourage behavioral changes as part of a continuous monitoring of this chronic condition; at times the patient will need stronger doses, and at times the patient will be able to function independently. Health practitioners in the field of obesity should expect a patient to have "flare-ups" or lapses in weight management over time. Without outside intervention, flare-ups can turn into severe relapses.[63] With continuous monitoring, a lapse stays smaller, more contained. The dieter and post-dieter may have many, many lapses—and interventions—until they gain confidence that indeed, they can get back on track. The health professional's job is to intervene, to help them get back on track, and to continue to support them so they can continue to manage their weight. Like hypertension patients who forget to take medication or deny their condition, obese patients may forget to modify their behavior and their environment unless health professionals continue to encourage and support the maintenance of their eating management skills.

Using Different Tools

A weight management center must be a "focuser"—a place where the patient can be redirected and supported to stay on track as well as a place for treatment of flare-ups. Therefore, the curriculum should include information and training that can be translated into different scenarios: for the patient who needs to understand nutrition better in order to eat healthier food; for the dieter who lost 20 lbs initially but has not been able to lose the other 30; for the patient who has lost 40 and regained 30; for the patient who is losing weight consistently and may be getting reckless, and finally, for weight maintenance.

Weight loss is predicated upon a simple, mathematical equation: if calorie consumption is less than calorie expenditure, weight loss will occur. Tools are creative ideas designed by the patient and the health professional to bring support and direction to the weight loss program. Tools are tangible action steps that help a person reach a goal.

If the tool is helpful, it will help set up roadblocks to make it harder to break the improved food and exercise patterns the patient has set. Much eating and overeating occurs when the patient loses focus and becomes fatigued at the difficulty of the process.

A diet is a tool. If a patient adheres to the policies of the diet, the patient will lose weight. But if a patient cannot follow one diet, then the health practitioner needs to be flexible enough to develop a different diet with the patient.

Food records are also a tool. For some people, keeping food records reduces their intake.[64] For others, they have no effect. Therefore, the feat is not in using food records; the feat is in finding a tool that is effective. For example, if a patient forgets to write down the food eaten, or if the daily calories continuously exceed the person's maintenance needs, then food records are not a good tool to help manage weight.

The practitioner must be creative, develop and try ideas until the correct match is made. If food records seem viable even though they seem ineffective in the traditional way, they can be used for calorie recording, rating hunger and satiety, and used at specific times to help the patient focus on snacking or after-dinner eating. Recording feelings about food is helpful.

The two patient examples, Jane F. and Jerry S. have both had success with tools. When Jane became bored with her food choices, she made a grid, looking at which foods she really enjoyed eating, and which of them were low calorie vs high calorie. What she found was that most of the foods she ate were not delicious at all, but mediocre, whether they were high or low fat, high or low calorie. She began to add more foods to her list of edibles, particularly those that were delicious but low fat and low calorie. She also omitted a lot of foods that she found mediocre such as low-fat ice cream and certain frozen foods. This was a wonderful tool for her to use to reduce total calories by increasing the foods she actually enjoyed more but which she didn't overeat.

Jerry S. was different. He was too afraid of food to add enjoyable foods. Instead, when he returned from formula to eating regular food, he tested his hunger by eating only half of whatever was on his plate, leaving the table for five minutes, and making a decision away from the table about whether he was hungry for more food.

"Try a tool," health practitioners should tell the patients. "If it doesn't work, try another." The point of trying is twofold: it helps the patient take action, which in itself is motivating and, if the idea is effective, the patient will have taken one more step toward to reaching that goal.

WEIGHT MAINTENANCE

The inability to maintain weight loss has been well-documented since 1959[65] when it was found that 95% of post-dieters returned to their pre-diet weights within five years. Yet, almost four decades later, the causes of weight recidivism remain elusive. Before the 1970s there was little data about long-term weight maintenance[66,67] and treatment was limited to the weight loss phase only. Furthermore, most weight loss data showed small weight loss. In the past 20 years weight loss treatments in combination with behavior therapy have been more successful during the weight loss phase.[68] However, maintenance of that weight loss continues to be all but impossible.[69] Weight management centers are beginning to offer more maintenance support, but not enough. Programs have changed from offering no maintenance, and then very short post-treatment sessions, to the current average length of 12 to 18 months. In one study summarizing data accumulated from controlled trials, the average length of follow-up increased from 15.5 weeks to 44 weeks (see Table 15–2).[70]

Although weight losses have increased because of VLCDs and longer treatments,[70] and weight maintenance has improved first-year maintenance statistics with a combi-

Table 15–2 Summary Analysis of Selected Studies from 1974–1990 Providing Treatment by Behavior Therapy and Conventional Reducing Diets

	1974	1978	1984	1985–1987	1988–1990
Number of studies included	15	17	15	13	5
Sample size	53.1	54.0	71.3	71.6	21.2
Initial weight (kg)	73.4	87.3	88.7	87.2	91.9
Length of treatment (wk)	8.4	10.5	13.2	15.6	21.3
Weight loss (kg)	3.8	4.2	6.9	8.4	8.5
Loss per week (kg)	0.5	0.4	0.5	0.5	0.4
Attrition (%)	11.4	12.9	10.6	13.8	21.8
Length of follow-up (wk)	15.5	30.3	58.4	48.3	53.0
Loss at follow-up (kg)	4.0	4.1	4.4	5.3	5.6

Source: Reprinted with permission from T.A. Wadden and S.J. Bartlett, Very Low Calorie Diets: An Overview and Appraisal, in *Treatment of the Seriously Obese Patient,* T.A. Wadden and T.B. VanItallie, eds., p. 65, © 1992, Guilford Press.

nation of behavioral and cognitive restructuring, diet, exercise, and social support,[71,72] five-year follow-up results remain discouraging. Longer-term programs remain almost nonexistent[3] as do their follow-up statistics.[70] And what is available is vague at best. Sporadically recorded weights do not lend insight into what may have occurred in between collected weights.[73] Follow-up weights are often measured annually (or less often). Bjorvell and Rossner[67] looked at weights over 10 years, but follow-up data was based on a 6-month follow-up, and then 2, 4, and 10 years, with no description of what occurred in between. In our center, some weight regain can actually be considered appropriate. After the barrage of short-term maintenance follow-up reports that show weight recidivism,[74-76] it is surprising that some people still expect weight maintenance to result in a flat weight graph. If obesity is a chronic disorder, then flare-ups will occur. Changes in socioeconomic factors, marriage, goal weight, support, etc., all seem to affect outcome.[77-79] This may mean that clinical interventions must occur more quickly, and that the health practitioner must be more aggressive about suggesting treatment at the time of small increases in weight.

What is weight maintenance? The term may perpetuate the all or nothing thinking that is so common among dieters. Asking someone to maintain weight loss without fluctuations is tantamount to asking a person with diabetes to show no fluctuations in blood sugar no matter what the situation.

Much is made of high recidivism rates,[80] the dismal failure of diets,[81] and how weight maintenance should be rethought.[72] Though the diet business has taken advantage of cultural ideals of thinness, weight loss for obesity remains crucial in order to alleviate many of the health risk factors associated with overweight.[82]

So what should the health practitioner do? Just as with any chronic disorder, instead of looking so bleakly at recidivism, practitioners must redefine their criteria for success. Does any weight regain during maintenance mean failure? What if the patient has regained 35 kg but is still 10 kg less than the initial weight? And what if concomitant risks are still reduced even if weight regain is substantial?

There is no accurate definition of weight maintenance, thereby making it difficult to measure success accurately. Weight maintenance is generally discussed, in terms of weight only. What does it mean to maintain weight loss? If it is to keep weight stable, within what range? Consider Jerry S. seven years later. Originally he lost 100 lbs on formula. After seven years, he has gained 50 lbs. Is he a failure or a success? True, he is 50 lbs heavier, but he is also 50 lbs lighter than he was when he began the program. Isn't Jerry a success compared with even the five-year statistics? And shouldn't the counselor work with him so that he understands that success, accepts it, and works to maintain his current 50-lb weight loss?

When the authors review our own long-term data of people who have been coming regularly to weight-maintenance classes, we see what one might expect in successful maintainers—weight fluctuations, usually within manageable ranges. (See Figure 15–3.)

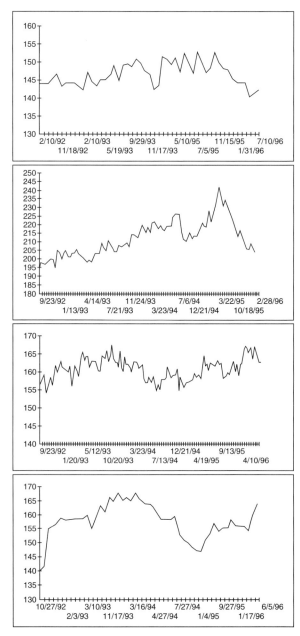

Figure 15–3 Examples of typical maintenance weights over four years post weight loss. Weights are on the vertical axis.

Each fluctuation is individual: some post-dieters regain immediately after weight loss is complete; some maintain their weight within 2 lbs for three years and then regain some weight; some have stable months and some have substantial weight increases during short periods of time. Although patients should be expected to try to lose weight when their weight increases, their primary goal should be not to gain more weight.

CONCLUSION

It is impossible with a condition like obesity, whose management is predicated on the equation energy intake = energy expended, not to expect life changes to interfere with newly formed eating and exercise patterns. The formerly obese person may create new and more supportive ways to live, but flare-ups can take many shapes and require cooperative monitoring and management.

Some weight gain is implicit in this disorder. Practitioners must become more effective in developing problem-solving skills with patients that support return for periodic checkups and interventions.[83] For example, a patient who was an avid exerciser found that when her work hours were increased dramatically due to a job promotion, this caused a disruption in her pattern that she couldn't quite correct.

Although lean people may not realize the difficulty in modifying food and exercise patterns to fit into changing lifestyles, for the formerly obese, it is like re-creating the wheel. As Jane F. said after four years in maintenance, "I play tennis three times, sometimes four times a week, two hours a day. I walk on the other days. Then I eat half a loaf of bread. So I'm gaining weight . . . am I going to do this for the rest of my life?" Yes, practitioners have to say. And then practitioners must offer them encouragement and tools to help them get back on track.

How do you explain, as another subject said, "that after three years I have gone through many stressful situations and I was shocked that I could take a step back and say I didn't deal with them using food. You don't feel deprived, you just feel noble. And it's all working. . . . Then, in some other place, for some other reason, you say 'what a wonderful excuse for me to fall off the wagon' and you do."

Perri et al[71] have shown that consistent contact of almost any kind helps reduce the risk of complete weight recidivism. Weight-maintenance support should be offered literally, not figuratively, for a lifetime. It should not be a reiteration of a diet, as much as a focus on everyday life and the integration of old and new policies so that successful dieters can be refocused and reminded of helpful behaviors that can help them keep their weight within a manageable range.

Weight management programs must have long-term maintenance support groups, but they must also define weight maintenance in terms that include more than just keeping weight off, such as maintenance of healthy behaviors. If the weight management center's definition of weight maintenance includes some weight gain, then weight-maintenance success will mean weight that is kept within a manageable but fluctuating range. This changes the whole premise of maintenance and gives the patient room to make mistakes and get back on track. It is critical for patients to understand that lapsing is appropriate and expected. It's how quickly they get back on track that is important.

The definition of weight maintenance should also include health status compared to the patient's health status at entry into the program. Are lipids still lower even though some weight has been regained? Is blood pressure lower? Is the person still exercising? Has the patient had fewer sick days?

What about longer-term support groups? After almost four decades of studies, have practitioners only moved from thinking that the formerly obese need no post-diet treatment to thinking that 1 year or even 18 months is enough? It may be that for every program offering weight loss, a coordinated post-dieting management program must also be offered—and that it should be offered for as long as the patient will attend regular monitoring sessions for support.

Furthermore, the outlook on post-dieting may become brighter if, instead of weight maintenance, practitioners and patients call it Healthstage, to encourage a healthier lifestyle including, but not limited to, weight management. As was stated so aptly by the Institute of Medicine's book on evaluating approaches to treat obesity, "We recommend that weight-loss programs evolve into weight-management programs and be judged more by their effects on the overall health of participants than by their effects on weight alone."[22]

REFERENCES

1. Kuczmarski RJ, Flegal KM, Campbell SM, Johnson CL. Increasing prevalence of overweight among US adults. National Health and Nutrition Examination Surveys. 1960–1991. *JAMA.* 1994;272:205–211.

2. VanItallie TB, Lew EA. Assessment of morbidity and mortality risk in the overweight patient. In: Wadden TA, VanItallie TB, eds. *Treatment of the Seriously Obese Patient.* New York: Guilford Press; 1992:3–11.

3. Robison JI, Hoerr SL, Strandmark J, Mavis B. Obesity, weight loss, and health. *J Am Diet Assoc.* 1993;93:445–449.

4. Willett WC, Manson JE, Stamfer MJ, et al. Weight, weight change, and coronary heart disease in women; risk within the "normal" weight range. *JAMA.* 1995;273:461–465.

5. Pi-Sunyer FX. Short-term medical benefits and adverse effects of weight loss. *Ann Intern Med.* 1993;119:722–726.

6. Zhang Y, Proenca R, Maffel M, Barone M, Leopold L, Friedman JM. Positional cloning of the mouse obese gene and its human homologue. *Nature.* 1994;372:425–432.

7. Pelleymounter MA, Cullen MJ, Baker MB, et al. Effects of the obese gene product on body weight regulation in ob/ob mice. *Science.* 1995;269:540–543.

8. Wilson GT. Behavioral treatment of obesity: thirty years and counting. *Behav Res Ther.* 1994;16:31–75.

9. Wadden TA, Sternberg JA, Letizia KA, Stunkard AJ, Foster GD. Treatment of obesity by very low calorie diet, behavior therapy, and their combination: a five-year perspective. *Int J Obes.* 1989;13:39–46.

10. Prochaska JO, DiClemente CC, Norcross JC. In search of how people change. *Am Psychol.* 1992;47:1102–1114.

11. NIH Technology Assessment Conference Panel. Methods for voluntary weight loss and control. *Ann Intern Med.* 1992;116:942–949.

12. Blackburn GL. Comparison of medically supervised and unsupervised approaches to weight loss and control. *Ann Intern Med.* 1993;199:714–718.

13. Heymsfield SB, Jain P, Ortiz O, Waki M. Cardiac structure and function in markedly obese patients before and after weight loss. In: Wadden TA, VanItallie TB, eds. *Treatment of the Seriously Obese Patient.* New York: Guilford Press; 1992:136–161.

14. Metropolitan Life Insurance Company. 1983 height and weight tables. *Stat Bull Metro Insurance Co.* 1984;64:2–9.

15. Manson JE, Willett WC, Stamfer MJ, et al. Body weight and mortality among women. *N Engl J Med.* 1995;333:677–685.

16. Garrow JS. Introduction. *Treat Obesity Seriously.* Edinburgh, Scotland: Churchill Livingstone; 1981:1.

17. Nonas CA, Aronoff NJ, Pi-Sunyer FX. Dietary strategies for weight loss. *Endocr Prac.* 1995;1:28–286.

18. Bjorntorp P. Regional fat distribution: implications for type II diabetes. *Int J Obes.* 1992;16: S19–S27.

19. Telch CF, Agras WS. The effects of a very low calorie diet on binge eating. *Behav Ther.* 1993;24:177–194.

20. Wooley SC, Garner DA. Obesity treatment: the high cost of false hope. *J Am Diet Assoc.* 1991;91:1248–1251.

21. Drewnowski A. Toward safe weight loss: recommendations for adult weight loss programs in Michigan. Task Force to Establish Weight Loss Guidelines. Petersmarck KA, ed. East Lansing, MI: Michigan Health Council; 1990.

22. Institute of Medicine, National Academy of Sciences. *Weighing the Options.* Washington DC: National Academy Press; 1995.

23. Seidell JC. Regional obesity and health. *Int J Obes.* 1992;16:S31–S34.

24. Yang MU, VanItallie TB. Effect of energy restriction on body composition and nitrogen balance in obese individuals. In: Wadden TA, VanItallie TB, eds. *Treatment of the Seriously Obese Patient.* New York: Guilford Press; 1992:83–106.

25. Mirvis DM. The significance of a prolonged Q-T interval. *Hosp Prac.* 1986;45–54.

26. Towbin J. Clinical implications of basic research. *N Engl J Med.* 1995;384–385.

27. Life Sciences Research Office. *Research Needs in Management of Obesity by Severe Caloric Restriction.* Washington, DC: Federation of American Societies for Experimental Biology; 1979. FDA 223-75-2090.

28. Foster GD, Wadden TA, Peterson FJ, Letizia KA, Bartlett SA, Conill AM. A controlled comparison of three very-low-calorie diets: effects on weight, body composition, and symptoms. *Am J Clin Nutr.* 1992;55:811–817.

29. Harris HA, Benedict FG. *A Biometric Study of Basal Metabolism in Man.* Washington, DC: Carnegie Institute; 1919. Publication 279.

30. Franz MJ, Horton ES, Bantle JP, et al. Nutrition principles for the management of diabetes and related complications. *Diabetes Care.* 1994;17:490–511.

31. National Research Council. *Recommended Dietary Allowances.* 10th ed. Washington, DC: National Academy Press; 1989.

32. VanItallie TB. The dietary treatment of severe obesity. In: Hamner JE III, ed. *The 1988 Distinguished Visiting Professorship Lectures.* Memphis, TN: University of Tennessee Press; 1989:33–44.

33. Rasmussen, A. The relationship between Qt_c changes and nutrition during weight loss after gastroplasty. *Acta Medica Scandinavica.* 1985;217:271–275.

34. VanItallie TB. Liquid protein mayhem. *JAMA.* 1978;240:140–141.

35. Vasquez JA, Morse EL, Adibi SA. Effect of dietary fat, carbohydrate and protein on branched-chain amino acid catabolism during caloric restriction. *J Clin Invest.* 1985;76:734–743.

36. Surgeon General's Report and Recommendations. Washington, DC: US Government Printing Office; 1988. DHHS Publication (PHS) 88-50211, Appendix C.

37. Stone, BG, Ansel HJ, Peterson FJ, Gebhard, RL. Gallbladder emptying stimuli in obese and normal-weight subjects. *Hepatology.* 1992;15:795–798.

38. Levinson DE, Fromm H. Ten grams fat per day may keep gallstones away. *Gastroenterology.* 1993;104:1880–1881.

39. Weinsier RL, Bacon JA, Birch R. Time-calorie displacement diet for weight control: a prospective evaluation of its adequacy for maintaining normal nutritional status. *Int J Obes.* 1983;7:539–548.

40. Pi-Sunyer, FX. Obesity. In: Rajek RD, ed. *Conn's Current Therapy.* Philadelphia: WB Saunders; 1994:546–551.

41. Wilson GT, Nonas CA, Rosenblum GD. Assessment of binge eating in obese patients. *Int J Eating Dis.* 1993;13:25–33.

42. Spitzer RL, Devlin M, Walsh BT, et al. Binge eating disorders: a multisite field trial of the diagnostic criteria. *Int J Eating Dis.* 1991;11:191–203.

43. Wadden TA, Bartlett SJ. Very low calorie diets: an overview and appraisal. In: Wadden TA, VanItallie TB, eds. *Treatment of the Seriously Obese Patient.* New York: Guilford Press; 1992:65.

44. Wing RR, Marcus MD, Salata R, et al. Effects of a very-low-calorie diet on long-term glycemic control in obese type II diabetics. *Ann Intern Med.* 1991;151:1334–1340.

45. Hyman FA, Sempose E, Saltsman J, Glinsmann WH. Evidence for success of caloric restriction in weight loss and control. *Ann Intern Med.* 1993;119:681–687.

46. Chernoff R, Lipschitz DA. Nutrition and aging. In: Shils ME, Young VR, eds. *Modern Nutrition in Health and Disease.* Philadelphia: Lee & Febiger; 1988:982–1000.

47. Goldfarb, S. Dietary factors in the pathogenesis and prophylaxis of calcium nephrolithiasis. *Kidney Int.* 1988;38:544–555.

48. LaPorte DJ, Stunkard AJ. Predicting attrition and adherence to a very-low-calorie diet: a prospective investigation of the Eating Inventory. *Int J Obes.* 1990;14:197–206.

49. Jeffrey RW, Wing RR, Thorson C, et al. Strengthening behavioral interventions for weight loss: a randomized trial of food provision and monetary incentives. *J Consult Clin Psychol.* 1993;61:1038–1045.

50. Aronoff NJ, Geliebter A, Hashim SA, Zammit, GK. The relationship between daytime and nighttime food intake in an obese night-eater. *Obes Res.* 1994;2:145–151.

51. Ferster CB, Nurnberge JI, Levitt EF. The control of eating. *J Math.* 1962;1:87–109.

52. Considine RV, Considine EL, Williams CJ, et al. Evidence against either a premature stop codon or the absence of obese gene mRNA in human obesity. *J Clin Invest.* 1995;95:2986–2988.

53. Walston J, Silver K, Bogardus C, et al. Time of onset of non-insulin dependent diabetes mellitus and genetic variation in the B3-adrenergic-receptor gene. *N Engl J Med.* 1995;333:343–347.

54. Bjorntorp P. Regional fat distribution—implications for type II diabetes. *Int J Obes.* 1992;16:S19–S27.

55. Leibel RL, Rosenbaum M, Hirsch J. Changes in energy expenditure resulting from altered body weight. *N Engl J Med.* 1995;332:673–674.

56. Fried SK, Russell CD, Grauso NL, Brolin RE. Lipoprotein lipase regulation by insulin and glucocorticoid in subcutaneous and omental adipose tissues of obese women and men. *J Clin Invest.* 1993;92:1–8.

57. Kern, PA, Ong JM, Saffari B, Carty J. The effects of weight loss on the activity and expression of adipose-tissue lipoprotein lipase in very obese humans. *N Engl J Med.* 1990;322:1053–1059.

58. Guy-Grand B. Long-term pharmacological treatment of obesity. In: Wadden TA, VanItallie TB, eds. *Treatment of the Seriously Obese Patient.* New York: Guilford Press; 1992:456–482.

59. Spitz A, Heymsfield S, Blank RC. Drug therapy for obesity: clinical considerations. *Endocr Prac.* 1995;1:274–279.

60. Kogon MM, Krauchi K, et al. Psychological and metabolic effects of dietary carbohydrates and dexfenfluramine during a low-energy diet in obese women. *Am J Clin Nutr.* 1994;60:488–493.

61. VanItallie TB. Introduction. *Metabolism.* 1995;44:1–3.

62. Russell RM. Nutrition. *JAMA.* 1995;273:1699–1700.

63. Marlatt GA, Gordon J. *Relapse Prevention.* New York: Guilford; 1985.

64. Heger JB, Trumble TL, Kalyandrug S. Attitudes of overweight women toward keeping written food records. *J Am Diet Assoc.* 1991;9:A–54.

65. Stunkard A, McLaren-Hume M. The results of treatment for obesity. *Arch Intern Med.* 1959;103:79–85.

66. Bjorvell H, Rossner S. Long-term treatment of severe obesity: four-year follow-up of results of combined behavioural modification programme. *Br Med J.* 1985;291:379–382.

67. Bjorvell H, Rossner S. A ten-year follow-up of weight change in severely obese subjects treated in a combined behavioural modification programme. *Int J Obes.* 1992;16:623–625.

68. Wadden TA, Bell ST. Understanding and treating obesity. In: Bellack AS, Hersen M, Kazdin AE, eds. *International Handbook of Behavior Modification and Therapy.* 2nd ed. New York: Plenum; 1990.

69. Wadden TA, Stunkard AJ, Liebshutz J. Three-year follow-up of the treatment of obesity by very low calorie diet, behavior therapy and their combination. *J Consult Clin Psychol.* 1988;56:925–928.

70. Brownell KD, Wadden TA. Etiology and treatment of obesity: understanding a serious, prevalent and refractory disorder. *J Consult Clin Psychol.* 1992;60:505–517.

71. Perri MG. Improving maintenance of weight loss following treatment by diet and lifestyle modification. In: Wadden TA, VanItallie TB, eds. *Treatment of the Seriously Obese Patient.* New York: Guilford Press; 1992:456.

72. Perri MG, McAllister DA, Gange JJ, Nezu AM. Effects of four maintenance programs on the long-term management of obesity. *J Consult Clin Psychol.* 1988;56:529–534.

73. Brownell K. Relapse and the treatment of obesity. In: Wadden TA, VanItallie TB, eds. *Treatment of the Seriously Obese Patient.* New York: Guilford Press; 1992:441.

74. Hovell MF, Koch A, Hofstetter R, et al. Long-term weight loss maintenance: assessment of a behavioral supplemented fasting regimen. *Am J Public Health.* 1988;78: 663–666.

75. Andersen T, Stokholm KH, Backer OG, Quadde F. Long-term (5 year) results after either horizontal gastroplasty or very-low-calorie diet for morbid obesity. *Int J Obes.* 1988;12:277–284.

76. Holden JH, Darga LL, Olson SM, et al. Long-term follow-up of patients attending a combination very-low calorie diet and behaviour therapy weight loss programme. *Int J Obes.* 1992;16:605–613.

77. Wolfe BL. Long-term maintenance following attainment of goal weight: a preliminary investigation. *Addict Behav.* 1992;17:469–477.

78. Kayman S, Bruvold W, Stern JS. Maintenance and relapse after weight loss in women: behavioral aspects. *Am J Clin Nutr.* 1990;52:800–807.

79. Dubbert PM, Wilson GT. Goal setting and spouse involvement in the treatment of obesity. *Behav Res Ther.* 1984;22:227–242.

80. Kramer FM, Jeffery RW, Forster JL, Snell MK. Long-term follow-up of behavioral treatment for obesity: patterns of weight regain among men and women. *Int J Obes.* 1989;13:123–136.

81. Brownell KD, Marlatt GA, Lichtenstein E, Wilson GT. Understanding and preventing relapse. *Am Psychol.* 1986;41:765–782.

82. Goodrick KG, Foreyt JP. Why treatments for obesity don't last. *J Am Diet Assoc.* 1991;91:1243–1247.

83. Brownell KD, Rodin J. The dieting maelstrom. Is it possible and advisable to lose weight? *Am Psychol.* 1994;49:781–791.

CHAPTER 16

The Role of Diet and Exercise in Weight Management

Wayne C. Miller
Alice K. Lindeman

WEIGHT REDUCTION DIETS OVER THE PAST 40 YEARS

Of the two main components in weight management, diet has a longer history than exercise. This chapter reviews some of that history including the goals of diet and exercise, their effectiveness in practice, and contemporary aspects such as the anti-dieting movement.

As stated by the California Dietetic Association in its 1988 review of weight control approaches, a weight reduction diet should:

- satisfy all nutrient needs except energy
- meet individual tastes and habits
- minimize hunger and fatigue
- be readily obtainable and socially acceptable
- favor the establishment of a changed eating pattern
- be conducive to improvement of overall health.[1]

Throughout the years, dietitians and nutritionists have advocated weight loss through a balanced, energy-controlled diet in conjunction with lifestyle changes, to produce moderate consistent weight loss. Although this may be the healthiest way to lose weight, it is not necessarily the way the public wishes to lose weight.

Approaches to weight loss through dieting have undergone quite a metamorphosis over the past 40 years. Diets to reduce weight can be classified by their degree of energy restriction and by their contribution of macronutrients. Table 16–1 gives energy and macronutrient breakdown of weight reduction diets typical of their era. During the late 1950s and early 1960s, total starvation was used to reduce the weight of the massively obese. Drenick et al[2] showed a 1.0 kg/day weight loss in obese men during the initial week, with a decrease to 0.5 kg/day

Table 16–1 Distribution of Calories in Popular Diets Over the Past 40 Years

Diet	Calories	% Carbohydrate	% Protein	% Fat
High protein, low carbohydrate (1960s–early 1970s)				
Atkins[5,6]	2136	5	23	72
Stillman[6,7]	1304	7	45	48
Protein-sparing modified fasts (1970s)				
Last chance diet[6,8]	300–400	100		
Commercial very-low-calorie diets (1980s)				
Optifast[9]	450	29	60	4
	800	50	35	15
HMR[10]	500	58	40	2
	800	49	40	18
Commercial prepackaged diets (1980s–early 1990s)				
Nutri/System[11,12]	1200	60	20	20
Jenny Craig[11,13]	1100	60	20	20
Low-fat diets (1990s)				
Pritikin[6,14]	1200	65	25	10
T-Factor Quick Melt[15]	1200/1700	60	24	16

after one month of fasting. Although this method did produce rapid weight loss and could be conducted with relative ease under medical supervision, fasting did have serious side effects, i.e., significant loss of lean body mass and electrolytes, especially potassium, and some deaths.[2–4]

In the late 1960s and early 1970s focus was placed on high-protein diets to reduce weight. Diets promoted by Atkins[5] and Stillman and Baker[7] provided significant protein and fat to not only prevent muscle catabolism, but also contributed to a "ketogenic" state with its associated appetite suppression. The significant carbohydrate restriction did produce rapid weight loss through loss of glycogen stores and diuresis, and possibly decreased energy intake associated with the lack of variety in the diet. As soon as the dieters reintroduced carbohydrate, some weight was gained due to refeeding edema. Some unfortunate side effects of the high-protein, low-carbohydrate diet included nausea and hyperuricemia associated with the ketosis, and fatigue associated with the depleted glycogen stores.[16]

In the mid-1970s very-low-calorie liquid diets became commercially available. Studies on semistarvation noted that administering even small amounts of protein during a fast could dramatically reduce protein and potassium losses observed in total starvation, but at the same time, one could produce the same rapid weight loss seen in total starvation.[3,8,17,18] These diets were known as protein-sparing modified fasts, or liquid protein diets. Unfortunately these diets were not as safe as initially thought. Fifty-eight deaths in 1977 and 1978 had been reported of persons having followed the liquid protein diets for weight reduction. Researchers from the Food and Drug Administration and the Center for Disease Control investigated the pattern of these deaths. Common to all deaths were the facts that the subjects had been markedly obese at the onset of dieting, had prolonged use of extremely low-calorie diets (300 to 400 kcal/day) and experienced significant weight loss. Death, due to ventricular arrhythmia, was independent of the presence of medical supervision, daily potassium supplementation, and biological quality of the protein used. These findings were contrary to the initial thought that death was attributed to inadequate potassium intake, and/or that the protein used in the formulas, either collagen or gelatin, was of poor biological quality. The researchers concluded that the use of these very-low-calorie weight reduction regimens should be terminated until further studies could assure their safety.[8]

A second generation of very-low-calorie diets became popular in the early 1980s. These commercial formula products, including Optifast[9] and HMR,[10] were embedded in a program of medical supervision, patient support sessions and counseling for weight maintenance after initial loss. Potential clients were screened for eligibility according to age, degree of overweight, preexisting medical conditions, and commitment to the lifestyle to lose and keep off the excess weight. Clients were initially only offered 450 to 500 calorie programs. Later, 800 calorie diets were considered more appropriate for men and those women who wanted to be more active. Costs for such programs ranged from $250 to $3000, depending on the weight loss desired. If the obesity was considered health debilitating, program costs could be covered by health insurance.[11]

Meanwhile, low-calorie balanced diets were literally being packaged and sold to dieters. Such franchises as Nutri/System[12] and Jenny Craig Weight Loss Centers[13] offered clients prepackaged foods, exercise and nutrition counseling, along with group support with a physician's approval for participation. Follow-up monitoring and counseling programs were offered for weight maintenance. To join such programs cost $29 to $300, with mandatory prepackaged food purchases averaging $70/week.[11]

In the early 1990s the commercial dieting industry came under close scrutiny by its consumers and the federal government. In September 1990, congressional hearings on the diet industry reviewed all aspects of the weight loss industry, but focused especially on advertising and promotional materials considered by some as false and deceptive. There was criticism that the diet industry was not providing accurate information to the public about the rate of weight loss for its clients nor how long clients were able to maintain the weight loss. As a result of these hearings, the Federal Trade

Commission stipulated that weight loss companies were to substantiate their weight loss claims with objective scientific studies, to state the average length of time customers maintained weight loss, and to include a disclaimer in their promotional information that many dieters find weight loss only temporary.[11]

Many commercial weight loss programs still exist in the 1990s, but with significantly more individualized offerings. The liquid formula diet programs now offer options for clients to consume liquid meal replacements and/or prepackaged foods. Clients can now consume from 500 to 1300 calorie plans. Most programs now emphasize exercise and behavior change as critical components to weight loss and maintenance.[11]

In 1989 the Surgeon General's Report on Nutrition and Health, and the National Research Council's Diet and Health Report stressed the role of reducing body weight and dietary fat intake as a means of disease prevention.[19,20] At the same time, the food industry introduced reduced-fat and fat-free versions of foods that were formerly only available in moderate- to high-fat levels. New fat-restricted diets became numerous and popular. Pritikin,[14] who pioneered stringent low-fat diets (<10%) in the late 1970s as a part of a lifestyle to decrease the risks of degenerative diseases, became popular in the late 1980s. In 1989 Katahn[15] introduced consumers to the T-Factor diet, a plan to reduce weight with a dietary intake of no more than 20% fat. The diet promoted counting fat gram intake and disregarding energy intake. Confirmation that fat restriction enhanced weight loss was reported by Kendall and colleagues[21] at Cornell University. Non-obese women (average weight 62 kg) were free to choose ad libitum from diets of 35% to 40% fat or 20% to 25% fat. Both the high-fat and low-fat consumers ate the same gram weight of food. However, the low-fat consumers averaged significantly greater weight loss on the low-fat diet (0.23 kg/wk) than those on the high-fat diet (0.11 kg/wk.) The low-fat consumers also averaged 500 calories less per day than the high-fat consumers. The researchers concluded that the results indicated that body weight could be lost by merely reducing the fat content of the diet without the necessity of voluntarily restricting food intake. The researchers did not, however, indicate if weight loss was due to eating less fat or to eating less calories. In the Women's Health Trial Feasibility Study, a low-fat dietary intervention study to prevent breast cancer, Sheppard and others[22] found that after one year, obese women (>150% ideal body weight) who had decreased fat intake from 39.2% to 21.6% total calories lost 3.1 kg of body weight. The controls, from the same original pool of candidates, only slightly modified fat intake, from 38.9% to 37.3%, and experienced a 0.4 kg loss during the year. Through multivariate analysis it was found that the weight loss was best predicted by reduction in dietary fat contribution to the diet, rather than the total energy intake. See Chapter 10 on diet composition and regulation of energy intake.

The American public today has embraced the concept that low-fat diets can induce weight loss. However, it is unclear whether such severe restrictions as those promoted by Pritikin[14] and Ornish[23] (i.e., only 10% of calories from fat) promote more weight loss than those containing 20% to 30% fat. Furthermore, since the early 1990s when many of these low-fat diets were studied and heavily promoted there has been an abundance of low-fat and fat-free calorie-rich snack foods on the market, such as crackers, cookies, candy, cake, and frozen desserts. The concern now is that dieters consuming these low-fat snacks could still over-consume energy while controlling fat intake.

WEIGHT MAINTENANCE AFTER WEIGHT REDUCTION

Recent research indicates that fat restriction is critical not only for weight reduction, but especially for weight maintenance. Current evidence suggests that the body is not "energy blind," i.e., all energy nutrients contribute equally to energy balance. There appear to be separate regulators of carbohydrate, protein, and fat metabolism. Astrup and Raban[24] propose that energy balance can only be achieved by macronutrient balance. In turn, achievement of macronutrient balance requires that the net oxidation of each macronutrient equals the average amount of the same macronutrient in the diet. Overconsumption of fat, for example, to the point that its ingestion exceeds the body's ability to oxidize it, could then lead to lipid storage, regardless of the total energy intake. Based mainly on animal research by Flatt,[25] this concept has recently been applied to postobese individuals. Current thought is that genetically predisposed individuals may have an impaired capacity to oxidize dietary fat, and thus when consuming a high-fat diet, have a tendency to store body fat in the absence of hyperphagia.[24,26–29]

To investigate the level of dietary fat intake in which preferential lipid deposition may occur in humans, Astrup and colleagues[28] matched nine formerly obese women with genetic predisposition to obesity to never-obese controls and fed them all diets of varying fat intake. The subjects ate isocaloric diets of 20% fat (low fat), 30% fat (medium fat), and 50% fat (high fat) for three days prior to and the day of a 24-hour respiratory chamber stay. After adjusting the 24-hour energy intake to equal output, Astrup and colleagues found that in all subjects consuming the 20% or 30% fat diets there was no difference in macronutrient (carbohydrate and fat) oxidation. However, those formerly obese women who had consumed the 50% fat diet were unable to increase the ratio of fat to carbohydrate oxidation appropriately, resulting in a positive (+11.0 g/day) fat balance. This inability to adequately oxidize fat was not observed in the never-obese women. The formerly obese, unlike the controls, also experienced an increased 24-hour energy expenditure with the low-fat diet. The authors concluded that independent of energy balance, an increase in dietary fat content to 50% fat results in preferential fat storage, impaired suppression of carbohydrate oxidation, and decreased energy expenditure in formerly obese women. Raban and others[26] found an altered fat oxidation in formerly obese women in response to a single high-fat meal. Compared to controls, previously obese women with a familial history of obesity had a 2.5 greater suppression of postprandial fat oxidation when fed a 50% fat meal.

In these cases, it appears that previously obese subjects, especially those with a genetic predisposition to obesity, can adequately oxidize dietary fat until the contribution of the fat reaches 30% of total caloric intake. Perhaps the ceiling for tolerance may be higher, but it is clear that at 50% fat, a preference for lipid storage occurs. Caution must be exercised in interpreting these results, as the experiments were conducted over only a few days. It is not clear if prolonged intake of high-fat diets, though energy controlled, can result in greater fat deposition in those genetically predisposed to obesity. But one can consider that by maintaining a moderately low-fat diet of 20% to 30% fat may help control regain of body fat in formerly obese individuals. Severe fat restriction, i.e., 10% to 20% fat, does not appear to have added benefit. Such severe restriction may actually encourage poorer adherence because of the associated cost, lack of variety, and boredom with food choices.

THE ROLE OF EXERCISE IN WEIGHT MANAGEMENT

Only in the last 20 years has the medical community recognized the critical role of exercise in weight control. In 1975, *Harrison's Principles of Internal Medicine*,[30] a highly respected medical reference, stated that although exercise was a good method to increase energy loss for weight reduction, it was very difficult to induce obese subjects to exercise, particularly for any length of time. Though excellent for the psyche and the circulation, exercise was deemed minimal in its overall caloric effect, when compared to a reduction in energy intake. Medicine has certainly changed its stand! The 1991 edition of the same book states that exercise has a place in any weight reduction program; incorporation of regular exercise into the overall weight reduction program will improve the chances that the patient will maintain the weight loss.[31]

The purpose of exercise is to promote strength, muscular endurance, flexibility, cardiorespiratory endurance, maintenance or enhancement of lean muscle mass, and increased motor skill performance. Any or all of these components of fitness can promote emotional and psychological well-being.[32] Exercise is described in terms of its mode, frequency, duration, and intensity. Each of these variables must be considered when designing an effective exercise program to promote weight loss. The American College of Sports Medicine provides some guidelines for exercise prescription for obesity reduction and weight maintenance.

- Goal: increase caloric expenditure.
- Mode: first choice is walking. Alternative modes include stair climbing, cycling, and water exercise.

- Intensity should be at the low end of target heart rate range, i.e., 50% to 60% VO_2max.
- Duration sufficient to cause expenditure of 200 to 300 kcal/session.
- Frequency should be a minimum of three times a week.

The guidelines also offer the following exercise precautions for the obese:

- Avoid stress on joints.
- Choose a setting that minimizes social stigma.
- Monitor muscle soreness and orthopaedic problems.[33]

Because obese individuals are at an increased relative risk for orthopaedic injury, most individuals are encouraged to maintain a lower intensity, longer duration of exercise in order to meet the energy expenditure goal of 200 to 300 kcal/session. Cross-training (rotation of exercise modalities) may be encouraged to prevent injuries and to enhance motor skill development. With development of skill, confidence, strength, and cardiovascular endurance, exercise programs should be manipulated to promote a high total caloric expenditure of 300 to 500 kcal/session, or 1000 to 2000 kcal/wk.[33]

Many obese individuals have had a long sedentary lifestyle and many have had poor experiences with exercise in the past. In addition to medical clearance to exercise, ideally the obese should begin their exercise program under the guidance of an exercise professional, either with a supervised group exercise program or an experienced personal trainer. Under such supervision, past negative experiences can be overcome and current strengths and interests can be emphasized. In addition, the individual attention can encourage the advancement to higher-intensity exercise, and incorporating higher energy expenditure activities into everyday life. The needs and goals of the obese can be matched with the exercise program to achieve long-term weight management, and the incorporation of exercise as an integral part of a healthy lifestyle.[32–34]

COMBINING DIET PLUS EXERCISE TO LOSE WEIGHT

Research studies conducted in the early 1970s confirmed that reduction in body fatness in overweight or obese individuals could be achieved through exercise without concurrent energy restriction. The fat loss was often small, occurring after a significant amount of low-intensity exercise.[35–39] Zuti and Golding[40] conducted one of the early studies combining diet and exercise to reduce weight. Women judged to be 20 to 40 lbs overweight were placed on weight-maintenance diets. They were then randomly placed on one of three regimens: 500 calorie deficit by diet alone; 250 calorie deficit by diet plus 250 calorie deficit through exercise; or 500 calorie deficit achieved through exercise alone. The exercise programs were supervised and careful food and exercise records were maintained. After 16 weeks, there was no difference in total weight loss (10.6 to 12.0 lb) but there was a difference in body composition. The exercise and combination groups increased lean body weight (+2.0 and +1.1 lb, respectively) where the diet alone group lost lean mass (–2.4 lb). The exercise groups also lost greater fat weight (–12.6 lb exercise alone, –13.1 lb combination) than those who only dieted (–9.3 lb). From the results of this and previous studies, the role of exercise in preserving or enhancing lean body mass for weight loss became evident.[35–40] Combining restricted energy intake with exercise may enhance fat loss more than just exercise alone.

Historically, and as advocated by the American College of Sports Medicine, low-intensity, long-endurance training has been advised for the obese person. Such programs are promoted because they are safe and the proportion of lipid in the fuel oxidized at low intensity is thought to be greater than during high-intensity efforts.[33,35,41] Tremblay and others[35] question the endorsement of low-intensity exercise to promote fat loss. They found that lean, previously sedentary subjects who completed a 15-week high-intensity, interval training program lost greater subcutaneous fat than a comparable group of 17 who completed a 20-week moderate-intensity endurance program. This greater fat loss occurred despite the fact that the longer endurance training cost twice as much energy as the shorter interval training program, and was conducted at an intensity considered optimal to promote fat loss. Based on animal models and previous similar studies on humans, the authors believe that high-intensity exercise has an enhancing effect on postexercise lipid utilization, therefore causing a greater overall body lipid utilization. Clinically, they caution others to use high-intensity exercise prudently with obese clients who may not be used to exercise. In such cases, low-intensity exercise is the safest. However, as the individual's fitness level improves, one may want to substitute vigorous exercise for the low-intensity workout, to promote greater fat utilization and a greater gain in strength.

When designing an exercise and diet program to promote weight loss, one needs to match the exercise and diet options with the individual's physical and financial limitations, level of motivation, preexisting medical conditions, past history of weight loss attempts, and current goals. A great deal of time must be spent initially in mutually deciding the best course of action. A partnership based on trust (by the client) and competence (by the counselor) can promote an emotionally and physically healthy lifestyle.

EFFECTIVENESS OF DIET AND EXERCISE IN WEIGHT MANAGEMENT

The use of diets and exercise in the treatment of obesity is being challenged today by the public and a growing number of health care professionals, as well as obesity researchers.[42] The challengers argue that diets are at best ineffective, and many times harmful.[43-45] The supporters contend that the commonly cited 95% failure rate for dieting is based on weak data that are more than 35 years old.[46] They further contend that the body of weight loss literature is based on a subpopulation of obese people who seek clinical help from hospital- or university-based programs, and that these people do not represent the entire obese population.[46] The issue becomes even more confusing when the scientific community itself cannot determine at what threshold of obesity health risks increase[47] or whether the disease to be treated is really obesity, or dieting itself.[42] Furthermore, in order to come to a consensus on whether or not diet and exercise are effective in the treatment of obesity, researchers must come to an agreement as to which outcome variables or criteria represent effective treatment.[48]

The physiological, psychological, and social pressures to be slim and fit have caused a heightened preoccupation and dissatisfaction with body size, which has led many to try any new weight loss promotion available.[49] Indeed, dieting occurs across all weight categories for both men and women.[49] Each individual may have a different weight loss objective, but the immediate measurable outcome variable is the same. For example, the morbidly obese may want to lose weight to reduce disease risk; the person with low self-image may want to lose weight in an attempt to build self-esteem; and the unfit individual may want to lose weight to increase functional capacity. Regardless of whether the individual objectives in this example are reasonable, the outcome variable is the same for each person: weight loss. One can see how this common outcome variable of weight loss easily becomes the central focus for intervention, while the original objectives disappear. Thus, weight loss alone should be avoided as a standard for success.[48] However, a paradox emerges when the scientific community recognizes that weight loss itself should not be used as a success criteria, but then favors using other measures of body size such as body mass index (BMI), percentage of excess weight, and body fat content.[48] On the other hand, those of the antidieting movement fuel the fire, by continually focusing on the ineffectiveness of obesity intervention techniques in changing body size; while refusing to recognize the enormous public health cost of excess body weight.[46,50] With this in mind, the remainder of this chapter will be devoted to presenting the data on both sides of the effectiveness issue, and designing reasonable health intervention strategies for the overweight individual.

Effectiveness Claims from the Scientific Community

Obesity researchers have been fighting an uphill battle ever since Stunkard and McLaren-Hume concluded in 1959 that dieting was ineffective for 99% of those in a hospital nutrition clinic in terms of weight loss maintenance and including 4% who gained back more than they lost.[45] Later studies seemed to confirm that clinical intervention for the obese was ineffective.[51,52] However, during the 1970s and 1980s the use of very-low-calorie diets (VLCDs) became popular and the research review by Wadden[53] demonstrated that weight loss in these VLCD programs amounted to 20 kg following 12 to 16 weeks of dieting, with a maintained weight loss of 10 to 13 kg after 1-year follow-up. Individual reports vary in their success claims, and it is difficult to interpret their results because dropout ratios can be as high as 80% in some programs.[54] For example, one report claimed that 30% of women and 58% of men who completed the VLCD maintained their weight within 4.5 kg of goal weight for 18 months postprogram.[55] Although these numbers are optimistic, the overall analysis of the program is not impressive. First, 25% of the patients were unable to adapt to this approach and dropped out within the first three weeks. Approximately 62% of the men and only 18% of the women who remained in the program after the first three weeks achieved their goal weight. However, only 58% of the men who achieved their goal weight and only 35% of the women who achieved their goal weight maintained their reduced body weight within 4.5 kg of their goal for 18 months. In other words, only 6% of the women and 36% of the men who entered the program were successful in reaching and maintaining goal weights for 18 months.

Results from programs with more moderate dietary restrictions seem less promising than those from the VLCDs, if the sole outcome variable is weight loss. Patients on a conventional 1200 kcal/day reducing diet, combined with behavior modification, lose about 8.5 kg in 20 weeks and maintain about two thirds of this weight loss for one year.[53] As follow-up is extended over time, body weight continues to rise and baseline weight is reached within five years of therapy.[56,57] Again, individual study results vary, but their overall effectiveness as measured by weight loss is relatively small.

Programs that employ some type of dietary restraint along with nutrition education and/or behavior modification have received praise over the past several years because of their theoretical self-empowerment capabilities. During the average 18-week behavior modification program, one can expect to lose about 10 kg, of which 66% can be maintained for one year.[58] However, further monitoring shows a 95% relapse within two years of treatment.[57] Similarly discouraging results have been seen with more broadly based programs such as community programs, worksite interventions, and home correspondence.[59] Initial weight loss in these programs is minimal, and outcome after one to three years negligible. More recent behavioral programs focusing on modifying diet composition rather than caloric restriction have shown weight losses of 7 to 9 kg in six months, but it is too early to tell whether these changes will last.[60–62] Moreover, these newer programs are considered lifestyle modifications rather than diet and exercise programs.[63]

Energy expenditure is opposite diet on the energy balance. Resting metabolic rate, which takes up a majority of the daily energy expenditure, is not easily manipulated. However, it is rather easy to increase daily exercise energy expenditure. Exercise has been used for years as an adjunct to diet in obesity intervention, but most of the guidelines for exercise prescription in the obese population are based on assumptions or data that were collected on populations other than the obese. Two of the earliest studies on prescribed exercise and weight loss revealed that aerobic exercise was effective in reducing body weight in middle-aged men and women, and that most of the weight lost was fat weight.[64,65] Zuti and Golding[40] added to the understanding of diet and exercise interactions in weight loss therapy in their study of overweight women who were placed in one of three intervention groups: diet, exercise, or diet plus exercise. All three groups maintained the same energy deficit during the 16-week study (500 kcal), but the exercise and diet plus exercise groups lost more body fat than the diet alone group. These data suggest that exercise alone or in combination with diet is the preferred treatment for obesity.

Literature reviews on exercise and weight control vary in their approaches, but all basically reveal the same thing, that exercise effects on body weight are rather small, but significant. Weight loss of about 2 kg has been reported for various exercise programs of differing lengths.[66,67] Epstein and Wing[68] reported in their review that exercise causes body weight to decrease at a rate of about 0.1 kg/wk, and that people do not lose as much weight as would be expected from the prescribed exercise. Similar rates of weight loss were seen in the review by Wood et al.[69] These review papers as well as that of Ballor and Keesey[70] also indicate that the effectiveness of exercise for weight loss is directly related to the initial degree of adiposity and the volume of exercise completed.

The long-term effects of exercise in weight control seem to be the most promising, but the follow-up data for exercise intervention are scanty for the first one to two years after intervention and nonexistent after five years. One of these longer-term exercise studies compared the body weight changes of police officers who participated in an eight-week weight loss program.[71] These officers were divided into four diet groups, each receiving a different type of VLCD. Each of the four diet groups were subsequently divided into an exercising subgroup and a nonexercising subgroup. The exercisers participated in a supervised exercise program conducted three times each week. The program consisted of 35 to 60 minutes of aerobic activity, calisthenics, and relaxation techniques. Follow-up measurements were taken at 6 and 18 months after treatment. When the body weight changes for the diet groups were averaged and those for the diet plus exercise groups averaged, the diet plus exercise had a more pronounced effect on body weight than diet alone (Figure 16–1). Amazingly, there were no significant gains in body weight for those who exercised during the follow-up period. However, those who did not exercise gained about 60% of their weight back by 6 months posttreatment and gained 92% back by 18 months posttreatment.

King and Tribble[67] recently summarized the results of exercise intervention studies, although clear comparisons among studies cannot be made due to differences in methodology, length of intervention, and length of follow-up. Nonethe-

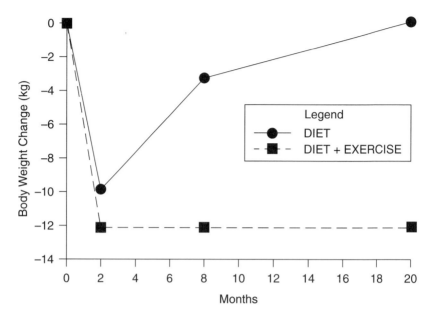

Figure 16–1 Average body weight changes for patients using diet alone, or diet and exercise 18 months posttreatment.

less, the four diet programs reviewed posted a mean weight loss at follow-up of 4.0 kg; the five exercise studies reviewed posted a 4.9 kg weight loss at follow-up, while the three diet plus exercise studies reported a 7.2 kg loss at follow-up. This review suggests again that exercise is important for weight loss and essential to reduced weight maintenance.

Almost completely ignored in the literature are data on self-help programs and people who make changes on their own. In fact, most of the weight loss methods used are not intensive face-to-face interventions, but low-cost alternatives that are primarily self-administered.[72] Results from one study illustrate the application of a self-administered program were recently reported.[60] Obese men (n = 14, percent body fat = 31.6 ± 2.1) and women (n = 21, percent body fat = 39.3 ± 1.2) were given a workbook detailing a behavior modification approach to weight loss that emphasizes self-monitoring of eating and exercise behaviors, and then sent home for six months to learn how to lose weight on their own. Subsequently, the obese adults in this study were able to teach themselves how to make positive changes in eating and exercise behaviors that produced significant decreases in body weight and body fat content. The group lost 8.1 ± 0.9 kg body weight, of which 6.4 ± 0.8 kg was fat, while reducing their fat intake (percent of daily energy intake) from 36.1 ± 1.0% to 27.9 ± 1.3% and increasing their carbohydrate intake from 45.7 ±

1.2% to 50.0 ± 1.7%. Exercise frequency increased from 1.5 ± 0.3 to 3.8 ± 0.4 days each week. Although these data look promising, two things must be remembered while interpreting the data in conjunction with other weight loss data. First, the focus of this program was not weight loss per se, but developing healthy eating and exercise behaviors, and thus, this program may be considered a lifestyle intervention rather than diet and exercise therapy for weight loss.[63] Second, the results are so new that long-term follow-up data are not yet available. Nonetheless, these data do suggest that some people can teach themselves how to make positive changes in eating and exercise behaviors that result in weight loss.

Along these same lines of thinking, Schachter[73] insinuates that obese people who cure themselves do not go to therapists and that the professional view of the intractability of obesity has been molded largely by that self-selected, hard-core group of people who, unable or unwilling to help themselves, go to therapists for help, thereby becoming the only easily available subjects for studies of recidivism and addiction. This concept is further supported by a survey of more than 20,000 readers from *Consumer Reports* magazine, where it was found that of those who reported losing a significant amount of weight (averaging 15 kg) and maintaining the loss, 72% had done so on their own, compared to 20% in commercial programs, 5% in hospital- or university-based programs, and 3% with diet pills.[46] The authors have observed something similar in their work over the years and propose the following model of how the overweight population may be subdivided into specific categories, shown in Figure 16–2.

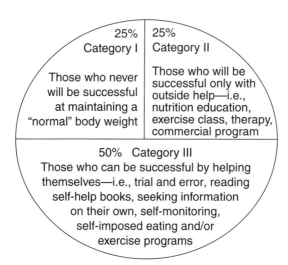

Figure 16–2 Categories of overweight individuals according to weight management success.

Figure 16–2 may help illustrate why Brownell[46(p340)] has stated in his editorial, "It is unfortunate but true that on the basis of current knowledge, it is simply not possible to say that the vast majority of weight loss attempts are or are not success-ful. In the absence of data on commercial programs, self-help programs, and people who make changes on their own, it would be inappropriate to argue that diets were effective. It is equally inappropriate to argue that all diets fail. This underscores the need for research on all approaches to weight loss." It may be that the weight loss data produced thus far by the scientific community represent a mixture of people coming from Categories I and II in Figure 16–2, and therefore, one would not expect reported success rates to be high.

Effectiveness Claims from the Industry

The weight loss industry is big business. Americans spend over $30 billion on weight loss products and services each year. Over the past few years this industry has been under heavy scrutiny from the public, media celebrities, and the scientific com-munity. This scrutiny has been levied in part because of claims of false advertising and fraudulent products. To examine the efficacy and safety of weight loss programs, the National Institutes of Health and the Food and Drug Administration requested data from the industry on the success of programs for use by persons with various degrees of obesity. A summary of the report compiled at the National Institutes of Health Technology Assessment Conference reveals a very dismal picture.[74] Material was received from only five companies, three representing nonphysician-directed programs and two representing physician-directed programs. For the nonphysician-directed programs, one company provided a study demonstrating reduced cardiovas-cular risk with short-term use of their program. Abstracts of research submitted by the same company were scientifically inadequate. The information provided showed that the studies had basic design problems including poor response rates to surveys, inad-equate follow-up to assess maintenance, high dropout rates for clinical trials, and insufficient group sizes to detect statistically significant differences.[74] The second company initially submitted four studies for review, but subsequently withdrew the studies. The third company submitted information for review that was inad-equate to evaluate the program's efficacy. For the physician-directed programs, one company submitted 55 publications that were well designed and well con-trolled, and where the data collected supported the study conclusions. These stud-ies revealed that many obese persons benefited from physician-supervised VLCDs in combination with behavior modification and exercise. Major benefits were reduced cardiovascular disease risk and better control of diabetes. The sec-ond company in this category submitted three published articles and several ab-stracts. Data from these showed beneficial metabolic and weight responses to the program, but further data were deemed necessary to draw conclusions.

The assessors concluded that VLCDs are helpful in obtaining and maintaining weight loss for two to three years in some persons when used in conjunction with behavior modification and an exercise program. They state that regardless of the products used, successful weight loss and control was limited and required individualized programs consisting of restricted caloric intake, behavior modification, and exercise.[74] However, these weak conclusions based on a paucity of data from a handful of companies are not representative of the industry as a whole. One must also remember that the conclusions drawn refer only to some people (possibly Categories II and III, Figure 16–2) and are dependent not only upon dieting, but also upon behavior modification and exercise, which most companies exclude from their programs. Table 16–2 makes a comparison among some of the most popular commercial weight loss programs offered publicly. One can easily see that most of these commercial programs do not meet the criteria upon which the

Table 16–2 Comparative Commercial Weight Loss Programs

	Nutri/System	Jenny Craig	Medifast	Optifast	Weight Loss Clinic	Health Mgmt Resources	Diet Workshop	Weight Watchers	Slim Fast	Physician's Weight Loss
Comprehensive behavioral approach										
Extensive exercise component										
Extensive individual counseling										
Liveable					X		X	X		
Contact with professionals			X	X	X	X				X
Maintenance plan	X	X	X	X	X	X	X	X		X
Supported by scientific research*										
Teach habit change										
Balanced meals			X			?	?	?		
Adequately trained staff		X				X	X			
Psychoeducational										

*Only one company provided significant scientific support for effectiveness, but the name of the company was kept anonymous in the NIH Technology Assessment Conference Report.[74]

Source: Reprinted with permission from F.N. Hyman et al., Evidence for Success of Caloric Restriction in Weight Loss and Control, *Annals of Internal Medicine,* Vol. 119, pp. 681–687, © 1993, American College of Physicians.

above conclusions were reached. Furthermore, the prudent consumer must determine if the programs listed in Table 16–2 (or other commercial programs) violate any of the guidelines for health promotion products and services established by the National Council Against Health Fraud (Exhibit 16–1).

Authorities Who Question the Effectiveness Claims

As seen in the preceding sections, the evidence to support the use of diet and exercise for the reduction of obesity is too elusive to be clearly interpreted. This

---

Exhibit 16–1 Guidelines for Evaluating Weight Loss Promotions

The National Council Against Health Fraud disparages commercial weight loss or control programs that:

1. Promise or imply dramatic, rapid weight loss (more than 1% of total body weight per week).
2. Promise diets that are extremely low in calories (below 800 calories per day; 1200 calorie diets are preferred) unless under the supervision of competent medical experts.
3. Attempt to make clients dependent upon special products rather than teaching how to make good choices from the conventional food supply.
4. Do not encourage permanent, realistic lifestyle changes including regular exercise and the behavioral aspects of eating wherein food may be used as a coping device. (Programs should emphasize changing the causes of overweight rather than simply the effect, which is overweight itself.)
5. Misrepresent salespeople as *counselors* supposedly qualified to give guidance in nutrition and/or general health.
6. Require large sums of money at the start or require that clients sign contracts for expensive, long-term programs.
7. Fail to inform clients about the risks associated with weight loss in general, or the specific program promoted.
8. Promote unproven or spurious weight loss aids such as human chorionic gonadotrophin hormone, starch blockers, diuretics, sauna belts, body wraps, passive exercise, ear stapling, acupuncture, electric muscle stimulating devices, spirulina, amino acid supplements, glucomannan, and so forth.
9. Claim that *cellulite* exists in the body.
10. Claim that use of an appetite suppressant or methylcellulose (a bulking agent) enables a person to lose body fat without restricting accustomed caloric intake.
11. Claim that a weight control product contains a unique ingredient unless it is unavailable in other weight control products.

Source: Reprinted from *Healthy Weight Journal* with permission from Frances M. Berg— National Coordinator of the Task Force on Weight Loss Abuse of the National Council Against Health Fraud.

elusiveness of the data has not discouraged those in favor of using diet and exercise for obesity treatment, but rather encouraged them to use diet and possibly exercise even more aggressively.[53,56] On the other side of the issue, a number of scientists support the notion of abandoning completely the use of energy-restrictive diets in obesity treatment, while using exercise only as a means to achieve health rather than weight loss.[44,75] Although this group has questioned the effectiveness of obesity treatment for over 15 years, their arguments have not been embraced, and health care professionals still vigorously promote weight loss as a means for achieving health.[75] Arguments from this group of challengers may be enlightening, and therefore, will now be presented.

A wake up call was given to the members of the American Dietetic Association in 1991 when David M. Garner, eating disorder specialist, stated

> It is difficult to find any scientific justification for the continued use of dietary treatments of obesity. Regardless of the techniques used, most participants regain the weight lost. The inevitability of this result is often obscured by the use of follow-up periods insufficient to capture the later phases of weight regain. No longer can we reasonably expect improved results with greater sophistication of techniques as was appropriate during the early period of development and refinement of behavioral technology.[76(pA152)]

Later Garner states, "The argument that health risk justifies treatment—in the absence of effective treatment—seems to me to be based upon flawed logic and is capricious. It doesn't make any sense that we should be trying to apply a treatment that's ineffective."[42(p109)]

The basic argument presented by those against using diet and exercise solely for weight reduction is that there is no substantial evidence supporting long-term effectiveness. A secondary issue is that there are several health risks associated with dieting and weight loss.[42,43,47,75,77] The issue of health risks associated with dieting, weight loss, and weight fluctuation remains controversial[77,78] and has been dealt with extensively elsewhere.[42] Therefore, the focus of this chapter will remain with the effectiveness claims. Practitioners will benefit from developing a view of obesity as a chronic disease and from considering whether management ought to be similar to that of any other chronic health problem. See Chapter 15 for a discussion of managing obesity as a chronic disease.

As seen previously in this chapter, even members of the NIH Technology Assessment Conference concluded that long-term weight loss following any type of intervention was limited to a small minority of the obese people studied.[54] However, it was suggested that further research be performed,[53,54,59,74,79] and that data from self-help programs, as well as commercial programs be obtained[46] before definite conclusions on effectiveness are made. Further defense for the lack of effectiveness data is the suggestion that obesity be categorized as a chronic disease, requiring continual treatment.[48,53,58,80,81] If obesity is categorized in this manner, then long-term effects following short-term intervention would certainly not be expected. Nobody expects chronic diseases like hypertension or diabetes to be cured through short-term intervention.[53,80] Wadden[53] even uses exercise as an example to support this suggestion. He states that even though it is well-established that aerobic exercise increases cardiovascular fitness, a six-month program of aerobic activity would not be expected to confer cardiovascular fitness three to five years later. Similarly, with obesity, intervention must be continual in order for the effect to be lasting. The logic behind this reasoning seems sensible, especially since diet interventions don't last and the strongest evidence for effective exercise intervention is that found in the studies where exercise was continued during the follow-up phase.

However, arguments against categorizing obesity as a chronic disease also seem logical. First, the weight loss literature fails to demonstrate large decreases in body weight, whether the intervention is short term or chronic,[54] so pushing for chronic intervention seems futile. Second, data from a few people who are successful in losing weight and maintaining a reduced weight do not justify the general use of dieting for the entire obese population. Third, one must consider a myriad of other implications before making this categorization. Some of these deal with the interests of the health care provider and some with the interests of the client. Bennett[82] expressed these implications concisely in a talk given to the National Association to Advance Fat Acceptance. He states that although there may be some psychological motivation for the fat person to accept the notion that he is a patient, that is, *ill*, from the physician's point of view there is a much greater incentive to medicalize the condition. By declaring fatness to be a disease, the physician annexes territory for his professional turf; he enlarges his area of presumed competence. For some physicians who specialize in bariatric medicine, this means new patients and a source of larger income. Now, once physicians have a disease to deal with (however they define it), they can start looking for a treatment or, preferably, a cure. This seems like a perfectly natural instinct. And, indeed, medical science has blessed us with a "cure" for obesity. The reducing diet is regarded as the cure for obesity, and virtually the entire medical research and treatment effort has been focused on dieting. Bennett continues his accusations by stating that the medical profession has created its own success story by first discovering a disease (obesity), then finding the cure (dieting). The cure is based on scientific principles derived from fundamental research. There is only one drawback: it doesn't work. Then who is to blame? The patients, of course.

The implications for the patients is that unlike most "sick" people, who get some benefit from the presumption of innocence that goes with having a disease, fat people have been subjected to a guilt trip—because they have a "disease" with a "cure" that doesn't happen to work for them. As a result, the blame is passed on to the patient. These latter accusations are confirmed by Goodrick et al.[83] who found that patients in VLCD programs greatly overestimate the success rate of the program and subsequently blame themselves for failure. This self-blame and failure leads obese persons to repeatedly diet in attempts to overcome their failure and increase their self-esteem.[43,49]

Hence, dieting itself has been implicated as being the real disease[42] and even as the cause of obesity.[84] Wooley[84] seriously questions dieting as the cause of obesity by citing the following evidence:

1. Non-dieters whose overeating is not preceded by a period of caloric restriction gain very little weight.
2. People re-feeding after weight loss gain weight very easily, and the regained weight is mostly fat.
3. Obese people gain weight much more easily than non-obese people.
4. Obese people almost always have a long history of dieting.

The overall position of those opposing dietary treatment of obesity may not be as unreasonable as sometimes portrayed. The summary statement of The American Dietetic Association portrays the position best:

> We fully recognize the complex and multidetermined nature of obesity and further recognize that discoveries in any number of areas might result in effective and appropriate treatment of some or all obese persons. However, at this time we can enhance the possibilities of meaningful scientific progress in other areas by reallocating resources currently invested in developing, applying, and studying dietary treatments that have little rational hope for success.[3(p768)]

Opposition to weight loss therapy is very strong when practices in the weight loss industry are discussed.[42,85,86] As presented earlier in this chapter, the weight loss industry has produced minuscule amounts of data to back up some of its unsupported effectiveness claims. The industry has not only been accused of failing to produce effectiveness data, but also has been accused of unethical practices. Some of the most common complaints registered against the industry are listed below.[42,85,86]

1. There are no standard licensing or certification requirements for the industry.
2. Potential risks to the client are sometimes known, but not disclosed.
3. Procedures and programs used in the industry are not validated.
4. Food, drug, and advertising laws related to weight loss are not enforced.
5. The industry is exploiting a situation where cultural norms are dramatically distorted in relation to biological reality.
6. The industry sells to people who do not need weight loss.
7. The industry is only interested in profit, not treatment.

8. Each new program promises results where others have failed.
9. There are no criteria to determine when the potential harm to consumers is severe enough to justify government intervention.

The net result of all these complaints is that consumers do not have the information they need to judge effectively the quality of the industry's products and services. See Chapter 21 on regulation of the weight management industry.

Organizations That Question the Effectiveness Claims

Founded in 1969, the National Association to Advance Fat Acceptance (NAAFA) is a human rights organization dedicated to improving the quality of life for fat people. NAAFA aims to eliminate discrimination based on body size as well as work to eliminate the oppression of fat people. So what are the indictments coming from NAAFA? The major indictment involves the political maneuvering used by many obesity researchers and the weight loss industry to serve their own interests. Smith, the executive director of NAAFA, claims that researchers on the NIH Task Force on the Prevention and Treatment of Obesity are biased because they are all either affiliated with commercial weight loss centers, weight loss research programs at universities, or receive research money from the commercial weight loss industry.[87] She further claims that because of this, obesity researchers may acknowledge the failure of diets, but respond by labeling fatness as a chronic condition requiring lifelong treatment. The media responds by saying, don't diet, just eat less and exercise more. The commercial weight loss industry responds by advertising that diets don't work, and then claim their diets are not diets, but rather lifestyle programs.[88]

The Association for Health Enrichment of Large People (AHELP) may not be as direct as NAAFA in its indictments, but similarly opposes the use of food restriction for weight loss, except where limited weight loss is essential in protecting someone from imminent life risk or permanent physical damage.[89] AHELP believes that research should be performed to uncover factors that both enhance and undermine the health of fat people, because weight reduction dieting is inappropriate and unhealthy.[89] Although NAAFA is not considered a scientific entity, and AHELP is too young to have any political clout in the scientific realm, other more established scientific organizations are questioning traditional weight loss therapy and proposing alternatives in weight management.

For example, members of the Society for Nutrition Education (SNE) are proposing a new division called Nutrition and Weight Realities.[90] This new division will help nutrition educators and dietitians incorporate the new *healthy weight* paradigm into their work. Even the American Dietetic Association (ADA) has taken a different stance than traditionally. In a 1994 ADA position statement on nutrition intervention in the treatment of eating disorders, the association recognizes that the vast majority of people who lose weight by dieting are unable to maintain the lower body weight without dramatically restricting energy intake and/or increasing exercise for the rest of their lives.[91] The association states that if changes in food- and weight-related behavior alone are the focus of treatment, interventions are likely to be counterproductive rather than therapeutic. Alternatively, the association suggests that most overweight women may benefit more from counseling about body image and about how to stop the pursuit of thinness than from weight loss therapy itself.[92]

BEHAVIORAL ASPECTS OF SUCCESSFUL WEIGHT MANAGEMENT

Although the majority of scientific evidence presented thus far suggests that diet and exercise intervention do not produce long-lasting weight control in the majority of treated individuals, one cannot refute the fact that there are some individuals who are successful at maintaining a reduced body weight. Even though the percentage of the obese population represented by the successful losers remains disputable, it seems prudent to examine how successful weight loss and control is established in this successful group. For discussion purposes, one must assume that the successful losers have the same barriers to weight loss and control as the unsuccessful (ie, genetics, slow metabolism, chronic dieting history, etc.). In other words, these successful losers must do something, or behave in a certain way that is different from the unsuccessful, which allows them to overcome the barriers to weight loss. (It is apparent that this assumption may be the underlying myth in the whole issue, in that the true difference between the successful losers and the unsuccessful might not be behavioral at all, but rather a physiological or genetic barrier that differentiates the unsuccessful by not allowing them to maintain weight loss, regardless of the behaviors imposed. However, this topic will be pursued because the assumption presented above is the same assumption found throughout the research literature on the effectiveness of behavioral aspects of weight management approaches.)

Colvin and Olson[93] studied the behaviors of men and women who were successful at maintaining a weight loss of at least 20% of original weight for a period of two years or more. Average weight loss for men was 35 kg, for women 24 kg, maintained for an average of six years. There was a gender difference in method of weight loss in that 85% of the men used diet plus exercise to lose weight, compared to only 5% of the women. However, 93% of the women used diet only to lose weight compared to only 8% of the men. In either case, dieting was an integral part of the weight loss therapy. Behaviors relevant to reduced weight maintenance were similar between the sexes, with 85% and 78% of men and women, respectively, increasing exercise, 77% and 66% increasing nutritional knowledge,

85% and 66% self-monitoring. These data are interesting in that they show successful weight loss through diet and exercise intervention, but it cannot be determined from which segment of the obese population these subjects were obtained (Figure 16–2). Moreover, no comparison can be made with unsuccessful people since no comparison group was included in the study.

More recently, Kayman et al[94] were able to make comparison measurements among successful female weight losers (maintainers), relapsers, and controls who never had a weight problem. Table 16–3 contains some data that were extracted from this study. There was a difference in method of weight loss between the maintainers and relapsers, with a greater percentage of the maintainers devising personal strategies and exercising compared to the relapsers. In contrast, a greater percentage of relapsers were depending upon external sources for weight loss success. The maintainers were very similar to controls in their methods of weight maintenance, in that they both exercised and used self-monitoring techniques to monitor body size and eating behaviors. Methods of coping were also different among the groups. The maintainers and controls tended to use various problem solving and coping techniques to deal with problems, whereas the relapsers tended to avoid dealing with their problems. The data from these two studies indicate a behavioral difference between successful weight losers and relapsers.

OVERWEIGHT AND OBESITY INTERVENTION STRATEGIES

It seems apparent that there is not enough data to support claims that diet and/or exercise are effective in long-term weight control for the majority of obese persons. The question of whether or not to pursue further research on diet and exercise as interventions for the obese remains controversial, but is not immediately relevant to the focus of this chapter. The questions that are relevant at this time are: (1) Should there be any intervention for the obese in light of the lack of successful intervention strategies? and (2) What intervention strategies should be used if intervention is deemed appropriate at all? The answer to the first question is that there should be some type of intervention for the obese, because of the well-recognized health risks associated with obesity. The fact that the point at which disease risk becomes increasingly associated with obesity is not well-defined[47] and may be found within a wide range of adiposity[47] should not deter the pursuance of health intervention strategies for the obese. Medical science cannot yet determine exactly how much dietary fat, how much smoking, how much inactivity, or what the exact values for blood pressure are that place a person at increased risk for cardiovascular disease; but this does not prevent health professionals from designing intervention strategies aimed at reducing cardiovascular disease. Indeed, dietary fat reduction, cessation of smoking, increased activity, and controlled hypertension are suggested not only for those diagnosed with cardiovascular disease,

Table 16–3 Comparison of Weight Control Behaviors Among Overweight Women Who Either Relapsed or Maintained, and Normal-Weight Controls

	Relapsers	Maintainers	Controls
How reduced			
Devised a personal eating plan	39%	73%	
Attended Weight Watchers	43%	10%	
Attended other programs or groups	29%	10%	
Exercised	36%	76%	
Followed the physician's orders	34%	20%	
Took pills or shots	47%	3%	
How maintained			
Monitoring body weight		87%	76%
Exercising		83%	88%
Eating less		83%	73%
Watching intake		60%	50%
Reducing the intake of high-fat foods		57%	38%
Reducing the intake of high-sugar foods		57%	50%
Changing to good eating habits		57%	29%
Changing their attitude toward food		47%	9%
Knowing body size by feel of clothes		23%	29%
Not eating three meals per day		20%	38%
Coping with problems			
Escape, avoidance (drink, pills)	70%	33%	35%
Seek social support (talk)	38%	70%	80%
Self-control (without outside help)	13%	16%	43%
Problem solving/confronting	10%	95%	60%
Tension-reducing techniques	2%	17%	42%

Source: Adapted with permission from S. Kayman, W. Bruvold, and J.S. Stern, Maintenance and Relapse After Weight Loss in Women: Behavioral Aspects, *American Journal of Clinical Nutrition,* Vol. 52, pp. 800–807, © 1990, The American Society for Clinical Nutrition.

but for the whole population. Similarly, any general intervention strategy for the obese should be one that would be beneficial for the whole population. Since weight loss is not suggested for the entire population, it is suggested that weight loss or any parameter dealing with body size (i.e., BMI, percent body fat, percent of ideal weight, etc.) be eliminated, or at least de-emphasized as an outcome parameter in intervention strategies. As Smith states, "Researchers must stop asking, 'How can we make fat people thin?' and start asking, 'How can we make fat people healthy?' "[88(p53)] If health professionals adopt this new paradigm, then they will be better able to deal with the entire obese population represented in Figure 16–2, especially those in Category I. Furthermore, they will be better able to treat those with a distorted body image, who continually try to get into the lowest 10% of the weight distribution curve.[95] Accordingly, the question for intervention now becomes: What strategies are best suited for improving the health of obese people? It is our premise, as well as others,[54] that health risks associated with most forms of obesity are more directly related to lifestyle factors, such as excessive consumption of alcohol, dietary fat, and sugar, and low consumption of vegetables, grains, and fruits, as well as inadequate exercise than with their fatness per se.

QUESTIONS AND ANSWERS FROM CLIENTS AND COUNSELORS

From Clients

Is it better to diet first and then exercise, or do both at the same time?

It's best to combine diet and exercise. Exercise burns extra calories, takes time from your day (keeps you away from food), and can generally make you feel good about your day's accomplishments. Also, by exercising, you get the added benefit of maintaining or increasing your lean muscle mass. With diet alone, you lose fat as well as muscle mass, which may decrease your metabolic rate. This makes you a "calorie sponge" just ready for any extra calories to be deposited as fat.

Aerobic (continuous, moderate-intensity exercise, using large muscles for locomotion) also strengthens the heart, reduces blood cholesterol and blood pressure, and increases general fitness. It does not take a long time or lots of effort to see the initial changes. Muscle overloading exercise, such as interval workouts or strength training, tones muscle and adds to lean body mass, thus raising your metabolic rate. Combining a weight reduction diet with aerobic and strength training can improve fitness, increase muscle tone, lower fat mass, increase lean body mass, raise metabolic rate, and help you develop a healthier and happier lifestyle.

Should I eat the same on days I don't exercise as on the days I do? Or should I eat more on those days I exercise?

Try to eat the same every day, but pay attention to your body signals. The key to sticking with a diet and exercise program for either weight loss or maintenance is consistency. Be sure to cross-train, i.e., vary your exercise activities by walking one day, swimming the next, playing racquetball a third day, in order to prevent becoming bored with your exercise regimen. After all, we don't eat the same for every meal, every day. Why expect the same for exercise?

If you find yourself unable to exercise for several days due to illness, injury, or travel, then you may want to eat less on those days. After all, you will not be burning 300 or more exercise calories by being inactive. If travel is an issue, go for walks and explore your new surroundings. Many hotels also have fitness centers with treadmills and stationary bikes for their clients to use. Try them!

I find myself more hungry on the days I exercise. Is this normal? Do I have to worry about my blood sugar being too low?

The research on exercise and appetite is controversial. A normal physiological response by the body is that on a long-term basis, increased energy expenditure through physical activity is counterbalanced by an increased food intake. This is a natural adaptation the body makes to maintain normal body weight.

When beginning an exercise and diet program, many find that initially appetite is suppressed. This could be due to the low-intensity level of exercise suppressing the appetite, but also by the excitement and novelty of the adventure. Research has indicated that high-intensity exercise may not suppress hunger. So on days of intense training you may find yourself hungry. But you can also learn to ignore the hunger and revel in how good the workout felt.

During exercise, blood glucose does drop initially. The glucose is entering the muscle cells to provide energy for your workout. After a few minutes, your body adapts and mobilizes glucose from liver storage to bring your blood sugar back to normal. If you find yourself consistently a little lightheaded or woozy during a workout, then have some juice an hour before. The juice is easily absorbed and quickly converted to blood glucose. The other option to prevent wooziness is to schedule your workout within three hours after a carbohydrate-rich meal.

I've heard about the glycemic index of food, that it affects blood sugar and this somehow affects exercise. What is the glycemic index of food? Now that I'm active, do I need to be aware of this index?

People who should be most concerned with the glycemic index of food are persons with diabetes. The glycemic index tells us how food affects our blood sugar. Just because a food is sugary or sweet doesn't necessarily mean it will raise our blood sugar more than a slice of whole wheat bread. If you have diabetes, then you and your dietitian should discuss how various foods may affect your blood sugar and subsequently your exercise. If diabetes is not a concern, then you won't vary as much in your response to different foods. You should be aware, however, that sweet liquids such as punch, lemonade, soda, and juice are just sugar and water that are quickly absorbed and turned into blood glucose. We suggest you refrain from drinking lots of sweet drinks for an hour before a workout. An 8-oz glass is no problem, but two to three could cause a jump in your blood glucose.

Does it matter when I eat in relation to when I exercise? Will I burn more calories if I eat before or after my exercise bout?

These effects are very small. Eating and exercise increase metabolic rate independent of each other. The effect of doing them close together has little if any advantage.

I only want to burn fat. Why should I weight train, too?

Weight training helps maintain muscle mass when you lose weight. If you maintain your muscle mass, you maintain a higher metabolic rate and burn more calories at rest. You may also be pleasantly surprised by the way your body looks after only a few weeks of weight training as it becomes more toned. Because women don't "bulk-up" as easily as men, weight training produces a more smooth toned muscle. Weight training provides you with much more than tone and muscle. It adds variety to your workout, strength and density to your bones (if you're under 35), or maintains bone density (if you're over 35), adds a swagger to your walk, and confidence to your psyche.

Let's say I lose 25 lbs. Do I need to exercise more to get the same benefits I did at the heavier weight?

It takes more energy (calories) to walk at a given speed weighing 225 lbs than it does weighing 200 lbs. However, if with weight loss you have become more physically fit and can exercise more intensely, you may not need to spend more time exercising to get the same caloric expenditure. For example, a 225-lb woman who walks 3.5 mph for one hour expends about 625 calories. Through a diet and exercise program, she now weighs 200 lbs. She is more fit and can walk faster. At 200 pounds, walking 4.0 mph, she will expend the same 625 calories. So increased time is not necessary if the intensity increases. If the intensity stays the same, then she will have to exercise longer or more frequently.

How do I determine my ideal body weight?

Ideal body weight, goal weight, normal weight, recommended weight, etc., are all terms that have been associated with some numerical value coming from a bathroom scale, which is supposed to indicate health status or disease risk. Whether obesity is a health risk and to what extent varies among individuals. One must remember that health is not defined by weight, but by health status. *Healthy weight*, therefore, can exist within a large range that is defined by an individual's health status. Hence, the focus of attention should be the establishment of healthy eating and exercise behaviors. When healthy behaviors are maintained and health status improves, then one can be assured that a healthy weight has been achieved. See Chapter 1 for definitions of healthy weight.

What health risks have been associated with weight loss and weight cycling?

Too many to mention, but to name a few: gallstones, cardiac disorders, elevated cholesterol, anemia, edema, hair loss, diarrhea, amenorrhea, pancreatic complications, and death. However, we cannot yet determine who is at highest risk for these problems during dieting episodes, nor what proportion of dieters suffer from these health problems. Therefore, prudence would dictate a very conservative approach to any dieting attempt.

Regardless of the mode of exercise, is more exercise better?

Epidemiological studies have shown that more exercise is better. However, the biggest health benefit coming from exercise occurs when one moves from the sedentary state to moderate activity. An active lifestyle or moderate exercise program that can be sustained will ultimately be more beneficial than an intense short-lived program.

From Counselors

How do you decide which diet and exercise plan is best for your client?

Regarding exercise, you must find something your clients enjoy. If they don't like a certain activity, they will soon lose interest and drop out from the program. Also encourage cross-training, i.e., a few different activities. People who have had little success with exercise in the past may settle into just one mode of exercise and not think to try new challenges once they have mastered their chosen activity. If they have attained a certain level of fitness, they will soon be rewarded by learning and mastering a new skill.

A diet plan has to be one that will fit into the client's lifestyle but ensures the basics of nutritional adequacy and variety. Both client and practitioner must be willing to compromise to incorporate both diet and exercises changes into a new lifestyle.

Many people want spot reducing, e.g., women want to lose their hips. How is it best to answer their questions?

Be honest with them. If they have a gynoid-type obesity, they will probably always have that pear shape, even with weight reduction. It's just that the pear will be smaller with more gentle curves. Explain to them that fat is lost differently in all people, but exercising one specific body part will only affect the muscle exercised and not the fat that surrounds it. For example, doing 200 situps daily will cause the waistline to appear slimmer due to increased muscle tone and firmness of the abdomen, but the situps will not necessarily reduce the amount of fat around the waist.

I've heard that people expend significant energy even after exercising. I think this is called EPOC. What is it? Does it differ in obese or non-obese people? Does it differ by age or gender?

EPOC is the acronym for excess postexercise oxygen consumption. It relates to the increase in metabolic rate after exercise. Research is controversial on the length and magnitude of this elevation. Some researchers have shown that metabolic rate stays elevated for up to 12 hours postexercise, and accounts for as much as 40% of the energy expended during exercise. Other researchers indicate EPOC accounts for less than 10 extra calories and lasts less than one hour. EPOC may be related to one's lean mass. The more lean mass, the greater the EPOC. Since obese individuals generally have more muscle mass (associated with the need to have more strength to move a heavier body), EPOC may be of some value to them. Studies that compare the EPOC of lean vs obese people are sparse and controversial.

What advice should I give about cross-training or injury prevention? Some clients have a difficult time tolerating just one mode of exercise, while others want to try them all. Do we need to caution them about injury prevention based on their degree of overweight?

Injury prevention is a major concern for obese individuals. They have a higher risk of both heat intolerance and orthopaedic injuries. Intensity of exercise is always a concern. With higher-intensity exercise, the risk of injury increases. Obese individuals often have more knee, lower leg, and foot injuries resulting from weight-bearing exercises. If a motivated client wants to exercise almost every day, use cross-training to prevent overuse injuries. An exercise program that incorporates walking, stationary cycling, weight training, and swimming on occasion will help prevent boredom as well as injury. With hot and/or humid weather, reinforce the need to consume more fluids and lighten the exercise intensity. Clients may want to exercise indoors where air conditioning is available.

How do I keep my clients from focusing so much on weight and getting depressed with weight fluctuations of a pound or two?

It has been our experience that most clients begin a new diet/exercise program being narrowly focused on weight loss. Although they may say that the reason they want to lose weight is to improve health or disease risk status, this is usually just lip service. The problem is that body weight and body size have been so highly emphasized that the *health equation*, so to speak, has been reversed in most clients' minds. Most dieters think that healthy weight = healthy behaviors. In other words, they believe that if they could just arrive at an ideal body weight, then other aspects of their life would become healthier. In reality, healthy behaviors = healthy weight. Thus, the counselor's job is to help the client realize the true paradigm. This is difficult, but can be achieved. In short, the counselor must focus all of the attention on behaviors. All monitoring, measurements, evaluations, rewards, and incentives should deal with behaviors. Systematic weighing, goal weights, and rewards for weight loss should be abolished. Periodic weighing is recommended only with clinical discretion.

CONCLUSION

The following outline contains general intervention strategies for either improving or maintaining the health status of obese people. These guidelines should be implemented in explicit ways to meet the specific needs of each individual person, depending upon the therapeutic environment and resources available.

1. *Pre-screening or pre-evaluation.* Success rates for obesity intervention will be enhanced by obtaining a pre-intervention evaluation that identifies the client's history of previous weight loss behaviors, detects symptoms of disease risk associated with the client's condition, and discovers whether the client's search for treatment is triggered by psychological problems unrelated to obesity.[43,91,96,97] This pre-evaluation will help the therapist understand how the client's past behaviors, perceptions, expectations, and failures will affect current behavior-modifying attempts.[97] Assessing pre-existing conditions will not only ensure a safer intervention, but will also help the therapist determine which outcome variables are most appropriate for the client. By recognizing that seeking treatment for obesity may

be triggered by psychological problems not necessarily associated with obesity, the therapist can then begin to help the client separate food- and weight-related behaviors from feelings and psychological issues. This process involves helping the person separate her or his identity, feelings, and unresolved issues from the focus of food, hunger, and weight so that the two problems can be worked on separately.[91]

2. *Program design.* Determine which outcome variables are important for each client, and design a program accordingly. Success of the intervention is dependent upon achieving the desired outcome variables. Individual outcome variables can be determined during the pre-evaluation, and then used as indicators of the progress and success of the intervention.

3. *Exercise.* Developing a lifestyle of increased activity through exercise should be a top priority. The exercise prescription for each client should be individualized. Demanding that the client reach a target heart rate or intensity during the exercise session is not necessary to improve fitness and functional capacity in an obese, sedentary population.[98] Therefore, the focus of the exercise component should be helping the client become more active through frequent, regular exercise that is enjoyable. Aerobic exercise is generally preferred, but recent evidence suggests that similar benefits for the obese can be obtained from both aerobic and anaerobic exercise.[99]

4. *Normalized food intake.* Most clients will have a long history of abnormal eating ranging from bizarre combinations of foods and supplements to severe restrictions. The most common pattern of eating for the chronic dieter is the *all or none syndrome*, in which the patient wavers back and forth from unrestricted eating to severely restricted eating. Emphasis should be placed on gradually developing healthier eating behaviors in which foods are not labeled in absolutes like *good* or *bad*, but rather in terms of *more desirable, less desirable* or *more frequently consumed, less frequently consumed*. The pre-evaluation will help determine whether or not an eating disorder exists, and if psychotherapy should be an integral part of the therapeutic intervention.

5. *Psychological component.* Depending upon the pre-screening and evaluation, a psychological component should be designed for each client, which includes behavior modification suitable for the client and may include stress management, family support, family counseling, peer group support, or individual counseling.[96]

6. *Continuing care or maintenance plan.* Regardless of whether obesity is labeled a chronic disease or not, continual reinforcement of newly established behaviors is critical to long-term maintenance. The focus of the maintenance plan should not be body weight, but rather maintaining the healthier lifestyle established during therapy. The client should play an integral part in designing the maintenance plan, and should feel comfortable with its structure. The mainte-

nance plan may or may not include continual contact with the therapist. We have seen several clients self-monitor for over five years by individualizing a simple daily scoresheet designed to help the obese establish healthy eating and exercise behaviors.[100]

ACKNOWLEDGMENT

The authors wish to thank David Creel, MS, RD, for his assistance in generating and answering questions from both the client's and counselor's perspectives.

REFERENCES

1. Rock CL, Coulston AM. Weight control approaches: a review by the California Dietetic Association. *J Am Diet Assoc.* 1988;88:44–48.
2. Drenick EJ, Swendseid ME, Blahd WH. Prolonged starvation as treatment for severe obesity. *JAMA.* 1964;187:100–106.
3. Position of the American Dietetic Association. Very-low-calorie weight loss diets. *J Am Diet Assoc.* 1990;90:722–726.
4. Atkinson RL. Issues and opinions in nutrition. *J Nutr.* 1986;116:918–919.
5. Atkins RC. *Dr. Atkins Diet Revolution.* New York: Bantam Books; 1982.
6. Fisher MC, Lachance PA. Nutrition evaluation of published weight-reduction diets. *J Am Diet Assoc.* 1985;85:450–454.
7. Stillman IM, Baker SS. *The Doctor's Quick Weight Loss Diet.* New York: Dell Publishing Co; 1978.
8. Sours HE, Frattali VP, Brand CD, Feldman RA. Sudden death associated with very low calorie weight reduction regimens. *Am J Clin Nutr.* 1981;34:453–461.
9. Sandoz Nutrition, Inc. Minneapolis, MN.
10. Health Management Resources, Inc. Boston, MA.
11. Winners or losers? EN reviews the top weight-loss programs. *Environmental Nutr.* 1994;17:1,3.
12. Nutri/System, Inc. Horsham, PA.
13. Jenny Craig, Inc. Del Mar, CA.
14. Pritikin N. *The Pritikin Permanent Weight Loss Manual.* New York: Bantam Books; 1982.
15. Katahn M: *The T-Factor Diet.* New York: Bantam Books; 1989.
16. Zeman F. *Clinical Nutrition and Dietetics.* New York: Macmillan Publishing Co; 1991.
17. Apfelbaum M, Fricker J, Igoin-Apfelbaum L. Low- and very-low-calorie diets. *Am J Clin Nutr.* 1978;45(suppl):1126–1133.
18. Genuth SM, Castro J, Vertes V. Weight reduction in obesity by outpatient semistarvation. *JAMA.* 1974;230:987–1002.
19. *The Surgeon General's Report on Nutrition and Health.* Washington, DC: US Government Printing Office; 1988. Publication 88-50210.
20. National Research Council. *Diet and Health, Implications for Reducing Chronic Disease Risk.* Washington, DC: National Academy Press; 1989.

21. Kendall A, Levitsky DA, Strupp BJ, Lissner L. Weight loss on a low-fat diet: consequences of the imprecision of the control of food intake in human. *Am J Clin Nutr.* 1991;53:1124–1129.

22. Sheppard L, Kristal AR, Kushi LH. Weight loss in women participating in a randomized trial of low-fat diets. *Am J Clin Nutr.* 1991;54:821–828.

23. Ornish D. *Eat More, Weigh Less.* New York: Harper Collins; 1993.

24. Astrup A, Raban A. Obesity: an inherited metabolic deficiency in the control of macronutrient balance? *Eur J Clin Nutr.* 1992;46:611–620.

25. Flatt JP. Dietary fat, carbohydrate balance, and weight maintenance: effects of exercise. *Am J Clin Nutr.* 1987;45:296–306.

26. Raban A, Andersen HB, Christensen NJ, Madsen J, et al. Evidence for an abnormal postprandial response to a high-fat meal in women predisposed to obesity. *Am J Physiol.* 1994;267:E549–E559.

27. Astrup A. Dietary composition substrate balances and body fat in subjects with a predisposition to obesity. *Int J Obes.* 1993;17(suppl 3):S32–S36.

28. Astrup A, Buemann B, Western P, Toubro S, et al. Obesity as an adaptation to a high-fat diet: evidence from a cross-sectional study. *Am J Clin Nutr.* 1994;59:350–355.

29. Astrup A, Buemann B, Christensen NJ, Toubro S. Failure to increase lipid oxidation in response to increasing dietary fat content in formerly obese women. *Am J Physiol.* 1994;266:E592–E599.

30. Thorn GW, Cahill GF. Gain in weight. Obesity. In: Thorn GW, Adams RD, Braunwald E, Isselbacher KJ, et al, eds. *Harrison's Principles of Internal Medicine.* 8th ed. New York: McGraw-Hill; 1977.

31. Olefsky JM. Obesity. In: Wilson JD, Braunwald E, Isselbacher KJ, Petersdorf RG, et al, eds. *Harrison's Principles of Internal Medicine.* 12th ed. New York: McGraw-Hill; 1991.

32. Getchell B. *Physical Fitness: A Way of Life.* 4th ed. New York: Macmillan Publishing Co; 1992.

33. American College of Sports Medicine. *ACSM's Guidelines for Exercise Testing and Prescription.* 5th ed. Baltimore: Williams & Wilkins; 1995.

34. Williams MH. *Nutrition for Fitness and Sport.* 4th ed. Dubuque, IA: Brown & Benchmark; 1995.

35. Tremblay A, Simoneau J, Bouchard C. Impact of exercise intensity on body fatness and skeletal muscle metabolism. *Metabolism.* 1994;44:814–818.

36. Gwinup G. Effect of exercise alone on the weight of obese women. *Arch Intern Med.* 1975;135:676–680.

37. Leon A, Conrad JS, Hunninghake DM, Serfass R. Effects of a vigorous walking program on body composition, and carbohydrate and lipid metabolism of obese young men. *Am J Clin Nutr.* 1979;32:1776–1787.

38. Despres JP, Pouliot MC, Moorjani S, Nadeau A, et al. Loss of abdominal fat and metabolic response to exercise training in obese women. *Am J Physiol.* 1991;261:E159–E167.

39. Moody DL, Wilmore JH, Girandola RN, Royce JP. The effects of a jogging program on the body composition of normal and obese high school girls. *Med Sci Sports.* 1972;4:210–213.

40. Zuti WB, Golding LA. Comparing diet and exercise as weight reduction tools. *Physician Sports Med.* 1976;4:49–55.

41. Bouchard C, Despres JP, Tremblay A. Exercise and obesity. *Obes Res.* 1993;1:133–147.

42. Berg FM. *Health Risks of Weight Loss.* Hettinger, ND: Healthy Weight Journal; 1995:27–32.

43. Wooley SC, Garner DM. Obesity treatment: the high cost of false hope. *J Am Diet Assoc.* 1991;91:1248–1251.

44. Garner DM, Wooley SC. Confronting the failure of behavioral and dietary treatments for obesity. *Clin Psychol.* 1991;11:729–780.
45. Stunkard A, McLaren-Hume M. The results of treatment for obesity. *Arch Intern Med.* 1959;103:79–85.
46. Brownell KD. Whether obesity should be treated. *Health Psychol.* 1993;12:339–341.
47. Pi-Sunyer FX. Medical hazards of obesity. *Ann Intern Med.* 1993;119:655–660.
48. Atkinson RL. Proposed standards for judging the success of the treatment of obesity. *Ann Intern Med.* 1993;119:677–680.
49. Rodin J. Cultural and psychological determinants of weight concerns. *Ann Intern Med.* 1993;119:643–645.
50. Colditz GA. Economic costs of severe obesity. *Am J Clin Nutr.* 1992;55(suppl):503S–507S.
51. Wadden TA, Sternberg JA, Letizia KA, Stunkard AJ, Foster GD. Treatment of obesity by very low calorie diet, behavior therapy, and their combination: a five year perspective. *Int J Obes.* 1989;13(suppl 2):39–46.
52. Wadden TA, Stunkard AJ, Liebschutz J. Three-year follow-up of the treatment of obesity by very low calorie diet, behavior therapy and their combination. *J Consult Clin Psychol.* 1988;56:925–928.
53. Wadden TA. Treatment of obesity by moderate and severe caloric restriction: results of clinical research trials. *Ann Intern Med.* 1993;119:688–693.
54. NIH Technology Assessment Conference Panel. Methods for voluntary weight loss and control. *Ann Intern Med.* 1993;119:764–770.
55. Kirshner MA, Schneider G, Ertel NH, Gorman J. An eight-year experience with very-low-calorie formula diet for control of major obesity. *Int J Obes.* 1988;12:69–80.
56. Brownell KD, Jeffery RW. Improving long-term weight loss: pushing the limits of treatment. *Behav Ther.* 1987;18:353–374.
57. Kramer FM, Jeffery RW, Forster JL, Snell MK. Long-term follow-up of behavioral treatment for obesity: patterns of weight regain in men and women. *Int J Obes.* 1989;13:123–136.
58. Foreyt JP, Goodrick GK. Evidence for success of behavioral modification in weight loss and control. *Ann Intern Med.* 1993;119:698–701.
59. Jeffery RW. Minnesota studies on community-based approaches to weight loss and control. *Ann Intern Med.* 1993;119:719–721.
60. Miller WC, Eggert KE, Wallace JP, Lindeman AK, Jastremski C. Successful weight loss in a self-taught, self-administered program. *Int J Sports Med.* 1993;14:401–405.
61. Miller WC, Wallace JP, Eggert KE, Lindeman AK. Cardiovascular risk reduction in a self-taught, self-administered weight loss program called the nondiet diet. *Med Exerc Nutr Health.* 1993;2:218–223.
62. Stevens VJ, Rossner J, Hyg MS, et al. Freedom from fat: a contemporary multi-component weight loss program for the general population of obese adults. *J Am Diet Assoc.* 1989;89:1254–1258.
63. Ballor DL, Harvey-Berino J, Ades PA. A healthy lifestyle is the treatment of choice for obesity in coronary patients. *Cardiopulm Rehab.* 1995;15:14–18.
64. Oscai LB, Williams BT. Effect of exercise on overweight middle-aged males. *J Am Geriatric Soc.* 1968;16:794–797.
65. Woo R, Garrow JS, Pi-Sunyer FX. Voluntary food intake during prolonged exercise in obese women. *Am J Clin Nutr.* 1982;36:478–484.

66. Wilmore JH. Appetite and body composition consequent to physical activity. *Res Q Exerc Sport.* 1983;54:415–425.

67. King AC, Tribble DL. The role of exercise in weight reduction in nonathletes. *Sports Med.* 1991;11:331–349.

68. Epstein LH, Wing RR. Aerobic exercise and weight. *Addict Behav.* 1980;5:371–388.

69. Wood PD, Stefanick ML, Williams PT, Haskell WL. The effects on plasma lipoproteins of a prudent weight-reducing diet, with or without exercise, in overweight men and women. *N Engl J Med.* 1991;325:461–466.

70. Ballor DL, Keesey RE. A meta-analysis of the factors affecting exercise-induced changes in body mass, fat mass and fat-free mass in males and females. *Int J Obes.* 1991;15:717–726.

71. Pavlou KN, Krey S, Steffee WP. Exercise as an adjunct to weight loss and maintenance in moderately obese subjects. *Am J Clin Nutr.* 1989;49:1115–1123.

72. Jeffery RW, Gerber WM. Group and correspondence treatments for weight reduction used in the multiple risk factor intervention trial. *Behav Ther.* 1982;13:24–30.

73. Schachter S. Recidivism and self-cure of smoking and obesity. *Am Psychol.* 1982;37:436–444.

74. Hyman FN, Sempos E, Saltsman J, Glinsmann WH. Evidence for success of caloric restriction in weight loss and control: summary of data from industry. *Ann Intern Med.* 1993;119:681–687.

75. Wooley SC. Is self-acceptance a reasonable goal? In: Allison DB, Pi-Sunyer FX, eds. *Obesity treatment.* New York: Plenum Press; 1995:75–78.

76. Garner DM. Obesity treatment: more harm than good. *J Am Diet Assoc.* 1991;91(suppl):A152.

77. Pi-Sunyer FX. Short-term medical benefits and adverse effects of weight loss. *Ann Intern Med.* 1993;119:722–726.

78. Wilson GT. Relation of dieting and voluntary weight loss to psychological functioning and binge eating. *Ann Intern Med.* 1993;119:727–730.

79. Blair SN. Evidence for success of exercise in weight loss and control. *Ann Intern Med.* 1993;119:702–706.

80. Bray GA. Barriers to the treatment of obesity. *Ann Intern Med.* 91;115:152–153.

81. Perri MG, McAllister DA, Gange JJ, Jordan RC, McAdoo MG, Nezu AM. Effects of four maintenance programs on the long-term management of obesity. *J Consult Clin Psychol.* 1988;56:529–534.

82. Bennett W. Indictment of Dieting-III. Presented at National Association to Advance Fat Acceptance Convention; September 2, 1979; Columbus, OH.

83. Goodrick GK, Raynaud AS, Pace PW, Foreyt JP. Outcome attributions in a very low calorie weight loss program. *Int J Eating Dis.* 1992;12:117.

84. Wooley OW. Indictment of Dieting-II. Presented at National Association to Advance Fat Acceptance Convention; September 2, 1979; Arlington, VA.

85. Begley CE. Government should strengthen regulation in the weight loss industry. *J Am Diet Assoc.* 1991;91:1255–1257.

86. Lustig A. Weight loss programs: failing to meet ethical standards? *J Am Diet Assoc.* 1991;91:1252–1254.

87. Smith S. An indictment of the NIH. *Dimensions.* 1995;January:39–40.

88. Smith S. Building bridges in the movement between past and future. *Healthy Weight J.* 1995;9:53–54.

89. Association for the Health Enrichment of Large People. *Association Brochure.* Blacksburg, VA.

90. Society for Nutrition Education Steering Committee for Nutrition and Weight Realities. *Newsletter.* January; 1995.

91. American Dietetic Association. Position of the American Dietetic Association: nutrition intervention in the treatment of anorexia nervosa, bulimia nervosa, and binge eating. *J Am Diet Assoc.* 1994;94:902–907.

92. Miller J. New findings on obesity presented. *Psychiatric Times Med Behav.* 1992;38.

93. Colvin RH, Olson SB. A descriptive analysis of men and women who have lost significant weight and are highly successful at maintaining the loss. *Addict Behav.* 1983;8:287–295.

94. Kayman S, Bruvold W, Stern JS. Maintenance and relapse after weight loss in women: behavioral aspects. *Am J Clin Nutr.* 1990;52:800–807.

95. Wooley SC. Indictment of Dieting-I. Presented at National Association to Advance Fat Acceptance Convention; September 2, 1979; Arlington, VA.

96. Pace PW, Bolton MP, Reeves RS. Ethics of obesity treatment: implications for dietitians. *J Am Diet Assoc.* 1991:91;1258–1260.

97. Miller WC, Eggert KE. Weight loss perceptions, characteristics, and expectations of an overweight male and female population. *Med Exerc Nutr Health.* 1992;1:42–46.

98. American College of Sports Medicine. The recommended quantity and quality of exercise for developing and maintaining cardiorespiratory and muscular fitness in healthy adults. *Med Sci Sports Exerc.* 1990;22:265–274.

99. Swensen T, Miller WC, White T. Effect of aerobic- vs weight-training and a simple diet modification on body composition in overweight adults. *Med Sci Sports Exerc.* 1995;27(suppl):S169.

100. Miller WC. *The Non-Diet Diet: A Simple 100-Point Scoring System for Weight Loss Without Counting Calories.* Englewood, CO: Morton Publishing; 1991.

CHAPTER 17

Emotional Eating and Obesity: Theoretical Considerations and Practical Recommendations

Myles S. Faith
David B. Allison
Allan Geliebter

INTRODUCTION

Kummerspeck is a German word meaning "fat of sorrow." This term was used to describe the unexpected weight gain observed among some women during World War I.[1] These women either had uncertain and unpredictable lives, or had lovers who were killed in war. Thus, their weight gain was attributed to excessive emotional trauma.

Although most people are unaware of the term *kummerspeck,* many believe that obesity and emotional distress go hand in hand. This notion dates back at least to the turn of the 20th century[2] and remains popular today. Indeed, the belief that obese persons experience greater psychopathology than non-obese persons is common among lay persons as well as among physicians and other professionals.[3–6]

Thus, there has been a common cultural belief that overweight and obese individuals experience greater emotional disturbance than thinner individuals. Along these lines, many argue that obese persons are more likely than non-obese persons to overeat in response to emotional distress, and hence to put on weight.[7] According to psychodynamic theory, obesity results from the use of food as an emotional defense.[8–11] This theory is generally known as the *psychosomatic model of obesity* (PMO)[12] and is the focus of this chapter.

This chapter explores the issue of emotional eating and obesity. Throughout this chapter, the term "emotional eating" is used to represent eating in response to a range of negative emotions such as anxiety, depression, anger, and loneliness.

Although this term lacks precision and focuses primarily on negative affect, it is used in order to remain within the tradition of the PMO, which historically has not differentiated between specific emotions. Nonetheless, the authors hope that future studies will progress beyond such broad conceptualizations and address more specific psychological and physiological mechanisms.

This chapter is broadly partitioned into two sections: theoretical issues and practical recommendations. The section on theoretical issues begins by reviewing the traditional PMO, as well as its cognitive-behavioral variants. Data supporting the PMO are then reviewed and critiqued. This is followed by a discussion of possible subgroups of obese persons who might be more prone to emotional eating. These include restrained eaters, binge eaters, and carbohydrate cravers. In essence, this first section addresses the question, "Are obese persons more likely than non-obese persons to overeat when emotionally distressed?"

The second section of this chapter is more practical in nature, focusing on the assessment and treatment of emotional eating among obese persons. First, methods for assessing emotional eating are reviewed. Because most researchers and clinicians rely on self-report instruments, a list of available self-report measures and their psychometric properties is provided. Second, traditional cognitive-behavioral and alternative psychological approaches to the treatment of emotional eating among obese persons are reviewed. In essence, this section addresses the question, "How do researchers and clinicians assess and treat emotional eating patterns among obese persons?"

The chapter ends with some general suggestions for researchers interested in exploring an emotional eating–obesity relationship. Suggestions include exploration of the use of longitudinal research designs, the use of children as subjects in research programs, the integration of psychology and physiology, the effects of chronic stressors on eating behavior, and the effect of specific emotions on eating behavior.

EMOTIONAL EATING AND OBESITY: THEORETICAL PERSPECTIVES

The PMO: Theoretical Overview

The observation that stress-induced eating promotes obesity has existed for many years and has even been traced back to philosopher David Hume in the 18th century.[1] However, it was the psychoanalytic community's acceptance and perpetuation of the PMO that legitimized it as a scientifically credible theory in the 20th century.[8-11] Since that time, enthusiasm for the PMO has carried over to cognitive-behavioral theorists as well.[13] In essence, the PMO states that obesity largely results from excessive eating in response to negative emotions, such as anxiety, boredom, anger, and depression. At its core, the PMO posits that obese and non-obese persons have different eating patterns. Specifically, obese individuals are believed to overeat in response to emotional distress whereas non-obese individuals are believed to display better coping skills and not overeat in such situations.

Theoretical writings on the PMO can be traced throughout the 20th century[8–21] and are discussed in detail elsewhere.[22] Early psychodynamic proponents of the model argued that emotional eating represents a psychosexual fixation, typically at the oral stage of development. For example, Bychowski construed obesity in terms of weak ego strength: "Some of the striking characteristics of our patients may serve as an introduction. It is easy to see that their attitude to food and to eating differs from the usual one . . . they behave like an addict deprived of his drug. . . . Food means strength and serves to weaken the Ego."[9(p303)]

Summarizing Kaplan and Kaplan's literature review,[12] Slochower presented 27 common psychodynamic interpretations of excessive overeating by obese individuals.[19] Exhibit 17–1 presents this list, which clearly emphasizes poor ego functioning and an inability to tolerate emotional discomfort.

Exhibit 17–1 Psychodynamic Interpretations Associated with Overeating among Obese Individuals

1. Diminishing anxiety
2. Achieving pleasure
3. Achieving social success and acceptance
4. Relieving frustration and deprivation
5. Expressing hostility (conscious or unconscious)
6. Diminishing feelings of insecurity
7. Self-indulgence
8. Rewarding oneself
9. Expressing defiance
10. Submitting (e.g., to authority)
11. Self punishment in response to guilt
12. Diminishing guilt
13. Exhibitionism
14. Attaining attention and care
15. Justifying failure in life
16. Testing love
17. Counteracting a feeling of being unloved
18. Distorting reality
19. Identifying with a fat parent
20. Sedating oneself
21. Avoiding competition in life
22. Avoiding changing the status quo
23. Proving one's inferiority
24. Avoiding maturity
25. Diminishing fear of starvation
26. Consciously fulfilling the wish to become fat
27. Handling anxiety from infantile oral frustration

Source: Reprinted with permission from J.A. Slochowar, *Excessive Eating: The Role of Emotions and Environment,* pp. 13–14, © 1983, Plenum Publishing Corporation.

Recently, PMO doctrine has borrowed from cognitive and learning theories to explain underlying mechanisms.[13,18,23,24] In particular, cognitive theorists have borrowed Herman and Polivy's notion of dietary restraint to explain stress-induced eating among obese persons.[23,25,26] This model proposes that emotional distress can act as a disinhibitor, causing obese persons to deviate from dietary rules and consequently overeat. This issue will be discussed later in this chapter.

Before reviewing empirical support for the PMO, one point should be noted. Whatever its scientific merits, many lay individuals and health professionals appear to accept tenets of the PMO at face value. That is, the model appears to have strong social validity. To cite one example, in a survey of 200 Australian citizens, 17% of respondents attributed obesity to "emotional reasons." In contrast, only 4% attributed obesity to "heredity."[27] This finding is consistent with a vast literature documenting a pervasive anti-fat attitude in Western culture.[6,28–32] See Chapter 12 on social issues related to overweight and obesity. Thus, before reviewing any data on the PMO, it is important to acknowledge the prejudiced social milieu within which any research and clinical work must be conducted.

The Psychosomatic Model: Empirical Support

Critical reviews of the PMO have recently appeared in the psychological literature.[18,33,34] Two reviews focused on emotional eating and obesity among humans,[18,33] whereas the third reviewed both human and animal studies.[34] The present discussion will focus entirely on data from human studies.

Researchers have traditionally tested the PMO by using tightly controlled laboratory studies in which precise measures of food consumption were taken.[35–38] These studies generally followed the same experimental paradigm, differing mostly in their selection of independent variables (i.e., type of stressor) and/or dependent variables (i.e., type of food consumed in the study).

In the typical study, obese and non-obese subjects were brought into the laboratory to participate in a taste test of foods such as ice cream, crackers, cookies, or candy. Before eating, however, some subjects were subjected to physical or psychological stressors such as the threat of being shocked,[35,36] failure feedback,[38] or instructions to impress a strange man[39]; other subjects served as experimental controls and were not emotionally manipulated. The PMO predicted obese, but not non-obese individuals, would overeat in response to these stressors.

On balance, the data from these experimental studies provide only weak support for the PMO.[34] That is, there is no consistent pattern of overeating by obese persons in response to laboratory stressors. Some researchers argue that specific preconditions might be necessary to elicit the effect, including the induction of a *diffuse* anxiety state[19] or an effective *ego threat*.[40,41] Still, the balance of laboratory studies have not consistently detected greater emotional eating among obese than non-obese individuals.

The PMO has received greater support from studies using self-report measures of emotional eating.[42–50] Indeed, Ganley's review of the PMO literature found that reports of emotional eating were prevalent among all classes of overweight, from the mildly to the morbidly obese.[18] On the other hand, when Allison and Heshka reviewed the same literature, they concluded that the studies were either too methodologically flawed to yield definitive conclusions or did not actually measure emotional eating.[33] Thus, in contrast to Ganley's conclusions, this review found limited empirical support for the PMO. Similar conclusions were reached by Greeno and Wing, who found minimal evidence that obese persons as a single population display greater emotional eating tendencies than non-obese persons.[34]

Thus, taking both laboratory and questionnaire data into account, the PMO has not received strong support. However, recent data tentatively suggest that certain subgroups of obese persons might be more prone to emotional eating than others. These subgroups include restrained eaters, binge eaters, carbohydrate cravers, and emotional eaters as their own unique subgroup. The following sections review the evidence that these specific subgroups demonstrate greater emotional eating habits than other obese persons.

Dietary Restraint

Dietary restraint, or restraint for short, refers to the self-perception that one is intentionally eating less than desired, typically to lose or maintain weight. The bulk of the studies on restraint stem from the pioneering work of Herman and Polivy,[23,25] who initially conceptualized obese individuals as being restrained eaters chronically attempting to lose weight. Their research, in turn, was based on previous work by Schachter[35,51] and Nisbett.[52,53]

Through a series of creative laboratory studies, various researchers have characterized the eating behavior of the restrained eater.[54] A crucial finding has been that of *disinhibition*—the tendency of restrained individuals to lose their restraint in response to certain stimuli and eat more than they would otherwise eat under similar circumstances. Food intake during disinhibition can become quite large and might constitute a binge eating episode.[26] As related to the PMO, several researchers have demonstrated that negative affect can act as a disinhibitor for restrained eaters and consequently promote overeating.[55,56] Thus, to the extent that most obese individuals are restrained eaters, these findings would support the PMO.

However, the picture is not so simple. First, not all obese individuals show behavioral disinhibition when studied in the laboratory.[57,58] Those who demonstrate greater disinhibition tend to have greater histories of dieting and current dieting practices than those who fail to show disinhibition.[59,60]

The second concern is a methodological one. Most of the original studies showing disinhibition among restrained eaters used Herman and Polivy's Restraint Scale.[25] When statistically analyzed (principal component analysis), this scale has two to three factors: "concern with dieting," "weight fluctuation," and sometimes "binging/disinhibition."[61,62] However, studies using different restraint scales that do not measure weight fluctuation or disinhibition have not reliably found an association between restraint and disinhibited eating.[55,63,64] Thus, it might be erroneous to conclude that restraint per se causes eating disinhibition. Rather, disinhibition might be due to other factors, such as weight fluctuation, that are measured only by the Restraint Scale.

Finally, some studies suggest that restraint may not be a necessary precondition for emotional eating among obese binge eaters.[65–67] For these individuals, negative affect by itself appears sufficient to trigger emotional and binge eating. Of course, this finding poses a problem for the application of traditional restraint theory to obese binge eaters.

On balance, although restraint is a good predictor of disinhibition in response to emotional distress, this construct appears to be independent of body mass index.[34] That is, both normal-weight and overweight persons may be restrained eaters. Nonetheless, for clinicians interested in assessing restraint, there are instruments available including the Restraint Scale,[25] the restraint scale from the Three-Factor Eating Questionnaire,[68] and the restraint scale from the Dutch Eating Behavior Questionnaire.[69] These scales are easily administered and easily scored. Detailed reviews of these scales can be found elsewhere.[61,62]

Binge Eating Patterns Related to Emotional Eating

Another subgroup of obese individuals prone to emotional eating might be those who binge eat. Originating with Stunkard's classic article,[70] reports on binge eating among obese persons have mushroomed in recent years and have culminated in DSM-IV's Binge Eating Disorder (BED).[71–74]

Binge eating correlates positively with body weight among obese persons[75] and is common among persons enrolled in weight loss programs, with prevalence estimates ranging from 23% to 46%.[76,77] Recent studies explicitly using BED criteria report prevalences of approximately 30% among obese persons receiving treatment.[72,73] One of the more consistent findings to date has been the greater prevalence of psychopathology among obese persons who binge eat than those who do not.[76–83]

Three studies have documented an association between binge eating and emotional eating tendencies among obese persons.[65,84,85] Studying the emotional eating patterns of 19 women seeking treatment for binge eating, Arnow and colleagues used a variety of measures to assess subjects' thoughts, feelings, and physical sensations before, during, and following a binge.[65] Results indicated that negative affect was very common both before and after binge eating and somewhat less common during binges. For example, 100% of the subjects reported awareness of negative emotions both before and after binge eating episodes. Whereas emotions such as anger, anxiety, and depression were more common before binge eating, guilt was more common afterward.

More recently, Kuehnel and Wadden compared the eating self-efficacy of obese nonbingers, obese "problem eaters," and obese individuals meeting BED criteria.[85] Problem eaters were individuals who reported some binge eating but failed to meet full BED criteria. In this study, participants rated their eating self-efficacy, or their ability to avoid emotional eating. The researchers found that individuals with BED reported significantly poorer eating self-efficacy than nonbinging obese persons. The mean level of emotional eating for problem eaters did not significantly differ from either nonbinging obese persons or those with BED. Thus, emotional eating might be more problematic for obese persons with more severe binge eating tendencies.

Finally, Eldredge and Agras compared emotional eating patterns among three groups of patients enrolled in commercial weight loss programs across the country.[84] These three groups included patients with BED, patients with Eating Disorder Not Otherwise Specified (EDNOS), or patients with no eating disorders. The researchers found greater emotional eating among BED patients than among EDNOS or non–eating-disordered patients. Interestingly, body mass index was not significantly related to emotional eating, thus suggesting an association between emotional eating and disordered eating rather than between emotional eating and overweight.

Thus, available data suggest a consistent association between binge eating and emotional eating tendencies. For clinicians interested in assessing obese patients' binge eating tendencies, there are a variety of instruments available. These include the Binge Eating Scale,[86] the Questionnaire on Eating and Weight Patterns-Revised,[73] and the Binge Scale Questionnaire.[87] These and other instruments are reviewed elsewhere in greater detail (see Chapter 4).[88,89]

Carbohydrate Cravers

In a series of studies, Wurtman et al have investigated the theory that carbohydrate craving plays a role in human obesity.[90,91] The theory has also received much attention in the public media, especially after the publication of a popular diet book.[92] The biochemical underpinning for the theory derives from early studies of Fernstrom and Wurtman showing that in rats, brain levels of serotonin can be increased by feeding carbohydrates.[93,94] The presumed mechanism is that carbohydrate ingestion stimulates insulin release, which promotes a greater ratio of tryptophan to other large neutral amino acids that compete for the same transport system into the brain. Since tryptophan is the precursor for serotonin, the result is higher concentrations of brain serotonin. The increased brain serotonin is postulated to reduce additional carbohydrate intake, and a feedback loop is established that can regulate carbohydrate ingestion.

In humans, brain levels of serotonin cannot be measured in vivo, and thus the assumption that carbohydrate ingestion increases brain serotonin must be inferred from levels of tryptophan in the blood and their ratio to the other large neutral amino acids. In fact, in human obesity, the basal levels of tryptophan tend to be rather low,[95] which Wurtman et al suggest act to drive carbohydrate ingestion. However, even after ingesting carbohydrates, obese subjects show only a small or negligible change in tryptophan levels and their ratio, which argues against a regulatory process.[95]

Another problem with carbohydrate craving theory is that in rats, even a small amount of protein (5%) mixed in with the carbohydrate completely abolishes the augmenting effect on brain serotonin.[96] Indeed, there is often a small amount of protein found in carbohydrate foods and snacks. Moreover, in carbohydrate snacks, carbohydrate is often combined with fat, which Drewnowski et al have argued is more preferred than carbohydrate by obese individuals.[97]

The Wurtman group has also suggested that when obese carbohydrate cravers consume carbohydrates, they report improved mood and less fatigue, whereas obese non-cravers report feeling more depressed and more fatigued.[98] They suggest that for the cravers, ingestion of carbohydrates is a form of self-medication. Nevertheless, when given a choice of snacks, the non-cravers still consume 56% as carbohydrate-rich snacks.[98] If carbohydrate ingestion makes them feel bad, why would they choose it? There is also no evidence that carbohydrate cravers are more likely to be emotional eaters than obese non-cravers.

There is some evidence that individuals with Seasonal Affective Disorder (SAD) are more likely to overeat carbohydrate snacks during the winter when they feel depressed.[91] However, this tendency is equally as common among normal-weight and overweight persons with SAD. There is also no evidence that SAD is more common among obese persons, posing further difficulties for the theory.

Further evidence to support the carbohydrate craving theory is drawn from studies in which an appetite suppressant, fenfluramine, a serotonin reuptake inhibitor that leads to higher brain serotonin levels, is administered to obese subjects who prefer carbohydrate snacks.[99,100] A marked reduction in the intake of these snacks occurs, which presumably shows that raising serotonin levels inhibits ingestion of carbohydrates. However, fenfluramine also significantly reduces *total* calorie intake, including those from protein and fat. Therefore, the reduction of the permissive snack intake, which happens to be largely carbohydrate, does not necessarily support the model.

In sum, although the notion that carbohydrate craving, possibly in response to emotional states, could contribute to human obesity still has appeal as a theory and has stimulated much research, the evidence remains incomplete and unconvincing.

Emotional Eaters As Their Own Subgroup

Finally, instead of looking for restrained eaters, binge eaters, or carbohydrate cravers, one could simply look for those obese individuals who eat (or report eating) when emotionally distressed. Indeed, cluster analytic research by Schlundt and colleagues identified such a subgroup.[45] Deriving a five-category topology of obese female participants in a weight loss program, these researchers identified one category as "emotional eaters." Compared to other groups, these individuals reported greater eating in response to negative emotions, positive emotions, illness, depression, somatic symptoms, stimulus exposure, and social adjustment difficulties. Unfortunately, identifying a distinct subgroup of obese emotional eaters does not indicate why they eat when distressed or the underlying psychological or physiological mechanism. That is, to identify obese individuals as emotional eaters solely on the basis of that behavior is somewhat tautological and opens the door for more questions.

Summary

There is mixed evidence that certain subgroups are more likely to be emotional eaters than others. The data are especially tenuous for obese persons described as restrained eaters or carbohydrate cravers. On the other hand, there is evidence that obese persons who binge eat are also more likely to overeat when emotionally distressed. This finding has implications for clinicians when selecting their treatment plan for reducing emotional eating behavior. The next section addresses more practical issues related to the assessment and treatment of emotional eating behavior among obese persons.

ASSESSMENT AND TREATMENT OF EMOTIONAL EATING

Challenges in Assessing Emotional Eating

The first step in understanding emotional eating is a reliable and valid assessment. Unfortunately, this is often a challenging task for several reasons. First, emotional eating is a broad construct that includes eating in response to a range of negative and positive emotions, across a wide range of situational stimuli. For example, one person might overeat due to the chronic stress of divorce, while another might binge after an evening of laughter at a comedy club. Therefore, the assessment of emotional eating should be sensitive to a range of situational events and emotional reactions thereof.

Second, some individuals are ashamed of emotional eating episodes.[43,65] Indeed, obese dieters are more likely to experience negative emotions after experiencing a dietary lapse than after merely experiencing the temptation to eat.[101] Consequently, these individuals might be reluctant to share their experiences with clinicians or researchers.

Similarly, self-reported emotional eating can be confounded by social desirability, or the desire to give "appropriate" responses. To demonstrate this point, Allison and Heshkha instructed subjects to complete an emotional eating questionnaire as if they were an "emotionally disordered patient."[102] Compared to control subjects and those instructed to make a "good impression," these subjects reported significantly greater emotional eating tendencies. In a recent experimental study, researchers found that obese participants exposed to the PMO model from an "obesity expert" reported greater emotional eating episodes in five-day food diaries than obese participants not exposed to the model.[103] Furthermore, actual emotional eating behavior was enhanced in a laboratory taste test setting. Taken together, these studies suggests that therapist instructions can influence obese persons' reports of emotional eating and actual eating behavior.

Finally, some obese individuals experience alexithymia, or the inability to identify emotional states. Recent data suggest that this condition may be more common among binge eating than nonbinge eating obese persons.[104] Of course, the presence of alexithymia could compromise the integrity of one's assessment.

Clinical Reasons for Assessing Emotional Eating

The assessment of emotional eating has documented clinical utility. Specifically, several studies indicate that the mastery of emotional eating predicts better success in clinical weight loss trials.[105–108] For example, one study tracked 187 participants who had participated in a "weight slimming effort" organized by the British Heart Foundation. At one-year follow-up, the researchers discovered that changes in emotional eating tendencies predicted weight loss and success toward target weight over the previous year. Compared to obese participants who did not decrease emotional eating, those who did lost more weight and made more progress toward target weights. Participants who increased emotional eating tendencies were less successful in reaching target weights.

Furthermore, as indicated earlier, emotional distress appears to be a trigger to eat for some obese dieters. For example, Grilo et al used cluster analysis to identify the situational antecedents of dieting relapses and dieters' attempts to cope with temptations.[101] Using a sample of 57 obese Type II diabetics, the researchers identified three antecedent triggers: "mealtime," "upset," and "low arousal." Upset was primarily characterized by anger, as well as anxiety and depression in some individuals.

Specific Assessment Strategies

Three common strategies for the assessment of emotional eating among obese persons will be outlined and discussed: behavioral observation, self-report inventories, and food diaries.

Behavioral Assessment. It has been argued that the best way to study eating behavior is to observe what people eat and not what they say they eat. Indeed, creative strategies for measuring eating behavior in the natural environment have been developed.[109] These studies have measured eating behavior in environments such as cafeterias[110] and nursing homes.[111] Several studies have measured the amount of snacks dispensed from automated vending machines.[99] Of course, some researchers have challenged how well these types of measures generalize to the "real world."[112–116]

Direct behavioral observation has a number of advantages over other methods.[117] Unfortunately, direct behavioral assessment is too time consuming for most clinicians and too costly for most researchers.[118] Given this reality, many clinicians and researchers opted for self-report inventories to assess emotional eating among obese individuals.

Self-Report Inventories. Only in recent years have obesity researchers developed and validated self-report measures of emotional eating. Fortunately, most are brief and can be easily implemented by clinicians and researchers. Unfortunately, numerous "emotional eating" scales now appear in popular magazines, journals, and self-help books with little or no psychometric foundation. These scales should be used with extreme caution, if at all, and are not discussed in this chapter.

Table 17–1 presents a list of the most commonly used emotional eating inventories, along with some of their psychometric properties. Van Strien et al developed a 13-item emotional eating scale as part of their 33-item Dutch Eating Behavior Questionnaire.[69] This inventory has good psychometric features and has been studied cross-sectionally and longitudinally in samples of obese men and women.[69,119] According to its authors, the emotional scale can be factor analyzed into two factors: eating in response to specific negative emotions, and general negative arousal. Still, the authors recommend using the total scale score. Sample items include, "Do you have the desire to eat when you are irritated?" and "Do you have the desire to eat when you are anxious, worried, or tense?"

Schlundt and Zimering developed the Negative Emotions scale as part of the Dieter's Inventory of Eating Temptations.[120] This five-item scale presents respondents with five separate scenarios and requires them to rate the percent of time they would eat in those situations (e.g., "You just had an upsetting argument with a family member. You are standing in front of the refrigerator and you feel like eating everything in sight. What percent of the time would you find some other way to make yourself feel better?"). Schlundt provides normative data for normal-weight and overweight samples, as well as clinical and community samples.[121] The scale has good internal consistency and test-retest reliability.

Brownell developed an emotional eating scale as part of his Dieting Readiness Test.[122] Scale items were based on the author's clinical experiences and were strongly influenced by relapse prevention, social learning, and transtheoretical models.[123] The three-item Emotional Eating sub-scale requires respondents to an-

Table 17–1 Self-Report Emotional Eating Scales

Scale and Reference	Description	Psychometric Properties
Diet Readiness Test[122]	23-item scale measuring three dimensions of readiness to lose weight: motivation, commitment, and life circumstances. The instrument has six subscales: Goals and attitudes, Hunger and eating cues, Control over eating, Binge eating and purging, Emotional eating, and Exercise patterns and attitudes. The emotional eating scale has three items. Developed on clinical sample of overweight individuals.	Unavailable.
Dieter's Inventory of Eating Temptations[120]	30-item scale measuring situation-specific weight control abilities. The instrument taps six categories: Overeating, Resisting temptation, Food choice, Positive social eating, Negative emotional eating, and Exercise. The Negative emotional eating scale has five items. Most items were developed because of their ability to discriminate between overweight and normal-weight individuals.	α = .86–.87. TR = .92 over one week.
Dutch Eating Behavior Questionnaire[69]	33-item scale measuring dietary restraint, external eating, and emotional eating. Factor analysis of the scale yields four factors: Restraint, Emotional eating in response to diffuse feelings, Emotional eating in response to specific emotions, and External eating. Scale was developed on over 1,000 community members completing a survey.	α = .94 for combined emotional eating scale. α = .94 for diffuse emotions. α = .93 for specific emotions.
Eating Self-Efficacy Scale[107]	25-item scale measuring self-efficacy with regard to eating during (a) negative affect, and (b) socially acceptable circumstances. Negative affect scale has 15 items. Developed on college undergraduates, but used on several clinical samples.	α = .94 for Negative affect scale.

continues

Table 17–1 continued

Scale and Reference	Description	Psychometric Properties
Emotional Eating Scale[66]	25-item scale measuring three dimensions of emotional eating: Anger/frustration, Anxiety, and Depression. Developed and used on clinical samples of obese, binge eating women seeking treatment.	α = .81 for the Total scale. α = .78 for the Anger/frustration scale. α = .78 for the Anxiety scale. α = .72 for the Depression scale.
Mood Eating Scale[130]	20-item scale measuring general emotional eating patterns.	Not available.
Situational Appetite Measures[108]	30-item scale measuring urges to eat and expectation to control eating under five circumstances: Relaxation, Food Present, Hunger, Reward, and Negative Feelings. The Negative Feelings scale has five items. Developed on college undergraduates, but also used on clinical samples.	α >.90 for Negative Feelings scale. TR >.70 over four weeks.
Weight Efficacy Lifestyle Questionnaire[106]	20-item scale measuring eating self-efficacy as a function of five situational factors: Negative Emotions, Availability, Social Pressure, Physical Discomfort, and Positive Activities. Items were adapted from previous research and clinical experience. Developed on samples of clinical patients.	α = .87–.88 for Negative Emotions subscale.
Yale Eating Pattern Questionnaire[129]	70-item scale measuring nine dimensions of eating: Uninhibited, Oversnacking, Binging, Dieting, Satiation: Full, Satiation: Nausea, Satiation: Guilty, Attributions to physical causes of weight problems, and Attributions to emotional causes of weight problems. Attributions to emotional causes of weight problems is a 2-item scale. Developed on college undergraduates to assess multivariate nature of normal eating patterns.	α = .78.

Note: α = Cronbach's alpha; TR = Test-retest reliability.

swer on a 1 (Never) to 5 (Always) scale. One study used factor analysis to confirm the instrument's proposed three-factor structure: motivation, commitment, and life circumstances.[124] However, the scale failed to predict weight loss among participants in a randomized placebo-control trial. On the other hand, the instrument's emotional eating subscale correlated with reported weight fluctuation in a large sample survey.[125]

Several scales have been developed that measure self-efficacy rather than emotional eating per se. That is, they assess one's perceived ability to resist eating in response to negative emotions. One such scale is the Negative Affect scale of the Eating Self-Efficacy Scale,[107] a 15-item scale requiring respondents to rate the difficulty of controlling overeating in response to various emotions. Developed on a sample of undergraduates, the scale has excellent internal consistency and correlates positively with dietary restraint, reported previous dieting, and reported current dieting.[107]

A related scale is the Negative Emotional scale of the Weight Efficacy Lifestyle Questionnaire.[106] Items on this scale were initially derived from Condiotte and Lichtenstein's Smoking Confidence Questionnaire[126] and were subsequently administered to obese clients enrolled in various workplace and hospital weight loss programs. The four-item Negative Emotions scale has good internal consistency. It has also been used in several studies to predict weight loss among obese persons.[127,128]

Stanton et al developed the Situational Appetite Measure (SAM), which comes in two versions.[108] In one version respondents must rate the strength of their urge to eat in specific situations. In the second version, respondents indicate their self-efficacy, that is, the belief that they can control their eating in the same situations. When factor analyzed, the SAM yielded five factors including a separate Negative Emotions scale. The scale has good internal consistency and test-retest reliability. Developed on undergraduate students, separate norms are presented for men and women.

Kristeller and Rodin developed the Yale Eating Pattern Questionnaire on a sample of undergraduates.[129] The instrument has six subscales, one of which is "attributions to emotional causes of weight problems." This two-item scale asks respondents how important anxiety and stress, and depression, are in their weight problems. The scale has good internal consistency although it has not been tested on clinical samples of obese individuals.

Arnow and colleagues recently developed a 25-item inventory that taps eating in response to three dimensions of emotion: anger and frustration, anxiety, and depression.[66] These subscales have acceptable internal consistency coefficients and demonstrate appropriate correlations with several binge eating measures.

Finally, clinicians might consider the Mood Eating Scale, reprinted in Abramson's book on emotional eating.[130] This scale has 20 items and norms derived from undergraduates are provided for males and females. No other psychometric data are provided for this instrument.

Food Diaries. Food diaries can offer an individualized assessment of emotional eating tendencies and can be of great utility to clinicians working with obese clients. Exhibit 17–2 presents a sample food diary entry from one study conducted at the Obesity Research Center. Although food diaries have been in existence for many years, Schlundt and colleagues have recently developed a computerized self-monitoring system that has great utility for assessing emotional eating patterns.[121] In their paradigm, individuals keep detailed food diaries for several weeks that document the situational and emotional antecedents of all eating behaviors. This information is then integrated through special computer software that performs a functional analysis of eating behavior.

In many respects, food diaries seem ideal for clinicians working with individual clients. This strategy emphasizes the functional relationship between food and emotions, as well as the importance of individual differences. However, there is an important limitation to food diaries. Doubly-labeled water assessments of actual caloric intake confirm that obese people tend to underreport food intake when keeping food diaries.[131–134] Therefore, researchers and clinicians should be very careful, perhaps skeptical, when extracting caloric information from food diaries and might select an alternative assessment strategy if very accurate data are needed.

Treatment Strategies

Most contemporary cognitive-behavioral treatment programs address the issue of emotional overeating as part of their package.[135–140] An in-depth description of the cognitive-behavioral treatment of obesity is beyond the scope of this chapter, especially since treatment programs have become very comprehensive in recent years, including nutrition education, coping skills training, environmental restructuring, and exercise inducement.

Cognitive-behavioral principles can be applied to the issue of emotional eating. In practice, coping skills are taught to obese clients to teach them alternatives to eating when emotionally distressed. There are various behavioral and cognitive coping techniques, most of which seem to work equally well for coping immediately after dietary lapses.[141] Ultimately, clinicians working with individual clients might need to experiment in order to determine which strategies will work best for their individual clients. As described by Grilo et al,[101] common behavioral coping skills include stimulus control, restraint, alternative behaviors, and social support. Common cognitive coping skills include compensation plans, alternative thoughts, and thought consequences. Table 17–2 lists and briefly illustrates these coping techniques. There are no data documenting clinical superiority of one technique over another specifically for the reduction of emotional eating. Nonetheless, clinical experience suggests that methods of environmental management (i.e., stimulus control) are especially useful for intervention.

A useful resource for clinicians is Abramson's book on emotional eating, which contains separate chapters dealing with different emotions as they relate to over-

Exhibit 17–2 Sample Food Diary Entry Form from Obesity Research Center Self-Monitoring Booklet

Time_____ Date_____ Day (Mon Tues Wed Thur Fri Sat Sun)

MEAL (Breakfast AM-Snack Lunch AFT-Snack Supper EVE-Snack)

PLACE (Home Work Rest Social-Event Car Street Other)

People (Family Friend Alone Other)

Feelings (Check ALL that apply):

_____Depressed or Blue   _____Afraid
_____Worried   _____Nervous or tense
_____Angry   _____Upset
_____Irritable or Frustrated   _____Excited
_____Bored   _____Happy/Cheerful
_____Lonely   _____Hopeful
_____Neutral   _____Relaxed or Calm

Special or Noteworthy Events Before/During Eating? _____
_____
_____

Unplanned/Impulsive Eating (Y N)

Amount Eaten (Undereat Just-Right Overeat)

Binge Eating (Y N)

FOOD DESCRIPTION (including preparation and amount)
_____
_____
_____
_____
_____
_____
_____
_____

Source: Adapted with permission from D.G. Schlundt, Assessment of Specific Eating Behaviors and Eating Styles, in *Handbook of Assessment Methods for Eating Behaviors and Weight-Related Problems,* D.B. Allison, ed., pp. 241–302, copyright © by Sage Publications, Inc. Reprinted by permission of Sage Publications, Inc.

Table 17–2 Examples of Behavioral and Cognitive Coping Strategies for Managing Emotional Eating Tendencies

Behavioral Technique	*Example*
Stimulus Control	Keeping snack foods out of the house during period of chronic stress.
Restraint	Limiting food consumption when eating at a fun social event and feeling elated.
Alternative Behaviors	Learning relaxation as an alternative to eating when feeling increased tension.
Social Support	Giving a family member or weight loss companion a phone call to cope with feelings of hopelessness.
Cognitive Techniques	*Examples*
Compensatory Planning	Planning ahead to overeat on carrots, or fat-free snacks, instead of cookies during periods of stress.
Alternative Thoughts	Distracting oneself by thinking about work or other issues instead of eating when lonely.
Thought Consequences	Thinking about long-term consequences of overeating on general health.
Lapse Consequences	Considering how lapses will escalate and become harder to control unless emotional eating is initially halted.

Source: Data from C.M. Grilo, S. Shiffman, and R.R. Wing, Coping with Dietary Relapse Crises and Their Aftermath, *Addictive Behaviors,* Vol. 18, pp. 89–102, © 1993, Pergamon Press; S. Shiffman, Relapse Following Smoking Cessation: A Situational Analysis, *Journal of Consulting and Clinical Psychology,* Vol. 50, pp. 71–86, © 1982, American Psychology Association; and S. Shiffman, Coping with Temptations to Smoke, *Journal of Consulting and Clinical Psychology,* Vol. 14, pp. 261–267, © 1984 American Psychology Association.

eating.[130] Cognitive distortions that fuel emotional eating are discussed in detail, as well as the appropriate methods for disputing these thoughts. Based on the writings of Beck[144,145] and Ellis,[146,147] Abramson identifies 10 common cognitive distortions associated with emotional distress. These distortions include all or nothing thinking, overgeneralization, mental filtering, discounting the positive, jumping to conclusions, magnification, emotional reasoning, should statements, labeling, and personalization and blame. Descriptions of these distortions, as well as clinical strategies for changing them, can be found elsewhere.[148]

Recent data suggest that alternative treatment packages might be useful for obese persons who binge eat. Unlike traditional cognitive-behavioral approaches that specifically target eating behavior, these alternative interventions focus on general emotional well-being and ruptured interpersonal relations. For example, a recent study by Portzelius and colleagues compared a standard behavioral weight loss program with a modified behavioral program for obese women who binge eat.[149] Compared to the standard program, this modified program primarily stressed assertiveness training, problem solving, and self-monitoring of negative thoughts for issues other than food intake. That is, the management of stressful events and negative affect was emphasized, while a strict focus on eating behavior was deemphasized. Results indicated that this modified program tended to produce greater weight loss at post-test than the standard one for severe binge eaters. The superiority of this alternative intervention reached statistical significance at 12-month follow-up.

Furthermore, researchers at Stanford University have demonstrated the efficacy of Interpersonal Therapy (IPT) for reducing obese patients' binge eating behavior.[150] IPT theory postulates four interpersonal problems that promote overeating: grief and loss, interpersonal disputes, role transitions, and interpersonal deficits.[151] According to IPT theory, eating behavior will change as interpersonal difficulties are "worked through," even though eating behavior per se is not the focus of treatment. Indeed, data from the Stanford group are very encouraging and suggest an alternative treatment avenue for clinicians.

To summarize this second section, there are a variety of options for the assessment and treatment of obese persons' emotional eating tendencies. To assist clinicians, Exhibit 17–3 offers some general clinical recommendations. This list is based on the data reviewed in this chapter plus the authors' clinical experience. Again, the authors are unaware of any data demonstrating the superiority of one intervention strategy over others that are intended specifically for the reduction of obese persons' emotional eating habits. Consequently, therapists will need to decide on specific strategies based on the individual needs of their patients.

CONCLUSION

Following are some general suggestions for researchers interested in studying a possible association between emotional distress and obesity. Some of these suggestions are methodological and others are substantive.

1. *Greater use of within-subject, longitudinal research designs.* The majority of PMO research has taken one measurement of emotional eating per subject at only one point in time. Consequently, intraindividual variation in emotional eating behavior has often been ignored. However, emotional eating patterns might only be detectable through multiple assessments that would allow the modeling of change over time.[153] For example, imagine that obese and non-obese individuals do not differ in average food intake when anxious, but that obese individuals are more likely to experience phases of "yo-yo" dieting when anxious. Dynamic weight cycling phases such as these can only be detected by taking multiple assessments

Exhibit 17–3 Clinical Recommendations for the Assessment and Treatment of Emotional Eating among Obese Persons

1. Identify personal assumptions about emotional eating and obesity. Clinicians should not automatically assume that all obese persons seeking treatment overeat when experiencing negative affect. Such prejudices might be perceived by patients and bias the information given during clinical assessment, as well as patients' actual eating behavior. Assessments of emotional eating should be as objective as possible.

2. Conduct a functional analysis of emotional eating behavior. Clinicians should avoid the use of overly general, trait-level descriptions of eating behavior (e.g., "She's an emotional eater."). Instead, attention should be focused on the specific antecedents and consequences of eating behavior. Antecedents and consequences can be situational (rejection from friends) or emotional (anger at parent). Collect data from as many sources as possible (e.g., self-report, behavioral, significant others).

3. Identify the specific goals of intervention. Clinical goals can vary, including the reduction of emotional eating behaviors, the reduction of body weight, or the modification of life circumstances that promote overeating (e.g., poor interpersonal relations). Each one of these outcomes is very distinct and should be clearly identified at the beginning of intervention. It would be erroneous to assume that the resolution of interpersonal deficits will automatically reduce emotional eating. Similarly, the reduction of emotional eating does not necessarily promote weight loss. Consequently, primary goals must be delineated with patients.

4. Be consistent in the behavior targeted for change. Clinicians following the IPT model should stay focused on interpersonal issues and not haphazardly jump back to the micromanagement of discrete eating behaviors. The converse is also true. If no clinical improvement is detected after a number of sessions (e.g., 8 to 12), clinicians might then switch to a different treatment strategy. Agras and colleagues recently evaluated this type of therapeutic transition with obese binge eaters.[152]

over time. Interested readers might explore the aforementioned publications by Schlundt and colleagues and the use of nonlinear statistical models.

2. Greater use of children and adolescent subjects. There have been no controlled studies comparing the emotional eating habits of obese vs non-obese children, or the development of emotional eating habits among obese children and adolescents. Furthermore, the authors are unaware of any self-report emotional eating scales developed specifically for children. This could be a promising line of research, with studies focusing solely on children or on child-parent dynamics. Along these lines, a recent European study completed a 10-year follow-up of children who were either apparently neglected or not neglected by their parents.[154] Neglected children were 9.8 times more likely to become obese adolescents than non-neglected children, thus suggesting that environmental stressors might contribute to obesity development.

3. *More research on the interplay of psychological and physiological processes.* The traditional PMO posits that stress promotes obesity primarily via excessive food intake; however, some researchers argue that physiological processes might mediate the effects of stress.[155–159] Thus, arousal of the hypothalamic-adrenal axis, triggered by physical or psychological stress, might promote central fat accumulation. Several animal and human studies provide preliminary support for this hypothesis,[160–162] although more longitudinal research using human subjects is still warranted.

4. *More research on the effects of chronic stressors on body weight.* Laboratory investigations of the PMO have made extensive use of acute stressors such as the threat of shock, failure feedback, or having to give a video-recorded speech. However, these affect induction procedures might not generalize to chronic stressors such as unemployment, exposure to violence, or crowded living conditions. Controlled studies of the effects of chronic stress on eating have not been studied primarily because of ethical and practical constraints. However, some data support the notion that chronic stress might promote overweight. First, Greeno and Wing's review of the animal literature concluded that chronic stressors (e.g., crowded living quarters) might promote overeating and obesity, if not general oral behaviors such as gnawing, in animals.[34] Second, there is tentative evidence that exposure to war promotes weight gain in children. Specifically, Rumboldt and colleagues observed weight gains that were significantly greater than chance among elementary school children exposed to the war in Croatia.[163] Thus, there are some data that suggest the importance of studying the effects of chronic rather than acute stressors.

5. *Identification of specific negative and positive emotions promoting weight gain.* As Table 17–1 indicates, the PMO has traditionally given equal weight to all negative emotions in terms of their ability to promote weight gain. However, this assumption is challenged by recent data suggesting that anger and depression, but perhaps *not* anxiety, promote weight gain among obese binge eaters.[164] Researchers should be encouraged to develop more focused research questions and to study the effects of specific negative and positive emotions on eating behavior and weight change.

REFERENCES

1. Bruch H. *Eating Disorders.* New York: Basic Books; 1973.
2. Leven G. *L'obesite et son traitement.* Paris; 1905.
3. Bray GA, York B, DeLany J. A survey of the opinions of obesity experts on the causes and treatment of obesity. *Am J Clin Nutr.* 1992;55:151S–154S.
4. Liese BS. Physicians' perceptions of the role of psychology in medicine. *Prof Psychol Res Pract.* 1986;17:276–277.

5. Young LM, Powell B. The effects of obesity on the clinical judgments of mental health professionals. *J Health Soc Behav.* 1985;26:233–246.

6. Yuker HE, Allison DB. Obesity: sociocultural perspectives. In: Alexander-Mott L, Lumsden DB, eds. *Understanding Eating Disorders: Anorexia Nervosa, Bulimia Nervosa, Obesity.* Washington, DC: Taylor & Francis; 1994:243–270.

7. Friedman R, Shackelford A, Reiff S, Benson H. Stress and weight maintenance: the disinhibition effect and the micromanagement of stress. In: Blackburn GL, Kanders BS, eds. *Obesity Pathophysiology Psychology and Treatment.* New York: Chapman & Hall; 1994:253–263.

8. Alexander F. The influence of psychological factors upon gastrointestinal disturbances. *Psychoanal Q.* 1934;3:501.

9. Bychowski G. On neurotic obesity. *Psychoanal Rev.* 1950;37:301–319.

10. Hockman S. Mental and psychological factors in obesity. *Med Rec.* 1938;148:108.

11. Hamberger WW. Emotional aspects of obesity. *Med Clin North Am.* 1951;35:483–499.

12. Kaplan HI, Kaplan H. The psychosomatic concept of obesity. *J Nerv Ment Dis.* 1957;125:181–200.

13. Robbins TW, Fray PJ. Stress-induced eating: fact, fiction, or misunderstanding? *Appetite.* 1980;1:103–133.

14. Abraham K. A short study of the development of libido viewed in the light of the mental disorders. *Selected Papers.* London: Institute for Psychoanalysis and the Hogarth Press.

15. Shorvon JH, Richardson JS. Sudden obesity and psychological trauma. *Br Med J.* 1949;4634:951.

16. Burdon AP, Paul L. Obesity: a review of the literature stressing the psychosomatic approach. *Psychiatr Q.* 1951;25:568.

17. Auteri MC, Mendorla G., Zammataro M. Results of the sceno-test on inter-oral dynamics in obese children. In: Cacciari E, Laron Z, Raiti S, eds. *Obesity in Childhood: Proceedings of the Serona Symposia.* New York: Academic Press; 1978:17.

18. Ganley RM. Emotion and eating in obesity: a review of the literature. *Int J Eating Dis.* 1989;8:343–361.

19. Slochower J. *Excessive Eating: The Role of Emotions and Environment.* New York: Human Sciences Press; 1983.

20. Weinstein L, Pickens D. Emotions underlying obesity. *Bull Psychonomic Soc.* 1988;26:50.

21. Glucksman ML. Obesity: a psychoanalytic challenge. *J Academy Psychoanal.* 1989;17:151–171.

22. Slochower J. The psychodynamics of obesity. *Psychoanal Psychol.* 1987;4:145–159.

23. Herman CP, Mack D. Restrained and unrestrained eating. *J Pers.* 1975;43:647–660.

24. Leon GR, Roth L. Obesity: psychological causes, correlations, and speculations. *Psychol Bull.* 1977;84:117–139.

25. Herman CP, Polivy J. Restrained eating. In: Stunkard A, ed. *Obesity.* Philadelphia: Saunders; 1980:208–225.

26. Polivy J, Herman CP. Etiology of binge eating. In: Fairburn CG, Wilson GT, eds. *Binge Eating: Nature, Assessment, and Treatment.* New York: Guilford Press; 1993:173–205.

27. Harris MB, Hopwood J. Attitudes towards the obese in Australia. *J Obesity Weight Regul.* 1983;2:107–120.

28. Crandall CS. Prejudice against fat people: ideology and self-interest. *J Pers Soc Psychol.* 1994;66:882–894.

29. Crandall CS, Biernat M. The ideology of anti-fat attitudes. *J Appl Soc Psychol.* 1990;20:227–243.

30. Wadden TA, Stunkard AJ. Social and psychological consequences of obesity. *Ann Intern Med.* 1985;103:1062–1067.

31. Yuker HE, Allison DB, Faith MS. Methods for measuring attitudes and beliefs about obese people. In: Allison DB, ed. *Handbook of Assessment Methods for Eating Behaviors and Weight Related Problems.* Thousand Oaks, CA: Sage; 1995:81–118.

32. Fallon P, Katzman MA, Wooley SC. *Feminist Perspectives on Eating Disorders.* New York: Guilford Press; 1993.

33. Allison DB, Heshka S. Emotion and eating in obesity: a critical analysis. *Int J Eating Dis.* 1993;13:289–295.

34. Greeno CG, Wing RR. Stress-induced eating. *Psychol Bull.* 1994;115:444–464.

35. Schachter S, Goldman R, Gordon A. Effects of fear, food deprivation, and obesity on eating. *J Pers Soc Psychol.* 1968;10:91–97.

36. McKenna RJ. Some effects of anxiety level and food cues on the eating behavior obese and normal subjects: a comparison of the Schachterian and psychosomatic concepts. *J Pers Soc Psychol.* 1972;22:311–319.

37. Slochower J, Kaplan S, Mann L. The effects of life stress and weight on mood and eating. *Appetite.* 1981;2:115–125.

38. Baucom CH, Aiken PA. Effect of depressed mood on eating among obese and nonobese dieting and nondieting persons. *J Pers Soc Psychol.* 1981;41:577–585.

39. Ruderman A. Obesity, anxiety, and food consumption. *Addict Behav.* 1983;8:235–242.

40. Heatherton TF, Baumeister RF. Binge-eating as escape from self-awareness. *Psychol Bull.* 1991;110:86–108.

41. Heatherton TF, Herman CP, Polivy J. Effects of physical threat and ego threat on eating behavior. *J Pers Soc Psychol.* 1991;60:138–143.

42. Geliebter A, Aversa A. Eating in response to emotional states and situations in overweight, normal weight, and underweight individuals. *Int J Obes.* 1991;15:9.

43. Lingswiler VM, Crowther JH, Stephens MAP. Emotional reactivity and eating in binge eating and obesity. *J Behav Med.* 1987;10:287–299.

44. Lowe MR, Fisher EB. Emotional reactivity, emotional eating, and obesity: a naturalistic study. *J Behav Med.* 1983;6:135–149.

45. Schlundt DG, Taylor D, Hill JO, et al. A behavioral taxonomy of obese female participants in a weight-loss program. *Am J Clin Nutr.* 1991;53:1151–1158.

46. VanStrien T, Frijters JER, Roosen RGFM, et al. Eating behavior, personality traits and body mass in women. *Addict Behav.* 1985;10:333–343.

47. Wilson G. Eating style, obesity, and health. *Pers Indiv Diff.* 1986;7:215–224.

48. Hudson A, Williams SG. Eating behavior, emotions, and overweight. *Psychol Rep.* 1981;48:669–670.

49. Leon G. Personality, body image, and eating pattern changes in overweight persons after weight loss. *J Clin Psychol.* 1975;31:618–623.

50. Leon G, Chamberlin K. Emotional arousal, eating patterns and body image as different factors associated with varying success in maintaining a weight loss. *J Consult Clin Psychol.* 1973;40:474–480.

51. Schachter S, Rodin J. *Obese Humans and Rats.* Washington, DC: Erlbaum/Wiley; 1974.

52. Nisbett RE. Determinants of food intake in obesity. *Science.* 1968;159:1254–1255.

53. Nisbett RE. Hunger, obesity, and the ventromedial hypothalamus. *Psychol Rev.* 1972;79:433–453.

54. Lowe MR. The effects of dieting on eating behavior: a three-factor model. *Psychol Bull.* 1993;114:100–121.

55. Lowe MR, Maycock B. Restraint, disinhibition, hunger, and negative affect eating. *Addict Behav.* 1988;3:369–377.

56. Schotte DE, Cools J, McNally RJ. Film-induced negative affect triggers overeating in restrained eaters. *J Abnorm Psychol.* 1990;99:317–320.

57. Ruderman A, Wilson GT. Weight, restraint, cognitions, and counterregulation. *Behav Res Ther.* 1979;17:581–590.

58. Ruderman A, Christensen HC. Restraint theory and its applicability to overweight individuals. *J Abnorm Psychol.* 1983;92:210–215.

59. McCann KL, Perri MG, Nezu AM, Lowe MR. An investigation of counterregulatory eating in obese clinic attenders. *Int J Eating Dis.* 1992;12:161–169.

60. Lowe MR. Staying on versus getting off a diet: effects on eating in normal weight and overweight individuals. *Int J Eating Dis.* 1992;12:417–424.

61. Allison DB, Kalinsky LB, Gorman BS. A comparison of the psychometric properties of three measures of dietary restraint. *Psychol Assess.* 1992;4:391–398.

62. Gorman BS, Allison DB. Measures of restrained eating. In: Allison DB, ed. *Handbook of Assessment Methods for Eating Behaviors and Weight Related Problems.* Thousand Oaks, CA: Sage;1995:149–184.

63. Jansen A, Oosterlaan J, Merckelbach H, van den Hout M. Nonregulation of food intake in restrained, emotional, and external eaters. *J Psychopathology Behav Assess.* 1988;10:345–353.

64. Wardles J, Beales S. Restraint and food intake: an experimental study of eating behavior patterns in the laboratory and real life. *Behav Res Ther.* 1987;25:179–185.

65. Arnow B, Kenardy J, Agras WS. Binge eating among the obese: a descriptive study. *J Behav Med.* 1992;2:155–170.

66. Arnow B, Kenardy J, Agras WS. The Emotional Eating Scale: the development of a measure to assess coping with negative affect by eating. *Int J Eating Dis.* 1995;18:79–90.

67. Wilson GT, Nonas CA, Rosenblum GD. Assessment of binge eating in obese patients. *Int J Eating Dis.* 1993;13:25–33.

68. Stunkard AJ, Messick S. The Three Factor Eating Questionnaire to measure dietary restraint, disinhibition and hunger. *J Psychosom Res.* 1985;29:71–83.

69. VanStrien T, Frijters JER, Bergers GPA, Defares PB. The Dutch Eating Behavior Questionnaire (DEBQ) for assessment of restrained, emotional, and external eating behavior. *Int J Eating Dis.* 1986;5:295–315.

70. Stunkard AJ. Eating patterns and obesity. *Psychiatr Q.* 1959;33:284–292.

71. Brody ML, Walsh TB, Devlin MJ. Binge Eating Disorder: reliability and validity of a new diagnostic category. *J Consult Clin Psychol.* 1994;62:381–386.

72. Spitzer RL, Devlin M, Walsh BT, et al. Binge Eating Disorder: a multisite field trial of the diagnostic criteria. *Int J Eating Dis.* 1992;11:191–203.

73. Spitzer RL, Yanovski S, Wadden T, et al. Binge Eating Disorder: its further validation in a multisite study. *Int J Eating Dis.* 1993;13:137–153.

74. Yanovski S. Binge Eating Disorder: current knowledge and future directions. *Obes Res.* 1993;1:306–323.

75. Telch CF, Agras WS, Rossiter EM. Binge eating increases with increasing adiposity. *Int J Eating Dis.* 1988;7:115–119.

76. Marcus MD. Binge eating in obesity. In: Fairburn CG, Wilson GT, eds. *Binge Eating: Nature, Assessment, and Treatment.* New York: Guilford Press; 1993:77–96.

77. deZwann M, Mitchell JE. Binge eating in the obese. *Ann Med.* 1992;24:303–308.

78. Kolotin RL, Revis ES, Kirkley BG, Janick L. Binge eating in obesity: associated MMPI characteristics. *J Consult Clin Psychol.* 1987;55:872–876.

79. Wadden TA, Foster GD, Letizia KA, Wilk, JE. Metabolic, anthropometric, and psychological characteristics of obese binge eaters. *Int J Eating Dis.* 1993;14:17–25.

80. Marcus MD, Wing RR, Hopkins, J. Obese binge eaters: affect, cognitions, and response to behavioral weight control. *J Consult Clin Psychol.* 1988;56:433–439.

81. Fitzgibbon ML, Kirschenbaum DS. Heterogeneity of clinical presentation among obese individuals seeking treatment. *Addict Behav.* 1990;15:291–295.

82. Kanter RA, Williams BW, Cummings C. Personal and parental alcohol abuse, and victimization in obese binge eaters and nonbingeing obese. *Addict Behav.* 1992;17:439–445.

83. Yanovski SZ, Nelson JE, Dubbert, BK, Spitzer RL. Association of Binge Eating Disorder and psychiatric comorbidity in obese subjects. *Am J Psychiatry.* 1993;150:1472–1479.

84. Eldredge KL, Agras WS. Weight and shape overconcern and emotional eating in Binge Eating Disorder. *Int J Eating Dis.* 1997;19:73–82.

85. Kuehnel RH, Wadden TA. Binge Eating Disorder, weight cycling, and psychopathology. *Int J Eating Dis.* 1994;15:321–329.

86. Gormally J, Black S, Daston S, Rardin D. The assessment of binge eating severity among obese persons. *Addict Behav.* 1982;7:47–55.

87. Hawkins RC, Clement PF. Development and construct validation of a self-report measure of binge eating tendencies. *Addict Behav.* 1980;5:219–226.

88. Pike KM, Loeb K, Walsh BT. Binge eating and purging. In: Allison DB, ed. *Handbook of Assessment Methods for Eating Behaviors and Weight Related Problems.* Thousand Oaks, CA: Sage; 1995:303–346.

89. Wilson GT. Assessment of binge eating. In: Fairburn CG, Wilson GT, eds. *Binge Eating: Nature, Assessment, and Treatment.* New York: Guilford Press; 1993:227–249.

90. Wurtman RJ, Wurtman JJ. Carbohydrate craving, obesity and brain serotonin. *Appetite.* 1986;7:99–103.

91. Wurtman JJ. Depression and weight gain: the serotonin connection. *J Affective Disord.* 1993;29:183–92.

92. Wurtman JJ. *The Carbohydrate Craver's Diet.* Boston: Houghton Mifflin; 1983.

93. Fernstrom JD, Wurtman RJ. Brain serotonin content: increase following ingestion of carbohydrate diet. *Science.* 1971;174:1023–1024.

94. Fernstrom JD, Wurtman RJ. Brain serotonin content: physiological regulation by plasma neutral amino acids. *Science.* 1972;178:414–416.

95. Cabalerro B. Brain serotonin and carbohydrate craving in obesity. *Int J Obes.* 1987;11:179–183.

96. Fernstrom JD. Tryptophan, serotonin and carbohydrate appetite: will the real carbohydrate craver please stand up! *J Nutr.* 1988;118:1417–1419.

97. Drewnowski A, Kurth C, Holden-Wiltze J, Saari J. Food preferences in human obesity: carbohydrates versus fats. *Appetite.* 1992;18:207–221.

98. Lieberman HR, Wurtman JJ, Chew B. Changes in mood after carbohydrate consumption among obese individuals. *Am J Clin Nutr.* 1986;44:772–778.

99. Wurtman JJ, Wurtman R, Mark S, Tsay R, Gilbert W, Growdon J. d-Fenfluramine selectively suppresses carbohydrate snacking by obese subjects. *Int J Eating Dis.* 1985;4:89–99.

100. Wurtman JJ. Disorders of food intake: excessive carbohydrate snack intake among a class of obese people. *Ann NY Acad Sci.* 1987;499:197–202.

101. Grilo CM, Shiffman S, Wing RR. Relapse crises and coping among dieters. *J Consult Clin Psychol.* 1989;57:488–495.

102. Allison DB, Heshka S. Social desirability and response bias in self-reports of "emotional eating." *Eat Disord.* 1993;1:31–38.

103. Faith MS. *The Psychosomatic Model of Obesity: Psychological Distress or Experimental Artifact.* Hempstead, NY: Hofstra University; 1995. Dissertation.

104. deZwaan M, Bach M, Mitchell JE, et al. Alexithymia, obesity, and Binge Eating Disorder. *Int J Eating Dis.* 1995;17:135–140.

105. Blair AJ, Lewis VJ, Booth DA. Does emotional eating interfere with success in attempts at weight control? *Appetite.* 1990;15:151–157.

106. Clark MM, Abrams DB, Niaura RS, et al. Self-efficacy in weight management. *J Consult Clin Psychol.* 1991;59:739–744.

107. Glynn SM, Ruderman AJ. The development and validation of an eating self-efficacy scale. *Cognit Ther Res.* 1986;10:403–420.

108. Stanton AL, Garcia ME, Green SB. Development and validation of the Situational Appetite Measures. *Addict Behav.* 1990;15:461–472.

109. Stunkard AJ, Kaplan D. Eating in public places: a review of reports of the direct observation of eating behavior. *Int J Obes.* 1977;1:89–101.

110. Gates JC, Huenemann RL, Brand RJ. Food choices of obese and non-obese persons. *J Am Diet Assoc.* 1975;67:339.

111. Brown JE, Tharp TM, Dahlberg-Luby EM, et al. Videotape dietary assessment: validity, reliability, and comparison of results with 24-hour dietary recalls from elderly women in a retirement home. *J Am Diet Assoc.* 1990;90:1675–1679.

112. Meiselman HL. Methodology and theory in human eating research. *Appetite.* 1992;19:49–55.

113. Booth DA. Towards scientific realism in eating research. *Appetite.* 1992;19:56–60.

114. Kissileff H. Where should human eating be studied and what should be measured? *Appetite.* 1992;19:61–68.

115. Pliner P. Let's not throw out the barley with the dishwater: comments on Meiselman's "Methodology and theory in human eating research." *Appetite.* 1992;19:74–75.

116. Rolls BJ, Shide DJ. Both naturalistic and laboratory-based studies contribute to the understanding of human eating behavior. *Appetite.* 1992;19:76–77.

117. Wolper C, Heshka S, Heymsfield SB. Measuring food intake. In: Allison DB, ed. *Handbook of Assessment Methods for Eating Behaviors and Weight Related Problems.* Thousand Oaks, CA: Sage; 1995:215–240.

118. Allison DB, Allison R, Paultry F, Pi-Sunyer FX. Power and money: Designing statistically powerful studies while minimizing financial costs. *Psych Methods.* In press.

119. VanStrien T, Rookus MA, Bergers GPA, Frijters JER, et al. Life events, emotional eating and change in body mass index. *Int J Obes.* 1986;10:29–35.

120. Schlundt DG, Zimering RT. The Dieter's Inventory of Eating Temptations: a measure of weight control competence. *Addict Behav.* 1988;13:151–164.

121. Schlundt DG. Assessment of specific eating behaviors and eating styles. In: Allison DB, ed. *Handbook of Assessment Methods for Eating Behaviors and Weight Related Problems.* Thousand Oaks, CA: Sage; 1995:241–302.

122. Brownell KD. Dieting readiness. *Weight Control Digest.* 1990;1:5–9.

123. Rossi JS, Rossi SR, Velicer WF, Prochaska JO. Motivational readiness to control weight. In: Allison DB, ed. *Handbook of Assessment Methods for Eating Behaviors and Weight Related Problems.* Thousand Oaks, CA: Sage; 1995:387–430.

124. Fontaine KR, Cheskin LJ, Allison DB. Predicting treatment attendance and weight loss: Assessing the psychometric properties and predictive validity of the Dieting Readiness Test. *J Personality Assess.* 1997;68:172–182.

125. Foreyt JP, Brunner RL, Goodrick GK, Cutter G. Psychological correlates of weight fluctuation. *Int J Eating Dis.* 1995;17:263–275.

126. Condiotte MM, Lichtenstein E. Self-efficacy and relapse in smoking cessation programs. *J Consult Clin Psychol.* 1981;49:648–658.

127. King TK, Clark MM, Pera V. *History of sexual abuse and obesity treatment outcome.* Paper presented at the Annual Meeting of the Association for the Advancement of Behavior Therapy; 1994.

128. Kuntz CB, Ronan GF, Ronan DW, Johnson C. *Levels of obesity in women: a test of group differences in stress, self-efficacy, and problem-solving.* Paper presented at the 15th Annual Meeting of the Society of Behavioral Medicine; 1994.

129. Kristeller JL, Rodin J. Identifying eating patterns in male and female undergraduates using cluster analysis. *Addict Behav.* 1989;14:631–642.

130. Abrahamson E. *Emotional Eating: A Practical Guide to Taking Control.* New York: Lexington Books; 1993.

131. Bandini LG, Schoeller DA, Cyr HN, Dietz WH. Validity of reported energy intake in obese and nonobese adolescents. *Am J Clin Nutr.* 1990;52:421–425.

132. Klesges RC, Eck LH, Ray JW. Who reports dietary intake in a dietary recall? Evidence from the Second National Health and Nutritional Examination Survey. *J Consult Clin Psychol.* 1995;63:438–444.

133. Lichtman SW, Pisarska K, Berman ER, et al. Discrepancy between self-reported and actual caloric intake and exercise in obese subjects. *N Engl J Med.* 1992;327:1893–1898.

134. Schoeller DA. How accurate is self-reported dietary energy intake? *Nutr Rev.* 1990;48:373–379.

135. Agras WS. *Eating Disorders: Management of Obesity, Bulimia, and Anorexia Nervosa.* New York: Pergamon Books; 1987.

136. Brownell KD, Fairburn CG. *Eating Disorders and Obesity.* New York: Guilford Press; 1995.

137. Brownell KD, Wadden TA. Behavior therapy for obesity: modern approaches and better results. In: Brownell KD, Foreyt JP, eds. *Handbook of Eating Disorders.* New York: Basic Books; 1986:180–197.

138. Foreyt JP, Goodrick KG. Attributes of successful approaches to weight loss and control. *Appl Prev Psychol.* 1994;3:209–215.

139. Goodrick KG, Foreyt JP. Why treatments for obesity don't last. *J Am Diet Assoc.* 1991;91:1243–1247.

140. Wadden TA, VanItallie TB. *Treatment of the Seriously Obese Patient.* New York: Guilford Press; 1992.

141. Grilo CM, Shiffman S, Wing RR. Coping with dietary relapse crises and their aftermath. *Addict Behav.* 1993;18:89–102.

142. Shiffman S. Relapse following smoking cessation: a situational analysis. *J Consult Clin Psychol.* 1982;50:71–86.

143. Shiffman S. Coping with temptations to smoke. *J Consult Clin Psychol.* 1984;14:261–267.
144. Beck AT. *Cognitive Therapy and the Emotional Disorders.* New York: International Universities Press; 1976.
145. Beck AT, Rush AJ, Shaw BF, Emery G. *Cognitive Therapy for Depression.* New York: Guilford Press; 1979.
146. Ellis A. *Reason and Emotion in Psychotherapy.* Secaucus, NJ: Lyle Stuart; 1962.
147. Ellis A. *Humanistic Psychotherapy: The Rational-Emotive Approach.* New York: McGraw-Hill; 1973.
148. Freeman A, Simon KM, Beutler LE, Arkowitz H. *Comprehensive Handbook of Cognitive Psychotherapy.* New York: Plenum Press; 1989.
149. Portzelius LK, Houston C, Smith M, et al. Comparison of a standard behavioral weight loss treatment and a binge eating weight loss treatment. *Behav Ther.* 1995;26:119–134.
150. Wilfley DE, Agras WS, Telch CF, et al. Group cognitive-behavioral therapy and group interpersonal therapy for the nonpurging bulimic: a controlled comparison. *J Consult Clin Psychol.* 1993;61:296–305.
151. Wilfley DE, Grilo CM, Rodin J. Group psychotherapy for the treatment of bulimia nervosa and binge eating disorder. In: Spira JL, ed. *Group Therapy for the Medically Ill.* New York: Guilford Press; In press.
152. Agras WS, Telch CF, Arnow B, Eldredge K, et al. Does interpersonal therapy help patients with Binge Eating Disorder who fail to respond to cognitive-behavioral therapy? *J Consult Clin Psychol.* 1995;63:356–360.
153. Friedman MA, Brownell KD. Psychological correlates of obesity: moving to the next research generation. *Psychol Bull.* 1995;117:3–20.
154. Lissau I, Sorensen TIA. Parental neglect during childhood and increased risk of obesity in young adulthood. *Lancet.* 1994;343:324–327.
155. Bjorntorp P. The associations between obesity, adipose tissue distribution and disease. *Acta Med Scand.* 1988;723:121–134.
156. Bjorntorp P. Visceral fat accumulation: the missing link between psychological factors and cardiovascular disease? *J Intern Med.* 1991;230:195–201.
157. Bjorntorp P. Visceral obesity: a "civilization syndrome." *Obes Res.* 1993;1:206–222.
158. Bjorntorp P. The importance of body fat distribution. In: Brownell KD, Fairburn CG, eds. *Eating Disorders and Obesity.* New York: Guilford Press; 1995:445–449.
159. Rebuffe-Scrive M. Steroid hormones and distribution of adipose tissue. *Acta Med Scand.* 1988;723:143–146.
160. Moyer AE, Rodin J, Grilo CM, et al. Stress-induced cortisol response and fat distribution in women. *Obes Res.* 1994;2:255–262.
161. Rebuffe-Scrive M, Walsh UA, McEwen B, Rodin J. Effects of chronic stress and exogenous glucocorticoids on regional fat distribution and metabolism. *Physiol Behav.* 1992;52:583–590.
162. Shively CA, Clarkson TB. Regional obesity and coronary artery atherosclerosis in females: a non-human primate model. *Acta Med Scand.* 1988;723:71–78.
163. Romboldt M, Rumboldt Z, Pesenti S. The impact of war upon the pupils' growth in southern Croatia. *Child: Care, Health, and Development.* 1994;20:189–196.
164. Eldredge KL, Agras WS, Arnow B. The last supper: emotional determinants of pretreatment weight fluctuation in obese binge eaters. *Int J Eating Dis.* 1994;83–88.

CHAPTER 18

The Role of Pharmacological Agents in the Treatment of Obesity

L. Arthur Campfield

INTRODUCTION

Obesity is a major health problem throughout both the developed and developing world. It is a complex, multifactorial disease with an increasing prevalence. Countries in the Caribbean and other locations in the developing world are starting to see the incidence of obesity increase. Obesity is associated with significant chronic diseases (hypertension, non–insulin-dependent diabetes mellitus [NIDDM], hypercholesterolemia) as well as stroke, sleep apnea, and certain cancers. Obesity is a cause of significant morbidity and, in turn, is having an increasing negative impact on health care systems worldwide. Although treatments (e.g., diet, exercise, drugs) are available and most people can achieve medically significant weight loss (5% to 10% of initial body weight), long-term maintenance of that weight loss is, unfortunately, very rare. Thus, obesity remains a poorly managed chronic medical condition that is a major cause of morbidity and mortality.

Obesity is a multifactorial disease at the interface between the biology of body energy regulation and an environment (physical and sensory) that has been increasingly characterized as "hostile to good health" and even "obesifying" or promoting obesity.[1] Most Americans have access to a large and increasing variety of highly palatable food, with declining incentives and opportunities for physical activity. Today many important issues such as well-being, health, and self-esteem are closely associated with body weight. This focus on body weight has resulted in overt and covert discrimination against obese individuals.[2] See Chapter 12 on social aspects of overweight.

For these reasons, the need for improved medical management of obesity is clear. A large part of that improved management may result from successful implementation of the concept that pharmacological agents for the treatment of obesity should be used as adjuncts to diet and exercise to promote increased success at weight maintenance.

HUMAN OBESITY: INTERACTION BETWEEN GENETICS AND ENVIRONMENT

Obesity is defined by the degree of excessive accumulation of body fat. It is simple to state that obesity is a problem of excessive expansion of fat mass, but the expansion results from a complex and interesting interaction between genetic predisposition to increased metabolic efficiency and the regulation of energy balance. The most commonly accepted model for the genetics of human obesity involves an interaction of genetic predisposition and environmental factors. Claude Bouchard and other investigators have estimated the heritability of variations in distribution of body fat to be approximately 35%.[3] To this we could add up to 15% for the presence of "modifier genes" that make some individuals much more susceptible to gaining weight on a palatable high-energy diet than others. Thus, at least 50% of the problem is due to environmental and lifestyle factors. This component of the variance of body fat content is the one that can be moderated by obesity treatment through diet, exercise, and drug therapy. See Chapter 6 on the genetics of body fat.

The goal is to block the progression of and, in turn, reverse the pathophysiology of obesity by integrated, multimodal management. The evidence, particularly from the long-term follow-up of surgical intervention, is quite strong that these goals can be accomplished.[4,5] In recent years, additional, and quite compelling, evidence has emerged that obesity is a disease of biological dysregulation, particularly in the context of one's biology, one's genetics, and one's adaptation to what has been called an "obesifying" or "obese" environment. The steady-state body weight of an individual is thought to result from an integration of multiple biological factors, which are at least partially genetically determined.

Animal and clinical studies have shown that increases or decreases in body weight are resisted and corrected by robust physiological mechanisms.[6] Patients who continue to seek treatment after multiple weight regain following multiple periods of weight loss know this through personal experience. Recently, renewed interest and attention has been directed toward OB protein, the product of the obese gene in adipose tissue, that is secreted into the circulation and acts on the brain and provides a long-term signal for energy balance. It may play a role in this "resetting response" that is responsible for weight regain following weight loss.[7] See Chapter 7 on body weight regulation.

GOALS OF OBESITY TREATMENT AND MANAGEMENT

What are the goals of obesity treatment? Most academic and industrial researchers propose a multiple approach to this complex question. This chapter discusses the use of multiple pharmaceutical agents with more than one mechanism of action as adjuncts to diet and exercise. An array of medications, diets, and lifestyle changes are needed so that treatment options and programs can be tailored to individuals, either based upon how they became obese, their present life situation, or which treatment program is more likely to be achieved. As Hill et al[8] and others note, people must find an exercise that they like, and can do, if they are expected to do it for a long time. Implementing something as simple and logical as an exercise component in the majority of treatment programs will be a major innovation and will require a major effort because there is little evidence of success in sustaining exercise behavior.

Key to improving the health outcome of obesity treatment is improving the compliance of individuals to a decision that they have made to lose weight. They may have been motivated by a class reunion, marriage, marriage of a child, divorce, medical exam, or other reasons, but they have made a decision that they need to improve their health, and one of the best ways to improve their health is to lose weight. Assistance and support must be provided to help them become and remain successful in achieving and maintaining medically significant weight loss.

A major barrier to effective long-term treatment of obesity is often the extremely unrealistic weight loss goals of people who are highly motivated to undergo treatment. Practitioners may try to teach them that 10% weight loss leads to improved health, or may show them the Institute of Medicine report on *Weighing the Options,*[9] which documents studies supporting improved health benefits from small, but maintained, weight loss. Often, they are not satisfied. Communicating the health benefits of small, maintained weight loss will continue to be an important educational mission of all obesity management professionals.

Once it is accepted that practitioners need multiple treatment options that can be matched to patients, the question then becomes, what options are available? Some alternatives and options are shown in Exhibit 18–1. In the past, short-term treat-

---

Exhibit 18–1 Goals of Treatment: Intervention and/or Lifestyle Change

What is the most appropriate treatment?

Short-term intervention
Long-term intervention
Sustained lifestyle changes
Interventions leading to sustained lifestyle changes

For which patients?

Overweight or obese
Free from associated disease, or medically at risk
"Successful" dieters, or individuals refractory to dietary treatment

ment with centrally acting appetite suppressants was the standard of care.[10] However, the regulatory environment in many states and locales in the United States and the governments of other countries was unsupportive or, in fact, hostile to long-term pharmacological treatment of obesity. The landmark Weintraub innovation of using the combination therapy of fenfluramine/phenteramine has allowed many practitioners, researchers, and patients to gain experience with long-term drug treatment for obesity.[11,12] Anecdotal reports have indicated that many patients were helped by combined treatment with existing appetite suppressants, although appropriately controlled studies of combined drug treatment in large numbers of patients are just appearing in the literature. Many patients report that they have some degree of control over their appetite for the first time while on the Weintraub combination. The most effective alternative may be long-term interventions, well matched to individuals, that help them make and sustain healthy changes in their lifestyle.

Who should be treated? People who have obesity-related health risks and who have clinically significant symptoms should be treated first, but many other categories of obese individuals may need and receive important health benefits from sustained weight loss. Some of these categories are also shown in Exhibit 18–1. These are important issues that are just beginning to be discussed.[13,14] Perhaps specific antiobesity agents will be more appropriate for some subgroups of obese individuals and other agents will serve the needs of different groups.

What are the goals of treatment? One set of goals of treatment is shown in Exhibit 18–2. The first goal is to prevent further body weight gain. This is desirable and achievable through diet and exercise, and it can be helped by drug therapy. Before focusing on the maintenance of weight loss, obese individuals must first be able to avoid gaining more weight. When obese individuals enter a treatment program, their obvious intention is to lose weight. Thus, they should not be gaining weight during the treatment period, although this may occur. The next goal is to induce a 5% to 10% weight loss from the initial body weight. Most obese individuals can achieve this goal in a variety of treatment programs (e.g., very-low-calorie diets). The next, and most important, goal is to maintain the lower body weight. This maintenance is the major goal of the pharmacological treatment of obesity and it is the most difficult to achieve.

Exhibit 18–2 Potential Uses of an Antiobesity Agent

Prevention of weight gain
Induction of weight loss
Maintenance of weight loss
Improve compliance to diet
Reduction of associated risk factors (+/– weight loss)

LONG-TERM WEIGHT MAINTENANCE

What exactly is weight maintenance? The problem and possibilities are shown in Figure 18–1, which shows a schematic body weight profile of an obese individual who seeks treatment at an initial body weight. Following a period of successful caloric restriction and exercise program, body weight decreases to a minimum point at the end of treatment. The goal would be to maintain all or most of the weight loss that was achieved (line labeled "ideal" in Figure 18–1). Although this would be ideal, it is also considered by most researchers as unrealistic because the biological systems regulating body fat content and body energy balance actively resist any change from the pretreatment steady state. A similar consensus exists[13] that the complete regain of all weight lost over a period of one or two or three years is unacceptable (lines labeled "A" and "B").

Figure 18–1 also raises a problem of economics for clinical trials and, thus, for pharmaceutical companies and potential antiobesity drugs. A clinical trial of a proposed antiobesity drug trial has a finite length. If the trial ends before most subjects have regained all or most of the weight they initially lost (time T1 in Figure 18–1), the candidate drug may appear to promote weight maintenance. However, if the trial is continued until most of the subjects on the active drug have regained back to initial weight (Time T2 in Figure 18–1), that same drug may appear unable to promote weight maintenance. Since a trial that ends at time T2 will cost substantially more and may be less likely to show weight maintenance than a trial that ends at time T1, there

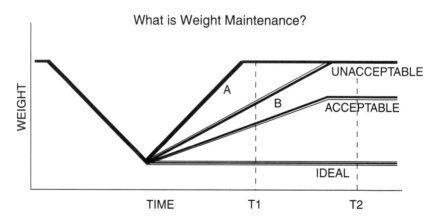

Figure 18–1 Idealized body weight curves of obese individuals undergoing weight loss and weight-maintenance treatment. The definition of minimally acceptable weight maintenance is the preservation of a negative non-zero differential in body weight at the end of active drug treatment. See text for additional details.

seem to be little incentive for the sponsor to continue the trial voluntarily. However, since the U.S. Food and Drug Administration (FDA) and European authorities have been actively encouraging longer clinical trials for new antiobesity drugs, (e.g., six-month, one-year, or two-year trials), patients and physicians will have drugs that have been evaluated for their weight-maintenance potential for one or two years and, ideally, for an additional extended period of posttreatment follow-up.

Given that extreme weight loss and its maintenance are either unrealistic or unacceptable, what are desirable and achievable goals? A negative difference in final body weight (and preferably body composition) from the initial body weight (and composition) at the beginning of the trials is an appropriate goal (line labeled "acceptable" in Figure 18–1). The author believes that a consensus exists that the preservation of a negative non-zero differential in body weight at the end of active drug treatment is minimally acceptable weight maintenance. However, a range of opinion exists within the research, industrial, and regulatory communities about the magnitude of the minimally acceptable weight differential.[14]

CONCEPT OF METABOLIC FITNESS: A MEDICALLY BASED ALTERNATIVE OUTCOME MEASURE

The author has proposed the concept of "metabolic fitness" as a medically based alternative outcome measure rather than body weight as the primary outcome measure for obesity treatment.[15,16] The idea is to not focus primarily on percentage body fat, body mass index (BMI), or body weight but instead to focus on, and to track, the metabolic health of obese individuals. The goal is to be "metabolically fit" and to achieve the absence of any metabolic or biochemical risk factor associated with obesity (Exhibit 18–3). Obese individuals might have 25% or 35% body fat, but if they do not have any risk factors and their biochemical values are within the normal range, it may not be urgent that they lose weight because their general health is probably fine. However, overweight individuals with only slightly elevated percentage body fat, but with one or more abnormal biochemical or other risk factors, may be in urgent need of losing weight to improve their already impaired health.

The concept of metabolic fitness is based upon, and strongly influenced by, biochemical and behavioral risk factors for cardiovascular disease that have been well-established by the Framingham longitudinal heart study.[17] Rather than lump all obese individuals into a single group that must lose weight, the metabolic fitness approach primarily focuses on the actual presence, or increased risk, of one or more obesity-associated disease indicators and views weight loss as a modality to improve metabolic health.

Other physicians and scientists in the obesity field have also advocated this idea or similar concepts, including the beneficial effects of exercise in improving meta-

Exhibit 18–3 Concept of "Metabolic Fitness" As an Alternate Outcome Measure

Definition of metabolic fitness: the absence of any metabolic or biochemical risk factor for diseases associated with obesity.

Metabolic fitness would correlate closely with general health and would improve with risk factor reduction.

Metabolic fitness may provide an alternative, medically oriented goal in the treatment of obesity that does not focus on weight.

Intervention options to improve metabolic fitness include (from most to least aggressive):

- medically significant reduction of risk factors
- restoration of abnormal risk factors to normal ranges
- reversal of "high normal" or "borderline" parameters
- prevention of risk factors in overweight individuals

Improvements in metabolic fitness, and, thus, in health status, may be independent of weight loss (or poorly correlated with weight loss).

bolic fitness.[18] Agreement appears to be growing about the validity of the metabolic fitness concept.[13]

Certainly, family history plays a role in increasing the risks of obesity and its impact on morbidity and mortality. If both parents of a child were obese and diagnosed with NIDDM, then that child has an increased risk of being obese and having NIDDM as an adult compared to another child without a family history of either obesity or NIDDM. An earlier and more aggressive intervention to prevent weight gain in the first child may be more appropriate than with the second child. Therefore, family history and genetic factors have a powerful influence on what the treatment should be and which outcome measure(s) should be used.

Within the concept of metabolic fitness there is a spectrum of intervention options ranging from mild to very aggressive (Exhibit 18–3). The first and most aggressive intervention would be to reduce significant and abnormal biochemical and behavioral risk factors that are already present. If an obese person has clinically significant hypertension, hypercholesterolemia, or glucose intolerance, then assistance and support are required to achieve weight loss and maintain that weight loss. This should aid in returning the abnormal biochemical parameters to normal levels.

A less aggressive approach would be to reduce the abnormal biochemical risk factors to within normal ranges. Another level of treatment would attempt to reduce high normal or borderline biochemical values to the middle of the normal range. The least aggressive intervention would prevent biochemical risk factors in the low to medium normal range from increasing to high normal values.

Improvements in biochemical risk factors may be dependent upon weight loss or they may be independent or poorly correlated with weight loss. For example, exercise may improve insulin sensitivity, reduce cholesterol levels, and reduce other cardiovascular risk factors without always inducing weight loss. On the other hand, during periods of rapid weight loss induced by very-low-calorie diets (VLCDs) uniform improvement of risk factors has been reported. Some studies also demonstrated an additional complexity in the weight-maintenance phase because risk factors increased in some patients, depending upon the rate at which weight was lost and the percentage of weight loss.[20]

If practitioners can help improve the health of individuals and take the focus away from body weight, percent body fat, or BMI, sustained change might be easier and patients might accept better health as a more realistic goal instead of success defined by dress or belt size or looking like a model on a magazine cover. An additional benefit of using metabolic fitness as the measure of success is that it is objective and can be viewed as such by both the health professional and the patient. The health professional can display the blood chemistry and blood pressure report graphically in the individual's chart and mark all the abnormal, high normal, and normal values at the beginning of treatment. During each visit, the individual's progress can be charted and as parameters move back toward the normal range, both the health professional and the individual can feel successful.

MULTIPLE DRUGS WITH DISTINCT MECHANISMS OF ACTION

A consensus is also emerging that multiple antiobesity drugs, with several distinct mechanisms of action, are not only desirable, but also needed and that combined or multiple drug treatment will play an increasingly important role in future obesity treatment.[21] At present, there is a small, but growing, set of appetite suppressants resulting from study of central nervous system (CNS) chemistry, including serotonin[22] and other monoamines. Soon combined serotonin and norepinephrine reuptake inhibitors[23] and inhibitors of lipid absorption[24] will be available, followed by other agents based on OB protein and OB-R receptor pathways and, hopefully, other human and mouse obesity genes.[7] Approval of the drugs currently under review or near submission to the FDA will enable the widespread implementation of multiple antiobesity drug treatment.

Another approach is treatment for a very long time, possibly for life, or at least intermittently during adult life. Treatment, or components of the treatment program, would be reinstituted when an individual gains weight or becomes less metabolically fit.

The risk-benefit and quality-of-life analyses of pharmacological treatment of obesity are also serious and important issues. Since the efficacy of current drugs for weight maintenance is not great and each drug has its own side effect profile, an argument can be made that the little bit of extra efficacy provided by the drug is not worth the potential risks. Yet there are health benefits from even small weight losses when maintained.[25] Therefore, a case can be made that the present antiobesity drugs make obese people healthier, and, in spite of the side effects, improve the quality of many lives. Vigorous discussion is needed to define, in objective and quantifiable terms, the minimum efficacy required to justify long-term, and possibly chronic, drug treatment for obesity. As new antiobesity drugs are approved, and gain the confidence of health professionals, intervention studies required to define the minimum efficacy will be performed. Incremental improvements in knowledge about the biology of obesity may lead to incremental improvements in efficacy and safety of new drugs. It is reasonable to expect that the next generation of antiobesity drugs will be an incremental improvement in efficacy, and perhaps, by two generations from now, efficacy will have increased so that risk-benefit and quality-of-life analyses will be greatly improved.

Paradigm Shift within the FDA

In the mid-1990s the FDA appears to have changed its expectations and perception of antiobesity agents. Previously, the FDA used precedent procedures in the review and evaluation of appetite suppressant antiobesity drugs in the CNS division. Procedures were based on what had been done before and each new drug was handled like those previously reviewed. The review of antiobesity agents was then moved into the endocrine and metabolic division, where multiple classes of drugs with innovative mechanisms are processed. The arguments of obesity researchers about the chronic nature of obesity, its strong association with other diseases, and the need for longer-term treatment are now considered. The FDA has proposed guidelines that clearly recognize the need for chronic therapy, long term efficacy, and promoting and demonstrating weight maintenance. The FDA is now prepared to review drugs that promote weight maintenance during long-term treatment.

The FDA has defined long-term treatment trials;[13] it expects at least 1500 obese patients to be exposed to all new antiobesity drugs for one year and at least 500 obese patients to be exposed to all new antiobesity drugs for two years. The FDA appears ready to approve drugs that demonstrate significant weight maintenance (at least 5% below initial body weight) with these patient exposures for two years. The FDA has also recognized that a drug that has a clinically important effect on an obesity-associated disease could have a higher risk-benefit ratio, yet be approved compared to another drug that promoted weight maintenance but failed to have a marked effect on an associated disease. If a sponsor is convinced that its drug will have a large, clinically important effect on reducing a comorbidity and states so prior to the large Phase III clinical trials in obese patients, and if they successfully demonstrate this effect on an associated condition, the FDA has proposed that this benefit may be included in the labeling of the approved product. The FDA appears to have given the pharmaceutical industry an opportunity to play an active role in obesity treatment and weight management.

Antiobesity Agents As Adjuncts to Diet and Exercise

About 10 years ago, emphasis in the pharmaceutical industry was on looking for the "magic bullet" to treat obesity. The dominant model for drug discovery was to find the molecule that would cure the defect and lead to normal body weight for all. However, apparently single magic bullets are not going to be found, but instead, multiple drugs acting through multiple mechanisms will be identified, and these agents are likely to be useful in combination with diet and exercise. Some scientists disagree and point to hypertension treatment as a model. Hypertension used to be treated with low-sodium diets, but now it is treated with a large number of drugs with distinct mechanisms of action.[21] Obesity, they argue, may require such an array of specific agents. On the other hand, obesity is very different. The major difference is that obesity is the result of biological dysregulation of energy balance at the interface between internal biology and the environment. Because it is essential for humans to ingest energy in the form of food, the management of NIDDM may be a better model for obesity treatment than hypertension.

Another important question relating to obesity treatment is: How long does someone have to maintain a reduced weight until their energy balance regulatory system resets to a new settling point? Few data on successful postobese individuals exist that may provide an answer to this question. Yet, it is reasonable to expect that individual differences exist, and that there are biological mechanisms that could be assessed in individuals undergoing the transition from a higher body fat content regulation point to a lower one. The answer to this question will require further research.

Need for New Research

One method of obesity research is to study animals' response to high-energy diets or experimental manipulations in order to understand the mechanisms that predispose animals to obesity. However, the most fundamental and important issues for researchers trying to develop improved treatments for obesity are the effects of interventions and the biological and psychological mechanisms that resist changes in body fat content. Instead of repeatedly inducing laboratory animals to become obese, studies should be directed at making obese animals to become leaner and to understand the mechanisms resisting and supporting these interventions.

Further research attention must be given to the goals of treatment, the assessment of interventions, and determining which interventions lead to medically significant outcomes (Exhibit 18–4). Careful longitudinal studies of subpopulations of obese individuals, when they can be defined, may provide a unique opportunity to answer these important issues. For example, studies of postobese individuals who have succeeded in weight maintenance, should help define what works and for how long it works. Likewise, studies of those who do not succeed in weight maintenance may provide valuable insights on what does not work for subgroups of individuals.

As is the case with almost all diseases, health workers require more information on almost every aspect of obesity. A critical need is research on interventions and outcomes. Investigators in basic and clinical research could design studies that would lead to improved treatment outcomes for obese patients. Carefully planned long-term follow-up of pharmacological interventions in different subpopulations may help define subpopulations that are particularly well-suited to a particular drug as well as those for whom the drug may not be optimal therapy.

As an example, consider the beta$_3$-adrenergic receptor mutation reported by three groups in the August 1995 *New England Journal of Medicine*.[26–28] These studies suggested that in the three populations studied, obese individuals who had

---

Exhibit 18–4 Need for New Research

Major efforts are currently focused on:

- etiology (genetics, mechanisms)
- consequences
- predictors of obesity

Increased attention must also be given to:

- goals
- assessment
- medical significance of therapeutic interventions in subpopulations of obese patients

More research is essential at all levels of analysis and all cells, tissues, organs, organ systems, and sites involved in the regulation of energy balance.

In addition, more research on interventions must be conducted and outcome assessment is essential.

Treatment will be improved if each basic and clinical investigator routinely asks:

"How will the results of this experiment improve the treatment of obese patients?"
"Can I increase the impact of the experiment with changes in design?"

the mutation in their $beta_3$-receptor had, on average, an earlier onset of Type II diabetes than those without the mutation. Assuming that a $beta_3$-selective adrenergic antiobesity drug actually existed and appeared to be efficacious, a clinical trial with a study population that was stratified by the presence of the $beta_3$-adrenergic receptor mutation might reveal that this drug was more efficacious for promoting weight maintenance in obese individuals with the mutation. Even if the efficacy was similar in obese individuals with and without the mutation, a case could be made for accepting a higher risk in those with the mutation who might have an earlier onset of Type II diabetes.

As additional obesity-associated human genes are identified, then populations of obese individuals in future clinical trials of antiobesity drugs can be genotyped at several loci associated with obesity. Ultimately, as the human genome map becomes more complete, genotyping may be an increasingly important component of antiobesity drug approval.

POPULATION-BASED AND INTERVENTION STUDIES

In comparing epidemiological and intervention studies in obesity research, consider the "J shaped curve" of morbidity or mortality as a function of average BMI. Increases in risk appear to occur as BMI increases and decreases, resulting in controversy about the optimal BMI for maximum health.[29] One may ask the following questions: How do these epidemiological studies relate to intervention trials? What impact do these studies have on the design of longitudinal studies? How can information from population studies help researchers design intervention trials that are relevant to the individual seeking treatment for obesity? One answer is to design studies in which individual and average BMI is decreased by intervention and the health consequences assessed, rather than asking whether health is improved when the average BMI of the population changes over time. In other words, to more specifically answer these questions, actual intervention is required. How do practitioners intervene to accomplish improved health? Diet and exercise alone do not work very well. Therefore, one approach is to add a pharmaceutical agent or a surgical procedure to the intervention. However, finding an effective pharmaceutical agent creates a "Catch-22" situation: an effective intervention is necessary to show the beneficial effects of weight loss, but to effect weight loss requires finding an effective antiobesity agent.

Intervention trials provide the scientific bases for the clinical judgments that result in the prescription of different treatments designed to achieve specific outcomes. Therefore, if lessons can be learned from epidemiological studies of obesity and then applied to design more informative intervention trials, then obese individuals can expect better outcomes from treatment and, thus, improved metabolic fitness and health. The obesity surgery community has provided ideal study populations. The Swedish Obese Study (SOS) is a good example.[4] Surgery, with its risks and benefits, was adopted as the intervention, and obese individuals were randomized to surgery or diet and exercise treatment groups. After five years of follow-up, the study has clearly shown that the metabolic fitness of previously obese individuals was improved, in the aggregate, after losing weight and maintaining the majority of the weight loss. Some obese individuals may have had only trivial improvements in metabolic fitness. Overall, however, previously obese populations were healthier after being at a lower average body weight for five years. Similar results have been reported by Pories and colleagues.[5] These important surgical interventions, compared to epidemiology research by itself, provide strong support for the health benefits of weight loss. The government of Sweden and pharmaceutical companies supported the SOS in search of answers helpful to all in the obesity community. Similar longitudinal weight-maintenance studies will continue to be helpful.

As more is learned about matching treatments to individuals, several additional questions arise. Some of these questions are shown in Exhibit 18–5. The Weintraub approach has also emphasized the idea that drug combinations might be more effective than one drug, that "drug holidays" might be beneficial for some patients, and that the treatment program may be modified over time in an attempt to maximize the health benefits for the patient. Therefore, instead of choosing one diet from menu A, one type and intensity of exercise from menu B, and one drug from menu C, we should try to match a specific treatment program to the indi-

---

Exhibit 18–5 Matching Treatments to Patients: Interface Between Behavioral and Medication-Based Approaches

Separate treatments combined in the same patient

Combination tailored to patients: "menu" approach

Integrated, multifaceted approach: medication supports behavioral change and helps patients to "learn to become successful" at sustaining beneficial voluntary behavioral and lifestyle changes

Questions:

Is dosing schedule for medication independent of diet and exercise aspects of the treatment program?

Could meal-contingent dosing increase compliance to diet?
Is once-a-day medication the appropriate goal?

How do ritual and routines associated with aspects of treatment affect compliance to diet and exercise as well as treatment outcome?

vidual that provides the best outcome for successful long-term weight maintenance. Weight maintenance longer than one to two years requires study and could be addressed through intervention trials as more effective pharmaceutical agents for obesity treatment become available. In fact, some issues related to long-term maintenance may even be addressed in the clinical trials conducted with antiobesity drugs in development.

When target profiles of new potential antiobesity drugs are discussed, marketing professionals within the pharmaceutical industry often express a preference for a once-a-day dosing schedule. This preference is based on the stated preference of patients for the convenience of once-a-day dosing. However, the same marketing professionals also find that obese individuals eagerly follow schedules to receive daily subcutaneous injections of a new potential treatment agent such as the OB protein (or leptin) regardless of convenience. These mixed messages from patients may result in lack of efficacious treatments and unknown drug requirements for sustained weight maintenance. Similar questions about the value of intensive insulin treatment for insulin-dependent diabetes mellitus (IDDM) patients were resolved recently. A comprehensive clinical trial, The Diabetes Control and Complication Trial (DCCT) clearly demonstrated that intensive insulin treatment involving multiple subcutaneous insulin injections based on fingerstick measurements of blood glucose concentration established markedly improved blood glucose control and halted the progression of diabetic complications in patients with IDDM.[30] Most experts in diabetes treatment expect similar clinical trials in NIDDM patients to also show a benefit from intensive management of blood glucose concentration.[31] Thus, multiple dosing each day may become the standard of care for NIDDM as it is now for IDDM. Therefore, if weight maintenance is shown to be best supported by multiple dosing each day with new antiobesity drugs, multiple dosing may also become the standard of care for obesity. In this case, the convenience of once-a-day dosing may be subordinated to improved efficacy resulting from multiple dosing each day.

An unfortunate lesson from the follow-up of the DCCT is that some of the patients are failing to maintain the same improved blood glucose control as they did during the trial.[31] Apparently these patients failed to actually integrate or incorporate the intensive glucose control schedule into their own daily routine. Perhaps, the trial was too "medicalized" with physicians, nurse practitioners, nurses, and dietitians in charge, leaving the patients only passively involved in the management of their diabetes? Or perhaps patients need the psychological benefits and reinforcement created by a constant, caring environment?

Whatever the reason, this failure to incorporate behaviors or skills necessary for these DCCT participants to manage their glucose levels offers an important lesson. In developing improved treatment programs, the aim should be to put the control of weight maintenance in the hands of the patient, rather than for health professionals to "dispense" treatment. By creating a caring environment of intermittent, long-term support, health professionals must encourage obese patients to take responsibility for influencing the management of their body weight and their health. Perhaps taking antiobesity medication three times a day may actually provide some advantages for treatment; particularly since most individuals eat three or more times a day. The ritual of taking a medication with meals might help one comply to diet by focusing attention on the altered eating habits and medication as integral parts of the treatment program. How to teach and support self-management of lifelong obesity is a challenge requiring continued research.

EXAMPLES OF ANTIOBESITY AGENTS

The following examples illustrate the types of antiobesity agents available or under development in the mid-1990s and some data from their development studies.

Dexfenfluramine (Redux®)

The FDA approved dexfenfluramine for the treatment of obesity in 1996 and it was launched under the tradename Redux®. Dexfenfluramine is a serotonin reuptake blocker that has been approved and used for several years in Europe and Canada. One key multicenter placebo-controlled, double-blind, clinical trial on which its European approval was based was the one-year INDEX trial published in 1989.[22] A summary of the key results of this trial is shown in Table 18–1. One feature of this trial was that the placebo group, which received the "standard" treatment used in each of the participating centers, had very good weight loss and reasonable weight maintenance for up to one year. The average difference in weight loss at 12 months between the dexfenfluramine and the placebo group was 2.7 kg or 3.1% of initial body weight. However, both groups showed significantly different weight change compared to initial weights. The efficacy of dexfenfluramine was also presented in terms of the percentage of patients that lost more than 10% of initial body weight (dexfenfluramine 34%; placebo 17%). Also noteworthy was that the dropout rate was smaller in the dexfenfluramine group than in the placebo group.

Orlistat (Xenical®)

Hoffmann-La Roche Inc. is developing a pancreatic lipase inhibitor, orlistat (Xenical®), which blocks the absorption of fat. Pancreatic lipase, which is an enzyme secreted from the exocrine pancreas into the lumen of the intestine, is required for the hydrolysis and absorption of dietary fat. Orlistat is a selective inhibitor of the lipase family of enzymes and does not affect the enzymes involved in protein digestion and absorption (Exhibit 18–6). Inhibition of pancreatic lipase

Table 18–1 Dexfenfluramine—The INDEX Trial (52-week weight loss trial in obese patients. Patients were dosed with 15 mg dexfenfluramine two times/day for 52 weeks.)

| | Weight Loss | | | |
| | (kg) | | (%) | |
	Dexfen	Placebo	Dexfen	Placebo
Weight loss	9.82*	7.15	10.3*	7.2
Difference	2.7*		3.1*	

	Dexfen	Placebo
Distribution of weight loss:		
>10% initial	34%*	17%
>10 kg	32%*	16%
Compliance:		
withdrawals	37%	45%
withdrawals for too little weight loss	49%	84%

Note: Dexfen = dexfenfluramine.
*Indicates statistically significant difference compared to the placebo group.
Source: Reprinted by permission from B. Guy-Grand et al., International Trial of Long-Term Dexfenfluramine in Obesity, *Lancet,* © by the Lancet Ltd.

with orlistat results in blocking the absorption of approximately one third of the dietary fat. The non-absorbed fat is excreted in the feces.

A 12-week placebo-controlled, double-blind, weight loss trial of orlistat has been conducted in obese patients.[24] Orlistat was given three times daily with meals. A statistically significant difference in weight loss between the placebo and orlistat-treated groups was observed (2.2 kg) and gastrointestinal side effects in the orlistat group were mild or transient in most patients (Table 18–2).

IDEALIZED TREATMENT MODEL: PATIENT-CENTERED CONTROL AND DECISION MAKING

An idealized treatment model that is testable may improve the outcome of obesity treatment. In this type of treatment program, several types of diets (with different energy contents) and different kinds of exercise programs (one activity or a combination with different workloads) would be matched to each obese individual. At an appropriate point in the treatment program, therapy with an antiobesity drug would be added (Exhibit 18–7). Drug treatment might be added when the

Exhibit 18–6 Selectivity of Orlistat Action on Digestive Enzymes

Pancreatic lipase (porcine, murine, human)	IC50 = 0.2–0.6 nmol/ml
Carboxylic-ester hydrolase (human)	
Gastric lipase (human)	
Lipoprotein lipase (bovine)	potent inhibitor
Hormone-sensitive lipase	
Trypsin (bovine)	
Chymotrypsin (bovine)	not affected
alpha-Amylase (porcine)	
Pancreatic phospholipase A2 (porcine)	

rate of weight loss due to the diet and exercise is decelerating or has reached a plateau or when weight regain is observed.

The treatment program for this patient would then continue but one or more of the components would slowly be decreased while keeping the patient at weight maintenance. For some patients, the amount of caloric restriction would be decreased, others would decrease the frequency or duration or the intensity of exercise, and a third group would decrease the dose or frequency of antiobesity medication or halt medication use altogether. By using these options, a treatment program for weight maintenance could be tailored to the needs and requirements of each patient through a collaborative process.

Table 18–2 Effects of Orlistat on Weight Loss (12-week weight loss trial among obese patients [BMI = 31.4 ± 2.5]. Patients were dosed with 120 mg orlistat three times/day while eating meals containing 30% calories as fat.)

	Weight Loss (kg)	
	Orlistat	Placebo
Absolute weight loss	4.74 ± 0.38	2.98 ± 0.38
Difference	1.75 ± 0.54*	

Note: GI side effects were noted in the orlistat group but were mild or transient in most patients; other side effects were minimal.

*Indicates statistically significant difference compared to the placebo group.

Source: Reprinted with permission from M.L. Drent et al., Orlistat (Ro 18-0647), A Lipase Inhibitor, In The Treatment of Human Obesity: A Multiple Dose Study, *International Journal of Obesity,* Vol. 19, pp. 221–226, © 1995, MacMillan Press.

Exhibit 18–7 Possible Strategy To Enhance Self-Efficacy for Weight Maintenance

---

Step 1: Combine three modalities or "tools" during the weight loss phase of a treatment program:

Diet
Exercise
An antiobesity drug

Step 2: One of the "tools" is then withdrawn during a supervised and supported weight-maintenance phase of the program.

Step 3: During weight-maintenance phase of a treatment program and after, the patient is instructed to add back the third "tool" when unacceptable weight gain occurs, and to continue its use until weight maintenance is restored.

In this way, individuals may feel that they:

have more control over their weight
may be more successful at responding to, and minimizing weight gain that often occurs following the end of closely supervised and supported weight management programs

---

After achieving weight maintenance with the less restrictive treatment program, closely supervised treatment would end and patients would be guided to manage their weight and improved metabolic fitness using the reduced program. By measuring their own weight at regular intervals they would have the ability to add back one, two, or three of the components of the maintenance program if they start to gain weight. This may mean doubling the caloric restriction, increasing exercise from twice a week to four times a week, increasing the dose of an antiobesity drug, or resuming the medication (if it has been discontinued) until weight maintenance is restored. In this way, the individual decides, based on weight gain, to follow the more restrictive treatment program in order to halt and reverse the gain. This approach would not only encourage more attention and and quick response to weight maintenance, but also would give patients control over the rate of weight regain.

It is reasonable to ask whether such a program would have a similar or improved outcome compared to current intervention practice. This, of course, is a question for future research. However, there are anecdotal reports that some people use the Weintraub regimen in connection with their health professional in exactly this way. By having even a minor control over the frequency and dose of their antiobesity medication, they have a "locus of control," in the psychological sense, over their hunger.

CONCLUSION

Many developments in obesity and weight management suggest a promising future. These include basic and clinical research focused on intervention, revised approaches in the pharmaceutical industry, revised views in the research community about intervention and weight maintenance, and an FDA philosophy receptive to innovative products. All may lead to the development of a safe, effective, multi-factorial treatment approach in which patients will learn to become successful at sustaining beneficial, voluntary behavioral and life-style changes. In such a treatment approach, pharmaceutical agents would not be the "end-all" or "be-all" but would be used to support, reinforce, and sustain desirable behavioral changes leading to improved health of obese patients. The patients that practitioners seek to serve expect no less.

REFERENCES

1. Pi-Sunyer FX. The fattening of America. *JAMA.* 1994;272:204.

2. Garner DM. Defining socially and psychologically desirable body weights and the psychological consequences of weight loss and regain. In: Allison DB, Pi-Sunyer FX, eds. *Obesity Treatment: Establishing Goals, Improving Outcomes, and Reviewing the Research Agenda.* New York: Plenum Press; 1995:27–33.

3. Bouchard C, Perusse L. Genetics of obesity. *Ann Rev Nutr.* 1993;13:337–354.

4. Naslund I. Effects of weight reduction on the somatic, psychological and social complications of morbid obesity. In: Angel A, Anderson H, Bochard C, Lau D, Leiter L, Mendelson R, eds. *Progress in Obesity Research: 7.* London: John Libbey and Co; 1996:679–686.

5. Pories WJ, Swanson MS, MacDonald KG, Long SB, et al. Who would have thought it? An operation proves to be the most effective therapy for adult-onset diabetes mellitus. *Ann Surg.* 1995;222:339–352.

6. Leibel RL, Rosenbaum M, Hirsch J. Changes in energy expenditure resulting from altered body weight. *N Engl J Med.* 1995;232:621–628.

7. Campfield LA, Smith FJ, Guisez Y, Devos R, Burn P. Recombinant mouse OB protein: evidence for a peripheral signal linking adiposity and central neural networks. *Science.* 1995;269:546–549.

8. Hill JO, Douglas HJ, Peters JC. Physical activity, fitness, and moderate obesity. In: Bouchard C, Shepard RJ, Stephens T, eds. *Physical Activity, Fitness, and Health: International Proceedings and Consensus Statement.* Champaign, IL: Human Kinetics; 1994.

9. Thomas PR. *Weighing the Options: Criteria for the Evaluating Weight-Management Programs.* Washington, DC: Food and Nutrition Board, Institute of Medicine, National Academy Press; 1995.

10. Scoville BA. Review of amphetamine-like drugs by the Food and Drug Administration: Clinical data and value judgments. In: Bray GA, ed. *Obesity in Perspective.* DHEW Publ no (NIH) 75–708. Bethesda, MD: DHEW; 1975:441–443.

11. Weintraub M. Long-term weight control study: parts I–VII. *Clin Pharm Ther.* 1992;51:581–641.

12. Weintraub M. Long-term weight control study: conclusions. *Clin Pharm Ther.* 1992;51:642–646.

13. North American Association for the Study of Obesity (NAASO). Guidelines for the approval and use of drugs to treat obesity. *Obesity Res.* 1995;3:473–478.

14. Atkinson RL, Hubbard VS. Report on the NIH workshp on pharmacologic treatment of obesity. *Am J Clin Nutr.* 1994;60:153–156.

15. Campfield LA. Simple solutions for complex problems? Occam's razor, the FDA, and the pharmacological treatment of obesity. Proceedings of Seminar on Human Obesity: Current Status of Scientific and Clinical Progress. Boston: Am Assn Advancement Science; 1993.

16. Campfield LA. Treatment options and the maintenance of weight loss. In: Allison DB, Pi-Sunyer FX, eds. *Obesity Treatment: Establishing Goals, Improving Outcomes, and Reviewing the Research Agenda.* New York: Plenum Press; 1995:93–95.

17. Lissner L, Odell PM, D'Agostino RB. Variability of body weight and health outcomes in the Framingham population. *N Engl J Med.* 1991;324:1839–1844.

18. Tremblay A, Despres JP, Maheux J. Normalization of the metabolic profile in obese women by exercise and a low fat diet. *Med Sci Sports Exer.* 1991;23:1326–1331.

19. Uusitupa MSJ, Laakso M, Sarlund J, Majunder H, Takala J, Penttila L. Effects of a very-low-calorie diet on metabolic control and cardiovascular risk factors in the treatment of obese non–insulin-dependent diabetics. *Am J Clin Nutr.* 1990;51:768–773.

20. Henry RR, Gumbiner B. Benefits and limitations of very-low-calorie diet therapy in obese NIDDM. *Diabetes Care.* 1991;14:802–823.

21. Bray GA. Drug treatment of obesity: The argument in favor. In: Allison DV, Pi-Sunyer FX, eds. *Obesity Treatment: Establishing Goals, Improving Outcomes, and Reviewing the Research Agenda.* New York: Plenum Press; 1995:175–179.

22. Guy-Grand B, Apfelbaum M, Crepaldi G, Gries A, Lefebvre P, Turner P. International trial of long-term dexfenfluramine in obesity. *Lancet.* 1989;2:1142–1144.

23. Bray GA, Ryan DH, Gordon D, Heidingsfelder S, Cerise F, Wilson K. A double-blind randomized placebo-controlled trial of sibutramine. *Obesity Res.* 1996;4:263–270.

24. Drent ML, Larsson I, William-Olsson T, et al. Orlistat (Ro 18-0647), a lipase inhibitor, in the treatment of human obesity: a multiple dose study. *Int J Obesity.* 1995;19:221–226.

25. Goldstein DJ. Beneficial health effects of modest weight loss. *Int J Obes.* 1992;16:397–415.

26. Clement K, Vaisse C, Manning BSJ, Basdevant A, et al. Genetic variation in the B_3-adrenergic receptor and an increased capacity to gain weight in patients with morbid obesity. *N Engl J Med.* 1995;333:352–354.

27. Walston J, Silver K, Bogardus C, Knowler WC, et al. Time of onset of non–insulin-dependent diabetes mellitus and genetic variation in the B_3-adrenergic-receptor gene. *N Engl J Med.* 1995;333:343–347.

28. Widen E, Lehto M, Kanninen T, Walston J, Shuldiner AR, Groop LC. Association of a polymorphism in the B_3-adrenergic-receptor gene with features of the insulin resistance syndrome in Finns. *N Engl J Med.* 1995;333:348–351.

29. Manson JE, Willett WC, Stampfer MJ, et al. Body weight and mortality among women. *N Engl J Med.* 1995;333:677–685.

30. American Diabetes Association. Position statement: Implications of the Diabetes Control and Complications Trial. *Clin Diabetes.* 1993;11:91–96.

31. Rubin RR, Peyrot M. Implications of the DCCT. *Diabetes Care.* 1994;17:235–236.

CHAPTER 19

Anthropometric Techniques for Identification of Obese Children: Perspectives for the Practitioner

Cara B. Ebbeling
Nancy R. Rodriguez

INTRODUCTION

Pediatric obesity is a major concern for nutritionists and other allied health professionals. Although obesity usually is not associated with mortality or overt physical morbidity in preadolescents, it represents a risk factor for several diseases later in life.[1] Given the potential for obesity to track from childhood into adulthood,[2–8] identification and treatment of obese children is important for prevention of adult disease.[9–11] Although several conventional assessment techniques such as weight-for-height (WH), body mass index (BMI), and triceps skinfold (TSF) are available, there is no consensus regarding a protocol for classifying preadolescents as obese.

This lack of consensus presents a challenge to the practitioner with respect to intervention. Misclassification of children as obese may have physiological as well as psychological consequences.[12–17] Physiologically, the effects of hypocaloric diet interventions on nutrient utilization and subsequent growth in obese children have not been clearly defined. Psychologically, there may be severe social ramifications for children who are identified as obese. Individuals encounter various degrees of prejudice and discrimination in social settings depending on their degree of obesity, and children are not immune to these situations.[18]

In the current health care environment, insurance coverage and reimbursement for services rendered dictate delivery of services. Enterprising approaches to managed care include the development of practice guidelines specific to chronic disease states as a basis for evaluating the impact and the cost-effectiveness of medical nutrition therapy (MNT).[19–23] Nutritional assessment is central to the diagnosis and documentation for comorbidity codes, intervention selection, and development of nutritional care plans.[21,23,24] Therefore, establishment of criteria for classifying children according to risk for obesity-related diseases is paramount to the eventual evolution of practice guidelines for pediatric obesity. This chapter provides an overview of classical norm-referenced techniques that have been used to identify children at risk for obesity-related diseases and summarizes data from one investigation that used criterion-referenced standards to evaluate these techniques.

PRACTICAL TECHNIQUES FOR ASSESSMENT OF OBESITY

Weight-for-Height

Given that weight and height are direct, reliable, and easily obtained measures, weight-for-height (WH) has been used extensively by practitioners to characterize growth patterns using growth curves available from the National Center for Health Statistics (NCHS).[25] This technique relies on the premise that during growth, weight and height should increase in proportion to one another. When weight gain is sustained at a greater rate than linear growth, the individual may be a potential candidate for intervention. In addition, gender-specific WH cutoff points coinciding with 120% of the median are often employed to identify children at risk for obesity and its related complications. However, the clinical utility of WH for assessment of body composition in obese children is limited given that NCHS growth curves were developed only for boys (90 to 145 cm tall) and girls (90 to 137 cm tall) in the specified height ranges[25] and that obese children tend to be taller than their non-obese counterparts.[26]

Body Mass Index

Body mass index (BMI; wt/ht^2, kg/m^2) is an alternative parameter that relies solely on weight and height measurements for assessing overnutrition in children. Correlation studies have demonstrated a relationship between BMI, adiposity, and risk factors for chronic diseases.[13,27] Although limited data are available with regard to a single cutoff point for defining obesity in preadolescents, BMI values approximating the 85th and 95th percentiles, which may be derived from the first National Health and Nutrition Examination Survey (NHANES I), have been recommended for use in clinical settings.[12,28,29]

Triceps Skinfold

Because triceps skinfold (TSF) reflects subcutaneous fat stores, it provides a more direct assessment of adiposity than either WH or BMI. Theoretically, the combination of TSF and WH will distinguish overweight children who carry excess fat from those who possess a more desirable body composition. Cutoff points corresponding to the 85th or 95th percentiles for TSF with respect to population data derived from NHANES I have been used to identify obese children.[30] However, compared to measurement of WH and BMI, obtaining a reliable TSF reading is more difficult and necessitates practice to develop skill and consistent technique.

Norm- vs Criterion-Referenced Approaches

As noted in the preceding discussion, norm-referenced approaches based on population data for WH ($\geq$120% of median), BMI ($\geq$85th or $\geq$95th percentile), or TSF ($\geq$85th or $\geq$95th percentile) often are used to identify obese children using the specified cutoff points.[30-34] Identification, therefore, is dependent on the weight distribution and fatness of a reference population. These cutoff points may not necessarily correspond to levels of adiposity associated with elevated risk for unfavorable health outcomes, thereby limiting clinical utility of the norm-referenced approach.[35,36]

In contrast, a criterion-referenced approach necessitates the development of cutoff points that are independent of a reference population and represent critical levels of body fat associated with increased risk for disease.[36,37] However, limited data are available to establish standards using this approach. Williams et al[36] were the first investigators to empirically define obesity in children by linking adiposity to risk factors for coronary heart disease. Cutoff points of 25% and 30% fat for boys and girls, respectively, were recommended given that these values were associated with elevated blood pressure and serum lipids. Because this association is clinically significant, these cutoff points recently were used to evaluate practical techniques incorporating WH, BMI, and TSF for assessing obesity in children.

EVALUATION OF PRACTICAL TECHNIQUES: CONTINGENCY ANALYSES

Practical techniques for classifying children aged six to nine years with regard to risk for obesity-related diseases were evaluated using a contingency analysis (unpublished data). That is, sensitivities, specificities, and predictive values were determined for the norm-referenced approaches listed in Exhibit 19–1 using the criterion-referenced cutoff points (i.e., 25% fat for boys, 30% fat for girls) recommended by Williams et al.[36] Sensitivity (Se) refers to the proportion of obese children who are correctly identified as obese using a designated cutoff point, and specificity (Sp) denotes the proportion of non-obese children who are correctly identified as non-obese. Positive (V+) and negative (V–) predictive values are the probabilities that children above or below a designated cutoff point are obese or

Exhibit 19–1 Conventional Techniques for Assessment of Obesity

---

1. WH ≥120% of median[a]
2. BMI ≥85th percentile[b]
3. TSF ≥85th percentile[b]
4. WH ≥120% of median[a] and TSF ≥85th percentile[b]

[a]Cutoff points established using NCHS growth curves.[25]
[b]Percentiles based on NHANES I data.[30]

---

non-obese, respectively. The clinical utility of techniques for identifying obese children is best indicated by positive predictive values that reflect information concerning both the techniques and populations under consideration. Thereby, positive predictive values denote the likelihood that a child will experience adverse health outcomes associated with obesity. Formulas used to calculate sensitivities, specificities, and predictive values are presented in Exhibit 19–2. Results of contingency analyses are shown in Table 19–1.

Exhibit 19–2 Sensitivity, Specificity, and Predictive Values

Sensitivity (Se)
- The proportion of obese children who are correctly identified as obese using a designated cutoff point
- $TP^a / (TP + FN^b)$

Specificity (Sp)
- The proportion of non-obese children who are correctly identified as non-obese using a designated cutoff point
- $TN^c / (TN + FP^d)$

Positive Predictive Value (V+)
- Probability that children above a designated cutoff point are obese
- $TP / (TP + FP)$

Negative Predictive Value (V–)
- Probability that children below a designated cutoff point are non-obese
- $TN / (TN + FN)$

[a]True positive.
[b]False negative.
[c]True negative.
[d]False positive.

Table 19–1 Results of Contingency Analyses Used to Compare Conventional Techniques Employing WH, BMI, and/or TSF with Criterion-Referenced Standards (25% fat for boys, 30% fat for girls)[a]

Technique	Se	Sp	V+	V–
Boys				
1. WH ≥120% of median	0.79	0.97	0.73	0.98
2. BMI ≥85th percentile	0.84	0.88	0.40	0.98
3. TSF ≥85th percentile	0.94	0.90	0.48	0.99
4. WH ≥120% of median and TSF ≥85th percentile	0.72	0.98	0.81	0.97
Girls				
1. WH ≥120% of median	0.92	0.95	0.53	0.99
2. BMI ≥85th percentile	1.00	0.86	0.36	1.00
3. TSF ≥85th percentile	0.97	0.88	0.41	0.99
4. WH ≥120% of median and TSF ≥85th percentile	0.92	0.98	0.74	0.99

[a]Body fat expressed as a percentage of total body weight was estimated using gender- and race-specific equations developed by Williams et al.[36] Subjects were children age six to nine years who participated in the second National Health and Nutrition Examination Survey (NHANES II).

In addition, receiver operator characteristic (ROC) curves were used to illustrate trade-offs between improving sensitivity or specificity when employing BMI or TSF to classify children as obese or non-obese. Curves were generated by plotting sensitivity as a function of [1—specificity] for a series of potential cutoff points for BMI and TSF (Figure 19–1). Each of the ROC curves has (1) a steep portion corresponding to an increase in sensitivity with essentially no change in specificity, (2) a flat region corresponding to an increase in specificity with essentially no change in sensitivity, and (3) a region of deflection between the two essentially linear portions of the curves.[38] To optimize both sensitivity and specificity, cutoff points typically are located near the deflection regions of the respective ROC curves. However, the most clinically relevant cutoff points may deviate from the points of maximum deflection because positive and negative predictive values, in addition to sensitivities and specificities, must be taken into consideration. Predictive values for selected points have been inserted for each respective curve. Asterisks denote reasonable cutoff points for appropriately classifying children with regard to obesity status.

While the method employing both WH and TSF yielded the highest positive predictive values (Table 19–1), the necessary exclusion of taller children from the analyses incorporating WH limited the utility of this technique. Classification of subjects according to obesity status using 85th percentiles for BMI and TSF furnished V+ ≤0.5. The cutoff points derived from ROC curves with respect to BMI (19.5 kg/m² for both genders) and TSF (17 mm for boys; 20 mm for girls) provided relatively high positive predictive values (Figure 19–1) and were comparable to values associated with respective 95th percentiles (Table 19–2). This latter observation supports the use of the 95th percentiles for BMI and TSF when identifying children at risk for obesity-related diseases. Although 85th percentiles have been used extensively,[30,31,33] authors have recommended definitions of obe-

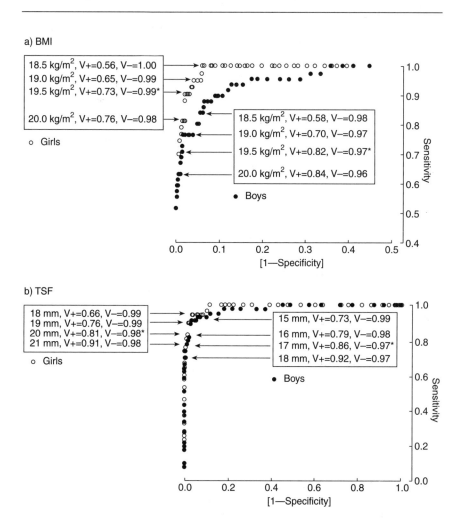

Figure 19–1 Receiver operator characteristic (ROC) curves for a) BMI and b) TSF.

Table 19–2 Comparisons among 85th and 95th Percentiles[a] and ROC Deflection Points for BMI and TSF

	BMI (kg/m²)			TSF (mm)		
Gender Age (yr)	85th percentile	95th percentile	ROC deflection region	85th percentile	95th percentile	ROC deflection region
Boys			19.5			17.0
6	16.6	18.0		11.1	14.1	
7	17.4	19.2		12.4	15.6	
8	18.1	20.3		13.7	17.2	
9	18.9	21.5		14.9	18.8	
Girls			19.5			20.0
6	16.2	17.5		13.4	15.6	
7	17.2	18.9		14.9	17.9	
8	18.2	20.4		16.4	20.2	
9	19.2	21.8		17.9	22.5	

[a]Percentiles based on NHANES I data.[30]

sity based on 95th percentiles to avoid misclassification of non-obese children as obese.[12,39,40] Indeed, cutoff points derived from ROC curves for BMI and TSF were more similar to values corresponding to 95th than to 85th percentiles and were better predictors of obesity. This recommendation is consistent with BMI criteria advocated by the Expert Committee on Clinical Guidelines for Overweight in Adolescent Preventive Services.[29]

The cutoff points determined from ROC curves are more conservative, compared to 95th percentiles, for younger than for older children (Table 19–2). A conservative approach is justified based on epidemiological data and clinical considerations. With respect to epidemiological data, the likelihood of becoming an obese adult who experiences obesity-related morbidities or mortality increases not only with increasing levels of adiposity but also for children in whom obesity persists with advancing age.[8] Clinically, given the potential physiological and psychological risks, as well as stigmatization, associated with an obesity classification, erroneous labeling of a non-obese child as obese may be associated with more severe consequences than misidentification of an obese child as non-obese.[18,39]

Compared to techniques employing percentiles, use of cutoff points based on inspection of ROC curves with consideration for predictive values are more attractive from theoretical and practical perspectives. Because body fat criteria associated with "silent" morbidities were used to calculate sensitivities and specificities for construction of ROC curves, the selected cutoff points with respect to BMI and TSF can be easily used to evaluate obesity status and assess risk for unfavorable health outcomes. Unlike conventional techniques, these cutoff points are independent of a reference population.

INCORPORATION OF PRACTICAL TECHNIQUES INTO ASSESSMENT PROTOCOLS

Practitioners must be confident in the criteria used to evaluate pediatric adiposity before initiating weight management protocols. While clinicians frequently use physical examination to identify obese patients who may benefit from an intervention program, numerous extraneous variables may affect a diagnosis based only on subjective evaluation.[41] Therefore, specific anthropometric criteria, in addition to routine dietary and biochemical assessments, should be included in the assessment protocol for determining whether a child is obese. When, given initial assessment data, a child is considered at risk for obesity-related diseases, more thorough dietary and biochemical assessments are warranted. As shown in this

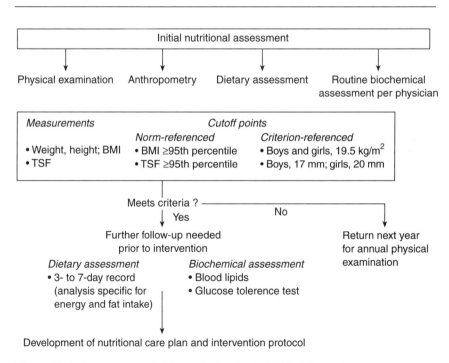

Figure 19–2 Assessment model for pediatric obesity highlighting anthropometry.

chapter, cutoff points for BMI and TSF that correspond to 95th percentiles for boys and girls should be applied when using a norm-referenced approach. When using a criterion-referenced approach, a BMI of 19.5 kg/m^2 for both genders and TSF values of 17 mm and 20 mm for boys and girls, respectively, are suggested at the present time. An assessment model that incorporates the data and recommendations summarized in this chapter is presented in Figure 19–2.

CONCLUSION

Additional research is warranted to validate the effectiveness of norm- and criterion-referenced approaches and to confirm the relationship between obesity criteria and morbidity. Specifically, randomized clinical trials and population-based studies must be designed to confirm the efficacy of these cutoff points for appropriate classification of children with regard to adiposity. When feasible, research designs should incorporate a current "gold standard" for assessment of body composition in obese children (i.e., dual-energy x-ray absorptiometry [DEXA]) to verify the applicability of these criteria for the practitioner. Because bioelectrical impedance analysis (BIA) is emerging as a practical tool for evaluation of body composition,[42] future research should also address the potential of BIA for the assessment of pediatric obesity using criterion-referenced standards.

REFERENCES

1. Pi-Sunyer FX. Health implications of obesity. *Am J Clin Nutr.* 1991;53:1595S–1603S.
2. Casey VA, Dwyer JT, Coleman KA, Valadian I. Body mass index from childhood to middle age: a 50-y follow-up. *Am J Clin Nutr.* 1992;56:14–18.
3. Clarke WR, Lauer RM. Does childhood obesity track into adulthood? *Crit Rev Food Sci Nutr.* 1993;33:423–430.
4. DiPietro L, Mossberg H-O, Stunkard AJ. A 40-year history of overweight children in Stockholm: life-time overweight, morbidity, and mortality. *Int J Obes.* 1994;18:585–590.
5. Must A, Jacques PF, Dallal GE, Bajema CJ, Dietz WH. Long-term morbidity and mortality of overweight adolescents: a follow-up of the Harvard Growth Study of 1922 to 1935. *N Engl J Med.* 1992;327:1350–1355.
6. Nieto FJ, Szklo M, Comstock GW. Childhood weight and growth rate as predictors of adult mortality. *Am J Epidemiol.* 1992;136:201–213.
7. Rolland-Cachera M-F, Deheeger M, Guilloud-Bataille M, Avons P, Patois E, Sempe M. Tracking the development of adiposity from one month of age to adulthood. *Ann Hum Biol.* 1987;14:219–229.
8. Serdula MK, Ivery D, Coates RJ, Freedman DS, Williamson DF, Byers T. Do obese children become obese adults? A review of the literature. *Prev Med.* 1993;22:167–177.
9. Endo H, Takagi Y, Nozue T, Kuwahata K, Uemasu F, Kobayashi A. Beneficial effects of dietary intervention on serum lipid and apolipoprotein levels in obese children. *Am J Dis Child.* 1992;146:303–305.

10. Strong WM, Deckelbaum RJ, Gidding SS, et al. Integrated cardiovascular health promotion in childhood: a statement for health professionals from the subcommittee on atherosclerosis and hypertension in childhood of the Council on Cardiovascular Disease in the Young, American Heart Association. *Circulation.* 1992;85:1638–1650.

11. Williams CL. Coronary heart disease prevention in childhood. Part I: background and rationale. *Med Exerc Nutr Health.* 1994;3:194–205.

12. Robinson TN. Defining obesity in children and adolescents: clinical approaches. *Crit Rev Food Sci Nutr.* 1993;33:313–320.

13. Ernst ND, Obarzanek E. Child health and nutrition: obesity and high blood pressure. *Prev Med.* 1994;23:427–436.

14. Hill AJ, Draper E, Stack J. A weight on children's minds: body shape dissatisfactions at 9-years old. *Int J Obes.* 1994;18:383–389.

15. Ohzeki T, Tachikawa H, Tanimoto K. Excessive food aversion, compulsive exercise and decreased height gain due to fear of obesity in a prepubertal girl. *Psychother Psychosom.* 1994;62:203–206.

16. Pflieger KL, Treiber FA, Davis H, McCaffrey FM, Raunikar RA, Strong WB. The effect of adiposity on children's left ventricular mass and geometry and haemodynamic responses to stress. *Int J Obes.* 1994;18:117–122.

17. Rumpel C, Harris TB. The influence of weight on adolescent self-esteem. *J Psychosom Res.* 1994;38:547–556.

18. Cassell J. Social anthropology and nutrition: a different look at obesity in America. *J Am Diet Assoc.* 1995;95:424–427.

19. Position of the American Dietetic Association: nutrition services in managed care. *J Am Diet Assoc.* 1996;96:391–395.

20. Laramee SH. Nutrition services in managed care: new paradigms for dietitians. *J Am Diet Assoc.* 1996;96:335–336.

21. Franz MJ. Practice guidelines for nutrition care by dietetic practitioners for outpatients with non-insulin-dependent diabetes mellitus: consensus statement. *J Am Diet Assoc.* 1992;92:1136–1139.

22. Franz MJ, Monk A, Barry B, et al. Effectiveness of medical nutrition therapy provided by dietitians in the management of non-insulin-dependent diabetes mellitus: a randomized, controlled clinical trial. *J Am Diet Assoc.* 1995;95:1009–1017.

23. Monk A, Barry B, McClain K, Weaver T, Cooper N, Franz MJ. Practice guidelines for medical nutrition therapy provided by dietitians for persons with non-insulin-dependent diabetes mellitus. *J Am Diet Assoc.* 1995;95:999–1006.

24. Schatz GB. Coding for nutrition services: challenges, opportunities, and guidelines. *J Am Diet Assoc.* 1993;93:471–477.

25. Hamill PVV, Drizd TA, Johnson CL, Reed RB, Roche AF, Moore WM. Physical growth: National Center for Health Statistics percentiles. *Am J Clin Nutr.* 1979;32:607–629.

26. Forbes GB. Nutrition and growth. *J Pediatr.* 1977;91:40–42.

27. Hammer LD, Kraemer HC, Wilson DM, Ritter PL, Dornbusch SM. Standardized percentile curves of body-mass index for children and adolescents. *Am J Dis Child.* 1991;145:259–263.

28. Lazarus R, Baur L, Webb K, Blyth F. Body mass index in screening for adiposity in children and adolescents: systematic evaluation using receiver operating characteristic curves. *Am J Clin Nutr.* 1996;63:500–506.

29. Himes JH, Dietz WH. Guidelines for overweight in adolescent preventive services: recommendations from an expert committee. *Am J Clin Nutr.* 1994;59:307–316.

30. Must A, Dallal GE, Dietz WH. Reference data for obesity: 85th and 95th percentiles of body mass index (wt/ht^2) and triceps skinfold thickness. *Am J Clin Nutr.* 1991;53:839–846.

31. Gortmaker SL, Dietz WH, Sobol AM, Wehler CA. Increasing pediatric obesity in the United States. *Am J Dis Child.* 1987;141:535–540.

32. Tiwary CM, Holguin AH. Prevalence of obesity among children of military dependents at two major medical centers. *Am J Public Health.* 1992;82:354–357.

33. Harlan WR, Landis R, Flegal KM, Davis CS, Miller ME. Secular trends in body mass in the United States, 1960–1980. *Am J Epidemiol.* 1988;128:1065–1074.

34. Wolfe WS, Campbell CC, Frongilla EA, Hass JD, Melnik TA. Overweight schoolchildren in New York State: prevalence characteristics. *Am J Public Health.* 1994;84:807–813.

35. Going S, Williams D. Understanding fitness standards. *J Phys Educ Recreation Dance.* 1989;60:34–38.

36. Williams DP, Going SB, Lohman TG, et al. Body fatness and risk for elevated blood pressure, total cholesterol, and serum lipoprotein ratios in children and adolescents. *Am J Public Health.* 1992;82:358–363.

37. Blair SN, Clark DG, Cureton KJ, Powell KE. Exercise and fitness in childhood: implications for a lifetime of health. In: Gisolfi CV, Lamb DR, eds. *Perspectives in Exercise Science and Sports Medicine: Youth, Exercise, and Sport.* Indianapolis, IN: Benchmark Press; 1989:401–430.

38. Browner WS, Newman TB, Cummings SR. Designing a new study: III. Diagnostic tests. In: Hulley SB, Cummings SR, eds. *Designing Clinical Research. An Epidemiologic Approach.* Baltimore: Williams and Wilkins; 1988:87–97.

39. Troiano RP, Flegal KM, Kuczmarski RJ, Campbell SM, Johnson CL. Overweight prevalence and trends for children and adolescents: the National Health and Nutrition Examination Surveys, 1963 to 1991. *Arch Pediatr Adolesc Med.* 1995;149:1085–1091.

40. Guo SS, Roche AF, Chumlea WC, Gardner JD, Siervogel RM. The predictive value of childhood body mass index values for overweight at age 35 y. *Am J Clin Nutr.* 1994;59:810–819.

41. Eck LH, Ray JW, Klesges RC, Relyea GE, Hackett-Renner C. Physicians' diagnosis of obesity status in NHANES II. *Int J Obes.* 1994;18:704–708.

42. Goran MI, Driscoll P, Johnson R, Nagy TR, Hunter G. Cross-calibration of body-composition techniques against dual-energy X-ray absorptiometry in young children. *Am J Clin Nutr.* 1996;63:299–305.

CHAPTER **20**

Childhood and Adolescent Weight Management

Debra K. Brown

INTRODUCTION

In the 10 years since Gortmaker and Dietz published their shocking data regarding the increasing prevalence of childhood obesity in America,[1] obesity rates have continued to climb and with them a slow but steady progression of public and professional attention to the problem.

While variations in measurement definitions raise questions about exact prevalence figures,[2] the most current estimates from the National Health and Nutrition Examination Survey (NHANES) report that obesity among youth in America has increased noticeably since the 1960s with the steepest rise from 1976 (NHANES II) through 1991 (NHANES III) as can be seen in Figures 20–1 and 20–2.

Using the 95th percentile for body mass index (BMI), approximately 11% of the two age groups are currently obese. If the 85th percentile is used, the figure rises to 22%.[3] Of particular concern is the slower and more progressive rise in the younger age group.

Childhood obesity tracks into adulthood with concomitant increases in morbidity and mortality. Estimates are that 25% to 50% of obese children and adolescents become obese adults.[4,5] The Harvard Growth Study shows that overweight in adolescence is a more powerful predictor of some health risks than overweight in adulthood.[6] The National Task Force on the Prevention and Treatment of Obesity recognizes obesity as a chronic lifelong disease with significant effects on future health, increasing the risk of cardiovascular disease, diabetes, stroke, certain types of cancer, osteoarthritis, sleep apnea, and gallstones.[7] Increased amounts of visceral fat, hyperinsulinemia, and hyperlipidemia are being found in obese adolescents, thus making them targets for cardiovascular disease as adults.[8] More immediate and perhaps more serious are the psychosocial consequences of excess weight for the growing child or adolescent.[9] Children as young as age six are de-

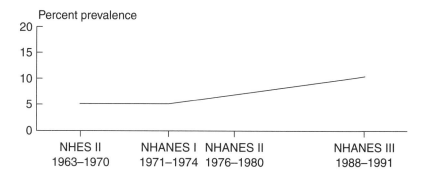

Figure 20–1 Overweight prevalence ages 6–11. *Source:* Reprinted from Center for Disease Control and Prevention, National Center for Health Statistics.

scribed negatively by their peers and social isolation is often the result.[10,11] Adolescents often experience rejection, which can have very real consequences such as lowered college acceptance rates, fewer opportunities for marriage, and lower financial remuneration in the job market.[12]

Compared to treatment of obesity in adults, treatment efforts with children have shown more promise. Most of this chapter is devoted to management and prevention approaches and guidelines. In particular, behavioral and dietary change methods are presented, with an emphasis on innovative, practical, and valid methods and ideas for developing and strengthening pediatric weight management options. A further objective is to stimulate research and more innovative intervention strategies.

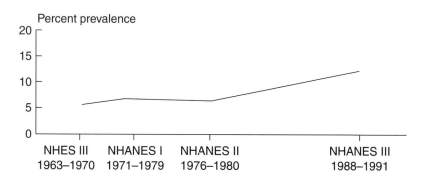

Figure 20–2 Overweight prevalence ages 12–17. *Source:* Reprinted from Center for Disease Control and Prevention, National Center for Health Statistics.

CONTRIBUTORS TO PEDIATRIC OBESITY

Many factors contribute to the recent increase of overweight in American youth (also see Chapters 3, 6, 10, and 12). The role of genetics is significant.[13] Most experts agree that parental-child obesity outcomes are indicative of both genetic and environmental influences.[3,14] Studies of the body mass index (BMI) of adopted children have shown a higher correlation to the weight of the biologic parents and siblings than to the adopted family members. A weak influence of the shared family environment has also been observed. These authors suggest that a genetic influence as strong as that observed in adults is expressed by seven years of age.

Increasing evidence indicates that obesity finds its genetic expression in energy metabolism and is site- and tissue-specific.[14] For example, it is known that fat patterning is determined genetically.[15] Truncal fat deposition in adults is associated with many disease states including hyperlipidemia, hypertension, insulin resistance, and diabetes.[16] For those treating children it is important to note that the deposition of central body fat occurs in adolescence and may thus be a causal factor in both adult obesity and increased risks of future morbidity and mortality.[8] Therefore, early identification and treatment of this significant risk factor in this age group may decrease future health risks.

In addition to early adolescence, other critical periods for obesity development are the intrauterine period and early infancy and the period of adiposity rebound (five to seven years of age).[17] All three periods have both genetic and environmental origins and may be important as targets for intervention efforts. Further research to support this theory is needed; recently, for example, the theory of the intrauterine period has been disputed.[18]

Although genetic factors are important, current thinking leans toward the role of environmental factors in positive energy balance. Modifiable components such as food intake and physical activity may play a larger role than was once thought.[20] Dietary data from surveys conducted in the mid-1970s compared to those in the early 1990s show similar overall mean energy intakes for children under 12 years of age but marked increases for adolescent females. A small decline in fat intake in all age groups has also been noted.[19] This latter point is surprising given the continued abundance of high-fat foods and the resulting preference for these foods among today's youth.[3] One explanation may be the underreporting of dietary intake. Both children and adults have been known to underreport intake by as much as 40%.[20] Therefore, the current outcome of positive energy balance that may be responsible for increased rates of obesity may thus be more related to the underestimating of dietary intake than to a decrease in energy efficiency as has been postulated by some.[15]

Another explanation that seems reasonable is a decrease in energy output. American children are certainly becoming less active. Participation in physical education classes has declined dramatically while engagement in sedentary activities such as television viewing, video games, and computers is on the rise.[21] The negative impact of television viewing in particular has been examined. A linear relationship exists between the prevalence of obesity in younger age groups and the number of hours of television viewed per day.[15] In addition to encouraging sedentary activities, television may also encourage the consumption of high-fat, low-nutrient foods through food advertisements.[15] Additionally, there is some evidence suggesting that television viewing slows the metabolic rate.[22,23]

The complete effect of this inactive lifestyle on adiposity has not yet been determined. Powerful social forces are often overlooked but may play a role in negative energy balance. American children are playing outdoors less due to a myriad of reasons including safety concerns, lack of recreational programs and supervision, and scarcity of playgrounds. As more women work outside the home, "latch-key" children are left after school locked in houses unable to engage in outdoor activities. The use of the doubly-labeled water technique to study the role of total energy expenditure in the development and maintenance of obesity shows that total energy expenditure in younger children is approximately 25% lower than current energy intake recommendations.[24] Are energy recommendations too high given lower levels of childhood activity? A related question is: If calorie recommendations were lowered, would the risk of children consuming insufficient food to meet other nutrient needs increase?

The weight status of parents in relation to their offspring has also been studied. Two decades ago the likelihood of childhood overweight was estimated at about 80% among offspring from two overweight parents, and at less than 10% from two normal-weight parents.[25] More recently, a "preobese" state is evidenced by studies like those of Roberts et al,[26] which report lower total energy expenditure and higher percentages of obesity among infants of overweight mothers. The majority of current studies show a lower total energy expenditure among children with either one or both parents obese, a risk factor for development of later obesity.[24]

Another study examined both the modifiable factors, dietary intake and physical activity, as well as the nonmodifiable, parental weight status. Both were associated with increases or decreases in the body mass index in preschooolers studied.[27] Factors found to have a statistical significance were a smaller number of overweight parents, decreases in fat intake, and higher levels of aerobic and leisure activity. The surprising outcome of the study was that the variables that could be modified accounted for more of the variance in changes in body mass index than those that could not be modified, pointing to the possible value of behavioral interventions at earlier ages.

PEDIATRIC OBESITY ASSESSMENT

Growth

The assessment of pediatric obesity is a complex task involving growth, diet patterns, nutritional and medical status, and activity. Because children are growing, it is difficult to obtain clear-cut definitions of degree of overweight. Practitioners generally use methods based on weight and height measurements as compared to a standard, usually the National Center for Health Statistics (NCHS) growth charts,[28] body mass index percentiles,[29] and skinfold measurement percentiles.[30] Although there may be both positive and negative aspects of each classification method, some system of categorization is essential for targeting intervention strategies. For example, a mildly overweight child may need only a small degree of intervention such as family nutrition counseling whereas a more severely obese child may require a more comprehensive dietary and behavioral approach. More than one assessment method may be used, such as relative weight and triceps skinfold to quantify the degree of overweight. An overview of current pediatric obesity assessment methods can be seen in Table 20–1.

At most pediatric centers, the assessment interview begins with an evaluation of previous growth patterns using age-specific growth charts. This method provides

Table 20–1 Pediatric Obesity Assessment Methods and Reference Standards

Method	Definition	References
Triceps skinfold measurements	TSF >95th percentile NHANES I data	Must et al[30]
Body mass index	BMI >95th percentile NHANES I data	Must et al[30]
Relative weight	Mildly obese: 120% to 149% of IBW* Moderately obese: 150% to 199% of IBW Severely obese: >200% of IBW	Suskind et al[58]
Growth charts	Body weight increases of >2 major percentile channels (NCHS growth charts)	Alemzadeh & Lifshitz[31]

*Ideal body weight (IBW) is defined as the 50th percentile of weight for children of the same height, age, and sex.

the clinician with a way to establish the presence of obesity accurately and detect its onset. The authors recommend instituting intervention strategies at the first sign of an increase in weight percentiles, preferably before the age of adiposity rebound (five to seven years) or puberty, two critical periods for adiposity development.[32]

Illustrated in Figures 20–3 and 20–4 are examples of two common growth patterns in obese children. Figure 20–3 represents a pattern of "constitutional" overweight, which has been defined as a body weight progression that is constant throughout childhood but is one or two percentile channels greater than the height.[31] In our example, the major weight progression was constant throughout at two major percentiles above that of the height. Even though the relative weight is

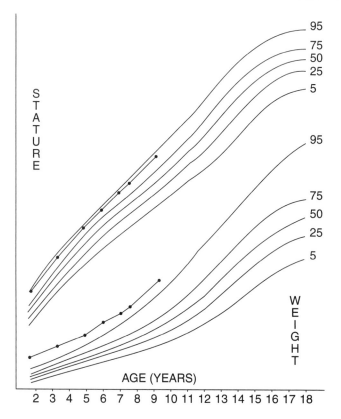

Figure 20–3 Growth chart illustrating pattern of constitutional overweight. *Source:* Reprinted with permission from R. Alemzadeh and F. Lifshitz, Childhood Obesity, in *Pediatric Endocrinology,* 3rd Edition, F. Lifshitz, ed., Figure 1, p. 754, by courtesy of Marcel Dekker, Inc., New York, NY, 1996.

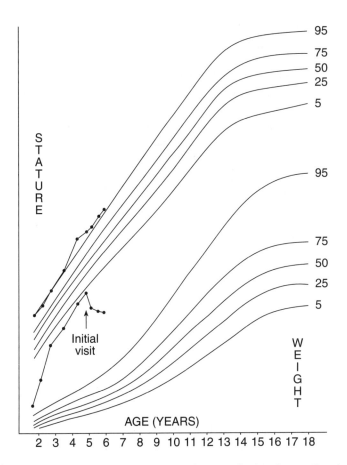

Figure 20–4 Growth chart illustrating pattern of severe obesity. *Source:* Reprinted with permission from R. Alemzadeh and F. Lifshitz, Childhood Obesity, in *Pediatric Endocrinology,* 3rd Edition, F. Lifshitz, ed., Figure 2, p. 755, by courtesy of Marcel Dekker, Inc., New York, NY, 1996.

138%, constituting a moderate degree of obesity, this child may not be truly obese by body composition standards. A balance and adjustment has been achieved in the maintenance of body weight that may be "normal" for this child. Figure 20–4, on the other hand, represents a pattern of severe or morbid obesity with a sudden acceleration at three years of age. Since this is earlier than the average age of adiposity rebound, intervention at three years of age might have lessened the continued weight gain. Previous research has shown that constitutional patterns of growth are encountered in approximately 25% of adolescents with excess body weight for height.[33] Therefore, health workers should use caution in the evaluation process, employing further measures of body composition before a management plan is formulated.

Another important part of the growth evaluation is to determine the age of obesity onset. This measure, along with the severity of obesity, usually predicts future health risks.[4] Yearly rates of weight change in relation to height should also be reviewed, especially in the year before the initial interview. It is helpful to explain normal rates of gain to the family and to compare differences between the growth rate of their child and rates on the growth chart. For normal-weight children an estimate of the expected gain can be achieved by using the widely utilized National Center for Health Statistics (NCHS) growth charts, although these were not derived from longitudinal studies.[34] One simply calculates the amount of weight the child should have gained according to the gains in height for the time period in question if the weight and height had remained within their previous percentile channels. For obese growing children, however, it is preferable to explain this to the parents using the concept of "the child growing into his or her weight." This is accomplished by achieving weight maintenance for a certain period of time rather than losing weight. Using the child's individual chart, the health practitioner can show this by pointing out the height percentile and then drawing a line horizontally across the growth chart from the present weight until it intersects the same percentile as the height on the weight chart. The length of time required to achieve the appropriate weight for height is then calculated by subtracting the current age from the age at which the intersection occurs.[35] For normal adolescents that do not have an endocrine disorder, it may be important to determine when and if peak height velocity has occurred. Girls experience this during early puberty and before menarch while for boys this happens later during mid to late puberty.[36] The growth potential can be estimated with bone age and pubertal staging. Pubertal stage is best assessed by an endocrinologist or adolescent medicine specialist by physical examination using the Tanner Staging schema.[37] If growth is almost completed, it is appropriate to emphasize weight loss rather than maintenance and a lower caloric intake can be prescribed. Further, a history of the highest and lowest weights achieved at the final height can be made. Finally, because it is widely accepted that the weight status of the parents affects obesity outcomes in children, it is valuable to assess the weight and health status of all family members.

Diet and Nutritional Status

Although records of dietary intake are an important component of assessment, obtaining the information is an imprecise and misleading task. Many use dietary records to obtain initial information about an individual's intake. However, this self-reporting method has been shown to be biased with a significant degree of underreporting and caution should be used when interpreting these data.[38]

The current "gold standard" for assessing both energy expenditure and dietary caloric intake is the doubly-labeled water technique.[39] This technique, which uses carbon dioxide production from two stable isotopes of water, measures the total energy expenditure from all sources over an extended time period. Caloric intake is estimated by subtracting from the caloric output from the total energy expenditure. A number of recent studies using this method have shown a poor correspondence of reported dietary intake and actual intake.[38] Although little research has yet been undertaken in children, underreporting has been documented in this age group as well as in adults. Therefore, estimating caloric requirements using dietary intake data is not recommended.[4]

Twenty-four hour recalls and food frequency checklists also are used to assess food intake. One goal in using them is to identify eating patterns and to obtain a general view of the usual intake rather than to obtain an exact accounting of calories. The main purpose of food frequency questionnaires is to identify foods of high caloric density that are frequently consumed. A second goal is to determine the general nutritional adequacy of the diet. In addition, a thorough review of beverage consumption is recommended because this often greatly contributes to the total caloric intake of obese children.[4]

Certain key nutrients that are underconsumed by American children and related to weight gain are also targeted for analysis. Iron and calcium have been shown to be lacking in the diets of obese children following short-term weight loss.[40] In the food frequency checklist, food sources of these two nutrients are assessed and if found lacking, counseling is provided to enhance their intake as part of the eating plan. Fruit and vegetable consumption is also assessed. Recently many national nutrition programs such as the "5-A-Day" have been launched with the goal of increasing the intake of these two food groups in children's diets.[41] The "5-A-Day" program illustrates a positive focus, "eat more apples and carrots" rather than a negative one such as, "cut down on french fries and donuts."[42]

MEDICAL ASSESSMENT

Three components of medical assessment are key when evaluating a child or adolescent with obesity. First, a thorough physical examination with special attention to growth parameters, skin manifestations, dysmorphic features, and body fat distribution should be performed as well as a fundoscopic exam. One important aim of this examination is to identify some of the possible pathological causes of obesity including endocrine and genetic entities such as Cushing's syndrome, hypoparathyroidism, Prader-Willi syndrome, or Bardet-Biedl syndrome, to name a few. In general, these conditions comprise less than 1% of the clinical manifestations of pediatric obesity and most are remarkable for some degree of delayed skeletal maturation and short stature in contrast to primary obesity where there is usually advanced maturation and increased or normal height.[4] Further investigations with laboratory analysis should follow when a particular diagnosis is suspected.[31]

Second, a thorough medical assessment includes a review of the comorbidities currently associated with the obesity in a particular individual. A careful review of cardiovascular, endocrine, gastrointestinal, pulmonary, musculoskeletal and neurological systems as depicted in Table 20–2 is a key component of the assessment. Appropriate referrals for further evaluation and management should be made if abnormalities are found.

Table 20–2 Medical Aspects of Pediatric Obesity

Review of Systems	Complications
Cardiovascular	Hypertension Hypercholesterolemia
Endocrine	Hyperinsulinism/insulin resistance Non–insulin-dependent diabetes mellitus Gynecomastia Decreased fertility Early puberty and menarche Hirsutism Acanthosis nigrans Advanced bone age Short stature Decreased testosterone
Gastrointestinal	Cholecystitis Steatohepatitis Reflux Abdominal pain
Pulmonary	Pickwickian syndrome Obstructive sleep apnea Primary alveolar hypoventilation Pulmonary function abnormalities
Musculoskeletal	Slipped capital femoral epiphysis Blount's disease Chronic ankle strain Delayed recovery time
Cardiovascular	Hypertension Hypercholesterolemia
Neurological	Recurrent headaches Pseudo-tumor cerebri

Source: Reproduced by permission of PEDIATRICS/*Pediatrics in Review*, Vol. 14, p. 341, Copyright 1993.

Finally, the medical assessment should include an evaluation of the risk for future morbidity based on family history, physical, and laboratory evaluation. In particular, cardiovascular disease, hypertension, and diabetes are associated with abnormalities in lipid and serum insulin levels and glucose tolerance in adolescents.[9,43] Routine preventive screening guidelines for adolescents have recently been developed that may be useful.[44] In these, adolescents with body mass indexes greater than the 95th percentile are considered frankly overweight and are recommended to be referred for in-depth medical follow-up. Anticipatory guidance with an emphasis on changes in lifestyle for the whole family should be provided if future health risks are suspected. The health practitioner should avoid using "scare tactics" with this population as there are some vulnerable adolescents who may be susceptible to the development of eating disorders.[9]

Some of the most commonly observed complications are hyperlipidemia, hypertension, and insulin resistance. A significant number of obese children have been recently reported to display signs of insulin resistance, which may be a precursor to adult-onset diabetes and cardiovascular disease.[8] Laboratory measures such as a lipid profile and thyroid test as well as a review of other clinically significant features such as an elevated waist-to-hip ratio and acanthosis nigrans, a brownish discoloration of the skin, are useful. More serious complications of obesity should also be assessed, including symptoms of sleep apnea and recurrent headaches, which may be symptomatic of a hypothalamic tumor.[4]

Activity and Body Composition

Assessment of activity levels in children participating in obesity programs is a difficult but important task. Again, both metabolic and environmental factors may be responsible for the reduced activity levels observed in American children today. Physical activity assessment tools vary but basically consist of three types: self-report questionnaires, exercise testing, and body composition and energy expenditure analysis. Some have questioned the validity and reliability of using self-report questionnaires with children.[45] However, because of low cost, ease of administration, and evidence that children as young as 10 years of age can provide reliable information, self-reports are used by many.[46] For program evaluation purposes, validity levels may be low. For clinical use, modifications of the questionnaire can be used to measure levels of physical activity in a general manner. Exercise testing provides a more concrete assessment tool and is comprised of tests of cardiorespiratory endurance, muscular strength and endurance, and muscular flexibility. Testing should be administered with the assistance of a trained exercise specialist. An easy method was developed as part of the Shape Down Program.[47] A three-minute modified step test is used to measure cardiovascular endurance; the sit and reach test for flexibility; and the modified sit-up for muscular strength. More in-depth measures of cardiorespiratory endurance are also available. For example, the M-PEP Moderate Progressive Exercise Program uses complex measures such as maximal oxygen uptake and isokinetic equipment.[48]

Measures of body composition and energy expenditure can provide an indirect measure of physical activity and dietary compliance, if performed both before and at the end of the intervention program. The authors recommend some assessment of body fat and fat-free mass as well as basal metabolic rate. Many practitioners and researchers currently employ bioelectrical impedance analysis (BIA) to measure body composition due to its relatively low cost, portability, and ease of administration.[49,50] It has also been shown to yield relatively high rates of validity when compared to more expensive methods. If this equipment is not available, one can measure several skinfolds sites using the Slaughter formula to determine total body fat.[51,52] (See Table 20–3.) A consistent technique and replication are important when performing the measurement of fat folds with either a caliper or BIA probe.

Measures of basal metabolic rate are easy to obtain using a metabolic cart or hood method. Studies have repeatedly shown that obese children and adults have higher or the same basal metabolic rates as their normal-weight counterparts due to increased lean body mass, and that moderate amounts of weight loss do not

Table 20–3 Prediction Equations for Children

Method	Ethnicity/Gender	Equation	Reference
SKF Σ triceps + calf	Black and white		
	Boys (all ages)	1. %BF = 0.735 (ΣSKF) + 1.0	Slaughter et al (1988)
	Girls (all ages)	2. %BF = 0.610 (ΣSKF) + 5.1	Slaughter et al (1988)
Σ triceps + subscapular (ΣSKF >35 mm)	Black and white		
	Boys (all ages)	3. %BF = 0.783 (ΣSKF) + 1.6	Slaughter et al (1988)
	Girls (all ages)	4. %BF = 0.546 (ΣSKF) + 9.7	Slaughter et al (1988)
(ΣSKF <35 mm)	Black and white		
	Boys (all ages)	5. %BF = 1.21 (ΣSKF) – 0.008 (ΣSKF)^2 + I	Slaughter et al (1988)
	Girls (all ages)	6. %BF = 1.33 (ΣSKF) – 0.013 (ΣSKF)^2 – 2.5	Slaughter et al (1988)
TEE	Younger children	7. TEE = 66 FFM + 11 HR + 0.74 REE – 1482 kcal/day	Goran (1995)

Note: TEE = total energy expenditure; FFM = fat free mass; HR = heart rate; REE = resting energy expenditure.
Source: Heyward VH, Stolarczyk LM, 1996; Goran MI, 1995.

produce changes in this measure.[24] Showing useful promise is the development of a formula that yields an estimate of total energy expenditure in children.[39] The formula is illustrated in Table 20–3.

Preliminary studies using this new formula show that actual total energy expenditure is 25% lower than that which had been previously recommended for this age group. Although most children appear to be active, they may not perform high-intensity exercise for long periods of time and the energy cost of playing may be less than was thought in the past.[24]

MANAGEMENT

Diet

Fortunately, dietary treatment of pediatric obesity has advanced in the last several years and now offers a variety of approaches. The choices range from very-low-calorie diets to general dietary guidelines and even further to the "nondiet approach." With children, one must consider several factors before deciding on the appropriate dietary plan. These include weight loss goals, age and developmental stage, educational level and abilities, and level of family functioning. The dietary program should be considered part of the total behavior change strategy and not as a separate entity in and of itself. Maintenance of positive results, the ultimate goal, can only be achieved if dietary changes are made within a comprehensive behavioral program.[53,54]

The traditional dietary treatment for pediatric obesity has been the balanced hypocaloric diet defined as between 1200 to 1500 calories daily with 50% to 55% coming from carbohydrate; 25% to 30% from fat; and 15% to 20% from protein.[55] Some have defined this as a reduction in caloric intake from 30% to 40% of usual intake.[56] The attainment of this lower calorie level is achieved in various ways including elimination of high-fat and calorically dense foods,[57] exchange lists,[58] and systems based on food groups of varying caloric density.[4] A balance of macronutrients and micronutrients is achieved by providing guidelines for age-related daily servings. A good example of the latter approach is "The Traffic Light Diet" in which foods are categorized as red, yellow, or green on the basis of their caloric and nutrient content.[40] Children are instructed to limit red foods (high-calorie) to a certain number weekly and to maintain nutrient balance by eating a certain number of servings from the four food groups or diet pyramid system. One advantage of this type of plan is that it offers choices among food lists of varying caloric density. Newer approaches consider that children prefer plans that allow choices rather than prescribed numbers of daily servings or other regimented plans.

In general, the hypocaloric diet is the best option when moderate weight loss is the goal. Since current research raises questions about the link between total caloric intake and adiposity, attention has turned to factors associated with diet composition. Several studies have shown that children of obese parents consume a larger percentage of their caloric intake from fat and less from fiber-containing foods.[59-61] In particular, the obesity status and fat intake of the mother have been implicated. Conclusions from these studies show that mothers may contribute to the development of obesity by influencing dietary fat intake and that overweight children may have increased taste preferences for high-fat foods. In addition, metabolically, fat utilization may be less efficient than carbohydrate utilization, requiring less energy for absorption and storage (see Chapters 9 and 10). Since a low-fat, high-fiber plan that includes fruits and vegetables is naturally incorporated within the structure of the hypocaloric diet, most diet programs include some attention to this feature. Taking these considerations in mind, a dietary program that examines the mother's and the family's eating habits as well as the child's seems appropriate. At the authors' center, general guidelines are given for lowering the fat content of the entire family's diet. Children are given menu options that are lower in fat while the mothers are taught appropriate cooking and shopping techniques. An example of a menu system is illustrated in Exhibit 20–1.

This kind of approach gives the child choices and some responsibility in food preparation and selection. The parent's role is supportive, directing food procurement and preparation activities and providing guidance. Research shows that restrictions imposed by parents in the food selection process in young children may result in a lessened ability to self-regulate and a higher risk of obesity development.[62] Therefore this program emphasizes the independence and responsibility of the child in the food selection process. At the same time, a less-restricted consumption of predominately carbohydrate-containing foods is allowed, thus diminishing the sense of dietary deprivation. A modest reduction in caloric intake is therefore achieved while preserving the child's natural desire for good-tasting foods.

In some clinics a more significant degree of weight loss is being promoted with use of the protein-sparing modified fast.[63] With this method, all children regardless of the initial degree of overweight are placed on a protein-sparing modified fast until the ideal body weight is achieved.[58] The diet consists of 2.0 grams of protein per kilogram body weight and 600 to 800 calories daily. Carbohydrate intake is limited to 20 to 25 grams in order to induce ketosis, a state which is monitored weekly by checking urinary ketone levels. This regimen also includes a daily potassium and multiple vitamin/mineral supplement. The length of time a child remains on such a diet varies between 10 and 20 weeks depending on the initial degree of obesity. At the end of this period, a balanced hypocaloric diet using the exchange system model is instituted. The program now known as the "Committed to Kids Pediatric Weight Management Program" also incorporates an excellent lifestyle management component with state-of-the-art exercise and be-

Exhibit 20–1 Menu Option Eating Plan

Design your own eating plan with the foods you like! Your nutritionist will assist you in deciding on portion sizes and amounts.

Breakfast

#1 Cereal _____	#2 Granola Bar _____	#3 Eggs _____
Fruit/Juice _____	Roll _____	Bagel/Bread _____
Milk _____	Fruit/Juice _____	Marg./Butter/
	Milk _____	Cr. Cheese _____
		Fruit/Juice _____
		Milk _____

Lunch

#1 Meat _____	#2 Salad _____	#3 Yogurt/
Starch _____	Soup _____	Cott. Cheese _____
Veg. _____	Bread/Roll _____	Fruit/Veg. _____
Fruit/Dess. _____	Bev. _____	Bev. _____
Bev. _____		

Dinner

#1 Meat _____	#2 Salad _____	#3 Yogurt/
Starch _____	Soup _____	Cott. Cheese _____
Veg. _____	Bread/Roll _____	Bread/Roll _____
Fruit/Dess. _____	Bev. _____	Fruit/Veg. _____
Bev. _____		Bev. _____

In-Between Foods

Time of Day	Food	Amount
_____	_____	_____
_____	_____	_____
_____	_____	_____
_____	_____	_____

havioral instruction. One-year results show that 66% of the initial 69 subjects who completed the one-year program maintained the initial 5% reduction in body weight at 52 weeks.[58] "Committed to Kids" now offers professional training instruction in its innovative multidisciplinary approach. While this method shows promise, more long-term follow-up studies are needed before it can be recommended as the standard dietary treatment. Data on those who have left the program and are not attending the maintenance program are essential, as well as tests that measure the psychological aspects of such a restrictive approach. For the time being, this diet may be more prudent to use with children or adolescents who have a serious health risk for which rapid weight reduction is essential. For younger children with a mild to moderate degree of overweight, weight maintenance while growth occurs is a reasonable goal and can be achieved with interventions that include modest reductions in caloric intake.

A diet high in dietary fiber is currently being used in the treatment of obesity. A larger fiber intake produces diets of reduced caloric density that produce a slower rate of food ingestion and increased satiety.[64] From an epidemiological perspective, obesity is rare among populations in developing countries where dietary fiber intake is high.[65] Although empirical data on the association between a low-fiber diet and increased obesity in children is needed, preliminary data from a large-scale longitudinal study of obesity in 9- and 10-year-old children suggests a correlation between a high-carbohydrate diet and a decreased risk of obesity. Since a higher carbohydrate diet usually implies a larger fiber and lower fat content, this association may be significant.[64]

The most sensible approach may be the promotion of increased amounts of fiber-containing foods as a public health policy. This would affect other aspects of children's health including heart disease and cancer prevention and improvements in gastrointestinal function and blood sugar control. Recently the American Health Foundation issued recommendations for dietary fiber intake in children older than two years of age, entitled the "Age Plus Five" program. Based on these recommendations, minimal fiber intake should range from 8 g in younger children to 25 g in older children, representing a significant increase from the present levels of intake.[66] These recommendations seem reasonable and their promotion should be encouraged by all those involved in the health care of children.

The Nondiet Approach

A movement currently in vogue for both adults and children is the "nondiet health enhancing paradigm" formally known as the antidiet approach. Supported by eating disorder specialists and nutritionists in both the United States and Canada, it appears to be gaining momentum through national health policies and congressional conferences.[67] The movement calls for wellness instead of weight loss, taking pleasure in eating rather than restraint, and self-acceptance in place of self-hate. Although controversial, it is important for health professionals to become aware of this approach as there are many aspects that may be useful for clinical practice.

In Canada, eating disorder specialists Janet Polivy and Peter Herman have led the movement for the past 16 years.[68] Canada now has a health policy promoting a broader range of healthy weights and a new program entitled "Vitality" that encourages more realistic weights and attitudes.[67] In addition, there are many popular treatment programs including Polivy's program, "Stop Dieting"[67] and "Teens & Diets: No Weigh," an innovative program for adolescents created by Canadian dietitian Linda Omichinski.[69,70] In the United States, psychologists Susan and Wayne Wooley have championed the movement. Their publications question the appropriateness of behavioral and dietary treatments in the face of evidence that these treatments are ineffective and may be a causal factor in the development of eating disorders.[71]

For the past 15 years there has been great concern about dieting in children starting with the publication of Ellyn Satter's books for parents on child feeding (see Resource List, Appendix 20–A). In her second book, *How to Get Your Child to Eat But Not Too Much,* responsibility is assigned to the child for making food choices. This was a revolutionary concept at the time it was presented and continues to be extensively used. Currently, Satter is promoting a new paradigm for child feeding that entrusts children to self-regulate their food intake.[72] Satter warns professionals that continuing to externally control children's food intake and activity may undermine natural food regulatory mechanisms, resulting in heavier children.

Another important contributor to the nondiet approach with children is Joanne Ikeda. Creator of "The California Model," Ikeda and other nutritionists in California became concerned about the rising number of overweight school-age children and the corresponding increases in eating disorders in this age group.[73] A multidisciplinary training program for child weight treatment was subsequently developed for the California schools; the popular "California Guidelines for Parents of Large Kids" are listed in Exhibit 20–2.

Am I Fat? Helping Young Children Accept Differences in Body Size, a book for health professionals and parents on the topic of size acceptance in younger children, was published in 1992 (see Resource List in Appendix 20–A). Unique features of the book are the encouragement of a "bias-free" school environment that discourages name-calling and the concept of promoting foods with a high nutrient density.

Exercise and Activity Guidelines

The effects of various types of exercise on children's weight have been studied. The different categories are: (1) aerobics: running and swimming; (2) calisthenics: sit-ups; and (3) lifestyle activities: taking stairs and walking. Weight loss and maintenance seem to be associated with programs that incorporate exercise as well as diet and those that promote lifestyle vs structured activities.[74] Research in adults has consistently shown that exercise that requires increased amounts of intensity are associated with lower adherence. Epstein and colleagues have demon-

Exhibit 20–2 California Guidelines for Parents of Large Kids

- Provide the child with lots of love and attention . . . don't pressure the child to lose weight.
- Have regular meals and snacks . . . try to discourage eating at other times.
- Let the child decide how much to eat . . . don't limit the amount of food a child can eat, or make a child "clean" the plate.
- Serve the same healthy food to all family members . . . don't put the child on a special low-calorie diet.
- Have appealing snack foods available like popcorn, frozen fruit juice bars, string cheese, and frozen low-fat yogurt . . . don't have lots of high-fat snack foods like chips, cake, pie, ice cream, cupcakes, and doughnuts.
- Expect the child to grow into his/her weight . . . don't expect the child to lose weight.
- Encourage the child to be more active by playing with toys like balls, frisbees, jump ropes, and bicycles, by joining a sports team, by taking gymnastics, swimming, tennis or other lessons, by walking the family dog, or by joining a 4-H club, Girl Scout, or Boy Scout troop . . . don't let the child spend a lot of time watching TV or playing video games.
- Go on family outings that include hiking, swimming, and going to parks and playgrounds where everyone can play actively . . . don't let your family become "couch potatoes"!

Source: Reprinted with permission from J. Ikeda, Promoting Size Acceptance for Children, in Children and Teens in Weight Crisis, *Healthy Weight Journal* (formerly *Obesity and Health*), F. Berg, ed., Summary Edition, p. 25, © 1996, *Healthy Weight Journal,* 402 S. 14th Street, Hettinger, ND 58639.

---

strated better long-term results with a lifestyle approach in obese children followed for a 10-year period.[75] In addition, reducing access to sedentary activities such as television viewing or computer games has shown some success. Reinforcements also play a role; in a recent study, maintenance of weight and loss of body fat was accomplished after one year when children received rewards for being more active.[76] In general, children have been shown to choose a more vigorous activity when there is more work required to be sedentary. An example of this would be offering the choice of doing chores before television watching is allowed or taking a walk. Thus, making exercise easier and sedentary activities harder to access should be incorporatated into the treatment plan.

The safety of using resistance exercise in children is questioned but is currently under study because of its effectiveness in adult programs.[77,78] Resistance exercise may increase lean body mass, thus inducing an increase in metabolic rate that promotes weight loss and improves body image. A one-year study of 15 preadolescent obese children in a moderate-intensity resistance training and behavioral program has recently reported the absence of accidents or injuries, good compliance, and improved maintenance of weight loss.[79] Thus, further attention should be given to this type of exercise in the weight management of children.

A program tailored to meet individual needs should be the mainstay of any intervention. In general, children in exercise programs that gradually increase strength and endurance experience enhanced skill development and fitness. A comprehensive physical skills assessment is recommended at the initial assessment. Professional supervision is essential with obese children, especially those at larger degrees of overweight. Often physical and coordination problems impair the overweight child's progress in regular structured exercise events. Because sedentary rather than high-energy activities are familiar and preferred among overweight children, individual encouragement and continuing support are needed to elicit participation.[49]

The most successful exercise programs for children incorporate many features. An emphasis on lifestyle and family activities, moderate strength training, and an increase in structured aerobic activities should be included. In the Kids Weight Down program, a behavioral approach is used that focuses on changing family activity patterns.

In addition, children receive incentives for increasing activity and for decreasing sedentary behavior such as television viewing; the child is asked to set goals and enter into a contractual agreeement with parents and staff as is illustrated in Exhibit 20–3. In addition, children receive points that represent rewards on a weekly basis for achieving these goals as is shown in Exhibit 20–4.

Community and population interventions are also important. In a recent Gallup Poll survey, only 28% of children stated that they participated in moderate physical activity at the level recommended in the Healthy People 2000 objectives for American children.[80] Currently only 36% of elementary and secondary schools offer daily physical education classes and less than 50% of these offer active types of events. Parents and health professionals need to promote increased fitness opportunities for children in their communities and schools. One example might be a campaign for more playgrounds or walking trails. In addition, governments must participate in health education efforts at the national level and continue to support initiatives to limit the negative influence of the media on children's health behaviors. A joint commitment from parents, health professionals, and state and federal governments seems essential to prevent further rises of weight in children.

School-Based Programs

The school is a potentially useful intervention site for the prevention and management of pediatric obesity. Since 95% of American children attend school and

Exhibit 20–3 Kids Weight Down Weekly Contract

Week _____

Activity Goal (choose one):

1. I will increase my activity by _____
   _____ times a week for _____ minutes.

   Examples: Walking to school, store, friend's house, riding bike, using exercise machine, doing exercise tape.

OR

2. I will limit my TV watching to _____ minutes each day.

Eating Goal (choose one):

1. I will replace _____ with _____ .
   (Red Light Food)   (Healthier Choice)

   Examples: Eat fruit instead of sweets, pretzels instead of chips, fat-free cheese instead of regular cheese.

OR

2. I will change the amount of food I eat by _____
   _____

   Examples: Taking smaller portions, splitting food with someone, not taking second servings.

OR

3. I will change when I eat by _____
   _____

   Examples: Eating only 3 regular meals, not snacking after dinner.

_____
Child

_____
Parent

therefore eat one or two meals and participate in physical education classes there, schools seem the logical place to implement health education efforts.[81] However, many other factors interfere. Reduced federal and state support and increased expenses prevent most schools from having adequate materials, personnel, or the training required to conduct either school-wide or high-risk obesity programs.[82]

Only a few school-based interventions report positive short-term results from using behavioral strategies and parental involvement.[83] Although significant treatment effects were observed, little is known about the maintenance of results from

Exhibit 20–4 Kids Weight Down Weekly Points System

Action	*Points*
Come to class on time and with records	5
Succeed at ACTIVITY GOAL	5
Succeed at EATING GOAL	5
Weight is same or lower than week before	10
BONUS: Keep eating/activity record for whole week	5

Rules
1. Parent and child will agree on one Activity and one Eating goal for the week.
2. Parents are responsible for monitoring whether kids reach goals.
3. Each week kids can win prizes by earning points:
    25 points = First Prize
    20 points = Second Prize
    15 points = Third Prize
4. Parent and child with most points by end of 10 weeks wins special prize!

Courtesy of Lisa Altshuler, Brooklyn, New York.

these programs. Similar inconclusive results have also been reported for school-based substance abuse programs.[84] School-wide general health education programs show only a slight positive effect on obesity levels in overweight participants. Analyses of specific program components are lacking and the curricula used may be too broad in scope to directly affect the obese child.[82]

School-based programs have potential if they include behavioral strategies. Parent involvement and continuing professional supervision and monitoring are essential components. Lacking the appropriate resources for this type of program, schools might better focus on improving the nutritional content of school meals and increasing the amount and intensity of physical education classes. Although the direct effects of these public health approaches on obesity levels would be difficult to measure, they would surely have an indirect effect.

Surgical and Pharmacological Approaches

Reports of gastric surgery as a treatment for the morbidly obese child or adolescent started to appear in the 1970s.[84,85] Children with medical complications of obesity or those who have failed previously with other treatments are being considered as candidates for this type of surgery.[86,87] To qualify, it is recommended that the child's relative weight is at least 180% of ideal body weight or the body mass index is well above the 95th percentile channel for the child's age.[86] No exact age limits have yet been specified but subjects in most reported studies range from 11 to 20 years of age.[88,89]

Two types of surgery are now available: the vertical banded gastroplasty and the Roux-en-Y gastric bypass.[15] Newer methods with fewer side effects are being used such as the adjustable silicone gastric band.[90] Older procedures produced many negative side effects, which have since been reduced in newer methods. In 1991, gastrointestinal surgery for severe obesity was approved by a NIH Consensus Panel for adults. Children and adolescents were not recommended for surgery as they had not been sufficiently studied.[91]

In adults, substantial weight loss has been reported with good post-surgery maintenance for as long as three years.[92,93] One summary of studies in children shows 80% to 90% maintenance of initial weight loss at three-year follow-up among 50% of patients.[86] Children with Prader-Willi syndrome have also been thought of as particularly good candidates for the surgery because of shortened life expectancy if their obesity is not treated.[94] Clinical results are positive for a small number of these children. However, others have experienced less successful outcomes with these patients.[15]

It is unfortunate that few studies document the psychological effects of radical treatments such as surgery in children and adolescents. Reports from studies of adults show improvements in many psychological measures following surgical intervention.[95] Obviously, this aspect should be more carefully examined in children. Complete psychological and nutritional assessments should be made before and after the procedure. Following the surgery, eating behaviors require close monitoring as excessive intake of high-calorie liquids or of soft foods and overeating result in vomiting, nausea, or the perforation of suture lines.[89,90]

Currently there is a flurry of research in the pharmacological treatment of obesity and new treatments have been recently approved and offered for adults.[96] Children have been infrequently studied, and reports of drug treatment with children are rare. In one experiment, 68 children treated with fenfluramine were studied for one year; results were measured against a placebo-treated group. Although there was greater weight loss and a lower drop-out rate in the drug-supplemented group, half of the subjects lost weight only for the first six months of treatment and then either regained or maintained the same weight in spite of continued drug administration.[97] Clearly, more research is needed before pharmacological agents can be considered a recommended weight management strategy for children.

CONCLUSION

For as long as he can remember, Johnny M. has been overweight. Lately the kids at school have begun teasing him and do not include him in many activities.

He would like to be more active and eat healthier foods but his school only offers physical education classes once a week, and he has to eat a lot of restaurant foods and the high-fat school lunch because his mother works and is unable to prepare healthier foods at home. To make matters worse, his Dad lives far away and cannot help either. What can he do?

Unfortunately, this scenario is typical for a growing number of children in America. Lacking resources or opportunities, children like Johnny continue on a path of increasing inactivity and a calorically dense diet that results in higher degrees of overweight. While it is easy to blame parents for setting poor examples or for carrying "pre-obese" genes, it may be more productive to take a broader view. Failures in many social and economic systems are equally responsible: schools, health care, and communities all play a role.

What can be done? Child and adolescent research in laboratory and practical settings is as essential as the promotion of community action. In addition, more comprehensive, prospective studies are needed. Targeted for study are neuro-endocrine cause-and-effect mechanisms, exercise expenditure among obesity phenotypes, and more long-term studies of the efficacy of specific program components.[98] Overall management issues that need further delineation include designing optimal dietary and activity programs and using effective behavioral, physiological, and pharmacological methods of weight control.

Clinic- and family-based programs that have proven to be effective must continue to be supported. In addition, intervention at earlier and critical ages in the life cycle is important. Dietary methods that are too restrictive or are insufficiently tested require caution, and behavioral approaches to changing eating and exercise patterns should command the health worker's primary attention.

REFERENCES

1. Gortmaker SL, Dietz WH, Sobol AM, Wehler CA. Increasing pediatric obesity in the United States. *Am J Dis Child.* 1987; 141:535–540.

2. Kuczmarski RJ. Trends in body composition for infants and children in the US. *Crit Rev Food Sci Nutr.* 1993;33:375–387.

3. Troiano RP, Flegal MK, Kuczmarski RJ, et al. Overweight prevalence and trends for children and adolescents. *Arch Pediatr Adolesc Med.* 1995;149:1085–1091.

4. Dietz WH, Robinson TN. Assessment and treatment of childhood obesity. *Pediatr Rev.* 1993;14:337–344.

5. Berenson GS, Sathanur R, Shrinivasan SR, et al. Obesity and cardiovascular risk in children. *Ann NY Acad Sci.* 1993;699:93–103.

6. Must A, Jaques PF, Dallal GE, et al. Long-term morbidity and mortality of overweight adolescents. *N Engl J Med.* 1992;327:1350–1355.

7. Hirsch J. Obesity prevention initiative. *Obes Res.* 1994;2:569–586.

8. Caprio S, Hyman LD, Mac Carthy S, et al. Fat distribution and cardiovascular risk factors in obese adolescents: importance of the intra-abdominal fat depot. *Am J Clin Nutr.* 1996;64:12–17.

9. Must A. Morbidity and mortality associated with elevated body weight in children and adolescents. *Am J Clin Nutr.* 1996;63:445S–447S.

10. Staffieri JR. A study of social stereotypes of body image in children. *J Pers Soc Psy.* 1967;7:101–104.

11. Stunkard A, Burt V. Obesity and body image: II. Age at onset of disturbances in the body image. *Am J Psychiatry.* 1967;123:1443–1447.

12. Gortmaker SL, Must A, Perrin JM, et al. Social and economic consequences of overweight in adolescence and young adulthood. *N Engl J Med.* 1993;329:1008–1012.

13. Bouchard C, Perusse L. Genetic aspects of obesity. *Ann NY Acad Sci.* 1993;699:26–35.

14. Sorensen TIA, Holst C, Stunkard A. Child body mass index—genetic and environmental influences assessed in a longitudinal adoption study. *Int J Obes.* 1992;16:705–714.

15. Dietz WH. Therapeutic strategies in childhood obesity. *Horm Res.* 993;3:86–90.

16. Wabitsch M, Hauner H, Heinz E, et al. Body-fat distribution and changes in the atherogenic risk-factor profile in obese adolescent girls during weight reduction. *Am J Clin Nutr.* 1994;60:54–60.

17. Dietz WH. Critical periods in childhood for the development of obesity. *Am J Clin Nutr.* 1994;59:955–959.

18. Allison DB, Paultre F, Heymsfield SB, Pi-Sunyer FX. Is the intra-uterine period really a critical period for the development of adiposity? *Int J Obes.* 1995;19:397–402.

19. Alaimo K, McDowell MA, Briefel RR, et al. Energy and macronutrient intakes of persons ages 2 months and over in the United States: third national health and nutrition examination survey, phase 1, 1988–91. *NCHS Advance Data.* 1994; 255.

20. Bandini L, Schoeller DA, Cyr HN, Dietz WH. Validity of reported energy intake in obese and nonobese adolescents. *Am J Clin Nutr.* 1990;52:421–425.

21. Heath GW, Pratt M, Warren CW, Kann L. Physical activity patterns in American high school students. *Arch Pediatr Adolesc Med.* 1994;148:1131–1136.

22. Klesges RC, Shelton ML. Effects of television on metabolic rates: potential implications for childhood obesity. *Pediatrics.* 1993;91:281–286.

23. Dietz WH, Bardoni LG, Morelli JA, et al. Effects of sedentary activities on resting metabolic rate. *Am J Clin Nutr.* 1994;59:556–559.

24. Goran MI, Figueroa R, Mc Gloin A, et al. Obesity in children: recent advances in energy metabolism and body composition. *Obes Res.* 1995;3:277–289.

25. Charney E, Goodman HZ, Mac Guide M, et al. Childhood antecedents of adult obesity: do chubby infants become obese adults? *N Engl J Med.* 1976;295:86–89.

26. Roberts SB, Savage J, Coward WA, et al. Energy expenditure and intake in infants born to lean and overweight mothers. *N Engl J Med.* 1988;318:461–466.

27. Klesges RC, Klesges LM, Eck LH, Shelton ML. A longitudinal analysis of accelerated weight gain in preschool children. *Pediatrics.* 1995;95:126–132.

28. Hamil PV, Drizd TA, Johnson CL, et al. Physical growth: National Center for Health Statistics percentiles. *Am J Clin Nutr.* 1979;32:607–629.

29. Hammer LD, Kraemer HC, Wilson DM, et al. Standarized percentile curves of body-mass index for children and adolescents. *Am J Dis Child.* 1991;145:259–263.

30. Must A, Dallal GE, Dietz WH. Reference data for obesity: 85th and 95th percentiles of body mass index (wt/ht^2) and triceps skinfold thickness. *Am J Clin Nutr.* 1991;53:839–846.

31. Alemzadeh R, Lifshitz F. Childhood obesity. In: Lifshitz F, ed. *Pediatric Endocrinology.* 3rd ed. New York: Marcel Dekker; 1996:753–774.

32. Dietz WH. Critical periods in childhood for the development of obesity. *Am J Clin Nutr.* 1994;59:955–959.

33. Pugliese M, Recker B, Lifshitz F. A survey to determine the prevalence of abnormal growth patterns in adolescence. *J Adolesc Health Care.* 1988;9:181–187.

34. Hamil PVV, Drizd TA, Johnson CL, et al. Physical growth: National Center for Health Statistics percentiles. *Am J Clin Nutr.* 1979;32:607–629.

35. Dietz WH. Childhood obesity. In: Suskind RM, ed. *Textbook of Pediatric Nutrition, Second Edition.* New York: Raven Press; 1993:279–293.

36. Lifshitz F, Cervantes CD. Short stature. In: Lifshitz F, ed. *Pediatric Endocrinology.* 3rd ed. New York: Marcel Dekker; 1996:1–18.

37. Tanner JM, Whitehouse RH, Marubini E, Resele L. The adolescent growth spurt of the boys and girls of the Harpenden Growth Study. *Ann Hum Biol.* 1976;3:109–126.

38. Lowe MR, Kopyt D, Buchwald J. Food intake underestimation: its nature and potential impact on obesity treatment. *Behav Ther.* 1995;19:17–20.

39. Goran MI. Methods of assessment of energy requirements. *Nutr Res.* 1995;15:115–150.

40. Valoski A, Epstein LH. Nutrient intake of obese children in a family-based behavioral weight control program. *Int J Obes.* 1990;14:667–677.

41. Krebs-Smith SM. Fruit and vegetable intakes of children and adolescents in the United States. *Arch Pediatr Adolesc Med.* 1996;150:81–86.

42. Subar AS, Heimendinger J, Krebs-Smith SM, et al. *5 a Day for Better Health: A Baseline Study of America's Fruit and Vegetable Consumption.* Rockville, MD: National Cancer Institute; 1992.

43. Caprio S, Hyman LD, Mc Carthy S, et al. Fat distribution and cardiovascular risk factors in obese adolescents; importance of the intra-abdominal fat depot. *Am J Clin Nutr.* 1996;64:12–17.

44. Himes JH, Dietz WH. Guidelines for overweight in adolescent preventive services: recommendations from an expert committee. *Am J Clin Nutr.* 1994;59:307–316.

45. Baranowski T. Validity and reliability of self-report measures of physical activity: an information processing perspective. *Res Q Exerc Sport.* 1988;59:314–327.

46. Sallis JF, Condon SA, Goggin KJ, et al. The development of self-administered physical activity surveys for 4th grade students. *Res Q Exerc Sport.* 1993;84:25–31.

47. Mellin L. *The Certificate of Advanced Clinical Training in Child and Adolescent Obesity Course Syllabus and Self-Assessment.* San Francisco: University of California; 1991.

48. Sothern M. *Committed to Kids Weight Managment Program Research Protocol.* Presented at the Committed to Kids Weight Management Training Program, New Orleans, LA; 1996.

49. Epstein LH. Exercise in the treatment of childhood obesity. *Int J Obes.* 1995;19:117–121.

50. Goran MI, Kaskoun MC, Carpenter WH. Estimating body composition of young children by using bioelectrical resistance. *Am Physiol Soc.* 1993:1776–1780.

51. Slaughter MH. Skinfold equations for estimation of body fatness in children and youth. *Hum Biol.* 1988;60:709–723.

52. Heyward VH, Stolarczyk LM. *Applied Body Composition Assessment.* Champaign, IL: Human Kinetics; 1996.

53. Altshuler L, Adesman A. Behavioral and developmental factors in atherosclerosis prevention. In: Jacob M, ed. *Atherosclerosis Prevention. Monographs in Clinical Pediatrics #4.* Philadelphia: Harwood Academic Pub; 1991:135–152.

54. Stunkard A. Diet, exercise and behavior therapy: a cautionary tale. *Obes Res.* 1996;4:293–294.

55. Epstein LH, Valoski A, Wing RR, McCurley J. Ten-year follow-up of behavioral, family-based treatment for obese children. *JAMA.* 1990;264:2519–2523.

56. Figueroa-Colon R, Franklin FA, Lee JY, et al. Feasibility of a clinic-based hypocaloric dietary intervention implemented in a school setting for obese children. *Obes Res.* 1996;4:419–429.

57. Cooperman N, Haast T, Skenker R. Adolescent obesity and cardiovascular risk: a rational approach to management. *Ann NY Acad Sci.* 1993;699:220–230.

58. Suskind RM, Sothern MS, Farris RP, et al. Recent advances in the treatment of childhood obesity. *Ann NY Acad Sci.* 1993;699:181–199.

59. Fisher JO, Birch LL. Fat preferences and consumption of 3- to 5-year-old children are related to parental adiposity. *J Am Diet Assoc.* 1995;95:759–764.

60. Eck LH, Klesges RC, Hanson CL, Slawson D. Children at familial risk for obesity: an examination of dietary intake, physical activity and weight status. *Int J Obes.* 1992;16:71–78.

61. Von Nguyen T, Larson DE, Johnson RK, Goran MI. Fat intake and adiposity in children of lean and obese parents. *Am J Clin Nutr.* 1996;63:507–513.

62. Johnson SL, Birch LL. Parent's and children's adiposity and eating style. *Pediatrics.* 1994;94:653–661.

63. Figueroa-Colon R, Von Almen TK, et al. Comparison of two hypocaloric diets in obese children. *AJDC.* 1993;147:160–166.

64. Kimm SY. The role of fiber in the development and treatment of childhood obesity. *Pediatrics.* 1995;96:1010–1013.

65. Kimm SY. The role of fiber in the development and treatment of childhood obesity. *Pediatrics.* 1995;96:1010–1013.

66. Williams CL, Bollella M, Wynder EL. A new recommendation for dietary fiber in childhood. *Pediatrics.* 1995;96:985–987.

67. Berg FM. Nondiet movement gains strength. *Obesity Health.* 1992;6:85–90.

68. Polivy J. Psychological consequences of food restriction. *J Am Diet Assoc.* 1996;96:589–594.

69. Omichinski L. Teens & Diets: No Weigh. *Healthy Weight J.* 1996;10:49–52.

70. Omichinski L, Harrison KR. Reduction of dieting attitudes and practices after participation in a non-diet lifestyle program. *J Can Diet Assoc.* 1995;56:81–85.

71. Garner DM. Confronting the failure of behavioral and dietary treatment for obesity. *Clin Psychol.* 1991;11:729–780.

72. Satter E. The new paradigm of trust. *Healthy Weight J.* 1995;9:110–111.

73. Ikeda JP. Impacting on pediatric obesity. *Ann NY Acad Sci.* 1993;699:273–274.

74. Epstein LH, Wing RR, Penner BC, Kress MJ. Effect of diet and controlled exercise on weight loss in obese children. *J Pediatr.* 1985;107:358–361.

75. Epstein LH. Methodological issues and ten-year outcomes for obese children. *Ann NY Acad Sci.* 1993;699:237–249.

76. Epstein LH. Effects of decreasing sedentary behavior and increasing activity on weight change in obese children. *Health Psychol.* 1995;1402:109–115.

77. *Guidelines for Exercise Testing and Prescription.* Philadelphia: American College of Sports Medicine; 1995.

78. Metcalf JA, Roberts SO. Strength training and the immature athlete: an overview. *Pediatr Nurs.* 1993;19:325–332.

79. Sothern M, Ewing T, Loftin M, et al. Resistance training in obese preadolescent children. *Exp Biol.* In review.

80. Borra ST, Schwartz NE, Spain CG, Natchiposky MM. Food, physical activity, and fun: inspiring America's kids to more beautiful lifestyles. *ADA Rep.* 1995;95:816–818.

81. Kanders BS. Pediatric obesity. In: Thomas P, ed. *Weighing the Options.* Washington, DC: National Academy Press; 1995:210–233.

82. Resnicow K. School-based obesity prevention: population versus high-risk interventions. *Ann NY Acad Sci.* 1993;699:154–166.

83. Murray DM, Pirie P, Luepker V, et al. Five and six year follow-up results from four seventh grade smoking prevention strategies. *J Behav Med.* 1989;12:207–218.

84. Rigg CA. Jejunoileal bypass for morbidly obese adolescents. *Acta Pediatr Scand (suppl).* 1975;256:62–63.

85. Soper RT, Mason EE, Printen KJ, Zellweger H. Gastric bypass for morbid obesity in children and adolescents. *J Pediatr Surg.* 1975;10:51–58.

86. Figueroa R, Spear B. *Etiology, Prevention, Diagnosis and Management of Obesity in Childhood and Adolescence.* Paper presented at the meeting Nutrition for Infants, Children and Adolescents. Birmingham, AL, February 1995.

87. Dietz WH. *Diet and Behavioral Strategies in Treating Childhood Obesity.* Paper presented at the meeting of the North American Association for the Study of Obesity, New Orleans, LA, October 1995.

88. Soper RT, Lewis JW. The morbidly obese young patient. In: Printen K, Griffin WA, eds. *Surgical Management of Morbid Obesity.* New York: Marcel Dekker; 1987:275–286.

89. Rand CSW, MacGregor AM. Adolescents having obesity surgery. *Southern Med J.* 1994;87:1208–1213.

90. Busetto L, Valente P, Pisent C, et al. Eating pattern in the first year following adjustable silicone gastric banding (ASGB) for morbid obesity. *Int J Obes.* 1996;20:539–546.

91. National Institutes of Health. Gastrointestinal surgery for severe obesity. *Ann Intern Med.* 1991; 115:956–961.

92. Brolin RE. Critical analysis of results: weight loss and quality of data. *Am J Clin Nutr.* 1992; 55:577S–581S.

93. Mason EE. Gastric surgery for morbid obesity. *Surg Clin N Am.* 1992;72:501–513.

94. Anderson AE, Soper RT, Scott DH. Gastric bypass for morbid obesity in children and adolescents. *J Pediatr Surg.* 1980;15:876–881.

95. Stunkard AJ, Wadden TA. Psychological aspects of severe obesity. *Am J Clin Nutr.* 1992;55:524S–532S.

96. Fixer N. Dexfenfluramine for weight maintenance. *Am J Clin Nutr.* 1992;56:1955–1985.

97. Pedrinola F, Cavaliere H, Lima N, Medeiros-Neto G. Is DL-Fenfluramine a potentially helpful drug therapy in overweight adolescent subjects? *Obes Res.* 1994;2:1–4.

98. Ikeda JP, Sigman-Grant M. NIH conference deals with children. *Healthy Weight J.* 1995;2:106–107.

Appendix 20–A

The Nondiet Approach Resource List

Good News for Big Kids. National Association to Advance Fat Acceptance. Pamphlet. NAAFA, 1900 K. St., #110, Sacramento, CA 95184 (1-800-422-1214; 916-558-6880; Fax: 916-558-6881).

Am I Fat? Helping Young Children Accept Differences in Body Size, by Joanne Ikeda, MA, and Priscilla Naworski, MS, CHES. 1992, softcover, 110 pages, $14.95. ETR Associates, PO Box 1830, Santa Cruz, CA 95061-1880.

If My Child Is Too Fat, What Should I Do About It? Booklet for parents by Joanne Ikeda, $1.50 each.

Children and Weight: What's a Parent to Do? and **Family Choices for Good Health.** Low-literacy booklets for parents by Joanne Ikeda and Rita Mitchell, $1.50 each. ANR Publications, University of California, 6701 San Pablo Ave., Oakland, CA 94608 (415-642-2431).

Children and Weight: What's a Parent to Do? 12-minute videotape, includes sample parent books. English and Spanish. $35. Visual Media, 1441 Research Park Drive, University of California, Davis, CA 95616.

How You Get Your Kid to Eat—But Not Too Much, by Ellyn Satter. Birth through adolescence, 1987, softcover, 396 pages, $14.95. Bull Publishing, Box 208, Palo Alto, CA 94302 (415-322-2855).

Child of Mine—Feeding with Love and Good Sense, by Ellyn Satter. Pregnancy through toddler stage, 1983, softcover, $14.95. Bull Publishing, Box 208, Palo Alto, CA 94302 (415-322-2855).

Feeding with Love and Good Sense, by Ellen Satter. Series of four 15-minutes videotapes about the feeding relationship for the infant, older baby, toddler, and the preschooler. $54.95 each, set of four tape, $164.95. Ellyn Satter Associates.

Feeding with Love and Good Sense Training Manual, 103 pages, $75.00, includes rights to reproduce teaching materials.

Ellyn Satter's Vision workshop, $375 reg. fee. Ellen Satter Assoc., 4226 Mandan Crescent, Madison, WI 53711 (1-800-808-7976; Fax 608-271-7976).

Teens & Diet—No Weigh: Building the Road to Healthier Living. A HUGS for Teens program franchised to licensed health professionals, by Linda Omichinski, RD. Eight lesson plans, scripts, and resources. Supported with Tailoring Your Taste, teen journal, parent guide handbook, 1995. HUGS International, Box 102A, RR3, Portage la Prairie, Manitoba, Canada R1N3A3 (204-428-3432; 1-800-565-4847; Fax: 204-428-5072).

Validity Leader's Kit. Contains Vitality health promotion materials that emphasize a fundamental shift from treatment to prevention of weight problems including overweight, underweight, eating disorders, weight preoccupation and negative body image, 1994. Health Services and Promotion, Health and Welfare Canada, 4th floor, Jeanne Mance Bldg., Ottawa, Ontario, Canada K14 1B4 (613-957-8331; Fax 613-941-2399).

Children and Teens in Weight Crisis, 3rd ed., by Frances M. Berg, 1955, softcover, Healthy Weight Journal, 402 South 14th Street, Hettinger, ND 58639 (701-567-2646; Fax 701-567-2602).

CHAPTER 21

Regulating the Weight Management Industry: Standards for Evaluating Weight Management Programs and Treatment Methods

Lori J. Silverstein
Sachiko T. St. Jeor

INTRODUCTION

The 1990s have been labeled the "Antidieting Decade,"[1] and much has been written about body weight acceptance and weight loss without dieting.[2] During this decade health workers have witnessed the decline of liquid fasting, a renewal of pharmacotherapy for obesity, and the development of a fat acceptance movement. Although it is still too early to sort out the events that will exert truly significant effects on the field of weight management, this tumultuous decade has also signaled the beginnings of regulation of commercial weight management.

One of the factors influencing the "antidieting" movement is that progress in obesity treatment has been slow. Professional treatment programs have limited success, and most experience extremely high rates of recidivism. On average, losses do not exceed 0.4 to 0.5 kg/wk; 15- to 20-week behavioral programs achieve only 8.5 kg losses; one third of the weight lost is regained within one year following treatment; and all of the weight lost is regained within five years in most individuals.[3] Little hard evidence exists to show the success of commercial and self-help weight loss programs and products[4] but this $2 billion industry flourishes. The limitations of current treatment are reflected in the National Health and Nutrition Examination Survey (NHANES) III data, which indicated that in the decade between surveys performed in 1976–1980 and 1988–1991, the prevalence of overweight increased 8%.[5]

In spite of the limitations of treatment and the antidieting movement, Americans continue to seek treatment from commercial and clinical providers, in part because of increasing evidence of the detrimental relationship of even small amounts of overweight to mortality.[6] Currently, 62% of men and 71% of women are dieting and these dieters include individuals who are underweight or normal weight as well as overweight.[7] Clearly, Americans are preoccupied with their weight and professionals are challenged to develop more effective treatment strategies that will maintain long-term health.

The medical community has been cautious in moving to models of weight loss requiring greater medical management, increased risk to the patient, and greater expense. The difficulties of dealing with weight management issues,[8] the feeling that weight gain is a personal moral failing[8,9] rather than a medical issue, and the development of a "weight loss industry" may have inhibited the progression of medical treatment for obesity. Surveys have shown that most individuals attempt to treat themselves and only a few (approximately 5% to 13% of the dieting population) seek professional advice or help through medical clinics.[7]

Recognition of the difficulty of managing obesity and its consequences has engendered many conferences, position papers, and reports and development of guidelines[10–18] pertaining to the evaluation and treatment of obesity and establishment of healthy weights and healthier-weight goals.[13,15–17] Table 21–1 summarizes conferences and position and guideline papers. The most significant of these to medical and commercial weight loss concerns is the *Weighing the Options*[10] (WTO) report from the National Academy of Sciences, which makes recommendations for clear criteria to evaluate approaches to preventing and treating obesity. The following section summarizes WTO and the salient points related to classifying, evaluating, and applying criteria to weight management programs.

WEIGHING THE OPTIONS

The Food and Nutrition Board of the Institute of Medicine, National Academy of Sciences, felt compelled for many years to develop criteria that could be used to evaluate options for treatment of obesity and overweight. Finally, in 1994, the National Academy of Sciences provided money for a one-year study with the following objectives[10(ppvii–viii)]: (1) identify direct measurements of outcomes of obesity treatment and prevention programs and their priorities and special uses; (2) identify program characteristics that should be specified and measured; (3) identify appropriate uses of direct measurements of outcomes of large-scale weight loss programs; (4) identify characteristics that contribute to clients' choices of programs and their outcomes with these programs; (5) identify the degree of weight loss needed to improve

Table 21–1 Summary of Assessment Conferences, Position Papers, and Guidelines Pertaining to Obesity Treatment

Agency	Source	Year	Summary
American Health Foundation	Report on the American Health Foundation Roundtable on Healthy Weight (Meisler JG, St. Jeor S.T. *Am J Clin Nutr.* 1996;63(suppl): 474S–477S)	1996	The Expert Panel on Healthy Weight was convened to define "healthy weight" and address the role of weight in fostering well-being and prevention of disease. The panel findings are as follows: • Overweight is epidemic in the United States • Most weight-related diseases are preventable • Action is needed to reduce health problems related to excess weight • A healthy weight below a body mass index (BMI) of 25 is recommended for adults • Adopt a healthy diet (fat, 25% of calories per day; fiber, 25 grams per day; no excess calories, particularly from sweets and alcohol); engage in regular physical activity • If you are above the Healthy Weight target, first try to achieve a healthier weight, which would be a reduction of up to 2 BMI units • If you have difficulty losing weight, maintain your current weight
United States Dept. of Agriculture/ Dept. of Health and Human Services	Dietary Guidelines	1995	Message emphasizes weight maintenance. No ranges are given but a chart illustrates weight according to risk. New guideline states "Balance what you eat with physical activity. Maintain or improve your weight." The following recommendations are made to individuals who need to lose weight: • Eat less fat and control portion sizes • If you are not physically active, be more active throughout the day; maintain activity for 30 min most days of the week • A safe rate of weight loss is 1/2 to 1 lb per week

continues

NAASO	The NAASO Position Paper on Approval and Use of Drugs to Treat Obesity (*Obes Res.* 1995;3:473–478)	1995	The panel answered questions on the use of drug therapy for treatment of obesity and summarized as follows: • As little as a 10% loss of initial body weight is medically significant • Drugs should be considered effective if they aid in weight losses and maintenance of 5% to 10% • Candidates with central obesity may be considered at lower BMI • A drug that reduced comorbidities with or without weight loss would be considered valuable • Further studies are needed on safety of long-term use • If drug helps continued maintenance, it should be considered effective • Individuals appropriate for drug therapy include those with significant health risk from obesity, with comorbidities, those requiring surgery whose weight places them at high risk, those for whom weight loss attempts have been unsuccessful but are at increased risk because of their obesity • Drug therapy should always be an adjunct to diet, exercise, and behavior modification
American College of Sports Medicine and Centers for Disease Control	Physical Activity and Public Health: A recommendation from the Centers for Disease Control and Prevention and the American College of Sports Medicine (*JAMA.* 1995;273:402–407)	1995	A concise public health message was developed and presented: • "Every US adult should accumulate 30 min or more of moderate-intensity physical activity on most, preferably all, days of the week."

Table 21–1 continued

Agency	Source	Year	Summary
AIN	Healthy Weight Guidelines—Report of the American Institute of Nutrition (AIN) Steering Committee on Healthy Weight (*J Nutr.* 1994;124:2240–2243)	1994	The major objective was to develop weight goals for healthy adults, age 21 and older, and provide a guideline for maintaining healthy level of body fat throughout the lifetime for primary prevention of obesity and obesity-related complications. • Committee preferred BMI criterion of 18 to 25 kg/m^2 with additional ranges of risk.
NIH	Voluntary Methods of Weight Loss and Control—NIH Technology Assessment Conference Panel (*Ann Intern Med.* 1993;119:764–770)	1993	Recommends principles that should be used to select a personal weight loss and control strategy. The fundamental principle is a lifetime commitment to changing lifestyle, behavioral responses, and dietary practices necessary to lose and maintain weight loss. The following guidelines are provided to aid in evaluation of weight loss programs: Information needed to evaluate a method or program • Percentage of all beginning participants who complete the program • Percentage of those completing the program who achieve weight loss • Proportion of weight loss that is maintained at 1, 3, and 5 years • Percentage of participants who experienced adverse medical or psychological effects and the kind and severity of these effects Additional information on program that should be obtained: • Relative mix of diet, exercise, and behavior modification • Amount and kind of counseling • Availability of multidisciplinary expertise • Training provided for relapse prevention • Nature and duration of maintenance phase • Flexibility of food choices and whether weight goals are set unilaterally or cooperatively with the program director

NIH	1992	Gastrointestinal Surgery for Severe Obesity: National Institute of Health Consensus Development Conference Statement (*Am J Clin Nutr*. 1992;55:615S–619S)	Panel recommended the following: • Patients seeking therapy for severe obesity for the first time should not be considered as surgical candidates • Gastric restriction or bypass could be considered for well-informed and motivated patients with acceptable operative risks • Candidates should be selected carefully with a multidisciplinary team evaluation, including medical, surgical, psychiatric, and nutritional expertise • Operation should be performed by surgeon with experience and in a clinical setting with adequate support for all aspects of management and assessment • Lifelong medical surveillance after surgical therapy necessary
Council on Scientific Affairs	1988	Treatment of Obesity in Adults (*JAMA*. 1988;260:2547–2551)	• Recommendations included height, weight, and skinfold measurements in clinical practice; definition of obesity as >20% of ideal body weight (IBW) from 1983 Metropolitan Life charts; develop concern with weight control early in life to prevent obesity; establish realistic weight goals • Specific recommendations were made with regard to diets, activity, behavior modification • Recommended the following criteria for evaluating a commercial program: First be evaluated by your physician Treatment should be preceded by medical and behavioral assessment The degree of obesity should be determined The treatment program should be long enough to effect changes in the patient's lifestyle Outcomes are the most important consideration

continues

Table 21–1 continued

Agency	Source	Year	Summary
International Congress of Obesity	Report to the International Congress on Obesity. Recommended therapeutic guidelines for professional weight control programs (Weinsier et al. *Am J Clin Nutr.* 1984;40:865–872)	1984	As early as 1984, professionals were calling for guidelines for weight control programs. The International Congress on Obesity recommended guidelines for diet, exercise, and behavioral therapy. • Diet: based on a sound scientific rationale; safe and nutritionally adequate; rate of weight loss of 1% body weight per week is appropriate; be practical and effective for the long term • Exercise: should promote increased energy expenditure; promote fat loss and maintenance of lean body mass; be safe for the individual; promote permanent increase in activity level within an individual's lifestyle; specific recommendations: 3 to 5 days/wk; 60% to 85% of maximum heart rate (HR); minimum 30 min; continuous aerobic activity; duration of program 15 to 20 weeks • Behavioral and psychological therapy: pretreat psychosocial problems; include therapeutic modalities for weight loss including self-monitoring, stimulus control, restraint and disinhibition, cognitive restructuring, psychosocial intervention in assertion training, and couples or family support

various health outcomes; and (6) develop a specific agenda for research where information concerning these topics is limited. The committee formed consisted of 10 researchers, all leaders in obesity research and management. The report was prepared for a large audience of professionals in the field of weight management and public health. The need for a book for the general public dealing with obesity and health was noted, as WTO is aimed at professionals.

Classifying Treatment Programs

Weighing the Options[10] classifies weight loss programs into three categories: do-it-yourself, nonclinical, and clinical (Table 21–2). Programs were also classified broadly by five treatment approaches: the calorie level of the diet portion and the inclusion or exclusion of formulated supplements; the presence or lack of behavioral therapy; the inclusion of behavioral and educational emphases on exercise; the adjunctive use of drugs; and surgical intervention. Table 21–3 summarizes different treatment components and recommendations for their application.

Program Components

Weighing the Options recommends that all treatment programs include attention to diet, physical activity, and behavior modification and that they incorporate improved outcome measures.

Balanced-Deficit Diet

These diets provide 1200 or more calories per day and meet the recommended dietary allowance (RDA) and minimum food group servings.[10(p81)] These diets do not require medical supervision unless an individual is under medical management for conditions that may be affected by weight loss.

Low-Calorie Diet

These diets provide 800 to 1200 calories per day and may use regular or prepackaged foods. Many commercial weight loss concerns utilize low-calorie diets and include fortified and formulated foods. Individuals may also follow low-calorie diets on their own, utilizing over-the-counter meal replacements and supplements available from the supermarket. These programs advise replacing one or more meals per day with the supplement but maintaining a minimum of one meal from regular food per day. Commercial programs providing low-calorie diets include Weight Watchers, Diet Workshop, Nutri/System, and Jenny Craig. Also, over-the-counter-products that tout programs with calorie levels in the 800 to 1200 range include Nestle's Sweet Success and Slim Fast. Low-calorie diets are safe for most individuals but for persons with comorbid conditions, dehydration, ketosis, and changes in medication requirements may necessitate physician supervision.

Table 21–2 Classification of Weight Loss Programs

Program Type	Program Specifics
Do-it-yourself	• Personally formulated low-calorie program • Guidance from published material (books, magazines) • Commercial products, diet aids, low-calorie foods, meal replacements • Group counseling • Community-based and worksite programs
Nonclinical	Commercial weight loss programs • Frequently franchised • May or may not be managed by licensed and/or qualified health care personnel
Clinical	Services provided by licensed professional • Working alone • Working in a multidisciplinary group Services may vary and include: • Very-low-calorie diet, behavior therapy, exercise, medical monitoring, nutrition counseling, psychological counseling, etc.

Source: Adapted with permission from *Weighing the Options: Criteria For Evaluating Weight Management Programs.* Copyright 1995 by the National Academy of Sciences. Courtesy of the National Academy Press, Washington, D.C.

Very-Low-Calorie Diet

Very-low-calorie diets provide less than 800 kcal/day and may be as low as 400 kcal/day. These modified fasts replace food with specially formulated supplements designed to minimize protein loss. Some programs are designed to place the patient into ketosis while others try to avoid ketosis by providing adequate carbohydrate.[19] Commercial programs include Medifast, Optifast, Health Management Resources, and New Direction. Very-low-calorie diets require medical supervision and, generally, a multidisciplinary team approach including dietitians, physicians, behaviorists, exercise physiologists, and nurses. Participation is usually limited to individuals with moderate to severe obesity or with comorbid states. Expected weight losses are much greater than with low-calorie diets (20 kg over 12 weeks vs 8.5 kg over 12 weeks).[10(p82)] These programs are expensive and most patients regain weight within five years.

Physical Activity

Physical activity is a frequently mentioned but seldom integral part of most programs. *Weighing the Options* recommends systematically planned and inte-

Table 21-3 Approaches to Treatment*

Strategy	Description	Assessment
1. Balanced-deficit diets	1200+ kcal/day usually nutritionally adequate. Average weight loss 0.25 kg/wk for every −500 kcal/day deficit.	Require little supervision for healthy individuals without underlying medical conditions. Group support and monitoring by a health care professional have been shown to yield better results.
2. Low-calorie diets	800 to 1200 kcal/day. Use regular foods, specially formulated or fortified products, and/or prepackaged foods; may require vitamin/mineral supplementation. Average weight loss of 0.5 to 1.5 kg/wk (8.5 kg over 20 weeks); most regain weight lost in 5 years.	Safe but need physician approval and supervision by a health care provider (especially for patients with comorbid conditions).
3. Very-low-calorie diets	<800 kcal/day = modified fast; replace usual food with supplements; based in hospitals or clinics; supply 45 to 100 g HBV protein (0.8 to 1.5 mg/kg % IBM), 100 g CHO minimum fat for EFA and RDAs of vitamins, minerals, and electrolytes. Average weight loss of 20 kg over 12 weeks, most regain weight lost in 5 years.	Medically supervised and administered by a multidisciplinary team. BMI >30 (moderate to severe obesity) who have failed at other Rx; may also be appropriate for BMI 27 to 30 who have comorbid conditions. Usually prescribed for 12 to 16 weeks; improvements noted in glycemic control, blood pressure, and cholesterol in approximately 3 weeks.
4. Pharmacotherapy (used in conjunction with calorie restriction, behavior modification, and increased activity/exercise)	Current recommendations include *phentermine*, a catecholaminergic agent (15 mg Ionamin) for appetite and *fenfluramine*, a serotonin agonist (20 mg Pondimin) for satiety. Weight loss averaged 0.23 kg/wk compared to placebo. Weight losses level off after 6 months; drugs help to maintain lower body weight.	Not all individuals respond to drug therapy; in some individuals when medication is discontinued, weight is regained. BMI of 30 or greater, patients who are medically at risk because of their comorbid conditions.

continues

Table 21-3 continued

Strategy	Description	Assessment
5. Gastric surgery (long-term commitment and follow-up; attention to diet, behavior modification, and activity/exercise)	Vertical banded gastroplasty Roux-en-Y gastric bypass Substantial weight losses occur within 12 months with some of the weight regained within 2 to 5 years. (Amount of weight loss is directly proportional to the degree of obesity—average of 50% of excess weight lost.) Estimates of 10% morbidity (leakage, stomal obstruction, marginal ulceration, anemia, neurological complications) and <1% mortality have been associated with gastric restrictive surgery.	Significant improvement in comorbid conditions. Risks include micronutrient deficiencies, "dumping syndrome," vomiting, and late postoperative depression. Patients who have failed with nonsurgical measures, who are well informed and motivated. BMI >40 (severe obesity) BMI 35 to 40 with high-risk comorbid conditions and/or physical problems.

*All approaches should include attention to diet, activity/exercise, and behavior modification for long term lifestyle changes. *Source:* Adapted from *Weighing the Options: Criteria For Evaluating Weight-Management Programs.* Copyright 1995 by the National Academy of Sciences. Courtesy of the National Academy Press, Washington, D.C.

grated physical activity intervention to increase energy expenditure and improve metabolic condition.[10(p83)] Current guidelines recommend 30 minutes of moderate activity daily.[18]

Behavior Modification

All obesity treatment programs should include behavior modification. The six major principles typically covered include self-monitoring, stimulus control, contingency management, stress management, cognitive-behavioral strategies, and social support. Behavioral principles are designed to improve patient adherence to healthy diet and exercise patterns.

Drug Therapy

Drug therapy for the treatment of obesity may be safe and appropriate for some people if used as an adjunct to diet, behavior modification, and exercise. It is unclear whether antiobesity drugs have been held to an unreasonable standard by medical and government bodies. *Weighing the Options* compares obesity as a disease to diabetes and hypertension and suggests that treatment options include drug therapy for longer than six months,[10(p84)] but few studies have examined this. Like any treatment involving increased complications, drugs should be considered for patients at greatest risk from their obesity, such as those with comorbidities and BMI greater than 30.[10(p88)]

Gastric Surgery

Vertical banded gastroplasty and Roux-en-Y gastric bypass are the two procedures currently approved for use. Gastric bypass produces greater long-term weight loss but has more complications than gastroplasty. Patients must have failed at nonsurgical methods of weight loss, be well-informed and motivated, and as suggested by the NIH Technological Conference,[14] have a BMI greater than 40 or medically significant comorbidities justifying surgery if BMI is less than 40. WTO reviews evidence regarding the success of surgical intervention.

The limited use of surgery as a treatment for obesity is attributed to the lack of understanding about the cost of obesity in terms of morbidity, mortality, and quality of life. Also, fears of the dangers, side effects, and lack of reimbursement are cited as responsible for the underuse of appropriate surgical treatment.

Evaluating Treatment Programs

Three criteria for evaluating weight management programs are discussed (Table 21–4). These criteria are based on a conceptual model that takes into consideration the individual, treatment options, and program outcomes.[10(pp92–93)]

Table 21–4 Criteria for Evaluating Weight-Management Programs

Program	Person
Criterion 1: The Match between Program and Consumer	
Who is appropriate for this program?	Should I be in this program, given my goals and characteristics?
Criterion 2: The Soundness and Safety of the Program	
Is my program based on sound biological and behavioral principles, and is it safe for its intended participants?	Is the program safe and sound for me?
Criterion 3: Outcomes of the Program	
What is the evidence for success of my program?	Are the benefits I am likely to achieve from the program worth the effort and cost?

Source: Reprinted with permission from *Weighing the Options: Criteria For Evaluating Weight Management Programs.* Copyright 1995 by the National Academy of Sciences. Courtesy of the National Academy Press, Washington, D.C.

Criterion 1: The Match between Program and Consumer

Using the model provided in WTO, the program and consumer must answer certain questions: Am I appropriate for this program? Is the program based on sound biological and behavioral principles and is it safe? Is the program sound and safe for me? Is the program successful? Are the benefits worth the effort and cost? The primary consideration in matching programs and consumers is assessing the degree of health risk and personal factors affecting choice by the individual. The assessment of health risk may be based on percent overweight, BMI, comorbidities, and location of adiposity.

Studies by Garrow[20] and Stunkard[21] are cited as the earliest efforts in "grading" obesity to facilitate matching treatment options. Using a classification based on percent overweight, Brownell and Wadden's stepped care decision model (Figure 21–1) is discussed.[22] This model takes into consideration risk from weight, and individual and program factors. Bray's model (Figure 21–2) classifies risk based on BMI and the presence or absence of complicating factors. The evolution of models for obesity treatment choice culminates in Blackburn's model, developed for the WTO report (Figure 21–3). In this model, risk assessment is based not only on degree of fatness and comorbidities, but location of adiposity, weight history, and weight cycling. Each step increases in degree of evaluation, medical monitoring, and risk to the patient. Failure at successful progress, which is defined as

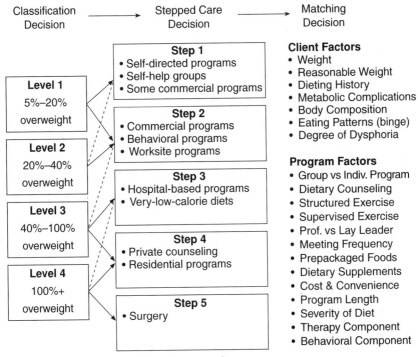

A conceptual scheme showing the three-stage process in selecting a treatment for an individual. The first step, the classification decision, divides individuals into four levels according to percentage overweight. These levels dictate which of the five steps would be reasonable in the second stage, the stepped care decision. This indicates that the least intensive, costly, and risky approach will be used from among alternative treatments. The third stage, the matching decision, is used to make the final selection of a program and is based on a combination of client and program variables. The dashed lines with arrows between the classification and stepped care stages show the lowest level of treatment that may be beneficial, but more intensive treatment is usually necessary for people at the specified weight level.

Figure 21–1 Conceptual scheme for matching individuals with treatments. *Source:* Reprinted with permission from K.D. Brownell and T.A. Wadden, The Heterogeneity of Obesity: Fitting Treatments to Individuals, *Behavior Therapy,* Vol. 22, pp. 153–177, copyright 1991 by the Association for the Advancement of Behavior Therapy. Reprinted by permission of the publisher.

cessation of weight gain, improved health, or a 2 kg/m² loss in BMI is an indication to proceed to the next step. Further goals of interventions include a 30% to 50% reduction of excess body fat and achievement of metabolic fitness.

Apart from theoretical models involving assessment based on medical criteria, three individual criteria may affect treatment decisions: personal, situational, and

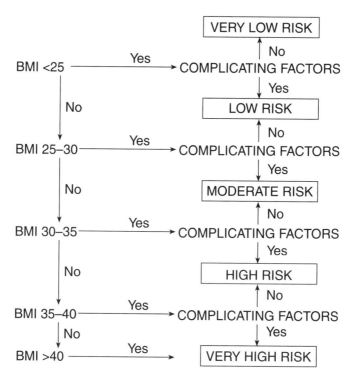

Figure 21–2 Risk classification based on body mass index. The presence or absence of complicating factors determines the degree of health risk. Complicating factors include an elevated waist-to-hip ratio, non–insulin-dependent diabetes mellitus, hypertension, hyperlipidemia, male sex, and age younger than 40 years. *Source:* Copyright © 1988, George A. Bray, M.D.

global factors; health status and weight-related risk factors; and information and guidance.[10(p100)] Personal factors include age, sex, and motivation. Situational factors can be altered by the individual. Global factors include cultural views about weight and environmental influences such as availability of weight loss programs in a region. Health status and weight-related risk are important motivators for some individuals while appearance is the primary motivator for many. Ideally, individuals choosing weight loss programs would do so according to their risk with appropriate assessment of comorbidities, family history, BMI, and visceral adiposity. Information and guidance come from the media, family and friends, and health care providers. One objective of WTO is to improve program disclosure, which would benefit the consumer by providing a more complete picture of program risks, benefits, and expected outcomes. Information and advertising from the media may provide helpful information and with advice from friends serves as the major determinant in program choice. By

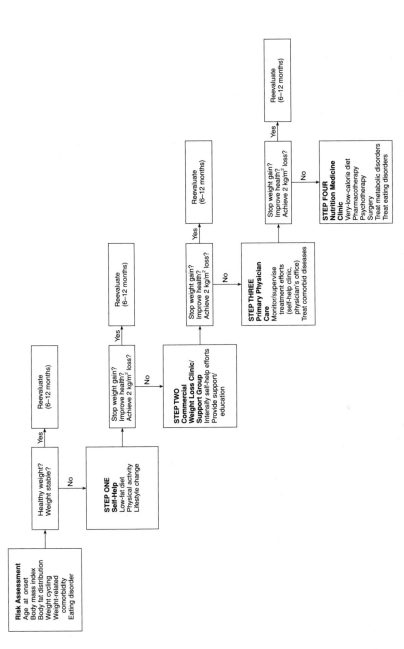

Figure 21-3 The Blackburn model. *Source:* Reprinted with permission from *Weighing the Options: Criteria For Evaluating Weight Management Programs.* Copyright 1995 by the National Academy of Sciences. Courtesy of the National Academy of Sciences, Washington, D.C.

improving program disclosure, consumers may be better able to make informed decisions, utilizing all sources of information.

Criterion 2: The Soundness and Safety of the Program

To ensure the safety and soundness of a program, WTO recommends that four areas be addressed: assessment of physical and psychological status; attention to diet; attention to physical activity; and ensuring program safety.[10(p102)]

Assessment of physical and psychological state: Minimally, WTO recommends that all individuals determine BMI and waist-to-hip ratio even if beginning a do-it-yourself program. Obese individuals should have a physical exam that includes measurement of blood pressure, blood glucose, and cholesterol as checks of comorbid conditions. Psychological evaluation should include screening for bulimia, binge eating, and depression, which may require special treatment.[10(p103)] Weighing the Options recommends that individuals beginning a do-it-yourself or nonclinical program answer the following questions[10(p104)]: (1) What is my overall state of health? (2) Do I have any weight-related comorbidities? (3) Are there risk factors in my family history that would indicate high risk of obesity-associated problems and/or comorbidities? (4) Do I have any medical problems that should be resolved before attempting weight loss? (5) Is it an appropriate time for me to lose weight? (6) Do I have an eating disorder? (7) What are my capacities and opportunities for restructuring my personal environment to succeed at weight loss? (8) What are my short- and long-term weight loss goals? (9) Am I ready to make a long-term commitment to a new lifestyle of healthful eating and regular physical activity? Weighing the Options recommends the Dieting Readiness Test[22] to assess motivation, commitment, and life circumstances, factors important to success of a diet program.

Diet: Guides to adequate diet are discussed in WTO[10(p107)] and include the Food Guide Pyramid,[23] the Recommended Dietary Allowances (RDAs),[24] the Dietary Guidelines,[25] the National Cholesterol and Education Program,[26] and the Institute of Medicine guide.[27] Dietary recommendations for weight loss are summarized as follows: (1) decrease total energy intake; (2) decrease alcohol and foods of minimal nutritional value such as fats and simple sugars; (3) consume adequate protein; (4) include all major food groups; and (5) seek the advice of a health care provider if the diet contains less than 1200 kcal/day.[10(p111)] Programs should be held accountable for any claims regarding weight loss rate and number of calories, provide medical monitoring when appropriate, provide accurate descriptions of the composition of prescribed diets, give attention to normalizing long-term eating patterns, and ensure that meal patterns and eating patterns take age, sex, ethnicity, and other social factors into consideration.

Activity: Weighing the Options discusses physical activity and benefits and barriers to promoting physical activity in obese individuals. Recommendations include a gradual increase in physical activity, with walking listed as the most feasible mode for most adults to obtain exercise. Also, developing a realistic goal that takes into consideration individual differences and sustainability of the exercise program should be a priority in any sound weight loss program.[10(p115)]

Program safety: Do-it-yourself and nonclinical programs must be safe for clients, while clinical programs must be as safe as reasonably possible considering the increased morbidity of individuals in clinical programs. Programs must provide detailed information about risks and monitor clients with obesity-related comorbidity. At-risk groups such as children and adolescents require consultation with a physician. Rapid weight loss is associated with increased risk of gallstones and psychological distress, emphasizing the importance of assessing the safety of a program before participating.

Criterion 3: Outcomes of the Program

The predictors of weight loss and maintenance are discussed as a prelude to presenting a new perspective on outcome assessment. *Weighing the Options* promotes a different view of appropriate outcome measures than previously held: long-term weight loss; improvement in comorbidities; improvement in health practices; and monitoring of adverse effects resulting from the program[10(p131)] (Table 21–5). Weight loss alone is an inadequate outcome measure for a program.

Table 21–5 Weight Management Outcome Criteria

Criteria	Successful Outcome
Long-term weight loss	• Loss of ≥5% body weight or loss of 1 BMI unit for 1 year or more
Improvement in comorbidities	• Improvement in one or more comorbidities (i.e., lower blood pressure to <140/90, cholesterol <200 mg/dL, triglyceride <225 mg/dL) to be objectively evaluated by a health care provider
Improved health practices	• Obtain health-related knowledge • Good eating habits—meet Food Guide Pyramid 4 of 7 days per week • Regular physical activity: 30 min per day moderate activity • Obtain regular medical attention • Improve self-esteem and self-care attitudes
Monitoring adverse effects	• Question self (program participant) about changes in health • Note adverse changes in health

Source: Reprinted with permission from *Weighing the Options: Criteria For Evaluating Weight Management Programs.* Copyright 1995 by the National Academy of Sciences. Courtesy of the National Academy Press, Washington, D.C.

The Weighing the Options Model (Figure 21–4) illustrates the comprehensive application of each criterion in the evaluation and reevaluation process.

Evaluating a Program by Applying WTO's Criteria

To aid in evaluation, WTO recommends that programs collect data as summarized in Exhibit 21–1. Claims should be made based on the data collected, reducing misleading testimonials. Programs must disclose information such as goals statements, staff credentials, a description of the client population and their success rate, full disclosure of costs for the length of the program and a statement of recommended medical procedures. The usefulness of WTO can be seen through some hypothetical case studies.

Case 1: Moderate Obesity

The individual seeking treatment is a 42-year-old white female who has a BMI of 33 and a long weight loss history that includes balanced-deficit diets with meal replacements and a very-low-calorie-diet. At least 10% of starting weight was lost with each attempt but maintained only two to four months each time. She has a positive family history for cardiovascular disease and non–insulin-dependent diabetes mellitus (NIDDM). She has never exercised regularly. This individual has chosen to evaluate a program that includes drug therapy and is run through a medical clinic.

The first step in evaluation is to apply Criterion 1: the match between the program and consumer. A BMI of 33, family history of comorbidities, and an exten-

---

Exhibit 21–1 Collection of Data by Weight Management Programs

Attendance
- Number of clients in first treatment session
- Number of clients in second treatment session
- Number at 1, 3, 6, and 12 months

Anthropometrics
- Height, weight, BMI, waist-to-hip ratio of clients at first and second session
- Change at 1, 3, 6, and 12 months by race, age, sex, starting BMI

Completion rate
- Percent of clients who complete treatment
- Percent of clients who re-enroll in same program

Source: Reprinted with permission from *Weighing the Options: Criteria For Evaluating Weight Management Programs.* Copyright 1995 by the National Academy of Sciences. Courtesy of the National Academy Press, Washington, D.C.

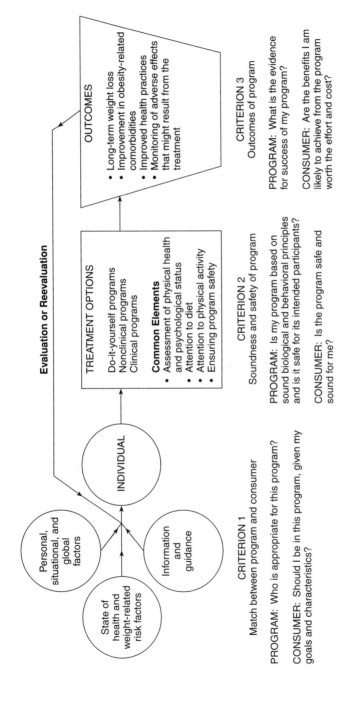

Figure 21-4 The Weighing the Options Model. *Source:* Reprinted with permission from *Weighing the Options: Criteria For Evaluating Weight Management Programs.* Copyright 1995 by the National Academy of Sciences. Courtesy of the National Academy Press, Washington, D.C.

sive weight loss history place this individual in a high-risk category of obesity. Drug therapy may be appropriate depending on her motivation and environmental influences such as availability of an acceptable program.

Criterion 2 (the soundness and safety of the program) must be addressed. As a part of a clinical program, a complete physical is required of all participants. During the physical, the questions related to overall health, comorbidities, family history, pre-existing medical problems, and eating disorders are asked. Unfortunately, this program does not have personnel to evaluate eating environment, readiness to diet, and other psychological factors that are important predictors of program success. Also, the following are lacking: prescribed diets and dietary monitoring, built-in maintenance program, integrated activity program, and closed group sessions.

Criterion 3 (the outcomes of the program) is then evaluated. Unfortunately, this clinic has not collected data on attendance, but has only records of weight loss over time.

Given the shortcomings of this program, the client has chosen to go elsewhere—to a clinic providing stronger behavior and lifestyle management and which offers drug therapy as an adjunct to weight management, in contrast to the clinic reviewed, which offers drug therapy as primary treatment.

Case 2: A 10-lb Goal

In another hypothetical case, a 22-year-old female college graduate with a BMI of 26 evaluates an over-the-counter meal replacement. Her goal is to lose 10 lbs. Starting with Criterion 1 (the match between program and consumer), her risk from her overweight is low. She is without family history or comorbidities, and has never attempted weight loss. Her motivation stems primarily from dissatisfaction with appearance. She is healthy, exercises regularly, and her weight gain occurred during college. According to Bray's model (Figure 21–2), she is low risk and according to Blackburn (Figure 21–3), is at step one (self-care) in the stepped care treatment model.

Criterion 2 (the soundness and safety of the program) is then assessed. As described in the literature accompanying the meal replacement, two beverages and a normal meal are recommended. The RDAs for major nutrients are met and the diet is suggested to last no more than three weeks. The calorie level can drop below 1200 kcal/day if the meal is not carefully designed, which is a shortcoming of the diet. Also, this individual has not assessed her own BMI and weight loss goals. Criterion 3 (outcomes of the program), cannot be assessed, the data neither collected nor effectiveness adequately addressed in a research context. Given that this is a first weight loss attempt, the program, with its recognized inadequacies, may be appropriate for this individual.

The criteria defined in WTO can be used to broadly evaluate any weight management program and, from an individual's standpoint, may be used to assess whether a program is acceptable. The major shortcoming of the criteria is that they must be applied rigorously and, perhaps, by professionals. Many forces work against individuals' ability to objectively evaluate a program for themselves; the power of the media, compelling advertising, and common willingness to extend responsibility for one's own health to a health care provider, have moved federal, state, and local governments toward regulation of the weight loss industry.

NEW DIRECTIONS IN REGULATION

The call to regulate the weight loss industry by the government may be made on the grounds of economic efficiency and consumer demand.[28] Economic efficiency is undermined by the inability of consumers to judge the quality of the industry's product. Many dieters overestimate the success of programs and believe they as individuals bear sole responsibility for program failure, leading to an inaccurate perception of the weight loss industry. Protective regulations would address the adverse side effects and potential risks associated with some programs. Emery et al[29] point to the fraudulent practices rampant in the industry—false claims, lack of provider credentials, false promises, and lack of physician supervision—as indications for government regulation.

Arthur Frank[10(pp234–235)] believes that voluntary accreditation for commercial weight loss programs would improve care provided by the industry. He proposes a national commission to formulate standards of care, to characterize the types of services provided, and to establish a governmental accrediting agency. The National Commission then closes down following completion of these tasks. Programs would pay for certification and require periodic recertification. The system would provide guidelines for consumers in selecting programs. Voluntary regulation, as Dr. Frank describes, places the onus of responsibility on the consumer to support programs that adhere to guidelines of the regulatory agency, in spite of the media and other external pressures involved in program selection.

On a federal level, the Federal Trade Commission (FTC) and the Food and Drug Administration (FDA) have enforcement capabilities and have used them to regulate, in the case of the FTC, commercial weight loss programs, and in the case of the FDA, weight loss products and drugs.[28] Two states and one city (New York State, Michigan, and New York City) have tried to regulate weight loss concerns.

Federal Regulation

In 1991, the FTC filed charges against the manufacturers of Optifast, Medifast, and Ultrafast, alleging that claims made about long-term effectiveness were deceptive.[30] Orders proposed by the FTC set requirements for claims: (1) claims about amount of weight lost must be based on a sample of all patients who have entered the program, or all persons who entered and completed the entire program or a portion thereof (where the claim only relates to such persons); (2) claims that weight loss is long term must be based on the experience of patients followed for at least two years after they complete the program; (3) claims that weight loss is maintained permanently must be based on a period of time generally recognized by experts as sufficient for such a claim, or for a period of time demonstrated by reliable survey evidence to permit such a prediction; (4) claims that patients have successfully maintained weight loss must include disclosures of the average weight loss maintained by those patients and how long they have maintained the loss, as well as the statement, "For many dieters, weight loss is only temporary." The FTC also brought action against five major nonclinical diet programs accusing them of misleading advertising.[31] These companies were accused of engaging in deceptive advertising by making unsubstantiated weight loss and maintenance claims and using unsubstantiated testimony of consumers and typical consumer experience to represent all program participants. The Acting Director of the Bureau of Consumer Protection stated that the cases were "designed to restore truth-in-advertising" to diet programs and provide consumers with "more realistic information about what they'll get for the more than $2 billion they spend each year on memberships in weight loss programs."

The Food and Drug Administration is also active in regulating some aspects of the weight loss industry. In 1992, the FDA banned 111 diet pill ingredients not generally recognized as safe and effective for over-the-counter sales.[32] The FDA has also been responsible for approval or lack of approval of antiobesity drugs.

Most recently, phentermine and fenfluramine were allowed limited (12 weeks) use in combination for obesity treatment. Weintraub's work[33] provided encouraging results that prompted support for limited use of these drugs. Dexfenfluramine was approved for use by the FDA but has been in use to treat obesity in Europe for many years and is available in 65 countries.[34] In May 1996, dexfenfluramine became available in the United States. (See Chapter 18.) The FDA review of olestra, a food additive designed to replace fat in many products, has received media attention,[35] and olestra-containing products are appearing in the marketplace.

State Regulation

On the state level, movement to regulate the prescription of anorectics and to regulate weight loss programs has occurred. Regulation of drugs for non-indicated uses falls to state medical and pharmacy boards. The American Society of Bariatric Physicians surveyed state medical boards in 1995 regarding rules and regulations for the dispensing of anorectic drugs. Of the 42 states that replied, 14 states had some type of restriction on the use of Schedule II and IV anorectic agents in the treatment of obesity. Restriction ranged from limitations on time or refills to disallowing any anorectic agent use. The Medical Board of the Commonwealth of Massachusetts was the most restrictive in that they prohibited the prescription of anorectics to treat obesity.[36] In an amendment to this regulation, physicians may petition for a waiver to allow use of a drug for its anorectic effect in a clinical research trial.

New York State, New York City, and Michigan have all held hearings on weight loss programs. In New York State, initiatives affecting weight loss services went before the legislature.[37,38] The bills were designed to provide consumers with guidance when choosing weight loss services and products and to provide oversight of weight loss services and products. Weight loss programs would have to be registered with the Department of State and provide information about their program, products, qualifications of personnel, success rates, and any reports of medical problems. All programs offering or advertising weight loss services would have to provide the following information to consumers: (1) WARNING! Rapid weight loss of more than one and a half to two pounds per week may cause serious health problems. (2) Consult with your physician before starting any weight loss program or using any diet medications or formulas. (3) Long-term weight control is the safest and most important goal of any diet program. Permanent lifestyle changes such as eating nutritious foods and increasing physical activity help promote long-term weight loss according to medical experts. (4) Ask the people providing or selling you weight loss advice or diet products, medications, or formulas about their qualifications and training in nutrition and health.

In 1993 the city of New York moved to regulate the weight loss industry. The Department of Consumer Affairs investigated diet programs and found them dangerous and deceptive; this led to the development of a rule governing weight loss providers.[39] The rule requires the following: (1) A "weight loss provider" is defined as any person or business entity who or which is primarily engaged in the business of offering services to consumers to assist them in losing weight. (2) It is a deceptive practice for a weight loss provider to quote a consumer a fixed or estimated cost for a weight loss program that is being recommended for the particular consumer without separately stating any additional charges the consumer may have to pay to purchase products, services, supplements, or laboratory tests that are part of such program. (3) It is a deceptive practice for a weight loss provider to recommend a weight loss program to a particular consumer without also disclosing the actual or estimated duration of the program. (4) It is a deceptive trade practice for a weight loss provider to make any oral or written statement, visual description, or other representation of any kind, including any advertisement, which statement, description, or representation has the capacity, tendency, or effect of leading consumers to believe that the use of a product or treatment, or participation in a program, will result in weight loss unless the weight loss provider conspicuously posts the following statement in each of its weight loss establishments: "1. Warning: Rapid weight loss may cause serious health problems. (Rapid weight loss is weight loss of more than 1½ pounds to 2 pounds per week or weight loss of more than 1 percent of body weight per week after the second week of participation in a weight loss program.) 2. Only permanent lifestyle changes—such as making healthful food choices and increasing physical activity—promote long-term weight loss. 3. Consult your personal physician before starting any weight loss program. 4. Qualification of this provider's staff are available on request. 5. You have a right to: i. Ask questions about the potential health risks of this program, its nutritional content, and its psychological-support and educational components; ii. Know the price of treatment, including the price of any extra products, services, supplements and laboratory tests; and iii. Know the program duration that is being recommended for you." (5) The above statement must be posted in a notice to the public at every temporary or permanent location of the weight loss provider. The notice must be conspicuously posted in every room in which a presentation is made, or in which a product or treatment is offered for sale, by the weight loss provider. The notice must be printed in letters in at least 36 point bold face type on a sign at least 22 inches by 34 inches in size. The sign shall be entitled "Weight Loss Consumer Bill of Rights," which shall be printed in letters of 60 point bold face type. (6) All the educational and professional experience of the weight loss provider's staff must be made available upon the request of any person. (7) Every weight loss provider shall produce and distribute to all consumers who inquire about its weight loss program a palm-sized card entitled "Weight Loss Consumer Bill of Rights," which shall contain the same information contained in the poster described above. (8) Every weight loss provider shall post the "Bill of Rights" sign which shall be provided by the Department of Consumer Affairs, and shall reproduce and distribute the palm-sized "Bill of Rights" card in every location in which its program or product is promoted, presented, or sold, and the weight loss provider must cause the posting of such sign and the distribution of such card by every agent, representative, franchisee, and independent contractor at every location in which such agent, representative, franchisee, or independent contractor promotes, presents, or sells the weight loss provider's program or product.

Michigan also set guidelines for the weight loss industry (Exhibit 21–2). In 1987, the Task Force to Establish Weight Loss Guidelines was formed. The Task Force believes that weight loss clinics and programs are in the business of health care and, as such, should meet certain standards of care.[40] The Task Force made specific recommendations in the areas of screening, staffing, disclosure, weight goals and rate of loss, diet, exercise, and behavior modification.[40] The guidelines were designed to protect consumers[41] and grew out of concern among health professionals following seven deaths in Michigan due to liquid diets in the late 1970s.

CONSUMER ACTIVITIES

The small advances made in developing successful treatment, regulating the weight loss industry, and recognizing obesity as a serious disease, do not match the extent and cost of obesity in the United States. The American Obesity Associa-

Exhibit 21–2 Recommendations for Adult Weight Loss Program

Screening	The client should be screened to verify that there are no medical or psychological conditions that would make weight loss inappropriate. The client's level of health risk should be identified: low risk, moderate risk, or high risk.
Level of Care	The weight loss program should provide the level of care appropriate to the client's level of health risk: level of care 1, 2, or 3.
Individualized Treatment Plans	Factors contributing to the client's weight status should be identified. These factors serve as the basis of each client's individualized weight loss plan, which includes the weight goal and plans for nutrition, exercise, behavioral change, medical monitoring or supervision, and health supervision.
Staffing	Weight loss service providers should be trained and supervised adequately for the level of health risk of clients receiving care.
Full Disclosure	The client should give informed consent, having been informed of potential physical and psychological risks from weight loss and regain, likely long-term success of the program, full cost of the program, and credentials of the weight loss care providers.
Reasonable Weight Goal	The weight goal for the client should be based on personal and family weight history, not exclusively on height and weight charts.
Rate of Weight Loss	The advertised and actual rate of weight loss, after the first two weeks, should not exceed an average of 2 lbs/wk.
Calories per Day	The daily calorie level should be adjusted so that each client can achieve but not exceed the recommended rate of weight loss. The daily caloric intake should not be lower than 1000 calories at level 1, 800 calories at level 2, and 600 calories at level 3. If the daily calorie level is below 800 calories, additional safeguards should be in place.
Diet Composition	Protein: between 0.8 and 1.5 g per kilogram of goal body weight, but no more than 100 g of protein per day. Fat: 10% to 30% of calories as fat. Carbohydrate: at least 100 g per day for level 1; at least 50 g per day for level 2.
Nutritional Adequacy	Fluid: at least 1 quart of water daily. The food plan should allow the client to obtain 100% of the recommended dietary allowances (RDA). If nutrition supplements are used, nutrient levels should not greatly exceed 100% of the RDA.
Nutrition Education	Nutrition education encouraging permanent healthful eating patterns should be incorporated into the weight loss program.
Formula Products	The food plan should consist of a variety of foods available from the conventional food supply. Formula products are not recom-

continues

Exhibit 21–2 continued

	mended for the treatment of moderate obesity and should not be used at low-calorie formulations without specialized medical supervision.
Exercise Component	The weight loss program includes an exercise component that is safe and appropriate for the individual client. The client is screened for conditions that would make medical clearance before exercise appropriate. The client is instructed to recognize and deal with potentially dangerous physical responses to exercise. The client works toward 30 to 60 minutes of continuous exercise five to seven times per week, with gradual increase in intensity and duration.
Psychological Component	Behavior modification techniques appropriate for the specific client should be taught.
Appetite Suppresants	Appetite suppressant drugs are not recommended and should not take the place of changes in diet, exercise, and behavior.
Weight Maintenance	A maintenance phase is included in the treatment program.

Health Care Levels

Level 1: Low-risk clients have no known health problems that, in the judgment of the personal physician, require direct medical monitoring during weight loss. It is the responsibility of weight loss providers to exclude moderate-risk or high-risk clients, unless they have specific clearance from their own physicians. Providers should preferably be health professionals but could be specially trained lay leaders. The essential components of nutrition, exercise, and behavior change should be approved by appropriate health professionals.

Level 2: Moderate-risk clients have medical conditions that could be complicated by weight loss or the treatment program. Medical monitoring is essential; a health care team is recommended.

Level 3: High-risk clients have severe, life-threatening conditions necessitating direct medical supervision during weight loss. Care is best provided in a hospital inpatient setting or an outpatient clinic staffed by an interdisciplinary team specializing in the treatment of obesity.

Evaluation of health status, rather than weight, should be the key factor in deciding level of care. Admitting high-risk clients to programs while failing to provide necessary health services is irresponsible and dangerous.

Weight loss is not appropriate for clients who are pregnant, suffer from anorexia or bulimia or psychological problems that may be aggravated by a weight loss program, are of normal weight or below, or who have low motivation or unrealistic expectations.

Source: Reprinted with permission from the Michigan Health Council, *Towards Safe Weight Loss,* p. 5, 1990, Michigan Department of Public Health.

tion (AOA) is currently being formed in response to the discrimination experienced by obese individuals and also in response to the lack of insurance reimbursement for obesity treatment or federal funding for obesity research.[42]
The AOA has several purposes:

1. Education:
   a. To educate obese people and the general public about obesity
   b. To educate health professionals to improve care for obese people
   c. To educate government officials and legislators about the need for more obesity research and about the negative impact of current laws and policies on obesity and obese people
   d. To educate insurance companies and third-party payers about the importance of payment for obesity treatment and prevention efforts
2. Political and social action:
   a. To lobby local, state, and federal legislatures to change laws and policies that have a negative impact on obese people
   b. To lobby for better health care policies for obesity
   c. To lobby for increased funding for obesity research by the National Institutes of Health (NIH)
   d. To encourage insurance companies to provide coverage for obesity treatment
   e. To point out discrimination against obesity where it exists
3. Research:
   a. To promote increasing the proportion of federal research funding devoted to obesity
   b. To raise funds for medical schools, research foundations, and individual scientists for increased obesity research
4. Prevention: To encourage the public, health care professionals, and governments to support efforts to prevent obesity, especially in children
5. Economic: To negotiate with companies, individuals, and governments to provide better service and to improve the economic status of obese people.

CONCLUSION

Recognition of obesity as a disease and acceptance and adoption of medical models for treatment may have a great impact on obesity research and treatment. As with many chronic diseases, behavioral and lifestyle changes serve as the first phase of treatment. Educating the public about prevention of obesity and treatment with diet and exercise will remain the most important tools of treatment. Personal responsibility remains a critical component in the success of any prevention and treatment effort. The more education the public has about obesity, its causes and its treatment, the more likely it becomes that individuals will accept some of the responsibility for the success of their treatment. Programs, clinics, and companies providing weight loss products and services must also accept responsibility for treatment success. Adequate evaluation of treatment options is a first step in improving the treatment of the disease of obesity. Regulation of the multibillion dollar weight loss industry may be necessary to force commercial concerns into accountability. Until obesity treatment is recognized as safe and effective, reimbursement will remain poor. Formation of the AOA will hopefully catalyze a nationwide examination of American opinions about the disease of obesity and of the role of health-workers in improving treatment options.

REFERENCES

1. Brownell KD. Whether obesity should be treated. *Health Psychol.* 1993;12:339–441.
2. Polivy J, Herman CP. Undieting: a program to help people stop dieting. *Int J Eating Dis.* 1992;1:261–268.
3. Wadden TA. The treatment of obesity. An overview. In: Stunkard AJ, Wadden TA, eds. *Obesity: Theory and Therapy.* 2nd ed. New York: Raven Press; 1993:197–217.
4. Consumer Reports Editorial Board. Rating the diets. *Consumer Reports.* 1993;June:353–357.
5. Kuczmarski RJ, Flegal KM, Campbell SM, Johnson CL. Increasing prevalence of overweight among US adults. *JAMA.* 1995;272:205–211.
6. Manson JE, Willett WC, Stampfer MJ, et al. Body weight and mortality among women. *N Engl J Med.* 1995;33:677–685.
7. Levy AS, Heaton AW. Weight control practices of US adults trying to lose weight. *Ann Intern Med.* 1993;119:661–666.
8. Bray GA. Barriers to the treatment of obesity. *Ann Intern Med.* 1991;115:152–153.
9. Maiman LA, Wang VL, Becker MH, et al. Attitudes toward obesity and the obese among professionals. *J Am Diet Assoc.* 1979;74:331–336.
10. Food and Nutrition Board. Institute of Medicine. *Weighing the Options: Criteria for Evaluating Weight Management Programs.* Washington, DC: National Academy Press; 1995.
11. National Institutes of Health Technology Conference Panel. Methods for voluntary weight loss and control: technology assessment conference statement. *Ann Intern Med.* 1993;119:764–770.
12. North American Association for the Study of Obesity. Guidelines for the approval and use of drugs to treat obesity. *Obes Res.* 1995;3:473–478.
13. Council on Scientific Affairs. Treatment of obesity in adults. *JAMA.* 1988;260:2547–2551.
14. National Institutes of Health. Gastrointestinal Surgery for Severe Obesity. National Institutes of Health Consensus Development Conference Statement. March 25–27, 1991. *Am J Clin Nutr.* 1992;55:615S–619S.
15. Meisler JG, St Jeor ST. Report on the American Health Foundation Roundtable on healthy weight. *Am J Clin Nutr.* 1996;63(suppl):474S–477S.
16. US Department of Agriculture, Agricultural Research Service, Dietary Guidelines Advisory Committee. Report of the Dietary Guidelines Advisory Committee on the Dietary Guidelines for Americans, 1995, to the Secretary of Health and Human Services and the Secretary of Agriculture.

17. Blackburn GL, Dwyer J, Flanders WH, et al. Report of the American Institute of Nutrition (AIN) Steering Committee on Healthy Weight. *J Nutr.* 1994;124:2240–2243.

18. American College of Sports Medicine and Centers for Disease Control. Physical activity and public health: a recommendation from the Centers for Disease Control and Prevention and the American College of Sports Medicine. *JAMA.* 1995;273:402–407.

19. Friedman RB. Very low-calorie diets. How successful? *Postgrad Med.* 1988;83:153–161.

20. Garrow JS. *Treat Obesity Seriously: A Clinical Manual.* New York: Churchill Livingstone; 1981.

21. Stunkard AJ. The current status of treatment for obesity in adults. In: Stunkard AJ, Stellar E, eds. *Eating and Its Disorders.* New York: Raven Press; 1984.

22. Brownell KD. Dieting Readiness. *Weight Control Digest.* 1990;1:5–10.

23. United States Department of Agriculture. *United States Department of Agriculture's Food Guide Pyramid.* Washington, DC: USDA Human Nutrition Information Service; 1992. Home and Garden Bulletin 252.

24. National Research Council. *Recommended Dietary Allowances.* 10th ed. Report of the Subcommittee on the Tenth Edition of the RDAs, Food and Nutrition Board, Commission of Life Sciences. Washington, DC: National Academy Press; 1989.

25. United States Department of Agriculture and Department of Health and Human Services. *Dietary Guidelines for Americans.* 3rd ed. Washington, DC: Government Printing Office; 1990.

26. National Cholesterol Education Program. *Second Report of the Expert Panel on Detection, Evaluation, and Treatment of High Blood Cholesterol in Adults.* National Heart, Lung, and Blood Institute, National Institutes of Health. Bethesda, MD: US Department of Health and Human Services; 1993. NIH Publication no. 93-3095.

27. Woteki CE, Thomas PR, eds. *Eat for Life: The Food and Nutrition Board's Guide to Reducing Your Risk of Chronic Disease.* Washington DC: National Academy Press; 1992.

28. Begley CE. Government should strengthen regulation in the weight loss industry. *J Am Diet Assoc.* 1991;91:1255–1257.

29. Emery EM, McDermott RJ, Ritter GP. Toward a policy of regulation of the weight loss industry. *J Health Educ.* 1991;22:150–153.

30. Berg FM. Three companies charged with false, deceptive claims. *Obes Health.* 1992;6:9,16.

31. Bureau of National Affairs. Two diet companies contest FTC claims; three others resolve false ad charges. *Bureau of National Affairs Antitrust and Trade Regulation Report.* 1993;65:460.

32. Berg FM. FDA bans diet pill ingredients after nearly 20 years. *Obes Health.* 1992;6:10–11.

33. Weintraub M. Long-term weight control study: conclusions. *Clin Pharmacol Ther.* 1992;51:642–646.

34. Merchcatie E. Panel deadlocks on safety, not efficacy, of Dexfenfluramine. *Fam Pract News.* 1995; Dec 15:33.

35. Lemonick MD. Is America ready for fat-free fat? *Time.* 1996;Jan 8:52–54,58–61.

36. Commonwealth of Massachusetts, Board of Registration in Medicine, Gitlin P, chair. *Massachusetts' Regulation of Physicians' Ability to Prescribe Anorectics.* Regulation 243 CMR 2.07 (21); 1988.

37. New York State Assembly. *Memorandum in Support of Legislation.* Assembly Bill A.6703-a. Weight Loss Program and Product Registry. 1993–1994.

38. New York State Assembly. *Memorandum in Support of Legislation.* Assembly Bill 6701-b. Weight Loss Program and Product Information. 1993–1994.

39. Berg FM. New York City takes a first step in industry regulation. *Obes Health.* 1993;7:52–53, 59.

40. Drewnowski A, chair. Task Force to Establish Weight Loss Guidelines, Michigan Health Council. *Toward Safe Weight Loss. Recommendations for Adult Weight Loss Programs in Michigan.* Lansing, MI: Michigan Department of Public Health; 1990.

41. Berg FM. Michigan sets guidelines for weight loss industry. *Obes Health.* 1991;5:27–29.

42. American Obesity Association. Board of Directors Meeting, October 15, 1995, Baton Rouge, LA.

CHAPTER 22

Design and Analysis of Obesity Treatment and Prevention Trials

David B. Allison
Joseph C. Cappelleri
Kenneth M. Carpenter

A statistician and a journalist were to be executed. Each was granted a last wish. The statistician requested the opportunity to report on his latest research findings. The jailer said he would arrange a seminar for the next Tuesday afternoon. Upon hearing this, the journalist said that his final request was to be executed on Tuesday morning.

Witmer

INTRODUCTION

The ill-fated journalist above expresses the sentiments of many when it comes to statistics. Nevertheless, the ubiquity of statistics in science suggests that a thorough grasp of the matter is essential for any contributor or consumer of research. Moreover, a thorough understanding of design and analysis issues enhances one's ability to conceptualize and test meaningful hypotheses, lending a greater richness and joy to the research enterprise. This chapter is intended to help investigators understand statistics and their use in obesity research and hopefully will not prompt too many requests for immediate execution.

This chapter addresses several aspects of designing obesity research and analyzing the resulting data. Countless books have been written about experimental design and statistical analysis, and it is obvious that all of that information cannot be covered here. This chapter focuses on specific issues that are especially timely or of particular interest to obesity researchers. The statistical and mathematical level is light, but some familiarity with basic statistics is assumed. The chapter is divided into four main sections. The first three are "experimental design options," "power analysis," and "data analysis issues." The section on data analysis briefly highlights some commonly occurring issues in obesity research. The fourth topic

557

is "meta-analysis." Meta-analysis is increasingly used in general and has recently begun to be used in obesity research. Meta-analysis is a powerful technique but, like many new and powerful methods, it is frequently misused and misunderstood. Many clinicians and researchers in the field of obesity may be unsure of how to read and interpret a meta-analysis, and this discussion explains both.

EXPERIMENTAL DESIGN OPTIONS

Within the empirical method are both observational (sometimes called correlational) studies and experimental studies. Although both kinds of studies are essential to scientific progress, experimental studies generally play a greater role in the evaluation of treatments and therefore this section will focus on them.

Some authors reserve the label "experiment" only for those studies in which observations (subjects) are *randomly* assigned to different levels of treatment. This chapter uses a broader definition in which an experiment is defined as any study in which the experimenter manipulates the independent variable, even if assignment is not random. Four kinds of experiments are discussed: randomized clinical trials (RCTs), quasi-experiments, cutoff-based designs, and single-case designs.

Randomized Clinical Trials

Randomized clinical trials (RCTs) are generally considered the soundest of experimental designs. This is because randomization is the only method that controls for the effects of both known and unknown variables. Because of their methodological rigor, RCTs have an unparalleled ability to convince other scientists and policy makers of treatment efficacy and safety.[1] The use of RCTs is recommended over alternative designs whenever possible. Nevertheless, there are situations where RCTs are impractical or impossible. In those situations, several other designs have been proposed[2-5] and some are reviewed below.

The conduct of RCTs will not be extensively discussed here because the issues are numerous and many are well known (for a more general review, see Meinert[6]). However, one issue, the actual process of randomization deserves attention.

Process of Randomization

The ability to draw valid conclusions (i.e., unbiased estimates of treatment effects) from an RCT is based upon the implementation of a *true* randomization procedure.[7] Consequently, the methods by which individuals or groups are assigned to a particular treatment (i.e., randomization) are of importance when evaluating the overall efficacy and generalizability of an intervention. This underscores the importance of conceptualizing the randomization procedure as a process.[8] This perspective differs from the view of randomization as the end state or outcome of a recruitment procedure that can be demonstrated by the lack of significant differences among treatment groups on various pretreatment characteristics.

A particular random assignment procedure is a probabilistic mechanism that ensures that the *expected values* of all variables and statistics are equivalent among treatment groups.[3,9] The fact that the probability of being assigned to a particular treatment is equal across all subjects provides a means by which, in the long run, subject idiosyncrasies and possible systematic biases in subject placement can be controlled for (i.e., equally distributed among all treatment conditions).[10] Thus, randomization guards against possible ad hoc decisions that may distort or restrict the ability to draw valid conclusions (viz., treatment effect estimates are unbiased).

The specific design in which random assignment is employed should be dependent upon theoretical considerations (e.g., what variables are of interest and what should be controlled for), practical constraints (e.g., number of subjects available, ethical considerations in treatment provision), and the hypothesis being tested. While it is beyond the scope of this chapter to detail all design specifications,[11] random assignment can be employed in designs in which all extraneous variables (known and unknown) are controlled for (completely randomized designs) or in designs in which specific extraneous variables are included within the experiment (factorial designs). In the latter, a stratified randomization procedure can be employed in which subjects are grouped by a particular criteria and randomly assigned to a treatment condition.[12] For example, a researcher may have theoretical reason to believe a particular weight reduction program may have differential impact on individuals within a certain weight class (i.e., slightly overweight, overweight, obese). Thus, subjects may be recruited from several weight classes. However, within each weight class subjects are randomly assigned to the treatment conditions.

There are numerous randomization strategies available to the researcher depending on the particular research design. If specific patient characteristics are not directly being controlled for, unstratified randomization procedures (unrestricted randomization) can be used.[13] However, such procedures require large sample sizes, which may be prohibitive in the typical RCT. Guyatt et al[14] outline procedures for randomized trials employing single-subject methodology. Restricted randomization (random permuted blocks) procedures are useful if equal sample sizes among treatment conditions are preferred.[13,15] Stratified randomization schemes are preferred when specific subject factors are being controlled for.[15] Furthermore, stratified designs can employ both restricted and unrestricted randomization schemes.

The randomization procedure can be facilitated with the use of random number charts,[11] random number generators,[16,17] or random permutations tables.[18] Zelen[5] offers a randomization scheme to be used in conjunction with possible difficulties associated with informed consent decisions. Specifically, subjects may refuse to participate in an RCT when informed of a random assignment to treatments. Together, such procedures help ensure that placement decisions are random and are not influenced by experimenter biases.

Whatever method of randomization is employed, it is crucial that it be adhered to throughout the assignment phase. Deviations from the protocol can severely confound the study even under the best intentions by introducing possible systematic biases. Consider the following example.

In the classic critique of a milk study, by a Guiness Brewery employee (W.S. Gosset, better known by his pseudonym "Student" and the t-test), the detrimental effects of deviating from a random assignment procedure were demonstrated.[19] In 1930, Scotland's Department of Health evaluated the effects of raw or pasteurized milk on the weight and height of children in Lanarkshire schools. In total, 20,000 (5,000 per milk group and 10,000 no-milk controls) children from 67 schools were recruited (the kind of power many researchers dream of!). The actual placement of students into the milk or control groups was to be conducted by teachers using a ballot or alphabetical system. However, to the extent that teachers thought the various groups were "unbalanced" (a greater proportion of undernourished children in the control) others could be substituted to equate the groups. Unfortunately, this post hoc adjustment introduced a bias by which sympathetic and concerned teachers assigned a greater proportion of undernourished children to the milk conditions. Thus, the control group consisted of children who were superior in measurements of both height and weight. The introduction of this systematic group difference prohibited a valid estimation of the effect of milk on children's height and weight despite the considerable time and effort expended.

The employment of a haphazard placement system is not a proxy for a randomization scheme. The assignment of subjects based upon an "every other" volunteer method or "day of the week assignment" does not rule out the possibility that various situational or individual variables associated with the order of presentation are related to the criterion variable(s) of interest.[20,21] Furthermore, such procedures potentially violate the assumption of independent assignment and limit the use of randomization models employed in many statistical procedures.[4,22] Thus, such relationships may introduce a bias into an experimental design that detracts from the conclusions that can be drawn.

The random assignment of subjects to a particular treatment condition is an important methodological consideration within an RCT. As such, the method by which random assignment is implemented should be clearly delineated within the method section of a clinical trial. This facilitates the overall evaluation of an empirical report for threats to both internal and external validity.[3] Unfortunately, this delineation is usually the exception, not the rule. For example, a (haphazard) selection of 16 empirical investigations mentioning randomized placement published in the *International Journal of Obesity* between 1992–1995, indicated that 0% specified the procedure by which the assignment was made including, unfortunately, our own.[23]

Quasi-Experiments

Often, in applied research, strict randomization is not an option. Constraints on the use of random assignment can involve physical, political, ethical, and economic issues. Furthermore, frequently encountered difficulties such as subject refusal, attrition, and nonresponding (particularly in survey research) can result in the introduction of systematic biases into what was initially a randomized design. As such, numerous studies fall within the realm of quasi-experiments.

Some would argue that the randomized experiment is the *sine qua non* of epistemological advancement. However, the pervasiveness and inevitability of the quasi-experimental design supports the attention devoted to the various methodological approaches associated with its use. Unfortunately, the ubiquity of the design does not detract from its limitations. Specifically, the quasi-experiment often fails to persuade the scientific community of the validity of the conclusions derived from its use. This is primarily attributed to the inability of a quasi-experiment to definitively control for, or rule out, alternative explanations for the observed relationships.

When evaluating a quasi-experimental design a common approach is a post hoc statistical adjustment of group differences. This is often facilitated by the employment of regression analysis (usually ordinary least squares regression [OLS]) in which the control variables of interest are entered in the equation prior to the evaluation of the "treatment effect" or an analysis of covariance (ANCOVA). Such procedures, while intuitively appealing, are problematic for several reasons.

First, strong theoretical guidance may suggest the source of group nonequivalency; however, it is often the case that such variables were not assessed. Thus, proxy variables may be substituted for the construct of interest. However, the use of such proxy variables can severely bias the estimate of the true treatment effect.[22] An example of this procedure can be found in studies assessing the effect of obesity on mortality. Specifically, to ascertain the effect of obesity it is important to control for preexisting disease differences among lean and obese subjects. However, such data are not always available. In such cases studies may exclude inviduals who have demonstrated early mortality (i.e., those who die before some specified time period). The use of early mortality is thus employed as a proxy for preexisting disease, which could bias the estimated effects of obesity.

Second, it is quite often the case that the source of nonequivalency (or bias) is unknown. Thus, statistical attempts to equate groups often fail to correct for all possible biases or systematic differences that detract from the overall validity of the conclusions derived from the study. Furthermore, if no attempt is made to adjust for the nonrandom nature of the assignment phase, severe distortions in the estimated treatment effect can occur.

The use of ANCOVA to "adjust" for group differences obtained by a *non-randomized* assignment procedure (quasi-experiments) can introduce both statistical and interpretive complications. Most important, the use of ANCOVA to correct group differences can lead to biased treatment estimates.[24] Issues related to the use of ANCOVA are outlined in numerous texts.[8,11,24] In a more conceptual framework, Lord demonstrated that the use of ANCOVA to adjust for differences in preexisting natural groups (i.e., sex) can often lead to contradictory conclusions (Lord's Paradox).[25] This paradox was demonstrated in an example in which sex differences in pretreatment weight were "controlled" for in the evaluation of a programmatic dietary change. Specifically, the use of ANCOVA resulted in the finding that boys demonstrated greater weight gain then girls when initial weight differences between the sexes were adjusted for. However, a second analysis comparing the average or mean weight of each sex at both times (that is, at the beginning and the end of the school year) indicated no difference in the average weight for both groups. Thus, although both analyses were correct, they yielded quite contrary conclusions. While offering no concrete explanation for such a paradox, Lord indicated that the use of such statistical corrections is dependent upon certain logical prerequisites.[26] Thus, the applicability of such an "equivalency" procedure is dependent upon both statistical and logical criteria, not frequently met in the quasi-experimental design. However, given the relative limitations of quasi-experimental designs there are several resources that can assist the researcher in extracting the most valid conclusions from such investigations. Achen[22] provides a detailed exposition of statistical methods that can be used for quasi-experiments, which address the limitations of traditional regression procedures. Cook and Campbell[3] offer both methodological and statistical approaches to the conduction and evaluation of quasi-experimental designs. Furthermore, the use of cutoff-based designs,[2] although not strictly a randomized procedure, allows the researcher to obtain unbiased estimates of a treatment effect.

Cutoff-Based Designs

Cutoff-based designs have been proposed to balance ethical and scientific concerns when not all patients can be randomized.[27–29] They deserve consideration particularly when the disease is potentially life threatening and when there is strong a priori (though not conclusive) evidence that the test treatment is superior to the control treatment. The cutoff-based design incorporates a need-based and clinically valid numerical covariate, as a measure of the baseline degree of severity of illness, by which patients are assigned either automatically or randomly to treatments. An example of such an assignment covariate is body mass index. Outcomes can be either continuous or discrete, such as body mass index at follow-up, serum lipid concentration, and mortality status (dead, alive).

Regression-Discontinuity Design

A cutoff-based design can have varying amounts of randomization, from none to randomization of almost all of the enrolled sample. The cutoff design with no randomization is known as the regression-discontinuity design.[3,27,30–33] It has been classified as a quasi-experimental design[3] and has been applied mainly to topics in the social sciences.[34] Figure 22–1 depicts a hypothetical application of a regression-discontinuity design with the cutoff at a baseline body mass index (BMI) of 35 kg/m^2 and body mass index at follow-up (say, one year later) as the outcome. All obese patients with a BMI equal to or greater than the cutoff value of 35 kg/m^2 (i.e., the more severely obese) are automatically assigned to surgical (test) treatment, and all obese patients with values less than 35 kg/m^2 (i.e., the less severely obese) are automatically assigned to conventional (control) treatment. The rationale is that patients who are less severely obese are receiving the best known (standard) treatment they would have received anyway and that patients who are more severely obese are in

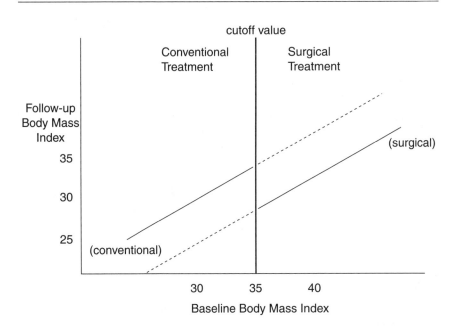

Figure 22–1 A regression-discontinuity design with a five-point treatment effect.

greater need of the potentially greater benefit from surgical treatment and, by implication, are more willing to incur its potential risks or side effects.

The solid lines in Figure 22–1 represent the fitted linear regression lines of BMI at follow-up onto BMI at baseline. This figure shows a treatment effect of 5 kg/m²: the outcome scores of the surgically treated group are lower by an average of 5 kg/m² from where they would be if the subjects had received conventional treatment. The dashed lines represent the expected (extrapolated) linear regression lines if patients in each group had been given the other treatment instead. The amount of the discontinuity (or "jump") at the cutoff value gives the estimate of treatment effect. Hence the term "regression-discontinuity" design.

Cutoff-Based Randomized Clinical Trials

Whenever feasible, cutoff-based designs should incorporate as much randomization as allowed so that they can benefit from the desirable scientific properties of randomization. Cutoff-based designs in which some patients are randomized and others are assigned to a particular treatment by cutoff assignment have been labeled as cutoff-based randomized clinical trials (RCTs).[28,29] Because it has features of both the regression-discontinuity design and the randomized design, the cutoff-based RCT can be classified as both a quasi-experimental design and a randomized design. Like all cutoff-based designs, cutoff-based RCTs involve the assignment of treatments on the basis of need and willingness to incur potential risk. At the same time, they capitalize in part on the more precise (i.e., lower standard error) estimate of treatment effect found in the traditional RCT, where all patients are randomized.

Using the principles depicted in Figure 22–1, Figure 22–2 shows one variation of a cutoff-based RCT. Obese patients with a BMI less than 35 kg/m² (the least severely obese) are automatically assigned to conventional treatment; patients with a BMI more than 40 kg/m² (the most severely obese) are automatically assigned to surgical treatment; and patients with values between 35 and 40 kg/m² inclusive (the moderately obese) are randomly assigned to either treatment. Such a cutoff-based RCT, with two cutoff points, was undertaken by Havassy and colleagues at the University of California at San Francisco (unpublished data). They used a composite indicator for severity of cocaine addiction to determine whether persons dependent on cocaine who were assigned to inpatient rehabilitation showed more improvement than they would if they received outpatient (less intensive) rehabilitation.

Figure 22–3 shows another variation of a cutoff-based RCT, with one cutoff value. Obese patients with a BMI less than 35 kg/m² are assigned to conventional treatment, while patients with a BMI equal to or greater than 35 kg/m² are randomized to either surgical treatment or conventional treatment. In cutoff-based RCTs, no extrapolated line is needed for the randomized portion of patients.

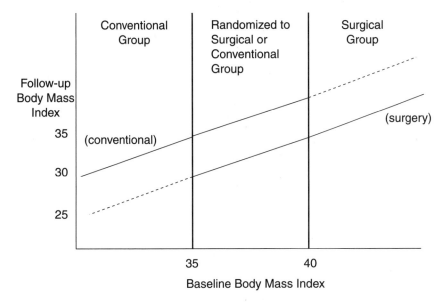

Figure 22–2 A cutoff-based RCT (two cutoff values) with a five-point treatment effect.

Methodological Issues

Cutoff-based designs can provide an unbiased estimate of treatment effect if, in addition to the assumptions required for completely randomized experiments, two conditions hold. One condition is that all patients be assigned to the treatment indicated by the baseline assignment variable, which must be included in the statistical analysis. The assignment rule must be followed without exception. Like randomized experiments, cutoff-based designs are potentially amenable to causal inference because treatment assignment is known perfectly. In the randomized experiment, prognostic factors are expected to be equivalent between the treatment groups, so that a statistically significant difference between treatments can be attributed to the tested intervention. In cutoff-based designs, the treatment groups are deliberately partitioned, but no selection bias is expected as the factors that make the difference between groups are controlled or adjusted for in the analysis by the addition of the baseline covariate into the statistical model. Furthermore, incorporating the complete knowledge of the assignment process via the baseline covariate into the model does not allow for random measurement error in the baseline covariate and its accompanying regression to the mean to bias the estimate of treatment effect.[3,30,34]

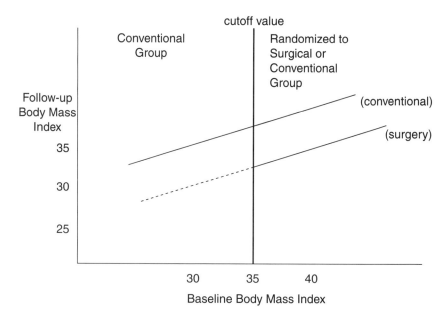

Figure 22–3 A cutoff-based RCT (one cutoff value) with a five-point treatment effect.

The other requirement for an unbiased treatment estimate is that the true functional relationship between baseline covariate and outcome measure be modeled correctly. A polynomial regression approach has been recommended.[2] (Figures 22–1 through 22–3 assume a linear form.) Unlike randomized experiments, where data are available for both treatment groups across the entire range of the baseline covariate, cutoff-based designs require the extrapolation of the regression line for a treatment group into the baseline-outcome region where there are no data. Correctly modeling the functional form, which cannot be empirically ascertained, justifies such an extrapolation. Cappelleri and Trochim[2] provide guidelines for the statistical analysis of cutoff-based designs.

The built-in correlation between the baseline covariate and the treatment group variable in cutoff-based designs makes them less efficient, with a larger standard error of the treatment estimate than randomized designs (where this correlation is expected to be zero) with the same sample size. This means that, everything else being the same, the statistical power (i.e., the probability of achieving statistical significance given that there is a treatment effect) is always lower in a cutoff-based design than in a randomized design with the same number of patients. Everything else being the same, a cutoff-based design with more randomization has more statistical power than a cutoff-based design with less randomization.

Depending on its amount of randomization, a cutoff-based design requires up to 2.75 times as many patients as a randomized design to achieve the same level of statistical power.[35,36] The larger sample size requirement in a cutoff-based design should be taken into account when considering it as an alternative to a randomized experiment.

Another consideration is that patients and their physicians must be informed about the general method of treatment delivery. Such informed consent means that the treatment administered to the patient may be known by the project staff, the patient, and the physician. This will make the trial largely unblinded and open to the possibility of observation bias.[37] But, unlike many pharmaceutical studies, many nutritional investigations are unblinded anyway, as when a surgical intervention is compared against a conventional intervention. Thus, when unblindedness is unavoidable, regardless of the design implemented, the cutoff-based design does not add to the drawback of unblindedness.

Despite their limitations, the cutoff-based design—especially the cutoff-based RCT—is among the strongest alternatives to the randomized design. The randomized design is clearly the method of choice. The cutoff-based design is not intended to replace the randomized design, but is offered as a useful design option when randomization cannot be applied to all subjects. As such, a comparison and evaluation with designs other than the fully randomized design would make for a more fair assessment. Although many kinds of quasi-experiments exist,[3] cutoff-based designs stand out because of the relatively high quality of causal inference they allow.

Single-Case Designs

Single-case designs (SCDs; also known as "single-subject designs" and "N-of-1 trials") are widely used in the fields of psychology and education and are the dominant mode of inference in applied behavior analysis. To a large extent, the use of these designs grew out of the writings of Skinner[38] and Sidman.[39] Although these designs have their roots in psychology, they are used in many contexts[42] including education,[41] rehabilitation,[42,43] sport and athletic performance,[44–46] and medicine.[14,47–49] SCDs have also been used to investigate obesity-related issues.[50–57] Thorough discussions of the various SCDs can be found in Barlow and Hersen[58] and Kazdin.[59]

Figure 22–4 is an example of a SCD from De Luca and Holborn.[51] De Luca and Holborn actually studied six individuals. For expository purposes, results for only one are presented here. The particular SCD used is the changing criteria design.[60] In this study, the investigators assessed the effects of variable-ratio reinforcement on the exercise behavior of an obese boy. As can be seen in Figure 22–4, there is a dose-response relationship between the reinforcement ratio (the independent vari-

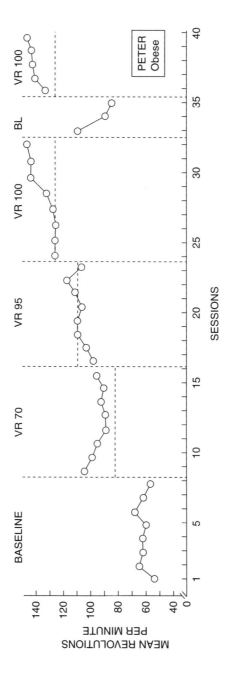

Figure 22–4 Single-case study example of variable-ratio reinforcement on bicycle exercise behavior of an obese boy. *Source:* Adapted from R.V. DeLuca and S.W. Holborn, *Journal of Applied Behavioral Analysis*, Vol. 25, pp. 671–679, © 1992, Society for the Experimental Analysis of Behavior, University of Kansas.

able) and revolutions pedaled per minute (the dependent variable). This demonstration of systematic within-person covariation between the manipulated independent variable and dependent variable is the essence of the SCD.

In the SCD, the subject truly serves as his or her own control. Instead of assigning multiple subjects to two or more conditions, the experimenter assigns multiple time points to two or more conditions within a single subject. In many cases, to improve generalizability or enhance the strength of inference, one SCD will include several individuals.

SCDs generally (though not always) ask a different question than group designs ask. The group design essentially asks "What is the *average* or *expected* effect of receiving treatment A vs receiving some other treatment or no treatment at all?" In contrast, the SCD design essentially asks "What is the effect of receiving treatment A vs receiving some other treatment or no treatment at all *for this individual?*" Thus, these designs are especially useful in clinical research where one is interested in evaluation of therapy for individual patients.[61]

Generalizing from the individual studied to other individuals is a problem in SCDs. Nevertheless, SCDs do contribute to the scientific literature and can be cumulated with meta-analytic techniques,[62-64] enhancing one's ability to make more general statements about average effects.

Special Issues in SCDs

There are several issues that users of SCDs should be aware of. First, SCDs work best with dependent variables that can change rapidly from one observation period to the next with little carryover effects. Body weight is not a good example of such a variable; it changes slowly and obviously carries over from day to day. Variables such as exercise behavior, caloric intake, blood pressure, and hunger are much better candidates.

A second issue concerns the possibility of trends in the time series. To the extent that any systematic trends are present in the subject's behavior, they may mimic treatment effects.[65] Although there are many ways to address this potential confound, perhaps the best is to ensure that time periods are randomly assigned to experimental conditions.[14,65-67]

A third problem that is intertwined with the problems of trends and carryover effects is the problem of autocorrelation. Autocorrelation occurs when subsequent scores on a variable can be predicted from previous scores on that variable. When autocorrelation occurs in the residuals of the model fitted to the dependent variable in a SCD, it causes the calculated standard errors of statistics to underestimate the actual standard errors. (This assumes that the autocorrelation is positive, which is the more common case. Negative autocorrelation will cause standard errors to be overestimated.) This in turn causes the p-values of the obtained results to be underestimated. Thus, conventional tests of statistical significance cannot generally be used with

SCDs. Instead, techniques that test for and/or take autocorrelation into account must be used. The analysis of SCDs is a subject of considerable discussion.[68,69] Although visual inspection, that is, simply making a judgment based on looking at a graph such as Figure 22–4, is the most common method of analysis of SCDs, visual inspection has been shown to be both unreliable and biased.[42] Unfortunately, a discussion of methods for analyzing SCDs is beyond the scope of this chapter. For detailed discussions see Kratochwill and Levin[68] and Gorman and Allison.[70]

POWER ANALYSIS

This section briefly highlights the importance of statistical power, defines basic terms and concepts, and discusses the implementation of power analysis.

Cohen[71] published an influential article indicating that most psychological studies were conducted with inadequate power. Subsequently, other investigators[72,73] also found this problem and found that it is not limited to psychological research. Consequently, researchers have become aware of the necessity of designing studies with sufficient power. It has even been argued that conducting studies with insufficient power is unethical. Such studies are likely to provide misleading information (i.e., they will contain many Type II errors) and they arguably waste subjects' time and research resources.* Alternatively, it can be argued that in some situations, due to the rarity of subjects, the expense of the experimental protocol, or similar limiting factors, it is simply not possible to conduct certain studies with adequate power. Such studies may still be justifiable on the grounds that future meta-analyses (see below) may still be able to draw firm and valuable conclusions by pooling the results of several small studies.

To provide a context for this discussion, the authors conducted an impromptu "power survey" of articles from the *International Journal of Obesity, Obesity Research,* and the *International Journal of Eating Disorders.* We haphazardly (but not randomly) selected two issues of each journal from 1994 and examined each of the 34 data-based obesity related articles involving human subjects that were included. For each article, we recorded sample size and used PowPal software[74] to calculate the power to detect significant effects at the .05 (two-tailed) level. We calculated power for "small," "medium," and "large" effects, defined as r's of .10, .30, and .50, respectively, following the guidelines of Cohen.[75]

In this power survey, sample sizes ranged from 10 to 3671 with a mean of 431. Across studies, the average power to detect small, medium, and large effects was .32, .72, and .90, respectively. If one uses 80% power as a definition of "acceptable" power, then 15%, 52%, and 71% of studies had acceptable power to detect small, medium, and large effects, respectively. Of course, these numbers should

---

*Type II errors will be defined in greater detail later. Briefly, the type II error occurs when the null hypothesis is false but one fails to reject the null hypothesis.

only be taken as approximations because they do not take into account the many study factors that could either increase power (e.g., well-chosen covariates) or decrease power (e.g., measurement error). Nevertheless, they suggest that, as in other fields, many studies in obesity research lack adequate power to detect anything less than large effects. This is unfortunate because large effects are the exception rather than the rule.

To appreciate the implications of this result, consider the example of the thermic effect of food (TEF). Numerous studies have been done to test whether obesity is associated with a lower TEF and results have generally been equivocal and difficult to interpret. Ravussin and Swinburn[76] list 46 studies of the association between obesity and TEF of which 28 (61%) showed a blunted response among the obese and the remainder showed no significant difference. When discussing this literature, Ravussin and Swinburn state:

> many factors influence the thermic effect of food: the test meal size and composition, the palatability of the food, and the time of the meal, as well as the subject's genetic background, age, physical fitness, and sensitivity to insulin. These influences plus the technical aspects such as the position of the subject and the duration of measurement mean that the thermic effect of food is the most difficult and the least reproducible component of daily energy expenditure to measure.[76(p102)]

Thus, one would expect that any effect of obesity that existed would not account for an overwhelming proportion of variance in TEF and power would therefore be low in small studies. Indeed, the average sample size of the 46 studies listed was 22. Because 61% of the studies did find a significant effect in the same direction, we estimated the size of effect that would have 61% power with an N of 22. The answer is an effect that accounts for 25% of the variance or an r of .50. Thus, the TEF studies may only appear equivocal and inconsistent due to low power. That is, the results of the 46 studies are entirely consistent with the hypothesis that obesity status explains 25% of the variance in TEF, which many[75] would consider a relatively large effect.

A further discussion of power is primarily based on treatment-based research; the statistical issues are the same for both treatment and nontreatment-based research. Thus, any tables, software, or formulas presented here are applicable to treatment and nontreatment studies. Similarly, when referring to the strength of association between an independent and dependent variable, this chapter uses the generic term "effect size." For research involving observational data, one should simply substitute "association" or "relationship" where "effect size" appears in this chapter.

Basic Terms and Concepts

The Null Hypothesis. The null hypothesis (H_o) commonly states that the treatment has no effect. In other words, there is no systematic difference between treated and untreated subjects. A typical operational definition of H_o is that the population mean under treatment conditions is equal to the population mean under no treatment (or alternative treatment) conditions.

Type I Error. The null hypothesis is either true or it is not true. After analyzing the results of a study, researchers either conclude that the null hypothesis is true, or conclude that the null hypothesis is not true (in other words, researchers "fail to reject the null hypothesis" and "reject the null hypothesis," respectively). These two possible realities and two possible conclusions are displayed in a 2 by 2 table in Exhibit 22–1. Rejecting the null hypothesis when the null hypothesis is actually true constitutes a Type I error. The probability of making a Type I error (typically fixed at .01 or .05) is denoted α. A clear discussion of the meaning of α and p-values can be found in Abelson.[77]

Type II Error. Failure to reject the null hypothesis when the null hypothesis is actually false constitutes a Type II error. The probability of making a Type II error is denoted β.

Power. The probability of finding an effect given that an effect actually exists is power. Power is equal to one minus β. Many investigators consider .80 an "acceptable" level of power and .90 a "desirable" level.

Effect Size. Power values are conditional probabilities. In other words, the power of an experiment is the probability of finding a significant result given a particular population effect size. Effect size is an index of the magnitude of the effect produced by the independent variable or treatment. There are many ways to express effect size and one metric can almost always be converted to another. The

---

Exhibit 22–1 Outcomes of Inference in Statistical Hypothesis Testing

	REALITY	
	Null Is True	Null Is False
Null Is True	Correct Decision $1-\alpha$ Specificity	Type II error β 1-Sensitivity
CONCLUSION		
Null Is False	Type I error α 1-Specificity	Correct Decision Power $1-\beta$ Sensitivity

two most common measures of effect size are Cohen's[75] *d,* the difference between means divided by the pooled within-group standard deviation, and *r,* the correlation coefficient. For other metrics and translation formulas see Table 22–1.

Conducting a Power Analysis

Power analyses can be used to calculate power given sample size as the authors showed in the "power survey" above. However, the more common approach to power analysis is to decide on the desired level of power, the Type I error probability (α), and the hypothesized effect size, and then solve for the required sample size.[78] Sample size can be solved for through very crude but easy-to-use approximate formu-

---

Table 22–1 Conversion of Some Common Test Statistics to r_m and *d* Values

Statistic	r_m Value	d Value
t	$r_m = \dfrac{t}{\sqrt{t^2 + df}}$	$d = 2\,\dfrac{t}{\sqrt{df}}$
Z	$r_m = \dfrac{Z}{\sqrt{Z^2 + N}}$	$d = 2\,\dfrac{Z}{\sqrt{N}}$
$F\ (df_n = 1)$	$r_m = \sqrt{\dfrac{F}{F + df_d}}$	$d = 2\sqrt{\dfrac{F}{df_d}}$
$F\ (df_n > 1)$	$r_m = \sqrt{\dfrac{F\,df_n}{F\,df_n + df_d}}$	$d = 2\sqrt{\dfrac{df_n\,F}{df_d}}$
$X^2\ (df = 1)$	$r_m = \sqrt{\dfrac{X^2}{N}}$	$d = \sqrt{\dfrac{4X^2}{N - X^2}}$
$X^2\ (df > 2)$	$r_m = \sqrt{\dfrac{X^2}{N + X^2}}$	$d = 2\sqrt{\dfrac{X^2}{N}}$
r	$r_m = r$	$d = \sqrt{\dfrac{4r_m^2}{(1 - r_m^2)}}$
d	$r_m = \sqrt{\dfrac{d^2}{d^2 + 4}}$	$d = d$

Note: df_n = numerator df; df_d = denominator df.
Source: Reprinted with permission from R.D. Franklin, D.B. Allison, & B.S. Gorman, *Design and Analysis of Single Case Research,* Table 10–1, p. 345, © 1996, Erlbaum Publishing.

las,[79,80] somewhat more rigorous approximations,[81,82] computer simulations,[83] published tables, and published software. For most purposes, the last two methods offer the best combination of accuracy, flexibility, and ease of use. Unfortunately, no one table or one piece of software will typically meet all of an investigator's needs. Thus, it is best to maintain a library of tables and/or software for such use. Two tables are supplied here. Table 22–2 is a "table of tables," and lists various tables for power analysis and their unique features. Table 22–3 is especially useful for providing power and sample size estimates and is adapted from Friedman.[84] A power analysis and the use of this table are illustrated with an example.

An Example of Power Analysis

The authors were approached by a company that marketed an acupressure device for weight loss and asked to conduct a clinical trial to test its efficacy.[23] The design was a randomized two-arm study (treatment vs placebo). In determining the sample size, α was set at .05 and power was set at .80. To calculate an estimate of effect size, we first needed an estimate of the amount of weight the treatment group would lose over 12 weeks. The company had conducted a quasi-experiment pilot study and observed an average of 1.69 lbs over two weeks. Since past research has shown that weight loss curves follow a double exponential decay pattern with the rate of weight loss during the first two weeks being approximately twice that during subsequent weeks,[85] we extrapolated the rate of weight loss during the subsequent 10 weeks at a rate half that of the first two weeks. This yielded an expected weight loss of 5.91 lbs. Assuming the treatment group lost twice as much as the placebo group, the expected loss in the placebo group is 2.96 lbs. To estimate the within-group standard deviations, we assumed homoscedasticity and assumed that the ratio of means to standard deviations in the proposed study would be the same as we have observed in our other studies of moderate caloric restriction.[86] This yielded expected within-group standard deviations of 4.17. These values were then converted to an effect size estimate $(d)^{75}$ of .708 (i.e., (5.91–2.96)/4.17)).

Entering a d of .708 into Table 22–3, and interpolating, 33 subjects in each group (treatment and placebo) provide 80% power to reject the null hypothesis at the .05 level of significance. Thus a total of 66 subjects are required. Our past experience with clinical weight loss trials indicates that we can expect a 30% dropout rate. Thus, 66/(1–.30), or 95 subjects are required at initial recruitment. Since even numbers are required, 96 subjects were recruited.

DATA ANALYSIS ISSUES

Numerous issues and complexities in the analysis of data are of interest to obesity researchers. These issues are frequently the same issues that are of importance

Table 22–2 A List of Power Analysis Tables

Source	Application	Comments
Bartko et al[148]	Provides two extremely simple to use nomograms for calculating sample size for t-tests.	Nomograms available for both dependent and independent t-tests.
Bird & Hall[149]	Provides tables that are especially useful with multiple comparison procedures such as the Bonferroni and Scheffé.	
Freedman[147]	Presents tables of necessary sample size for use of the logrank test in survival analysis.	
Friedman[84]	Any analysis within the "general linear model."	The basis of Table 22–3 printed in this chapter.
Gatsonis & Sampson[150]	Multiple regression and correlation.	Exact sample size requirements meant to be an improvement over Cohen's[77] approximations.
Hinkle & Oliver[151]	Provides a table for the one-factor ANOVA design with two to eight levels.	A fairly limited range and number of effect sizes are incorporated.
Kraemer & Thiemann[152]	Presents a large "Master Table" covering various levels of α, β, and Δ where Δ is a measure of effect size (the intraclass correlation coefficient).	No estimates are provided for sample sizes less than 10.
Lipsey[153]	Provides power charts (curves) for one- and two-tailed tests for $\alpha = .01, .05, .10, .15,$ and $.20$.	May require some difficult "eyeball" interpolation.
Lui[154]	Presents very useful tables for determining necessary sample sizes for studies involving a dichotomous outcome.	Incorporates repeated measures designs and cost considerations.
Schoenfeld & Richter[155]	Provide easy-to-use nomograms when the dependent variable is time to an event (i.e., survival analysis).	
Shuster[156]	Used primarily for planning large clinical trials where outcome is time to an event (i.e., survival analyses).	Very extensive tables. Software is available to accompany the book and tables.

Table 22–3 Power, Degrees of Freedom, and Effect Sizes for Selected 2-tailed Significance Levels

Alpha = .05

Effect Sizes

Effect Measure	0.05	0.10	0.15	0.20	0.25	0.30	0.35	0.40	0.45	0.50	0.55	0.60	0.65	0.70	0.75	0.80	0.85	0.90	0.95
r_m	0.05	0.10	0.15	0.20	0.25	0.30	0.35	0.40	0.45	0.50	0.55	0.60	0.65	0.70	0.75	0.80	0.85	0.90	0.95
r^2	0.00	0.01	0.02	0.04	0.06	0.09	0.12	0.16	0.20	0.25	0.30	0.36	0.42	0.49	0.56	0.64	0.72	0.81	0.90
d	0.10	0.20	0.30	0.41	0.52	0.63	0.75	0.87	1.01	1.15	1.32	1.50	1.71	1.96	2.27	2.67	3.23	4.13	6.08
f	0.05	0.10	0.15	0.20	0.26	0.31	0.37	0.44	0.50	0.58	0.66	0.75	0.86	0.98	1.13	1.33	1.61	2.06	3.04
f^2	0.00	0.01	0.02	0.04	0.07	0.10	0.14	0.19	0.25	0.33	0.43	0.56	0.73	0.96	1.29	1.78	2.60	4.26	9.26

Power

	0.05	0.10	0.15	0.20	0.25	0.30	0.35	0.40	0.45	0.50	0.55	0.60	0.65	0.70	0.75	0.80	0.85	0.90	0.95
0.1	185	47	21	12	8	6	4	4	3	3	2	2	2	2	1	1	1	1	1
0.2	501	125	56	31	20	14	10	8	6	5	4	4	3	3	2	2	2	2	1
0.3	825	206	91	51	33	23	16	12	10	8	6	5	4	4	3	3	2	2	2
0.4	1165	291	129	72	46	31	23	17	13	11	9	7	6	5	4	3	3	2	2
0.5	1536	383	169	94	60	41	30	22	17	14	11	9	7	6	5	4	3	3	2
0.6	1957	488	215	120	76	52	38	28	22	17	14	11	9	8	6	5	4	3	3
0.7	2466	614	271	151	96	65	47	35	27	21	17	14	11	9	8	6	5	4	3
0.8	3136	781	345	192	121	83	60	45	34	27	22	17	14	11	9	8	6	5	3
0.9	4198	1045	461	257	162	111	80	60	46	36	28	23	18	15	12	10	8	6	4

Alpha = .01

Effect Sizes

Effect Measure	0.05	0.10	0.15	0.20	0.25	0.30	0.35	0.40	0.45	0.50	0.55	0.60	0.65	0.70	0.75	0.80	0.85	0.90	0.95
r_m	0.05	0.10	0.15	0.20	0.25	0.30	0.35	0.40	0.45	0.50	0.55	0.60	0.65	0.70	0.75	0.80	0.85	0.90	0.95
r^2	0.00	0.01	0.02	0.04	0.06	0.09	0.12	0.16	0.20	0.25	0.30	0.36	0.42	0.49	0.56	0.64	0.72	0.81	0.90
d	0.10	0.20	0.30	0.41	0.52	0.63	0.75	0.87	1.01	1.15	1.32	1.50	1.71	1.96	2.27	2.67	3.23	4.13	6.08
f	0.05	0.10	0.15	0.20	0.26	0.31	0.37	0.44	0.50	0.58	0.66	0.75	0.86	0.98	1.13	1.33	1.61	2.06	3.04
f^2	0.00	0.01	0.02	0.04	0.07	0.10	0.14	0.19	0.25	0.33	0.43	0.56	0.73	0.96	1.29	1.78	2.60	4.26	9.26

Power																					
0.1	670	167	74	42	27	18	14	10	8	7	5	4	4	3	3	2	2	2	2	2	1
0.2	1203	300	133	74	47	32	24	18	14	11	9	7	6	5	4	3	3	3	2	2	2
0.3	1683	419	185	103	66	45	33	24	19	15	12	10	8	7	5	4	4	3	3	2	2
0.4	2156	537	237	132	84	57	41	31	24	19	15	12	10	8	7	5	4	4	3	3	3
0.5	2651	660	292	162	103	70	51	38	29	23	18	15	12	10	8	6	5	5	4	4	3
0.6	3197	796	351	196	124	85	61	46	35	28	22	18	14	12	9	8	6	5	5	4	3
0.7	3839	956	422	235	148	101	73	55	42	33	26	21	17	14	11	9	7	6	6	5	4
0.8	4665	1161	512	285	180	123	88	66	51	40	32	25	20	17	13	11	8	7	6	6	4
0.9	5944	1479	653	363	229	156	112	84	64	50	40	32	26	21	17	13	10	8	8	6	5

Source: Adapted with permission from H. Friedman, Simplified Determinations of Statistical Power, Magnitude of Effect and Research Sample Sizes, *Educational Psychology Measurement*, Vol. 42, pp. 521–526, © 1982, Plenum Publishing Corporation.

to people conducting applied data analysis in other fields and are extensively discussed in several books.[87–89] This chapter will briefly mention several analytic issues of interest. These include the use of ratios, polychotomization of continuous data, the use of residuals from regression analysis, and the management of missing data. Furthermore, broader issues will be discussed, such as handling protocol violations in the analysis of clinical trials, methods for analyzing clinical trial data that go beyond the analysis of group means to examine heterogeneity of response, and the conduct of "sensitivity analyses."

Ratios

The use of ratios is common in obesity research. Frequently employed ratios include the waist-to-hip ratio, the activity factor (total energy expenditure/resting metabolic rate), body mass index, the subscapula to tricep-skinfold ratio, percent body fat, and percent fat in the diet. The use of such ratios as a "default strategy" should be seriously questioned. While there are circumstances under which ratios are appropriate and perform quite well, the indiscriminate use of ratios can introduce many potential problems. These problems include introduction of heteroscedasticity into the data, failure to fully control for effects, introduction of spurious correlations, and distortion of the distribution of variables. These issues are extensively discussed by Allison et al.[89]

Polychotomization

Many investigators find it simpler to deal with dichotomous or categorical data than continuous data and therefore polychotomize their continuous data prior to analysis. That is, they divide up their continuous variables into two or more discrete (i.e., nonoverlapping) categories and then test for differences among categories. For example, researchers investigating the effects of body mass index on mortality frequently divide BMI into quintiles and analyze the relative risk of mortality in each quintile. A second example involves researchers using median splits on the distribution of restrained eating scores in studies of human eating behavior and then testing for differences among people "high" and "low" in restraint. Such polychotomization of data is undesirable for several reasons. First, and perhaps most important, it either markedly reduces the power of statistical tests, which may result in increased Type II errors[91] or it can produce spurious relationships among variables, increasing Type I error rate.[92] Second, it can introduce residual confounding into the data when the continuous variable being polychotomized is being used as a control factor or covariate.[93] Finally, the polychotomization of continuous variables can markedly change interaction effects in ways that are not easily predicted.[94] Given these caveats, polychotomization offers a way of investigating the possibility of markedly nonlinear relations between continuous variables and therefore has quite a bit of merit as an exploratory technique. Nevertheless, there are other techniques that allow for the fitting of nonlinear relationships while maintaining the continuous scaling of the variables.[87] Thus, polychotomization of data may be useful for exploratory analyses although it is not recommended as a primary data analytic strategy.

Residual Analysis

The use of residuals from a regression analysis is also a common method in obesity research. For example, some investigators regress resting metabolic rate on lean body mass and calculate the residual from the regression line. This residual is then taken as an index of unusually high or low energy expenditure and is then used as a dependent or independent variable in subsequent analyses. Although this method has the advantage of simplicity, the regression coefficient estimated in this manner in the first regression is not necessarily an unbiased estimator. This method also affects the standard error of coefficients in subsequent analyses. Therefore, it is best to control for the variable of interest and the confounding variables in a single analysis rather than in this "stagewise" procedure.[95,96]

Missing Data

Missing data represents one of the most ubiquitous and complex problems presented to the applied data analyst. This is especially true in obesity research where both multivariate and longitudinal data are common. It is rare for any given subject to have complete data on all variables in a study that has many longitudinal measurements on many variables. There are many methods for handling missing data.[97] Methods include listwise deletion, pairwise deletion, various imputation strategies, multiple group structural equation modeling,[98] hierarchical linear modeling,[99] the use of the EM algorithm,[100] and other methods.[101] By far the most common approach appears to be listwise deletion. In listwise deletion any subject that does not have complete data for all variables required for an analysis is excluded from that analysis. This can have two unfortunate consequences. First, it forces the investigator to discard much data. Second, it can, under certain circumstances, lead to biased results. Therefore, investigators should explore more sophisticated missing-data strategies that make greater use of all of the available data. Although a complete discussion of these strategies is beyond the scope of this chapter, several useful discussions are available.[100,102,103]

Handling Protocol Violations in the Analysis

The essence of a carefully planned randomized controlled trial is to assess properly whether treatments differ with respect to primary outcomes. No matter how meticulously a trial is planned, it is almost inevitable that some patients (or investigators) will deviate from the protocol specifications. There are innumerable ways that protocol violations can adversely affect a proper assessment of treatment efficacy or toxicity. It is important to at least minimize bias of treatment comparisons from protocol violations that include ineligible patients; patient withdrawals and incomplete evaluations; and patients who do not comply with the randomly assigned therapy as evidenced by their later switching to the other therapy, a different therapy, or no therapy while enrolled in the study.

A consensus exists to avoid or minimize bias of treatment efficacy stemming from protocol violations: All patients should be analyzed according to the treatment to which they were randomly assigned regardless of their protocol violations. This approach is known as intention to treat—that is, analyze all patients by the way they are randomized. The intention-to-treat approach provides a more valid assessment of treatment comparisons because it is only at randomization that the treatment groups are expected to be equivalent, with any difference thereafter expected to be due to treatment. This approach takes into account actual clinical practice and whether offering a treatment is beneficial. Patient withdrawals, noncompliance with the assigned treatment, and losses to follow-up may relate to factors that distinguish treatments and affect the risk of the outcome. Failure to analyze data on all randomized participants could introduce substantial bias. While this approach is optimal to estimate the true effect, it can lead to a conservative underestimate of the true treatment effect, especially when treatment compliance is low or losses to follow-up are high.

An alternative approach is to analyze only those patients who receive the treatment according to protocol; patients who either withdraw or do not comply are not considered in the analysis. But this approach is more likely to distort treatment comparisons, by overestimating treatment effect. While it is possible to adjust for known confounders in the analysis, analyzing only these patients makes it impossible to regain the balance of unknown confounders between treatment groups that had been achieved originally through randomization.

Suppose that a randomized control trial involved the comparison of two types of diet rehabilitation (intensive, conventional) on subsequent coronary heart disease (yes, no), using the data in Table 22–4. Using the traditional 0.05 level of statistical significance, the initial interpretation is that conventional rehabilitation gives a significantly higher proportion of coronary heart disease than intensive rehabilitation (15/45 vs 6/46), with p-value equal to 0.02. However, suppose that data were later obtained on the 15 patients who withdrew from conventional treatment and 2 patients who withdrew from intensive treatment, and none of them had coronary heart disease. Including these patients in an intention-to-treat analysis produces no statistical evidence of a treatment difference (p-value = 0.10). With-

Table 22–4 Three Analyses of Hypothetical Data from a Randomized Control Trial

Coronary Heart Disease	Dietary Treatment		p
	Intensive	Conventional	
Analysis of data from cases in initial sample			
Yes	6	15	
No	40	30	
Total assessed	46	45	
Withdrawn patients	2	15	
Basis for comparison	6/46	14/45	0.020
Analysis of data from randomly assigned cases (intention to treat)			
Yes	6	15	
No	42	45	
Total randomized	48	60	
Basis for comparison	6/48	15/60	0.100
Analysis of data from cases actually treated			
Yes	6	15	
No	55	32	
Patients originally randomized to other treatment	15	2	
Incorrect comparison	6/61	15/47	0.004
Correct comparison	6/46	15/45	0.020

drawal from treatment, whatever the reason, should not preclude a patient from subsequent evaluations. Sackett[104] illustrates the same principle.

Fifteen patients randomized to conventional treatment later switched to intensive treatment and two patients randomized to intensive treatment later switched to conventional treatment; none of them had coronary heart disease. Reaching the same conclusion as the analysis based on compliers only (Table 22–4), the analysis based on treatment actually taken at follow-up gives a spurious benefit in favor of intensive rehabilitation (p-value = 0.004). Patients should be analyzed, therefore, according to the treatment to which they were randomized.

Because complete follow-up data are often not available, it is desirable to undertake supplemental analyses aimed at quantifying the degree of conservatism implied by the main analysis from intention to treat. One supplemental analysis should assume that none of the patients lost to follow-up has experienced the outcome. Another analysis may assume that all such patients have experienced the outcome, and another that they experienced the outcome at the same rate as the proportion of control patients under follow-up. Losses to follow-up are not a serious concern if alternative analyses reach the same conclusion and if they are not differential by treatment group. The best standard is to maintain high levels of compliance, keep losses to follow-up at a minimum, and collect complete information on all randomized patients. Methods for handling protocol violations and related issues in clinical trials can be found in several books.[6,105–108]

Going Beyond the Mean

The analysis of mean (i.e., average) differences among treatment and control groups is one common method of evaluating the efficacy of an intervention. However, the use of grouped data may obfuscate the effectiveness of the treatment on various subgroups of individuals. Thus, alternative methods of analysis that are based on individual cases may at times provide a more sensitive evaluation of the treatment effect.

One such analytic alternative, pattern analysis, was proposed by Holman.[109] The authors present a treatment assessment method employing an a priori criteria of treatment success. Individuals are then classified as "successes" or "failures" based upon the a priori standard. Following the individual classifications, the proportions of successes and failures between treatment and control groups are compared. This approach offers the advantage of assessing the treatment effect on an individual basis and challenges the researcher to conceptualize and incorporate a refined operational definition of a desired treatment outcome. Furthermore, the use of an a priori evaluation standard facilitates a more objective case assessment than the reliance on post hoc clinical judgments.

Extending the work of Holman et al,[109] Allison[110] outlines various considerations when employing pattern analysis. First, it is suggested that the researcher employ several definitions of success because the effectiveness of a treatment may be relative to the criteria employed. Thus, the incorporation of a range of success criteria may provide a better assessment of the sensitivity of the outcome given particular definitions of success. Second, the assessment of success does not provide information concerning negative treatment outcomes (iatrogenic failure). While it is important to assess the relative probability of a successful outcome given a treatment condition, it behooves the researcher to evaluate the relative probability of a failure or worsening of a condition. Overall, although the use of group mean evaluations will remain an analytic mainstay, the consideration of other analytic techniques that can further elucidate the effectiveness of interventions is recommended.

Sensitivity Analyses

The investigator is often confronted with several decisions associated with the data analytic procedures employed. Examples of such decisions include the exclusion or inclusion of outliers and the appropriateness of sample data transformations. Often there are no clear-cut decision rules or predictable outcomes. In such situations the use of "sensitivity analyses" is recommended.

Sensitivity analysis refers to the evaluation of a particular outcome given as a function of the specific analytic procedure employed. For example, a sensitivity analysis might evaluate the extent to which a particular outcome is dependent upon the inclusion or exclusion of data points or the use of a particular transformation. Thus, it is recommended that if one is unsure about whether to include outliers or not, analysis of the data with the outliers included and then excluded may facilitate the decision of whether or not to incorporate them. It is recommended that the researcher incorporate the results of the various analyses in the study report to provide the reader with a richer source to draw conclusions from.

META-ANALYSES

Investigators rely heavily on a literature review to define the present state of knowledge. In many areas, the literature has developed into a rapidly increasing body of published and unpublished studies. How can an obesity researcher quantify the effects of weight reduction from different diets based on studies with conflicting results? How can such information be combined to arrive at a general conclusion? Questions like these have increased the need for meta-analysis. While it can be applied to data of any sort, meta-analysis has been commonly used to combine results from different studies to draw conclusions about treatments. A special feature of meta-analysis, which distinguishes it from the traditional narrative review, is that the results from individual studies are integrated and quantified, rather than being based on judgment alone.

Meta-analysis has been used to address uncertainty when results disagree, to increase statistical power for primary outcomes and subgroups, to improve estimates of the size of effect, and to lead to new knowledge and questions.[111] The number of publications on meta-analysis has increased greatly over the last few years. There are several meta-analyses that address weight management issues.[112–116] and publications covering general meta-analytic issues.[117–120] Abramson[121] provides a chapter on meta-analysis with ample references and examples as well as a checklist showing how to evaluate a meta-analysis.

The discussion in this section is general, applying to obesity research as well as other areas. The focus here is how one can evaluate a meta-analysis of randomized (experimental) and nonrandomized (nonexperimental) studies aimed at comparing treatments. To evaluate a meta-analysis, one must evaluate (1) the identification, selection, and quality of the studies; (2) the extraction of data; (3) how the data were combined; and (4) how the results were analyzed. These four broad areas are interrelated. Figure 22–5 is a pictorial representation of these steps.

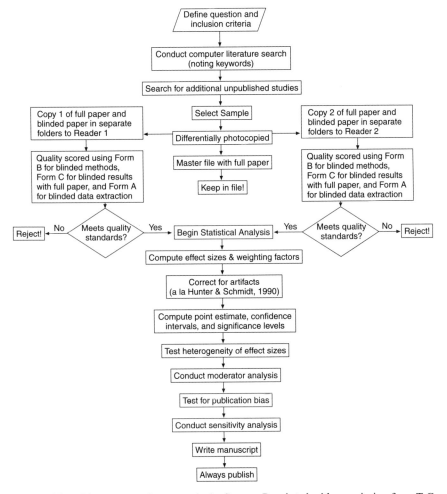

Figure 22–5 The process of meta-analysis. *Source:* Reprinted with permission from T.C. Chalmers and J. Lau, *Statistical Methods in Medical Research,* Vol. 2, No. 2, pp. 161–172, © 1993, Edward Arnold Publishers.

Identification, Selection, and Quality of Studies

After knowing the objectives and scope of the meta-analysis, the assessor of a meta-analysis should note how the studies were identified and selected. What is typically required is a systematic search of the literature using, for example, MEDLARS and *Current Contents.* These formal searches should be supplemented by informal searches through scanning the references of review articles and relevant studies. Unpublished studies, which tend to give negative or inconclusive findings, should be included whenever possible to overcome publication bias, which tends to exaggerate the overall treatment effect. One way to assess the possible bias due to the omission of unidentified studies is to calculate how many studies with no treatment effect are needed to change a combined result from significant to nonsignificant.[122] The larger the number of such studies, the smaller the impact of publication bias.

The issue of publication bias and a method for its detection are illustrated in Figure 22–6 taken from Allison, Faith, and Gorman.[123] Figure 22–6 shows the results (in terms of weight) of 68 trials of drug treatment of obesity plotted against $1/N^{.5}$, where N is the combined sample size of the study. The rationale for this analysis is that a treatment's effect size is normally distributed with a finite mean and variance and, as with any normal distribution, the mean and variance are independent. In other words, there is no reason why larger studies should obtain smaller or larger weight losses than smaller studies. However, larger studies will produce effect size estimates with smaller variances that are therefore more likely to be statistically significant even with a relatively small effect size (given that there is some non-zero population effect). In contrast, smaller studies are unlikely to have statistically significant results unless the effect size is very large. Because of the above relations, if significant findings are more likely to be published than

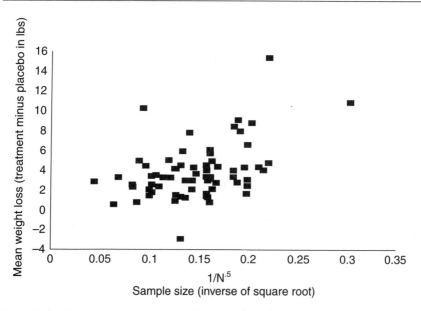

Figure 22–6 Meta-analysis of data from 68 obesity drug interventions illustrating misleading effect size estimates. *Source:* Reprinted with permission from D.B. Allison, M. Faith, and B.S. Gorman, Publication Bias in Obesity Treatment Research, *International Journal of Obesity,* Vol. 20, pp. 931–937, © 1996, Macmillan Press.

nonsignificant findings, across many studies, this will produce a positive correlation between effect size and its standard error (or $1/N^5$). As can be seen in Figure 22–6, such a positive association is present and is statistically significant. This suggests that there is publication bias with respect to trials of pharmacological treatment of obesity such that treatment outcome studies yielding statistically significant findings are more likely to be published. This implies that estimates of treatment efficacy based on average reported effect sizes in the literature are likely to be overestimates of actual treatment efficacy.

The selection of studies should be tied to the objectives of the meta-analysis. A broader objective will typically include more studies. If the question asked is whether weight reduction reduces cholesterol for patients of all ages, then more studies will be selected than if the researcher asked whether weight reduction reduces cholesterol in adolescents. A biased selection of studies will obviously lead to biased results. An objective, unbiased selection can be fostered by explicit inclusion and exclusion criteria that are completely independent of the results of the studies. Part III of *The Handbook of Research Synthesis*[124] is devoted to the identification and selection of studies.

The quality of a meta-analysis depends on the quality of its studies. Possible biases can be inherent in the studies themselves, before data extraction begins, especially in nonexperimental studies. The quality of the studies should be appraised in accordance with acceptable scientific principles generally regarded as important to make valid inferences. For example, studies can be classified and analyzed according to their study design: randomized studies with blinding (the most valid), randomized studies without blinding, observational studies, uncontrolled studies (the least valid). Randomized control trials that are combined have generally higher quality than nonexperimental studies in which non-randomly selected treatment groups are compared and combined. More complete follow-up information is a desirable feature. An analysis based on intention to treat gives more reliable information than on an analysis based on treatment actually received. It is worthwhile to determine whether measures of treatment effect have been adjusted for confounding when different patient characteristics exist between treatment groups in nonexperimental studies and how losses to follow-up on outcomes were handled for patients who did not continue with their randomized regimen in experimental studies.

Did the authors of the meta-analysis give sufficient attention to quality? Did they consider the potential problems of studies with poor quality? A reader of a meta-analysis should note what precautions were taken to appraise the quality among studies. These may include discarding all studies of poor quality, comparing the combined results with and without the studies of poor quality, and using statistical techniques that account for study quality. Critiques of quality assessment can be found in several publications.[39,125–127]

Extraction of Data

Having only one reviewer extract the data from studies may increase bias in the collection of data. It is preferable in most cases to have two or more reviewers extract data and to have their disagreements resolved by discussion. A critique of a meta-analysis should consider whether, to reduce possible bias, the authors used explicit guidelines in advance for extracting data on specific outcomes and potential risk factors. A meta-analysis that reports important data for each study not only unveils the data extraction for scrutiny but also allows the validation of the results. Any limitation on data extraction, whether or not mentioned in the article, must be considered when interpreting the results.

Meta-analyses of nonexperimental studies have often involved the pooling of two or more outcomes to arrive at an overall treatment effect. If different studies contribute different numbers of outcomes, studies with more relevant outcomes will have a greater overall impact on the results, which must be considered when interpreting results. Moreover, in multiple-treatment experimental and nonexperimental studies, where each study involves several types of exercise compared with a sedentary control, each treatment comparison is no longer independent. Because such independence is an assumption of statistical tests, the cautious reader should note how (if at all) the possible correlations among the estimated treatment effects were accounted for in the analysis. Gleser and Olkin[128] discuss methods of handling dependence among measures of effect.

Combining Results

A major issue in pooling data is whether the results of separate trials can be meaningfully combined. Meta-analysis has been criticized for mixing "apples and oranges"—that is, combining the results of studies that are so different that it is uncertain whether the results can be legitimately combined.[129–132] It is therefore essential to appraise the combinability and consistency of results. A narrowly defined inclusion criteria, consistent with the objectives of the meta-analysis, is a desirable way of evaluating whether the studies analyzed were similar enough to be pooled.

Related to combinability is the issue of heterogeneity of treatment effects across studies. A statistical test for heterogeneity[133] is one way to examine heterogeneity or consistency among study results. If this test gives a low p-value, for example, less than 0.10, possible explanations and complementary analyses should be explored. Because the test of heterogeneity has low statistical power for detecting true heterogeneity, however, a nonsignificant statistical finding should be interpreted cautiously. The issue here is not whether true heterogeneity exists but rather whether it is of substantial magnitude to qualify or adjust the results. Differences among studies in design, patient characteristics, and definition of outcomes are among the factors that can contribute to heterogeneity.

A graph of study treatment effects and a factor of interest, for instance, risk ratios and mean length of study follow-up, may prove informative. Another way to visually inspect heterogeneity in a meta-analysis comes from a cumulative meta-analysis where a cumulative, combined treatment effect appears for each study with all studies ordered by a factor of interest.[134] For example, the combined, cumulative odds ratios up to a given study, which is based on results from that study and all studies that proceed it in terms of year of publication, may provide insight on how the odds ratio (the treatment effect) changes cumulatively with year of publication (the factor of interest).

A judicious meta-analysis often involves the comparison of combined results with all studies and without studies thought to be different enough to affect the conclusions; an analysis that excludes such studies is known as a sensitivity analysis (see above). Finding out the results for relevant subgroups is another way to help decipher heterogeneity. When subsets of studies are compared, it should be made clear whether this was done to test a planned, a priori hypothesis or an unplanned, data-driven hypothesis. Subgroup analyses based on the former lead to more reliable inferences in a meta-analysis than those based on the latter.

In a meta-analysis of randomized control trials it is generally advisable to check for differences among control rates (i.e., the proportion of events in the control group). The control rate in a study can serve as a measure of the baseline risk of disease of patients in a study.[135,136] It may be linked to factors such as mean length of follow-up, definition and ascertainment of outcome, treatment protocol, and patient characteristics—factors that may lead to heterogeneity of study results. Careful reading of the characteristics of the randomized studies, coupled with their control rates, would probably clarify matters.

Heterogeneity can sometimes occur when adjusted treatment effects (adjusted for an important baseline covariate that is different between treatment groups) from some nonexperimental studies are combined with unadjusted (crude) treatment effects from other nonexperimental studies, arriving at a questionable overall estimate of treatment effect. A confounder is a variable that is related both to the treatment and, independently, to the outcome. A confounder can mask, diminish, reverse, or exaggerate an association between treatment and outcome. Empirical evidence of confounding in a study occurs when there is a marked difference between crude and adjusted estimates of treatment effect. Confounding is generally not a concern in a meta-analysis of randomized control trials, but must be addressed in a meta-analysis of nonexperimental studies.

Heterogeneity of results across studies may also express effect modification, which when spotted makes heterogeneity an asset rather than a liability. An effect modifier is a variable that modifies the association between treatment and outcome; as such, it has important clinical implications. Evidence of effect modification occurs when the association between treatment and outcome depends on the effect modifier, so the reporting of only one overall treatment effect can be misleading. The possibility of effect modifiers should be investigated in both a meta-analysis of experimental studies and a meta-analysis of nonexperimental studies.

Analyzing the Results

Valid techniques for pooling results of separate studies have one element in common: an estimate of treatment effect is calculated first for each study and then combined across studies. Simply lumping the numbers together, as if only one large study has been done, can be misleading. A reviewer of a meta-analysis should examine whether studies with more information or precision were given more weight; this is an optimal way to pool. Another consideration is whether the measure of effect chosen is consistent with the objectives of the meta-analysis. For example, ratio measures assess determinants of disease and the magnitude of the association between disease and treatment. Absolute differences in risk, on the other hand, deal with the public health impact that the treatments have on disease.

To help address concerns of combinability, two types of models have been devised in meta-analysis. In the fixed effects model, which leads to inferences only about the studies assembled, each study is assumed to have the same treatment effect and only within-study variability of treatment effect is considered. In the random effects model, which leads to inferences about all studies in a hypothetical population, each study can have a different effect that is randomly positioned about some central value, and both among-study and within-study variability of treatment effect are considered.

The random effects model is favored over the fixed effects model when there is a substantial amount of heterogeneity—that is, when there is no common measure of treatment effect across studies. Models for discrete data include the fixed effects Mantel-Haenszel procedure[137] and the random effects DerSimonian-Laird procedure.[138] For continuous data, effects sizes exist for fixed effects models[139] and random effects models.[140] A critique of a meta-analysis requires an understanding of the appropriate statistical methods of pooling, which can found in Hedges and Olkin[141] and Cooper and Hedges.[124]

Effect modifiers can be evaluated not only by comparing the treatment effects across the values of the suspecting effect modifier but also by meta-regression.[121,142–144] A reader of a meta-analysis should check whether a regression of treatment effects on a potential modifier was done. Or, for each subgroup or category of a potential effect modifier, whether the regression coefficient of treatment from the regression of outcome on treatment was tested as being different across subgroups. Alternatively, a reader could ask whether the coefficient of the interaction between treatment and modifier on outcome was included in a regression model, which also contains a treatment variable and a suspected effect modifier as predictors. If a regression model was employed, one should note how the suspected confounders, which can be controlled by adding them to the regression model, were handled. It is more desirable to weight each study in the meta-regression proportional to its precision (e.g., the inverse of the variance of a study's treatment effect) rather than weighting the studies equally. While potentially informative, the results of meta-regression based on covariates with aggregate numbers (e.g., group averages) should be interpreted as cautiously as other ecological investigations.[145,146]

The confidence intervals produced by statistical methods should be examined. The evaluator of a meta-analysis should decide whether the results were interpreted correctly and whether the conclusions were presented with appropriate reservations.

CONCLUSION

This discussion is by no means an exhaustive presentation of all design issues and data analytic strategies of interest to the obesity researcher. Nevertheless, it is hoped that this chapter provides useful information for obesity researchers that can be used to both strengthen their own research as well as their interpretations of others' data.

ACKNOWLEDGMENTS

Supported in part by National Institutes of Health grants DKY2618, DK26687, and R29DK47256-01A1 (D.B.A), grant R01 HS07782 from the Agency for Health Care Policy and Research, U.S. Public Health Services (J.C.C.), and grant MH13043 from the National Institute of Mental Health (K.M.C.).

The authors gratefully acknowledge Bernard S. Gorman, Myles Faith, and Elizabeth M. Kucera for their helpful comments and assistance in the preparation of this manuscript.

REFERENCES

1. Gilbert JP, Light RJ, Mosteller F. Assessing social innovations: an empirical basis for policy. In: Bennett CA and Lumsdaine AA, eds. *Evaluation and Experiment.* New York: Academic Press; 1975:39–193.

2. Cappelleri JC, Trochim WMK. An illustrative statistical analysis of cutoff-based randomized clinical trials. *J Clin Epidemiol.* 1994;47:261–270.

3. Cook TD, Campbell DT. *Quasi-Experimentation: Design and Analysis Issues in Field Settings.* Boston: Houghton-Mifflin; 1979.

4. Rubin DB. Estimating causal effects of treatments in randomized and nonrandomized studies. *J Educ Psychol.* 1974;66:688–701.

5. Zelen M. A new design for randomized clinical trials. *N Engl J Med.* 1979;300:1242–1246.

6. Meinert CL. *Clinical Trials: Design, Conduct, and Analysis.* New York: Oxford University Press; 1986.

7. Ederer F. Why do we need controls? Why do we need to randomize? *Am J Ophthalmol.* 1975;79:758–762.

8. Pedhazur EJ, Schmelkin LP. *Measurement, Design, and Analysis: An Integrated Approach.* Hillsdale, NJ: Lawrence Erlbaum; 1991.

9. Hsu LM. Random sampling, randomization, and equivalence of contrasted groups in psychotherapy outcome research. *J Consult Clin Psychol.* 1989;57:131–137.

10. Tukey JW. Tightening the clinical trial. *Controlled Clin Trials.* 1993;14:266–285.

11. Kirk RE. *Experimental Design: Procedures for the Behavioral Sciences.* 2nd ed. Pacific Grove, CA: Brook/Cole; 1983.

12. Lachin JM, Matts JP, Wei LJ. Randomization in clinical trials: conclusions and recommendations. *Controlled Clin Trials.* 1988;9:365–374.

13. Pocock SJ. Allocation of patients to treatment in clinical trials. *Biometrics.* 1979;35:183–197.

14. Guyatt GH, Heyting A, Jaeschke R, Keller J, Adachi JD, Roberts RS. N of 1 randomized trials for investigating new drugs. *Controlled Clin Trials.* 1990;11:88–100.

15. Lachin JM. Statistical properties of randomization in clinical trials. *Controlled Clin Trials.* 1988;9:289–311.

16. Rundell BA, Brown BW, Herson J. A randomization list generator for biomedical experiments. *Comput Prog Biomed.* 1982;14:171–174.

17. Ryan BF, Joiner BL, Ryan TA Jr. *Minitab Handbook.* 2nd ed. Boston: Duxbury Press; 1985.

18. Moses LE, Oakford RV. *Tables of Random Permutations.* Stanford, CA: Stanford University Press; 1963.

19. "Student." The Lanarkshire milk experiment. *Biometrika.* 1931;23.

20. Feder F. Why do we need controls? Why do we need to randomize? *Am J Ophthalmol.* 1975;79:758–762.

21. Wright IS, Marpel, CD, Beck DF. *Myocardial Infarction: Its Clinical Manifestations and Treatment with Anticoagulants.* New York: Grune and Stratton; 1954.

22. Achen CH. *The Statistical Analysis of Quasi-Experiments.* Berkley, CA: University of California Press; 1986.

23. Allison DB, Kreibich K, Heshka S, Heymsfield SB. A randomized placebo-controlled clinical trial of an acupressure device for weight loss. *Int J Obes.* 1995;19:653–658.

24. Reichardt CS. The statistical analysis of data from nonequivalent group designs. In: Cook TD, Campbell DT, eds. *Quasi-Experimentation: Design and Analysis Issues for Field Settings.* Boston: Houghton Mifflin; 1979:147–205.

25. Lord FM. A paradox in the interpretation of group comparisons. *Psychol Bull.* 1967;68:304–305.

26. Lord FM. Statistical adjustments when comparing pre-existing groups. *Psychol Bull.* 1979;72:336–337.

27. Trochim WMK. The regression-discontinuity design. In: Sechrest L, Perrin P, Bunker J, eds. *Research Methodology: Strengthening Causal Interpretations of Nonexperimental Data.* Washington, DC: US Public Health Service; 1991:119–139.

28. Trochim WMK, Cappelleri JC. Cutoff assignment strategies for enhancing randomized clinical trials. *Controlled Clin Trials.* 1992;13:190–212.

29. Cappelleri JC, Trochim WMK. Ethical and scientific features of cutoff-based designs: a simulation study. *Med Decis Making.* 1995;15:387–394.

30. Mohr LB. *Impact Analysis for Program Evaluation.* Chicago: Dorsey Press; 1988.

31. Berk RA, Rossi PH. *Thinking About Program Evaluation.* Newbury Park, CA: Sage Publications; 1990.

32. Coyle SL, Boruch RF, Turner CF, eds. *Evaluating AIDS Prevention Programs.* Washington, DC: National Academy Press; 1991.

33. Marcantonio RJ, Cook TD. Convincing quasi-experiments: the interrupted time series and regression-discontinuity designs. In: Wholey JS, Hatry HP, Newcomer KE, eds. *Handbook of Practical Program Evaluation.* San Francisco: Jossey-Bass; 1994:133–154.

34. Cappelleri JC, Trochim WMK, Stanley TD, Reichardt CS. Random measurement error doesn't bias the treatment effect estimate in the regression-discontinuity design: I. The case of no interaction. *Eval Rev.* 1991;15:395–419.

35. Goldberger AS. *Selection Bias in Evaluating Treatment Effects: Some Formal Illustrations.* Discussion paper 123–72. Madison, WI: Institute for Research on Poverty; 1972.

36. Cappelleri JC, Darlington RB, Trochim WMK. Power analysis of cutoff-based randomized clinical trials. *Eval Rev.* 1984;18:141–152.

37. Chalmers TC, Smith H Jr, Blackburn B, et al. A method for assessing the quality of a randomized control trial. *Controlled Clin Trials.* 1981;2:31–49.

38. Skinner BF. *Science and Human Behavior.* New York: The Free Press; 1953.

39. Sidman M. *Tactics of Scientific Research: Evaluating Experimental Data in Psychology.* New York: Basic Books; 1960.

40. Franklin RD, Allison DB, Gorman BS. *Design and Analysis of Single-Case Research.* Hillsdale, NJ: Erlbaum Publishing; 1997.

41. Sugai G. Single subject research in bilingual special education. *NABE: J Nat Assoc Bilingual Educ.* 1981;12:65–84.

42. Kearney S, Fussey I. The use of adapted leisure materials to reinforce correct head positioning in a brain-injured adult. *Brain Injury.* 1991;5:295–302.

43. Wagenaar RC, Van Wieringen PCW, Netelenbos JB, Meijer OG, Kuik DJ. The transfer of scanning training effects in visual inattention after stroke: five single-case studies. *Disabil Rehab.* 1992;14:51–60.

44. Kearns DW, Crossman J. Effects of a cognitive intervention package on the free-throw performance of varsity basketball players during practice and competition. *Percep Mot Skills.* 1992;75:1243–1253.

45. Rogers-Wallgren JL, French R, Ben-Ezra V. Use of reinforcement to increase independence in physical fitness performance of profoundly mentally retarded youth. *Percep Mot Skills.* 1992;75:975–982.

46. Williams JG. Effects of instruction and practice on ball catching skill: single-subject study of an 8-year-old. *Percep Mot Skills.* 1992;75:392–394.

47. Estrada CA, Young MJ. Patient preferences for novel therapy: an n-of-1 trial of garlic in the treatment for hypertension. *J Gen Intern Med.* 1993;8:619–621.

48. Johannssen T, Petersen H, Kristensen P, Fosstvedt D. The controlled single subject trial. *Scand J Prim Health Care.* 1991;9:17–21.

49. Senn S. Suspended judgement n-of-1 trials. *Controlled Clin Trials.* 1993;14:1–5.

50. Aronoff NJ, Geliebter A, Hashim SS, Zammit GK. The relationship between daytime and nighttime food intake in an obese night eater. *Obes Res.* 1994;2:145–151.

51. De Luca RV, Holborn SW. Effects of a variable-ratio reinforcement schedule with changing criteria on exercise in obese and nonobese boys. *J Appl Behav Anal.* 1992;25:671–679.

52. De Luca RV, Holborn SW. Effects of fixed-interval schedule of token reinforcement on exercise with obese and non-obese boys. *Psychol Rec.* 1985;35:525–533.

53. De Luca RV, Holborn SW. Effects of fixed-interval and fixed-ratio schedules of token reinforcement on exercise with obese and non-obese boys. *Psychol Rec.* 1990;40:67–82.

54. Aragona J, Cassady J, Drabman RS. Treating overweight children through parental training and contingency contracting. *J Appl Behav Anal.* 1975;8:269–278.

55. Smith GR, Medlik L. Modification of binge eating in anorexia nervosa: a single case report. *Behav Psychother.* 1983;11:249–256.

56. Zlachevsky-Ojeda AM. Anorexia nervosa: behavioral modification using a single case design. *Revista Chile Psicol.* 1981;4:21–25.

57. Agras WS, et al. Behavior modification of anorexia nervosa. *Arch Gen Psychiatry.* 1974;30:279–286.

58. Barlow DH, Hersen M. *Single Case Experimental Designs.* New York: Pergamon; 1984.

59. Kazdin AE. Single-case research designs. In: *Methods for Clinical and Applied Settings.* New York: Oxford University Press; 1982.

60. Hartmann DP, Hall RV. The changing criterion design. *J Appl Behav Anal.* 1976;9:527–532.

61. Ingelfinger JA. Has the treatment of the patient? Intrasubject and intersubject variability. In: Ingelfinger JA, ed, *Biostatisitcs in Clinical Medicine.* New York: Macmillian Publishing; 1983.

62. Allison DB, Gorman BS. Calculating and estimating effect sizes for meta-analysis: the case of the single case. *Behav Res Ther.* 1983;31:621–631.

63. Busk PL, Serlin RC. Meta-analysis for single-case research. In: Kratochwill TR, Levin JR, eds. *Single-Case Research Design and Analysis: New Directions for Psychology and Education.* Hillsdale, NJ: Lawrence Erlbaum; 1992:187–212.

64. Faith M, Allison DB, Gorman BS. Meta-analysis. In: Franklin RD, Allison DB, Gorman BS, eds. *Design and Analysis of Single-Case Research.* Hillsdale, NJ: Erlbaum Publishing; 1997:245–277.

65. Beasley M, Allison DB, Gorman, B. The potentially confounding effects of cyclicity: identification, prevention and control. In: Franklin RD, Allison DB, Gorman BS, eds. *Design and Analysis of Single-Case Research.* Hillsdale, NJ: Erlbaum Publishing; 1997:279–333.

66. Allison DB. When cyclicity is a concern: a caveat regarding phase change criteria in single-case designs. *Compr Ment Health Care.* 1992;2:131–149.

67. Edgington ES. Random assignment and statistical tests for one-subject experiments. *Behav Assess.* 1980;2:19–28.

68. Kratochwill TR, Levin JR. *Single-Case Research Design and Analysis.* Hillsdale, NJ: Lawrence Erlbaum; 1992.

69. Baer DM. Perhaps it would be better not to know everything. *J Appl Behav Anal.* 1977;10:167–172.

70. Gorman BS, Allison DB. Statistical alternatives. In: Franklin RD, Allison DB, Gorman BS, eds. *Design and Analysis of Single-Case Research.* Hillsdale, NJ: Erlbaum Publishing; 1997:159–202.

71. Cohen J. The statistical power of abnormal-social psychological research: a review. *J Abnorm*

Soc Psychol. 1962;65:145–153.

72. Rossi JS. Statistical power of psychological research: what have we gained in 20 years? *J Consult Clin Psychol.* 1990;58:646–656.

73. Sedlmeier P, Girgenzer G. Do studies of statistical power have an effect on the power of studies? *Psychol Bull.* 1989;105:309–316.

74. Gorman BS, Primavera LH, Allison DB. PowPal: software for generalized power analysis. *Educ Psychol Measur.* 1995;55:773–776.

75. Cohen J. *Statistical Power Analysis for the Behavioral Sciences.* Hillsdale, NJ: Lawrence Erlbaum; 1988.

76. Ravussin E, Swinburn BA. Energy metabolism. In: Stunkard AJ, Wadden TA, eds. *Obesity: Theory and Therapy.* New York: Raven Press; 1993.

77. Abelson RP. *Statistics as Principled Argument.* Hillsdale, NJ: Erlbaum Publishing; 1995.

78. Allison DB, Silverstein JM, Gorman BS. Power, sample size estimation, and early stopping rules. In: Franklin RD, Allison SD, Gorman BS, eds. *Design and Analysis of Single-Case Research.* Hillsdale, NJ: Erlbaum Publishing; 1997.

79. Lehr R. Sixteen S-squared over *D*-squared: a relation for crude sample estimates. *Stat Med.* 1992;11:1099–1102.

80. Dallal GE. The 17/10 rule for sample size determinations. *Amer Stat.* 1992;46:70.

81. Darlington RB. *Regression and Linear Models.* New York: McGraw-Hill; 1990:385–386.

82. Hays WL. *Statistics. 4th ed.* Philadelphia: Holt, Rinehart, & Winston; 1988.

83. Bradley DR. *Datasim.* Lewiston, ME: Desktop Press; 1989.

84. Friedman H. Simplified determinations of statistical power, magnitude of effect and research sample sizes. *Educ Psychol Measur.* 1982;42:521–526.

85. Forbes GB. *Human Body Composition. Growth, Aging, Nutrition, and Activity.* New York: Springer-Verlag; 1987.

86. Hoy MK, Heshka S, Allison DB, Grasset E, Blank B, Heymsfield SB. Reduced risk of liver function test abnormalities and new gallstone formation with weight loss on 800 calorie formula diets. *Amer J Clin Nutr.* 1994;60:249–254.

87. Cohen J, Cohen P. *Applied Multiple Regression/Correlation Analysis for the Behavioral Sciences.* 2nd ed. Hillsdale, NJ: Lawrence Erlbaum; 1983.

88. Collins LM, Seitz LA, eds. *Advances in Data Analysis for Prevention Intervention Research.* Washington DC: US Government Printing Office; 1994. National Institute on Drug Abuse Research Monograph 142.

89. Stevens J. *Applied Multivariate Statistics for the Social Sciences.* 2nd ed. Hillsdale, NJ: Lawrence Erlbaum; 1992.

90. Allison DB, Paultre F, Goran MI, Poehlman ET, Heymsfield SB. Statistical considerations regarding the use of ratios to adjust data. *Int J Obes.* 1995;19:644–652.

91. Cohen J. The cost of dichotomization. *Appl Psychol Measur.* 1983;7:249–253.

92. Maxwell SE, Delaney H. Bivariate median splits and spurious statistical significance. *Psychol Bull.* 1983;113:181–190.

93. Becher H. The concept of residual confounding in the regression models and some applications. *Stat Med.* 1992;11:1747–1758.

94. Veil HOF. Base-rates, cut-points, and interaction effects: the problem with dichotomized continuous variables. *Psychol Med.* 1988;18:703–710.

95. Bollen KA, Ward S. Ratio variables in aggregrate data analysis: their uses, problems, and alternatives. *Sociol Methods Res.* 1979;7:431–450.

96. Maxwell SE, Delaney H, Manheimer JM. ANOVA of residuals and ANCOVA: correcting an illusion by using model comparisons and graphs. *J Educ Stat.* 1983;10:197–209.

97. Allison DB, Gorman BS, Primavera LH. Some of the most common questions asked of statistical consultants: our favorite responses and recommended readings. *Genet Soc Gen Psychol Monogr.* 1993;119:153–185.

98. McArdle JJ. Structural factor analysis experiments with incomplete data. *Multivar Behav Res.* 1994;29:409–454.

99. Bryk AS, Raudenbush SW. *Hierarchical Linear Models: Applications and Data Analysis Methods.* Newbury Park, CA: Sage; 1992.

100. Little RJA, Rubin DB. *Statistical Analysis with Missing Data.* New York: Wiley; 1987.

101. Graham JW, Hofer SM, Piccinin AM. *Analysis with Missing Data in Drug Prevention Research.* Washington, DC: US Government Printing Office; 1994:13–63. National Institute on Drug Abuse Research Monograph 142.

102. Graham JW, Donaldson SI. Evaluating interventions with differential attrition: the importance of nonresponse mechanisms and the use of follow-up data. *J Appl Psychol.* 1993;78:119–128.

103. Rindskopf D. A general approach to categorical data analysis with missing data, using generalized linear models with composite links. *Psychometrika.* 1992;57:29–42.

104. Sackett DL. How to read clinical journals: I. Why to read them and how to start reading them critically. V. To distinguish useful from useless or even harmful therapy. *Can Med Assoc.* 1981;124:555–558, 1156–1162.

105. Pocock SJ. *Clinical Trials: A Practical Approach.* New York: John Wiley & Sons; 1983.

106. Shapiro SH, Louis TA. *Clinical Trials: Issues and Approaches.* New York: Marcel Dekker; 1983.

107. Friedman L, Furberg CD, DeMets DL. *Fundamentals of Clinical Trials.* 2nd ed. Littleton, MA: PSG Publishing; 1985.

108. Hennekens CH, Buring JE. *Epidemiology in Medicine.* Boston: Little, Brown and Company; 1987.

109. Holman SL, Goldstein DJ, Enas GG. Pattern analysis method for assessing successful weight reduction. *Int J Obes.* 1993;18:281–285.

110. Allison DB. Commentary on Holman, Goldstein, and Enas. *Int J Obes.* 1994;19:74–76.

111. Sacks HS, Berrier J, Reitman D, Ancona-Berk VA, Chalmers TC. Meta-analyses of randomised control trials. *N Engl J Med.* 1987;316:450–455.

112. Brown SA. Studies of educational interventions and outcomes in diabetic adults: a meta-analysis. *Patient Educ Counsel.* 1990;16:189–215.

113. Ballor DL, Keesey DL. A meta-analysis of the factors affecting exercise-induced changes in body mass, fat mass and fat-free mass in males and females. *Int J Obes.* 1991;15:717–726.

114. Brown SA. Meta-analysis of diabetes patient education research: variations in intervention effects across studies. *Res Nurs Health.* 1992;15:409–419.

115. Dattilo AM, Kris-Etherton PM. Effects of weight reduction on blood lipids and lipoproteins: a meta-analysis. *Am J of Clin Nutr.* 1992;56:320–328.

116. Ballor DL, Poehlman ET. Exercise-training enhances fat-free preservation during diet-induced weight loss: a meta-analytical finding. *Int J Obes.* 1994;18:35–40.

117. Wachter KW, Straf ML, eds. *The Future of Meta-Analysis*. New York: Russell Sage Foundation; 1990.

118. Cook TD, Cooper H, Cordray DS, et al. *Meta-Analysis for Explanation: A Casebook*. New York: Russell Sage Foundation; 1992.

119. Dickersin K, Berlin J. Meta-analysis: state-of-the-science. *Epidemiol Rev.* 1992;14:154–176.

120. Pettitti DB. *Meta-Analysis, Decision Analysis and Cost-Effectiveness Analysis*. New York: Oxford University Press; 1994.

121. Abramson JH. *Making Sense of Data*. 2nd ed. New York: Oxford University Press; 1994.

122. Orwin RG. A fail-safe N for effect size. *J Educ Stat.* 1988;8:157–159.

123. Allison DB, Faith M. Publication bias in obesity treatment trials? *Int J Obes.* 1996;20:931–937.

124. Cooper H, Hedges LV, eds. *The Handbook of Research Synthesis*. New York: Russell Sage Foundation; 1994.

125. Wortman PM. Judging research quality. In: Cooper H, Hedges LV, eds. *The Handbook of Research Synthesis*. New York: Russell Sage Foundation; 1994: 97–109.

126. Mohr D, Jadad AR, Nichol G, Penman M, Tugwell P, Walsh S. Assessing the quality of randomized controlled trials: an annotated bibliography of scales and checklists. *Controlled Clin Trials.* 1995;16:62–73.

127. Schulz KF, Chalmers I, Hayes RJ, Altman DG. Empirical evidence of bias: dimensions of methodological quality associated with estimates of treatment effects in controlled trials. *JAMA.* 1995;273:408–412.

128. Gleser LJ, Olkin I. Stochastically dependent effect sizes. In: Cooper H, Hedges LV, eds. *The Handbook of Research Synthesis*. New York: Russell Sage Foundation; 1994:339–355.

129. Goldman L, Feinstein AR. Anticoagulants and myocardial infarction: the problems of pooling, drowning, and floating. *Ann Intern Med.* 1979;90:92–94.

130. Wachter KW. Disturbed by meta-analysis? *Science.* 1988;241:1407–1408.

131. Thompson SG, Pocock SJ. Can meta-analyses be trusted? *Lancet.* 1991;338:1127–1130.

132. Greenland S. Invited commentary: a critical look at some popular meta-analytic methods. *Am J Epidemiol.* 1994;140:290–296.

133. Fleiss JL. *Statistical Methods for Rates and Proportions*. 2nd ed. New York: John Wiley & Sons; 1982.

134. Lau J, Antman EM, Jimenez-Silva J, Kupelnick B, Mosteller F, Chalmers TC. Cumulative meta-analysis of therapeutic trials for myocardial infarction. *N Engl J Med.* 1992;327:248–254.

135. L'abbe KA, Detsky AS, O'Rourke K. Meta-analysis in clinical research. *Ann Intern Med.* 1987;107:224–233.

136. Boissel J-P, Collet J-P, Lievre M, Girard P. An effect model for the assessment of drug benefit: example of antiarrhythmic drugs in postmyocardial infarction patients. *J Cardiovasc Pharmacol.* 1993;22:356–363.

137. Mantel N, Haenszel W. Statistical aspects of the analysis of data from retrospective studies of disease. *J Natl Cancer Inst.* 1959;22:719–748.

138. DerSimonian R, Laird NM. Meta-analysis in clinical trials. *Controlled Clin Trials.* 1986;7:177–188.

139. Hedges LV. In: Cooper H, Hedges LV, eds. *The Handbook of Research Synthesis*. New York: Russell Sage Foundation; 1994:285–299.

140. Raudenbush SW. In: Cooper H, Hedges LV, eds. *The Handbook of Research Synthesis.* New York: Russell Sage Foundation; 1994:301–321.

141. Hedges LV, Olkin I. *Statistical Methods for Meta-Analysis.* Orlando, FL: Academic Press; 1985.

142. Greenland S. Quantitative methods in the review of epidemiologic literature. *Epidemiol Rev.* 1987;9:1–30.

143. Thompson SG. Controversies in meta-analysis: the case of the trials of serum cholesterol reduction. *Stat Meth Med Res.* 1993;2:173–192.

144. Berlin JA, Antman EM. Advantages and limitations of metaanalytic regressions of clinical trials data. *Online J Curr Clin Trials.* 1994;3 (June 4) Doc. No. 134.

145. Langbein LI, Lichtman AJ. *Ecological Inference.* Newbury Park, CA: Sage Publications; 1978.

146. Morgenstern H. Uses of ecologic analysis in ecological research. *Am J Public Health.* 1982;72:1336–1344.

147. Freedman LS. Tables of the number of patients required in clinical trials using the logrank test. *Stat Med.* 1982;1:121–129.

148. Bartko JJ, Pulver AE, Carpenter WT. The power of analysis: statistical perspectives. Part 2. *Psychiatry Res.* 1988;23:301–309.

149. Bird KD, Hall W. Statistical power in psychiatric research. *Aust N Z J Psychiatry.* 1986;20:189–200.

150. Gatsonis C, Sampson AR. Multiple correlation: exact power and sample size calculation. *Psychol Bull.* 1989;106:516–524.

151. Hinkle DE, Oliver JD. How large should the sample be? A question with no simple answer? *Educ Psychol Measur.* 1983;43:1051–1060.

152. Kraemer HC, Thiemann S. *How Many Subjects? Statistical Power Analysis in Research.* Newbury Park, CA: Sage; 1987.

153. Lipsey MW. *Design Sensitivity: Statistical Power for Experimental Research.* Newbury Park, CA: Sage; 1990.

154. Lui K. Sample sizes for repeated measurements in dichotomous data. *Stat Med.* 1991;10:463–472.

155. Schoenfeld DA, Richter JR. Nomograms for calculating the number of patients needed for a clinical trial with survival as an endpoint. *Biometrics.* 1982;38:163–170.

156. Shuster JJ. *Practical Handbook of Sample Size Guidelines for Clinical Trials.* Boca Raton, FL: CRC Press; 1990.

Index